Directory of American Medical Education

2008–2009

AAMC President and CEO
Darrel G. Kirch, M.D.

Editor
Susan Monseur

Project Coordinator
TaNika Switzer

Acknowledgements

The association wishes to express appreciation to its staff members and to the deans of the medical schools and their representatives for their assistance in revising the information for this edition of the AAMC directory.

The entries appearing in this edition were updated in summer 2008 for the 2008-2009 academic year.

Orders

To order additional copies of this publication, please contact:

Association of American Medical Colleges
Section for Publication Orders
2450 N Street, NW
Washington, DC 20037

Phone: 202-828-0416
Fax: 202-828-1123

Price: $85, plus shipping
(Item Code: DAME08)

AAMC Members: $25, plus shipping
(Item Code: DAME08)

AAMC Members (Additional copies after the first copy): $10
(Item Code: DAME08)

See order form in this publication for ordering instructions.

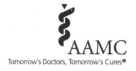

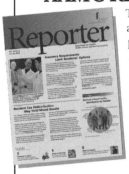
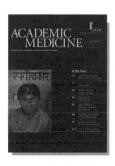

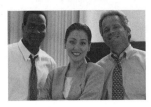

Employers
Target your recruiting and reach qualified candidates quickly and easily. Simply complete our online registration form and start posting jobs today!

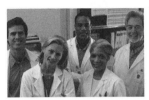

Job Seekers
Whether you're looking for a new job, or ready to take the next step in your career, we'll help you find the opportunity that's right for you.

CareerConnect

CareerConnect provides an online forum for medical schools and teaching hospitals to connect with the industry's best and brightest talent.

AAMC's exclusive niche community includes hundreds of accredited medical schools, teaching hospitals, and medical centers throughout the United States and Canada, as well as thousands of individuals within our academic and scientific societies and professional development groups.

For more information visit our Job Board at **www.aamc.org/careerconnect**

The Successful Medical School Department Chair: A Guide to Good Institutional Practice

A Manual for Medical School Deans, Teaching Hospital CEOs, Department Chairs, Search Committees, and Chair-Candidates.

The Successful Medical School Department Chair offers helpful advice, details good practice, and provides a wealth of sample documents and policies that can be adapted for local use. Each of the three modules is devoted to a different time period in the total career life of the medical school department chair.

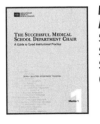

Module 1: Search, Selection, Appointment, Transition
$50 Member
$75 Non-Member Non-Profit
$100 Non-Member For-Profit
(Product ID CHAIR1)

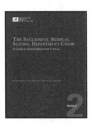

Module 2: Characteristics, Responsibilities, Expectations, Skill Sets
$50 Member
$75 Non-Member Non-Profit
$100 Non-Member For-Profit
(Product ID CHAIR2)

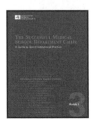

Module 3: Performance, Evaluation, Rewards, Mentorship
$50 Member
$75 Non-Member Non-Profit
$100 Non-Member For-Profit
(Product ID CHAIR3)

For a full listing of publications that are for sale and those that are free, please visit our Web site, **www.aamc.org/publications**.

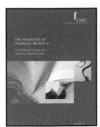

The Handbook of Academic Medicine: How Medical Schools and Teaching Hospitals Work
$25 Member/Non-Member
(Product ID HANDBOOK)

Medical schools and teaching hospitals can be complex, intimidating organizations, surely to those new to the enterprise, even to those who have made their careers within its walls. The Handbook of Academic Medicine describes this world of academic medicine, explaining what medical schools and teaching hospitals are, how they work and interrelate, and what prominent issues they face. The Handbook is a comprehensive reference source on the fundamentals of academic medicine.

The Handbook is essential reading for medical school and teaching hospital leaders, governing board members, university officials, members of the media, national and state legislators and staff members, Federal agency staff, and anyone who wants to know more about medical schools and teaching hospitals, their structure, financing, interrelationships, and programs - and the issues they and society face in preserving and enhancing their unique contributions to the national well-being.

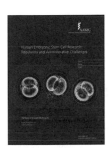

Human Embryonic Stem Cell Research: Regulatory and Administrative Challenges
2006
$25 Member/Non-Member
(Product ID STEMCELL06)

The Bush Administration has limited the federal funding of human embryonic stem (hES) cell research to those successful applications that utilize one or more of the 22 lines currently listed on the NIH Human Embryonic Stem Cell Registry. The derivation and use of hES cell lines developed after the Administration's August 9, 2001 policy declaration remains legal and there is no pending legislative or regulatory effort to prohibit their use. The AAMC sponsored a workshop on April 27, 2006 to discuss policy and administrative issues on how best to organize, monitor, document, and allocate costs for laboratories that utilize stem cell lines both listed and not listed on the NIH stem cell registry. This monograph summarizes the workshop discussions and provides additional background information on the topics considered.

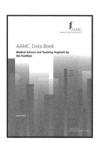

AAMC Data Book: Medical Schools and Teaching Hospitals by the Numbers 2008
May 2008
$70 Member
$120 Non-Member Non-Profit
$170 Non-Member For-Profit
(Product ID DATABOOK08)

The *AAMC Data Book*, a statistical abstract of U.S. medical schools and teaching hospitals, includes current and historical data on a comprehensive list of topics including: Applicants and Students, Faculty, Medical School Revenue, Tuition and Financial Aid, Graduate Medical Education, Teaching Hospitals, Faculty Compensation, Physicians, Biomedical Research, and reference data such as Price Indices.

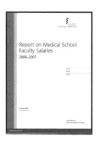

Report on Medical School Faculty Salaries 2006-2007
2008
$115 Member
$210 Non-Member Non-Profit
$350 Non-Member For-Profit)
(Product ID FACSAL08)

The Report on Medical School Faculty Salaries contains 33 tables that present the total income attributable to teaching, patient care, or research for full-time medical school faculty. The total income is broken out in a number of ways, such as by discipline, degree, region, and school ownership. The tables provide the 25th percentile and 75th percentile as well as the mean and median for each combination of faculty rank and faculty department/specialty. The number of faculty in each total income statistic is given also.

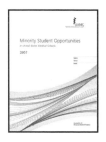

Minority Student Opportunities in United States Medical Schools
2007
$15 Member/Non-Member
(Product ID MSOUSMS07)

The information in this book is supplied by individual medical schools in response to a questionnaire from the AAMC's Division of Diversity Policy and Programs about minority student opportunities.

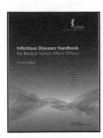

Infectious Disease Handbook for Medical School Student Affairs Officers (Second Edition)
December 2006
$25 Member
$35 Non-Member
(Product ID INFECDIS06)

This handbook is intended as a resource for those who are concerned about the transmission of infectious diseases in the health care setting. It is intended primarily for use by Student Affairs deans who are charged with the formulation and administration of policies related to medical student health. It contains information about common hospital-acquired agents, methods of transmission, risks of infectivity, and control/prevention procedures. Both risks to health care workers (HCWs) as a result of caring for infected patients and risks to patients from infected IICWs are discussed, where appropriate. Well-accepted infection control practices are presented, and areas of continued controversy are addressed.

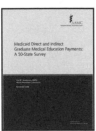

Medicaid Direct and Indirect Graduate Medical Education Payments: A 50 State Survey 2006
November 2006
$10 Member
$25 Non-Member Non-Profit
$50 Non-Member For-Profit
(Product ID MEDIGME06)

This publication provides the results of a 2006 survey of state Medicaid programs on their 2005 policies for financing direct graduate medical education costs, and indirect medical education costs, which reflect the higher patient care costs at teaching hospitals. The study reflects responses from all 50 states and the District of Columbia.

This survey was conducted for the AAMC by Tim Henderson, a noted Health Workforce consultant and is the third in a series of surveys intended to collect information on payment type, funding mechanisms and methodologies, and expenditure estimates. The previous studies were conducted in 1999 and 2003.

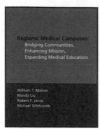

Regional Medical Campuses: Bridging Communities, Enhancing Mission, Expanding Medical Education
November 2006
$25 Member
$50 Non-Member
(Product ID BRIDGING06)

Regional Medical Campuses: Bridging Communities, Enhancing Mission, Expanding Medical Education is a reprinting of the 2003 AAMC monograph, the first comprehensive study of regional campuses at medical schools in the United States. This book examines the distinct educational benefits for medical students offered by regional clinical campuses. It also investigates the structure, organization, governance, leadership, and strengths and weaknesses of regional campuses.

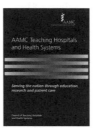

Teaching Hospitals and Health Systems: Serving the Nation Through Education, Research and Patient Care 2008
June 2008
$20 Member
$75 Non-Member
(Product ID COTHSERV)

This report provides an overview of the characteristics that uniquely distinguish teaching hospitals from other teaching and nonteaching hospitals. It includes charts and tables that compare Council of Teaching Hospitals and Health Systems (COTH) hospitals to other teaching and nonteaching hospitals in three categories (short-term, general, nonfederal hospitals; VA hospitals; and Children's hospitals).

Publication Order Form

Association of
American Medical Colleges
2450 N Street, N.W., Washington, D.C. 20037-1127
T 202 828 0400 **F** 202 828 1125
www.aamc.org

Item Code	Title	Quantity	Unit Price	Total

*Shipping/Handling

Within Continental U.S.:
$8.00 for first publication
$2.00 for each additional publication
Alaska and Hawaii:
$18.00 for first publication
$2.00 for each additional publication

Subtotal	
*Shipping/ Handling	
Total Amount Enclosed	

For international shipping rates, please visit our Web site or contact us by phone or email.

NAME

TITLE

INSTITUTION

ADDRESS

CITY   **STATE**   **ZIP**

PHONE   **E-MAIL ADDRESS**

PAYMENT

All orders must be accompanied by payment. Please make checks payable to AAMC. All payments must be in U.S. dollars, drawn on a U.S. bank. Prices are subject to change without notice.

❏ Check   ❏ Money Order   ❏ Mastercard   ❏ Visa   ❏ American Express

NAME OF CARD HOLDER_____

CARD NUMBER_____   **EXPIRATION DATE**_____

SIGNATURE_____

ORDER ONLINE	ORDER BY MAIL	ORDER BY PHONE
www.aamc.org	Customer Service & Order Fulfillment AAMC 2450 N Street, NW Washington, DC 20037	202-828-0416 **ORDER BY FAX** 202-828-1123

Questions? Call us at the number noted above, or email publications@aamc.org.

Contents

Alphabetical Listing of Medical Schools

MEDICAL SCHOOL MEMBERS
(Accredited by the Liaison Committee on Medical Education [LCME].
Preliminary and provisional accreditation are sufficient for eligibility.)

MEDICAL SCHOOL MEMBERS (Continued)

PROVISIONAL MEDICAL SCHOOL MEMBERS

AFFILIATE MEDICAL SCHOOL MEMBERS
(Jointly accredited by the LCME and the Committee on Accreditation of Canadian Medical Schools [CACMS])

PROVISIONAL AFFILIATE MEDICAL SCHOOL MEMBER

Geographical Listing of Medical Schools

UNITED STATES

Geographical Listing of Medical Schools

CANADA

Geographical Listing of Medical Schools

Association Organizational Structure and Activities

2008–2009

About the AAMC

Founded in 1876, the AAMC is a not-for-profit association representing all 130 accredited U.S. and 17 accredited Canadian medical schools; nearly 400 major teaching hospitals and health systems; 68 Department of Veterans Affairs medical centers; nearly 90 academic and professional societies, representing 125,000 faculty members; the nation's 75,000 medical students; and 106,000 resident physicians.

What We Do

The AAMC serves and leads the academic medicine community to improve the health of all. To fulfill this mission, the association focuses on nine strategic priorities:

- Serving as the voice and advocate for academic medicine on medical education, research, and health care
- Leading innovation along the continuum of medical education to meet the health needs of the public
- Facilitating development of a health system that meets the needs of all for access, safety, and quality of care
- Strengthening the national commitment to discovery that promotes health and enhances the treatment of disease and disability
- Leading efforts to increase diversity in medicine
- Being a valued and reliable resource for data, information, and services
- Helping our members identify, implement, and sustain organizational performance improvement
- Providing outstanding leadership and professional development to meet the most critical needs of our members
- Nurturing a culture at the AAMC that promotes excellence in service to our members and the public good.

Medical Education

Each year, more than 16,000 students graduate with an M.D. degree from AAMC-member medical schools, and over 100,000 resident physicians continue their training at teaching hospitals and associated community sites across the United States. The AAMC works to ensure that the medical education and advanced preparation of these new doctors meet the highest standards and keep pace with the changing needs of patients and the nation's health care system.

The Liaison Committee on Medical Education (LCME) is the U.S. Department of Education-recognized accrediting body for U.S. medical education programs leading to the M.D. degree. It also accredits M.D. programs in Canada, in cooperation with the Committee on Accreditation of Canadian Medical Schools. The LCME is jointly sponsored by the AAMC with the American Medical Association.

Medical schools and teaching hospitals, as well as the future physicians and medical scientists they train, rely on AAMC service programs, such as the admission test to medical school (the MCAT® examination), Web-based applications for medical school (AMCAS®) and residency programs (ERAS®), and the "Match," the annual process that matches graduating medical students with residency programs on behalf of the National Resident Matching Program.

Information and Data

The AAMC also provides leaders of medical schools and teaching hospitals with an extensive array of data to support their missions, including CurrMIT® (Curriculum Management & Information Tool), an online database for managing medical school curricula; the Medical School Profile System, a source of information about medical school revenues, expenditures, enrollments, faculty counts, and other operations; the Faculty Roster and FAMOUS (Faculty Administrative Management Online User System) interface, an online database of full-time, part-time, volunteer, and emeritus faculty appointments at U.S. medical schools; GME Track®, an online graduate medical education resource; clinical productivity benchmarking tools for faculty practice plans; and annual surveys of teaching hospitals and residents' and fellows' stipends.

Advocacy

As the leading voice of the academic medical community, the AAMC represents the interests of the nation's medical schools and teaching hospitals before Congress, federal regulatory agencies, and the executive branch on a wide range of issues, including Medicare and Medicaid funding; federal support for

About the AAMC

medical research and public health; federal student loan programs; health professions education funding; and veterans' medical care and biomedical research. Through various programs and initiatives, the AAMC also educates the public to build awareness of and support for the unique missions of the nation's medical schools and teaching hospitals.

Organization and Governance

Headquartered in Washington, D.C., the AAMC is guided by its five core constituent groups. Representatives elected from these five groups participate in the association's governing body, the AAMC Board of Directors. Following is a brief description of these five groups.

The *Council of Deans (COD)* represents the leaders of America's medical schools, providing medical school deans with a forum to discuss important issues, and offering services, information, and programs that advance their efforts.

The *Council of Teaching Hospitals and Health Systems (COTH)* comprises the leaders of America's major teaching hospitals and health systems. Participation in COTH is recognized throughout the world as a benchmark for excellence in patient care, research, and medical education.

The *Council of Academic Societies (CAS)* provides a forum for discussing and exchanging information of interest to medical school faculty and scientists involved in life sciences research, research training, and medical education.

The *Organization of Student Representatives (OSR)* represents the interests of students enrolled in the nation's medical schools.

The *Organization of Resident Representatives (ORR)* provides a venue for discussing issues of interest to resident physicians, and offers leadership opportunities for those interested in academic medical careers.

AAMC Services

Following is a list of major services the AAMC provides.

American Medical College Application Service (AMCAS®)—a not-for-profit, Internet-based application processing service for first-year applicants to U.S. medical schools.

AspiringDocs.org—a Web site and outreach campaign to increase diversity in medicine by encouraging well-prepared African American, Latino/a, and Native American students to apply to and enroll in medical school.

Careers in Medicine®—a print and Web-based career-planning program that helps medical students understand options in choosing a specialty and identifying residency programs that meet individual career objectives.

Electronic Residency Application Service (ERAS®)—an Internet-based service that enables medical students and graduates to transmit applications, transcripts, recommendations, and other supporting credentials to U.S. residency program directors.

FindAResident®—a year-round Web-based service that allows residents and residency programs to search for, and fill, open residency and fellowship positions.

FIRST for Medical Education—a program that offers a full range of Financial Information Resources, Services, and Tools for applicants, medical students, residents, advisors, and financial aid officers.

Medical College Admission Test (MCAT®)—the national standardized test used to assess medical school applicants' science knowledge, reasoning, and communications skills.

National Resident Matching Program (NRMP®)—an annual process that enables medical students and residency programs to match their preferences for each other as closely as possible.

Visiting Student Application Service (VSAS)—a brand-new AAMC application designed to make it easier for medical students to apply for senior electives at other U.S. medical schools. During the pilot year, 10 U.S. schools will exclusively use VSAS to accept elective applications.

For more information about these and other AAMC service programs, go to www.aamc.org/services.

AAMC Data

Key informational resources provided by the AAMC include:

CurrMIT® (Curriculum Management & Information Tool)—an online database to help medical schools

About the AAMC

organize, manage, and report on their curriculum. Faculty Roster and FAMOUS System—demographic data and the current appointments of full-time, part-time, volunteer, and emeritus U.S. medical school faculty.

GME Track®—a Web-based graduate medical education resource and resident and program database, jointly conducted with the American Medical Association.

MedEdPORTAL®—a resource designed to help faculty publish and share educational resources-focusing exclusively on the continuum of medical education and addressing the unique needs of medical educators.

Medical School Profile System (MSPS)—information on U.S. medical school revenues and expenditures, faculty counts, curricula, student enrollment, and student financial aid.

For more information about these and other AAMC data resources, go to www.aamc.org/data.

Professional Development

Fourteen AAMC professional development groups offer individuals at AAMC member institutions opportunities for information sharing, professional growth, and leadership.

Government Relations Representatives (GRR)
Graduate Research, Education, and Training Group (GREAT)
Group on Business Affairs (GBA)
Group on Educational Affairs (GEA)
Group on Faculty Affairs (GFA)
Group on Faculty Practice (GFP)
Group on Information Resources (GIR)
Group on Institutional Advancement (GIA)
Group on Institutional Planning (GIP)
Group on Regional Medical Campuses (GRMC)
Group on Research Advancement and Development (GRAND)
Group on Resident Affairs (GRA)
Group on Student Affairs (GSA)/Minority Affairs Section (GSA-MAS)
Women in Medicine (WIM)

For links to these groups, go to www.aamc.org/members.

Publications

The AAMC publishes a range of books, journals, reports, and other print and electronic resources, including the following:

Academic Medicine®, the monthly journal of the AAMC, publishes articles on the most pressing challenges facing the leaders of medical schools and teaching hospitals today. www.academicmedicine.org

Directory of Medical Education (DAME), a complete directory of association members and their key staff in U.S. and Canadian medical schools, teaching hospitals, and academic societies, along with a listing of the AAMC's organizational structure and key contacts.

Medical School Admissions Requirements (MSAR™), a comprehensive guide featuring the most up-to-date information about medical school entrance requirements, curriculum features, first-year expenses, financial aid, and application procedures.

Reporter, the AAMC's monthly news publication, covering major programs and initiatives at the AAMC and member institutions, as well as broader issues that affect the nation's medical schools and teaching hospitals. www.aamc.org/newsroom/reporter

STAT (Short, Topical and Timely), a weekly electronic newsletter featuring brief and immediate news bites about AAMC activities, as well as policy developments, initiatives, and data important to the academic medicine community. www.aamc.org/newsroom/aamcstat/aamcnews.htm

Washington Highlights, a weekly electronic newsletter focusing on key federal legislative and regulatory developments. www.aamc.org/advocacy/washhigh

On the Web

The AAMC Web site provides a rich source of data, information, and services, along with the latest association news, publications, and events.

To learn more about the association and its initiatives, visit **www.aamc.org**.

AAMC Board of Directors, 2008-2009

Chair
Elliot J. Sussman, M.D., M.B.A.
Lehigh Valley Hospital and
Health Network

Chair-elect
Deborah E. Powell, M.D.
University of Minnesota

Immediate Past Chair
Robert J. Desnick, Ph.D., M.D.
Mount Sinai School of
Medicine

President and CEO
Darrell G. Kirch, M.D.
Association of American
Medical Colleges

John D. Forsyth
Wellmark, Inc.

Kelli Harding, M.D.
Columbia University

Randall K. Holmes, M.D., Ph.D.
University of Colorado

Mark R. Laret
University of California,
San Francisco

Thomas J. Lawley, M.D.
Emory University

Steven Lipstein
BJC Healthcare

Jason P. Lott
University of Pennsylvania

J. Lloyd Michener, M.D.
Duke University

Lois Margaret Nora, M.D., J.D., M.B.A.
Northeastern Ohio
Universities

E. Albert Reece, M.D., Ph.D., M.B.A.
University of Maryland

Anthony A. Meyer, M.D., Ph.D.
University of North Carolina at
Chapel Hill

Peter L. Slavin, M.D.
Massachusetts General
Hospital

Valerie N. Williams, Ph.D., M.P.A.
University of Oklahoma

AAMC

2450 N Street, N.W. • Washington, D.C. 20037
Phone: 202-828-0400 • Fax: 202-828-1125

Office of the President

President and CEO
Darrell G. Kirch, M.D.
828-0460
dgkirch@aamc.org

Chief of Staff
Kathleen S. Turner
828-0463
ksturner@aamc.org

Deputy Chief of Staff
Jennifer M. Schlener
828-0466
jmschlener@aamc.org

Chief Legal Officer
Joseph A. Keyes Jr., J.D.
828-0555
jakeyes@aamc.org

Office of the Executive Vice President (OEVP)

Executive Vice President and Chief Strategy Officer
Carol A. Aschenbrener, M.D.
828-0665
caschenbrener@aamc.org

OEVP/Center for Workforce Studies

Director, Center for Workforce Studies
Edward Salsberg
828-0415
esalsberg@aamc.org

OEVP/Diversity Policy and Programs

Chief Diversity Officer
Charles Terrell, Ed.D.
862-6105
cterrell@aamc.org

Director of Research, Diversity Policy and Programs
Laura Castillo-Page, Ph.D.
828-0579
lcastillopage@aamc.org

OEVP/Membership and Constituent Services

Director, Membership and Constituent Services
Heather Brinton Parker
828-0427
hbrinton@aamc.org

Director of Meetings
Kirsten Olean
828-0479
kolean@aamc.org

OEVP/Organizational and Management Studies

Director, Organizational Learning and Research
William T. Mallon, Ed.D.
828-0424
wmallon@aamc.org

OEVP/Organizational Effectiveness

Director, Faculty Development and Leadership
Diane Magrane, M.D.
828-0575
dmagrane@aamc.org

Academic Affairs

Chief Academic Officer
John E. Prescott, M.D.
741-4758
jprescott@aamc.org

Academic Affairs/Accreditation

Senior Director, Accreditation Services and LCME Secretary
Dan Hunt, M.D.
828-0596
dhunt@aamc.org

Director, LCME Surveys and Team Training
Robert F. Sabalis, Ph.D.
828-0556
rsabalis@aamc.org

Academic Affairs/Medical Education

Senior Director, Continuing Education and Performance Improvement
David Davis, M.D.
862-6275
ddavies@aamc.org

Senior Director, Educational Affairs
M. Brownell Anderson
828-0562
mbanderson@aamc.org

Academic Affairs/MedEdPORTAL

Director, MedEdPORTAL
Robby Reynolds
828 0962
rreynolds@aamc.org

Academic Affairs/Student Affairs and Programs

Senior Director, Student Affairs and Programs
Henry Sondheimer, M.D.
828-0684
hsondheimer@aamc.org

Director, Careers in Medicine
George V. Richard
898-6223
grichard@aamc.org

Director, Student/Resident Debt Management Services
Julie A. Fresne
828-0511
jfresne@aamc.org

Health Care Affairs

Chief Health Care Officer
Joanne M. Conroy, M.D.
828-0493
jconroy@aamc.org

Senior Director, Health Care Affairs
Karen S. Fisher, J.D.
862-6140
kfisher@aamc.org

AAMC Senior Staff

Director and Regulatory Counsel
Ivy S. Baer
828-0499
ibaer@aamc.org

Director, Health Care Affairs
David Longnecker, MD
862-6113
dlongnecker@aamc.org

Director, Health Care Affairs
Sunny G. Yoder
828-0497
syoder@aamc.org

Biomedical and Health Sciences Research

Interim Chief Scientific Officer and Senior Director, Regulatory Affairs
Anthony J. Mazzaschi
828-0059
tmazzaschi@aamc.org

Senior Director and Regulatory Counsel
Susan Ehringhaus, J.D.
828-0543
sehringhaus@aamc.org

Advocacy and Voice

Advocacy and Voice/Communications

Chief Communications Officer
Elisa K. Siegel
828-0459
esiegel@aamc.org

Director and Managing Editor, *Academic Medicine*
Anne Farmakidis
828-0593
afarmakidis@aamc.org

Director, Institutional Advancement
Chris Tucker
828-0989
ctucker@aamc.org

Senior Director, Print and Electronic Publishing
Eric Weissman
828-0044
eweissman@aamc.org

Director, Public Affairs
Mary Jane Fingland
828-0983
mjfingland@aamc.org

Director, Public Relations
Retha Sherrod
828-0975
rsherrod@aamc.org

Advocacy and Voice/Government Relations

Senior Director, Government Relations
David Moore
828-0559
dbmoore@aamc.org

Director, Government Relations
Atul Grover, M.D., Ph.D.
828-0666
agrover@aamc.org

Mission Support

Chief Mission Support Officer
Robert F. Jones, Ph.D.
828-0520
rfjones@aamc.org

Mission Support/Administrative and Financial Services

Chief Finance and Administrative Officer
Barbara S. Friedman
828-0404
bfriedman@aamc.org

Controller
Daniel Berringer
862-6295
dberringer@aamc.org

Director, Business Development
Gabrielle Campbell
828-0643
gcampbell@aamc.org

Director, Business Services
Mark S. Wood
828-0450
mwood@aamc.org

Director, Financial Systems and Budget
Jeanne L. McCarroll
828-0451
jmccarroll@aamc.org

Senior Director, Human Resources
Donna Whitlock Stewart
28-0446
dwstewart@aamc.org

Mission Support/Information Technology

Chief Information Officer
Jeanne L. Mella
862-6173
jmella@aamc.org

Director, Enterprise Technology
Lee Leiber
862-6247
lleiber@aamc.org

Director, IT Service Portfolio
Greg Haywood
862-6172
ghaywood@aamc.org

Director, Software Applications Management
Albert Salas
828-0675
asalas@aamc.org

Director, Software Applications Management
Farideh Soltani
828-0987
fsoltani@aamc.org

Director, Enterprise Data Services
Kirke Lawton
828-0974
klawton@aamc.org

Mission Support/Medical School Services and Studies

Senior Director, Admissions Testing Services
Karen Mitchell
828-0500
kmitchell@aamc.org

AAMC Senior Staff

Director, AMCAS Programs
Stephen J. Fitzpatrick
828-0621
sfitzpatrick@aamc.org

Senior Director, Application Services
Moira Edwards
828-0058
medwards@aamc.org

Director, MCAT Development and Research
Scott Oppler
862-6073
soppler@aamc.org

Director, Medical School and Faculty Studies
Hershel Alexander
828-0649
halexander@aamc.org

Senior Director, Medical School Financial and Administrative Affairs
Jack Y. Krakower, Ph.D.
828-0654
jykrakower@aamc.org

Senior Director, Project Management office
Nicole Nitowski
862-6087
nnitowski@aamc.org

Senior Director, Special Studies
Paul Jolly Jr., Ph.D.
828-0642
pjolly@aamc.org

Director, Student and Applicant Studies
Gwen Garrison
862-6186
ggarrison@aamc.org-

AAMC Subject Listing

A

AAMC Data Book
Wendy Geraci
862-6101
wgeraci@aamc.org

AAMC Reference Center and Mary H. Littlemeyer Archives
Marian Taliaferro
828-0433
mtaliaferro@aamc.org

AAMC Reporter
Scott Harris
862-6284
sharris@aamc.org

AAMC STAT
Nicole Buckley
828-0041
nbuckley@aamc.org

Academic Medical Center Organization and Governance
William T. Mallon, Ed.D.
828-0424
wmallon@aamc.org

Academic Medicine
  Editorial
  Anne Farmakidis
  828-0593
  afarmakidis@aamc.org

  Subscriptions/Renewals
  Complimentary
  Subscription Publications
  828-0416
  publications@aamc.org

Paid Subscription
Lippincott Williams & Wilkins
Customer Service
800-638-3030
www.lww.com/customerservice

Academic Physician & Scientist
Scott Harris
862-6284
sharris@aamc.org

Accounting
Daniel Berringer
862-6295
dberringer@aamc.org

Accreditation of Continuing Medical Education
David Davis, M.D.
862-6275
ddavis@aamc.org

Accreditation of Medical Schools
Dan Hunt, M.D.
828-0596
dhunt@aamc.org

Robert F. Sabalis, Ph.D.
828-0556
rsabalis@aamc.org

Accreditation of Residencies (ACGME)
Sunny G. Yoder
828-0497
syoder@aamc.org

Ad Hoc Group for Medical Research
David Moore
828-0559
dbmoore@aamc.org

Admission Policies and Procedures
Henry M. Sondheimer, M.D.
828-0684
hsondheimer@aamc.org

  Holistic Review
  Ruth Beer Bletzinger
  828-0585
  rbletzinger@aamc.org

Admission Traffic Rules
Henry M. Sondheimer, M.D.
828-0684
hsondheimer@aamc.org

Advisor Information Service (AIS)
Stephen Fitzpatrick
862-0621
sfitzpatrick@aamc.org

Advisory Panel on Health Care
Joanne M. Conroy, M.D.
828-0493
jconroy@aamc.org

Advisory Panel on Research
Stephen J. Heinig
828-0488
sheinig@aamc.org

AIDS/HIV
Henry M. Sondheimer, M.D.
828-0684
hsondheimer@aamc.org

American Board of Medical Specialties (ABMS)
David Longnecker, M.D.
862-6113
dlongnecker@aamc.org

AMCAS (American Medical College Application Service) Policies, Procedures
Stephen Fitzpatrick
862-0621
sfitzpatrick@aamc.org

AAMC Subject Listing

AMCAS General Information
828-0600
amcas@aamc.org

Animals in Education and Research
Anthony J. Mazzaschi
828-0059
tmazzaschi@aamc.org

Legislation
Tannaz Rasouli
828-0057
trasouli@aamc.org

Annual Meeting
Heather Brinton Parker
828-0427
hbrinton@aamc.org

Applicant/Acceptance and Matriculation Data
Collins Mikesell
862-6080
cmikesell@aamc.org

Archives
Molly Alexander
862-6261
malexander@aamc.org

AspiringDocs.org
Ruth Beer Bletzinger
828-0585
rbletzinger@aamc.org

Elisa K. Siegel
828-0459
esiegel@aamc.org

Awards
Alpha Omega Alpha
Henry M. Sondheimer, M.D.
828-0684
hsondheimer@aamc.org

Award for Distinguished Research
Sandra D. Gordon
828-0472
sgordon@aamc.org

Caring for Community
Ally Anderson
828-0682
aanderson@aamc.org

David E. Rogers Award
Sandra D. Gordon
828-0472
sgordon@aamc.org

Flexner Award for Distinguished Service
Sandra D. Gordon
828-0472
sgordon@aamc.org

Herbert W. Nickens Award
Juan Amador
862-6149
jamador@aamc.org

Herbert W. Nickens Faculty Fellowships
Juan Amador
862-6149
jamador@aamc.org

Herbert W. Nickens Medical Student Scholarships
Juan Amador
862-6149
jamador@aamc.org

Humanism in Medicine Award
Ally Anderson
828-0682
aanderson@aamc.org

Denine Hales
828-0681
dhales@aamc.org

Spencer Foreman Award for Outstanding Community Service
Sandra D. Gordon
828-0472
sgordon@aamc.org

B

Biomedical Research Issues
Stephen J. Heinig
828-0488
sheinig@aamc.org

Legislation
David Moore
828-0559
dbmoore@aamc.org

Biosecurity Issues
Susan Ehringhaus, J.D.
828-0543
sehringhaus@aamc.org

Biotechnology Regulation
Stephen J. Heinig
828-0488
sheinig@aamc.org

Bioterrorism Preparedness Legislation
Tannaz Rasouli
828-0057
trasouli@aamc.org

Board of Directors
Kathleen S. Turner
828-0463
ksturner@aamc.org

Jennifer Schlener
828-0466
jschlener@aamc.org

Business Development
Gabrielle Campbell
828-0643
gcampbell@aamc.org

C

Career Advising for Medical Students
George V. Richard, Ph.D.
862-6223
grichard@aamc.org

Careers in Medicine Program
George V. Richard, Ph.D.
862-6223
grichard@aamc.org

Center for Workforce Studies
Edward Salsberg
828-0415
esalsberg@aamc.org

Clinical Research
Irena Tartakovsky, M.D.
862-6134
itartakovsky@aamc.org

Legislation
David Moore
828-0559
dbmoore@aamc.org

COD Fellowship Program
John E. Prescott, M.D.
741-0758
jprescott@aamc.org

Communications
Elisa K. Siegel
828-0459
esiegel@aamc.org

Compliance Officer Forum
Ivy S. Baer, J.D.
828-0499
ibaer@aamc.org

Conflict of Interest in Research
Susan Ehringhaus, J.D.
828-0543
sehringhaus@aamc.org

Congress, U.S.
David Moore
828-0559
dbmoore@aamc.org

Continuing Medical Education
David Davis, M.D.
862-6275
ddavis@aamc.org

Contracts
Gabrielle Campbell
828-0643
gcampbell@aamc.org

Council of Medical Specialty Societies (CMSS)
Atul Grover, M.D., Ph.D.
828-0666
agrover@aamc.org

Councils at the AAMC
Academic Societies (CAS)
Anthony J. Mazzaschi
828-0059
tmazzaschi@aamc.org

Deans (COD)
John E. Prescott, M.D.
741-0758
jprescott@aamc.org

Teaching Hospitals and Health Systems (COTH)
Joanne M. Conroy, M.D.
828-0493
jconroy@aamc.org

Criminal Background Checks
Henry M. Sondheimer, M.D.
828-0684
hsondheimer@aamc.org

Centralized Service for Medical Students
Stephen Fitzpatrick
862-0621
sfitzpatrick@aamc.org

Cultural Competence
Norma Poll, Ph.D.
862-6115
npoll@aamc.org

Ann Steinecke, Ph.D.
862-6296
asteinecke@aamc.org

Curriculum Management & Information Tool (CurrMIT)
CurrMIT Helpline
helpcurrmit@aamc.org

D

Databases on Medical Education
Curriculum Management & Information Tool (CurrMIT)
CurrMIT Helpline
helpcurrmit@aamc.org

Data Warehouse
Kirke Lawton
828-0974
klawton@aamc.org

Dean's Letter (Medical Student Performance Evaluation)
Henry M. Sondheimer, M.D.
828-0684
hsondheimer@aamc.org

Development Survey
Chris Tucker
828-0989
ctucker@aamc.org

Directory of American Medical Education
Susan Monseur
828-0489
smonseur@aamc.org

Disability/ADA
Medical Schools
Henry M. Sondheimer, M.D.
828-0684
hsondheimer@aamc.org

Medical College Admission Test
John Hosterman, Ph.D.
862-6190
jhosterman@aamc.org

AAMC Subject Listing

Diversity Research Forum
Laura Castillo-Page, Ph.D.
828-0579
lcastillopage@aamc.org

E

Education Programs
M. Brownell Anderson
828-0562
mbanderson@aamc.org

Electronic Communications
Eric Weissman
828-0044
eweissman@aamc.org

Electronic Residency Application Service (ERAS)
B. Renee Overton
828-0504
broverton@aamc.org

ERAS General Information
828-0413
ERASHelp@aamc.org

Enrollment/Graduation Data
Gwen Garrison, Ph.D.
862-6186
ggarrison@aamc.org

Executive Development Seminars for Associate Deans and Chairs
Carol A. Aschenbrener, M.D.
828-0648
caschenbrener@aamc.org

F

Facilities at the AAMC
Mark Wood
828-0450
mwood@aamc.org

Facilities at Medical Schools
Heather Sacks
862-6220
hsacks@aamc.org

Facts & Figures Data Series
Laura Castillo-Page, Ph.D.
828-0579
lcastillopage@aamc.org

Faculty Development and Leadership Programs (FD&L)
Carol A. Aschenbrener, M.D.
828-0648
caschenbrener@aamc.org

Faculty Forward Program
William T. Mallon, Ed.D.
828-0424
wmallon@aamc.org

Faculty Policies (Promotion and Tenure)
William T. Mallon, Ed.D.
828-0424
wmallon@aamc.org

Sarah Bunton, Ph.D.
862-6225
sbunton@aamc.org

Faculty Practice Plan Survey
Mary Patton
862-6297
mpatton@aamc.org

Faculty Practice Plans
Ivy S. Baer, J.D.
828-0499
ibaer@aaamc.org

Faculty Practice Solutions Center
Mary Patton
862-6297
mpatton@aamc.org

Faculty/Chair Recruitment
STARS Central
862-6239
starscentral@aamc.org

Faculty Roster
Hershel Alexander
828-0649
halexander@aamc.org

Faculty Salary Survey
Wendy Geraci
862-6101
wdesmarais@aamc.org

Faculty Vitae
Carol A. Aschenbrener, M.D.
828-0648
caschenbrener@aamc.org

Federal Budget
David Moore
828-0559
dbmoore@aamc.org

Fee Assistance Program (FAP)
Kelly Begatto
828-6003
kbegatto@aamc.org

Financial Aid
Legislation
J. Matthew Shick
862-6116
jmshick@aamc.org

Policies/Procedures and Indebtedness
Shelley J. Yerman
828-0539
syerman@aamc.org

Julie Fresne
828-0511
jfresne@aamc.org

FindAResident Service
Michelle Duafala
828-0626
mduafalla@aamc.org

FIRST for Medical Education
Julie Fresne
828-0511
jfresne@aamc.org

Fogarty International Clinical Research Scholars Support Center
Tanya Smith
828-0481
tsmith@aamc.org

Forum on Conflict of Interest in Academe (FOCI Academe)
Susan Ehringhaus, J.D.
828-0543
sehringhaus@aamc.org

Fraud and Misconduct in Research
Susan Ehringhaus, J.D.
828-0543
sehringhaus@aamc.org

Fulfilling the Promise Campaign
Elisa K. Siegel
828-0459
esiegel@aamc.org

Retha Sherrod
828-0975
rsherrod@aamc.org

G

Genetics Research
Stephen J. Heinig
828-0488
sheinig@aamc.org

GME Track
Jennifer Faerberg
862-6221
gmetrack@aamc.org

Governance of AAMC
Kathleen S. Turner
828-0463
ksturner@aamc.org

Government Relations
David Moore
828-0559
dbmoore@aamc.org

Graduate Medical Education
Administration
Sunny G. Yoder
828-0497
syoder@aamc.org

Accreditation
Carol A. Aschenbrener, M.D.
828-0648
caschenbrener@aamc.org

Curriculum
Alexis L. Ruffin
828-0439
alruffin@aamc.org

Financing
Karen S. Fisher, J.D.
828-0490
kfisher@aamc.org

Immigration
Sunny G. Yoder
828-0497
syoder@aamc.org

Legislation
Atul Grover, M.D., Ph.D.
828-0666
agrover@aamc.org

Christiane A. Mitchell
828-0461
cmitchell@aamc.org

Regulatory Payments
Karen S. Fisher, J.D.
828-0490
kfisher@aamc.org

Grants Administration
Leslye Fulwider
828-0646
lfulwider@aamc.org

Groups at the AAMC
Chief Medical Officers (CMO)
David Longnecker
828-0490
dlongnecker@aamc.org

Government Relations Representatives (GRR)
David Moore
828-0559
dbmoore@aamc.org

Graduate Research, Education, and Training Group (GREAT)
Jodi B. Lubetsky, Ph.D.
828-0485
jlubetsky@aamc.org

Group on Business Affairs (GBA)
Heather Sacks
862-6220
hsacks@aamc.org

Group on Educational Affairs (GEA)
M. Brownell Anderson
828-0562
mbanderson@aamc.org

Group on Faculty Affairs (GFA)
Valarie Clark
828-0586
vclark@aamc.org

Group on Faculty Practice (GFP)
Ivy S. Baer, J.D.
828-0499
ibaer@aaamc.org

AAMC Subject Listing

Group on Information Resources (GIR)
Morgan Passiment
828-0476
mpassiment@aamc.org

Group on Institutional Advancement (GIA)
Chris Tucker
828-0939
ctucker@aamc.org

Group on Institutional Planning (GIP)
Heather Sacks
862-6220
hsacks@aamc.org

Group on Regional Medical Campuses (GRMC)
M. Brownell Anderson
828-0562
mbanderson@aamc.org

Group on Research Advancement and Development (GRAND)
Stephen J. Heinig
828-0488
sheinig@aamc.org

Group on Resident Affairs (GRA)
Sunny G. Yoder
828-0497
syoder@aamc.org

Group on Student Affairs (GSA)
Henry M. Sondheimer, M.D.
828-0684
hsondheimer@aamc.org

GSA Minority Affairs Section (GSA-MAS)
Lily May Johnson
828-0573
lmjohnson@aamc.org

Juan Amador
862-6149
jamador@aamc.org

Women Liaison Officers (WLO)—Women in Medicine
Valarie Clark
828-0586
vclark@aamc.org

H

Health Care Disparities
Ann Steinecke, Ph.D.
862-6296
asteinecke@aamc.org

Health Care Improvement
Joanne M. Conroy, M.D.
828-0493
jconroy@aamc.org

Health Information Technology Legislation
Chistiane A. Mitchell
828-0461
cmitchell@aamc.org

Policy
Morgan Passiment
828-0476
mpassiment@aamc.org

Jennifer Faerberg
862-6221
jfaerberg@aamc.org

Health Professions Education Funding
Tannaz Rasouli
828-0057
trasouli@aamc.org

Health Professionals and Nursing Education Coalition (HPNEC)
Tannaz Rasouli
828-0057
trasouli@aamc.org

Health Professionals for Diversity Coalition (HPD)
Sarah Schoolcraft
828-0560
sschoolcraft@aamc.org

Health Services Research (HSR) Legislation
Tannaz Rasouli
828-0057
trasouli@aamc.org

HHS Office of Inspector General
Ivy S. Baer, J.D.
828-0499
ibaer@aamc.org

HIPAA
Ivy S. Baer, J.D.
828-0499
ibaer@aamc.org

Susan Ehringhaus, J.D.
828-0543
sehringhaus@aamc.org

Morgan Passiment
828-0476
mpassiment@aamc.org

Holistic Review Admission Policies and Procedures
Ruth Beer Bletzinger
828-0585
rbletzinger@aamc.org

Hospital Operations and Financial Data
LaTonya Ford
862-6192
lford@aamc.org

Hospital Payment Legislation
Atul Grover, M.D., Ph.D.
828-0666
agrover@aamc.org

Christiane A. Mitchell
828-0461
cmitchell@aamc.org

Regulatory (CMS)
Karen S. Fisher, J.D.
828-0490
kfisher@aamc.org

Ivy S. Baer, J.D.
828-0490
ibaer@aamc.org

Hospital Quality Alliance
Jennifer Faerberg
862-6221
jfaerberg@aamc.org

House Staff Salary and Benefits Survey and Data
LaTonya Ford
862-6192
lford@aamc.org

Human Resources (AAMC)
Donna Whitlock Stewart
828-0446
dwstewart@aamc.org

I

Industry/Academia/Government Relations
Stephen J. Heinig
828-0488
sheinig@aamc.org

Information Technology
Jeanne L. Mella
862-6173
jmella@aamc.org

Innovations in Medical Education (IME)
M. Brownell Anderson
828-0562
mbanderson@aamc.org

Caroline Ford Coleman
828-0412
ccoleman@aamc.org

Intellectual Property (AAMC)
Gabrielle Campbell
828-0643
gcampbell@aamc.org

Intellectual Property (and Public Policy)
Susan Ehringhaus, J.D.
828-0543
sehringhaus@aamc.org

Stephen J. Heinig
828-0488
sheinig@aamc.org

International Accreditation Issues
Carol A. Aschenbrener, M.D.
828-0648
caschenbrener@aamc.org

International Medical Education
M. Brownell Anderson
828-0562
mbanderson@aamc.org

Interprofessional Issues
Carol A. Aschenbrener, M.D.
828-0648
caschenbrener@aamc.org

J

Job Board
Pia Aladdin
828-0524
paladdin@aamc.org

Journal
Academic Medicine
Anne Farmakidis
828-0593
afarmakidis@aamc.org

L

Leader to Leader
Retha Sherrod
828-0975
rsherrod@aamc.org

Leadership Training and Development Program for Associate Deans and Chairs
Carol A. Aschenbrener, M.D.
828-0648
caschenbrener@aamc.org

Legal Counsel
Joseph A. Keyes Jr., J.D.
828-0555
jakeyes@aamc.org

Liaison Committee on Medical Education (LCME)
Dan Hunt, M.D.
828-0596
dhunt@aamc.org

Robert F. Sabalis, Ph.D.
828-0556
rsabalis@aamc.org

Librarian
Marian Taliaferro
828-0433
mtaliaferro@aamc.org

Loan Repayment Programs
Shelley J. Yerman
828-0539
syerman@aamc.org

Denine Hales
828-0681
dhales@aamc.org

Legislation
J. Matthew Shick
862-6116
jmshick@aamc.org

AAMC Subject Listing

Log-in
STARS Central
862-6239
starscentral@aamc.org

M

Mailing Labels
STARS Central
862-6239
starscentral@aamc.org

Matriculating Student Questionnaire (MSQ)
Gwen Garrison, Ph.D.
862-6186
ggarrison@aamc.org

Collins Mikesell
862-6080
cmikesell@aamc.org

MedEdPORTAL
Robby Reynolds
828-0962
rreynolds@aamc.org

Media Relations
Retha Sherrod
828-0975
rsherrod@aamc.org

Nicole Buckley
828-0041
nbuckley@aamc.org

Medicaid
Legislation
Christiane A. Mitchell
828-0461
cmitchell@aamc.org

Regulatory
Karen S. Fisher, J.D.
828-0490
kfisher@aamc.org

Medical College Admission Test (MCAT)
General Information
mcat@aamc.org
828-0690

Policy Research
Karen Mitchell, Ph.D.
828-0500
kmitchell@aamc.org

Scott Oppler, Ph.D.
862-6073
soppler@aamc.org

Test Administration
Michelle Sparacino
828-0603
msparacino@aamc.org

Medical Liability Reform
Christiane A. Mitchell
828-0461
cmitchell@aamc.org

Medical Minority Applicant Registry (Med-MAR)
Lily May Johnson
828-0573
lmjohnson@aamc.org

Angela R. Moses
862-6203
amoses@aamc.org

Medical Records Confidentiality:
Legislative
David Moore
828-0559
dbmoore@aamc.org

Tannaz Rasouli
828-0057
trasouli@aamc.org

Regulations
Susan Ehringhaus, J.D.
828-0543
sehringhaus@aamc.org

Ivy S. Baer, J.D.
828-0499
ibaer@aamc.org

Medical School Admission Requirements (MSAR)
Tami Levin
862-6084
tlevin@aamc.org

Medical School Admissions
Henry M. Sondheimer, M.D.
828-0684
hsondheimer@aamc.org

Medical School Application, Acceptance, and Matriculation Data
Collins Mikesell
862-6080
cmikesell@aamc.org

Medical School Graduation Questionnaire
Jason Cantow
828-0960
jcantow@aamc.org

M. Brownell Anderson
828-0562
mbanderson@aamc.org

Medical School Objective Project (MSOP)
M. Brownell Anderson
828-0562
mbanderson@aamc.org

Alexis L. Ruffin
828-0439
aruffin@aamc.org

Medical School Profile System
Katherine Brandenburg
862-6158
kbrandenburg@aamc.org

Medical Student Education Costs
Medical Schools
Robert F. Jones, Ph.D.
828-0520
rfjones@aamc.org

Students
Julie Fresne
828-0511
jfresne@aamc.org

Medical Students
Career Counseling, Health Services, Insurance, Disability
Henry M. Sondheimer, M.D.
828-0684
hsondheimer@aamc.org

George V. Richard, Ph.D.
869-6223
grichard@aamc.org

Medical Student Performance Evaluation (Dean's Letter)
Henry M. Sondheimer, M.D.
828-0684
hsondheimer@aamc.org

Medicare
Compliance
Ivy S. Baer, J.D.
828-0490
ibaer@aamc.org

Hospital Legislation
Atul Grover, M.D., Ph.D.
828-0666
agrover@aamc.org

Christiane A. Mitchell
828-0461
cmitchell@aamc.org

Hospital Payments
Karen S. Fisher, J.D.
862-6140
kfisher@aamc.org

Medicare Payment Advisory Commission (MedPAC)
Karen S. Fisher, J.D.
862-6140
kfisher@aamc.org

Physician Legislation
Christiane A. Mitchell
828-0461
cmitchell@aamc.org

Physicians Payment
Ivy S. Baer, J.D.
828-0499
ibaer@aaamc.org

Meeting Planning
Kirsten Olean
828-0479
kolean@aamc.org

Meeting Registration
Nathalie Tavel
863-6227
ntavel@aamc.org

Membership
Institutional
Kathleen S. Turner
828-0463
ksturner@aamc.org

Minority Faculty Development
Lily May Johnson
828-0573
lmjohnson@aamc.org

Laura Castillo-Page, Ph.D.
828-0579
lcastillopage@aamc.org

Minority Physician Database
Kehua Zhang, Ph.D.
828-0578
kzhang@aamc.org

Minority Student Data
Kehua Zhang, Ph.D.
828-0578
kzhang@aamc.org

Minority Student Medical Career Awareness Workshop and Recruitment Fair
Juan Amador
862-6149
jamador@aamc.org

Angela R. Moses
862-6203
amoses@aamc.org

Minority Student Opportunities in U.S. Medical Schools
Lily May Johnson
828-0573
lmjohnson@aamc.org

Mission-based Management
William T. Mallon, Ed.D.
828-0424
wmallon@aamc.org

N

National Institutes of Health Legislation
David Moore
828-0559
dbmoore@aamc.org

National Resident Matching Program (NRMP)
Mona Signer
828-0629
msigner@aamc.org

O

Organization of Resident Representatives (ORR)
Alexis L. Ruffin
828-0439
alruffin@aamc.org

Organization of Student Representatives (OSR)
Ally Anderson
828-0682
aanderson@aamc.org

AAMC Subject Listing

Denine Hales
828-0681
dhales@aamc.org

P

Patents and Licensing
Susan Ehringhaus, J.D.
828-0543
sehringhaus@aamc.org

Stephen J. Heinig
828-0488
sheinig@aamc.org

Patient Safety Legislation
Christine A. Mitchell
828-0461
cmitchell@aamc.org

Ph.D. Training and Postdoctoral
Jodi B. Lubetsky, Ph.D.
828-0485
jlubetsky@aamc.org

Tammi Simpson
828-0685
tsimpson@aamc.org

Physicians Payment
Legislation
Christiane A. Mitchell
828-0461
cmitchell@aamc.org

Regulatory
Ivy S. Baer, J.D.
828-0499
ibaer@aaamc.org

Physicians and Teaching Hospitals (PATH)
Ivy S. Baer, J.D.
828-0490
ibaer@aamc.org

Premedical Advising
Henry M. Sondheimer, M.D.
828-0684
hsondheimer@aamc.org

Premedical Student Questionaire (PMQ)
Gwen Garrison, Ph.D.
828-0186
ggarrison@aamc.org

Professionalism
M. Brownell Anderson
828-0562
mbanderson@aamc.org

Project Medical Education (PME)
Sallyann Bergh
862-6289
sbergh@aamc.org

Public Opinion Research
Elisa K. Siegel
828-0459
esiegel@aamc.org

Publication Orders
Customer Service Office
828-0416
publications@aamc.org

R

Research in Medical Education (RIME)
M. Brownell Anderson
828-0562
mbanderson@aamc.org

Caroline Ford Coleman
828-0412
ccoleman@aamc.org

Research Funding
Anthony J. Mazzaschi
828-0059
tmazzaschi@aamc.org

Legislation
David Moore
828-0559
dbmoore@aamc.org

Research Infrastructure and Instrumentation
Legislation
David Moore
828-0559
dbmoore@aamc.org

Regulation and Policy
Stephen J. Heinig
828-0488
sheinig@aamc.org

Residency Applications
Electronic Residency Application Service (ERAS)
B. Renee Overton
828-0504
boverton@aamc.org

National Resident Matching Program (NRMP)
Mona Signer
828-0629
msigner@aamc.org

Resident Education
Alexis L. Ruffin
828-0439
alruffin@aamc.org

Sunny Yoder
828-0497
syoder@aamc.org

S

STAT (Short, Topical, and Timely)
Nicole Buckley
828-0041
nbuckley@aamc.org

Stem Cell Research and Cloning
Anthony J. Mazzaschi
828-0059
tmazzaschi@aamc.org

Legislation
David Moore
828-0559
dbmoore@aamc.org

Student Affairs
Henry M. Sondheimer, M.D.
828-0684
hsondheimer@aamc.org

Student Records
Henry M. Sondheimer, M.D.
828-0684
hsondheimer@aamc.org

Danielle J. Gregory
828-0680
dgregory@aamc.org

Student Records System
Gwen Garrison, Ph.D.
828-0186
ggarrison@aamc.org

Subscriptions
Customer Service Office
828-0416
publications@aamc.org

Summer Medical & Dental Education Program (SMDEP)
Norma Poll, Ph.D.
862-6115
npoll@aamc.org

T

Technology Transfer
Susan Ehringhaus, J.D.
828-0543
sehringhaus@aamc.org

Stephen J. Heinig
828-0488
sheinig@aamc.org

Tool for Assessing Cultural Competence Training (TAACT)
Norma Poll, Ph.D.
862-6115
npoll@aamc.org

Ann Steinecke, Ph.D.
862-6296
asteinecke@aamc.org

U

"Underrepresented in Medicine" Definition
Ruth Beer Bletzinger
828-0585
rbletzinger@aamc.org

V

Veterans Affairs Issues
Legislation
J. Matthew Shick
862-6116
jmshick@aamc.org

Research Policy
Stephen J. Heinig
828-0488
sheinig@aamc.org

W

Washington Highlights/Headlines
David Moore
828-0559
dbmoore@aamc.org

Women in Medicine (WIM)
Valarie Clark
828-0586
vclark@aamc.org

www.aamc.org
Eric Weissman
828-0044
eweissman@aamc.org

AAMC Elected Leaders

Past Presidents

1876-79 J. B. Biddle
1879-81 Samuel D. Gross
1881-82 J. M. Bodine
1882-83 W. W. Seely
1890   Aaron Friedenwald
1890-94 Nathan S. Davis
1894-95 E. Fletcher Ingals
1895-96 William Osler
1896-97 J. M. Bodine
1897-98 James W. Holland
1898-99 Henry O. Walker
1899-00 Parks Ritchie
1900-01 Albert R. Baker
1901-02 Victor C. Vaughan
1902-03 William L. Rodman
1903-04 James R. Guthrie
1904-06 Samuel C. James
1906-07 George M. Kober
1907-08 Henry B. Ward
1908-09 Eli H. Long
1909-10 George H. Hoxie
1910-11 John A. Witherspoon
1911-12 William P. Harlow
1912-13 Egbert LeFevre
1913-14 E. P. Lyon
1914-15 Isadore Dyer
1915-16 Charles R. Bardeen
1916-17 John L. Heffron
1917-18 W. S. Carter
1918-19 William J. Means
1919-20 George Blumer
1920-21 William Pepper
1921-22 Theodore Hough
1922-23 Charles P. Emerson
1923-24 Irving S. Cutter
1924-25 Ray Lyman Wilbur
1925-26 Hugh Cabot
1926-27 Charles F. Martin
1927-28 Walter L. Niles
1928-29 Burton D. Myers
1929-30 William Darrach
1930-31 Maurice H. Rees
1931-33 Louis B. Wilson
1933-35 Ross V. Patterson
1935-36 John Wyckoff
1936-37 E. Stanley Ryerson
1937-38 Alan M. Chesney
1938-39 Willard C. Rappleye
1939-40 Russell H.
        Oppenheimer
1940-41 C. W. M. Poynter
1941-42 Loren R. Chandler
1942-43 Waller S. Leathers
1943-44 E. M. MacEwen
1944-45 Albert C. Furstenberg

1945-46 John Walker Moore
1946-47 William S. McEllroy
1947-48 Waller A. Bloedom
1948-49 J. Roscoe Miller
1949-50 Joseph C. Hinsey
1950-51 Arthur C. Bachmeyer
1951-52 George Packer Berry
1952-53 Ward Darley
1953-54 Stanley E. Dorst
1954-55 Vernon W. Lippard
1955-56 Robert A. Moore
1956-57 John B. Youmans
1957-58 Lowell T. Coggeshall
1958-59 John McK. Mitchell
1959-60 Thomas H. Hunter
1960-61 George N. Aagaard
1961-62 Donald G. Anderson
1962-63 John E. Deitrick
1963-64 Robert C. Berson
1964-65 George A. Wolf, Jr.
1965-66 Thomas B. Turner
1966-67 William N.
        Hubbard, Jr.
1967-68 John Parks

Past Chairs

1968-69 Robert J. Glaser
1969-70 Robert B. Howard
1970-71 William G. Anlyan
1971-72 Russell A. Nelson
1972-73 Charles C. Sprague
1973-74 Daniel C. Tosteson
1974-75 Sherman M.
        Mellinkoff
1975-76 Leonard W.
        Cronkhite, Jr.
1976-77 Ivan L. Bennett, Jr.
1977-78 Robert G. Petersdorf
1978-79 John A. Gronvall
1979-80 Charles B. Womer
1980-81 Julius R. Krevans
1981-82 Thomas K. Oliver, Jr.
1982-83 Steven C. Beering
1983-84 Robert M. Heyssel
1984-85 Richard Janeway
1985-86 Virginia V. Weldon
1986-87 Edward J. Stemmler
1987-88 John W. Colloton
1988-89 D. Kay Clawson
1989-90 David H. Cohen
1990-91 William T. Butler
1991-92 J. Robert Buchanan
1992-93 Spencer Foreman
1993-94 Stuart Bondurant
1994-95 Kenneth I. Berns
1995-96 Herbert Pardes
1996-97 Mitchell T. Rabkin
1997-98 Robert O. Kelley
1998-99 William A. Peck
1999-00 Ralph W. Muller
2000-01 George F. Sheldon
2001-02 Ralph Snyderman
2002-03 Theresa Bischoff
2003-04 Donald E. Wilson
2004-05 N. Lynn Eckhert
2005-06 Thomas M. Priselac
2006-07 Richard D. Krugman

Annual Awards and Lectures

Abraham Flexner Award for Distinguished Service to Medical Education

The Abraham Flexner Award for Distinguished Service to Medical Education was established in 1958 to recognize extraordinary individual contributions to medical schools and to the medical educational community as a whole. Recipients of this award have been:

1958	Joseph C. Hinsey	1975	Thomas Hale Ham	1991	Daniel C. Tosteson
1959	Alfred N. Richards	1976	Franz J. Ingelfinger	1992	August G. Swanson
1960	Herman G. Weiskotten	1977	Paul B. Beeson	1993	Robert G. Petersdorf
1961	Willard C. Rappleye	1978	Ivan L. Bennett, Jr.	1994	Richard S. Ross
1962	George Packer Berry	1979	Julius H. Comroe, Jr.	1995	Saul J. Farber
1963	Lowell T. Coggeshall	1980	William G. Anlyan	1996	Arthur C. Guyton
1964	Ward Darley	1981	Sherman M. Mellinkoff	1997	Edmund D. Pellegrino
1965	Jospeh T. Wearn	1982	Robert H. Ebert	1998	Joseph S. Gonnella
1966	James A. Shannon	1983	Julius R. Krevans	1999	Joseph B. Martin
1967	Stanley E. Dorst	1984	Robert J. Glaser	2000	Howard S. Barrows
1968	Lister Hill	1985	John A. D. Cooper	2001	Daniel D. Federman
1969	John M. Russell	1986	David E. Rogers	2002	Kelley M. Skeff
1970	Eugene A. Stead	1987	Frederick C. Robbins	2003	Kenneth M. Ludmerer
1971	Carl V. Moore	1988	Thomas H. Hunter	2004	Haile T. Debas
1972	William R. Willard	1989	Lloyd H. Smith, Jr.	2005	Georges Bordage
1973	George T. Harrell, Jr.	1990	James A. Pittman, Jr.	2006	Jordan J. Cohen
1974	John L. Caughey, Jr.	1991	Daniel C. Tosteson	**2007**	**David C. Leach, M.D.**

Alpha Omega Alpha Distinguished Teacher Awards

The Alpha Omega Alpha Distinguished Teacher Awards were initiated by AOA in the spring of 1988. The name of the award was changed in 1997 to the Alpha Omega Alpha Robert J. Glaser Distinguished Teacher Awards, in honor of Robert J. Glaser, M.D., long-time Executive Secretary of AOA. The establishment of these awards by AOA emphasizes the importance of recognizing those who devote their time and energy to the accomplishment of the educational mission of the medical schools. The selection committees for the awards are jointly appointed by the AOA and the Association of American Medical Colleges. Each U.S. and Canadian school of medicine may make one nomination annually. The purpose of these awards is to provide national recognition to faculty members who have distinguished themselves in medical student education. Recipients of this award have been:

1988	W. Proctor Harvey; Carson D. Schneck
1989	Jerome P. Kassirer; Cornelius Rosse
1990	Thomas H. Kent; David L. Sackett
1991	John P. Atkinson; William K. Metcalf
1992	David C. Sabiston; Robert L. Trelstad
1993	Kelley M. Skeff; Parker A. Small
1994	Jane F. Desforge; William E. Erkonen; Jose Ignacio; Guido Majno
1995	Pamela C. Champe; Phyllis A. Guze
1996	Ruth-Marie E. Fincher; Edward C. Klatt; Steven R. McGee
1997	George Libman Engel; William H. Frishman; Carlos Pestana; Michael S. Wilkes
1998	Bruce M. Koeppen; Daniel H. Lowenstein; Hugo R. Seibel; Mark H. Swartz
1999	Susan Billings; L.D. Britt; W. Patrick Duff; John T. Hansen

2000	Frank M. Calia; Cyril M. Grum; Ronald J. Markert; Jeanette J. Norden
2001	Walter J. Bo; J. John Cohen; Douglas S. Paauw; Steven E. Weinberger
2002	Lewis R. First; Faith T. Fitzgerald; Aviad Haramati; Ralph F. Jozefowicz
2003	Joel M. Felner; Barry D. Mann; Gabriel Virella; Lawrence Wood
2004	Linda S. Costanzo; Arthur F. Dalley: Steven L. Galetta; Charles H. Griffith
2005	Paul F. Aravich; David E. Golan; Louis N. Pangaro; Robert T. Watson
2006	Carmine D. Clemente; Molly Cooke; Helen Davies; Jeffrey Wiese
2007	**Robert M. Klein; John Nolte; Richard M. Schwartzstein; James L. Sebastian**

Annual Awards and Lectures

Award for Distinguished Research in the Biomedical Sciences

The AAMC Award for Distinguished Research in the Biomedical Sciences was established in 1981, continuing a tradition of honoring high caliber research begun in 1946 with the Borden Award. The award recognizes outstanding clinical or laboratory research conducted by a member of the faculty of a medical school, which is a member of the Association of American Medical Colleges. Recipients of this award have been:

1981	J. Michael Bishop	1990	Robert J. Lefkowitz	1999	Elizabeth H. Blackburn
1982	Raymond L. Erikson	1991	Sheldon M. Wolff	2000	Ferid Murad
1983	Philip Leder	1992	Bruce M. Alberts	2001	C. David Allis
1984	Michael S. Brown	1993	Bert Vogelstein	2002	Stanley Korsmeyer
	Joseph L. Goldstein	1994	Francis S. Collins	2003	Aaron J. Shatkin
1985	Eric R. Kandel	1995	Solomon H. Snyder	2004	Cynthia Kenyon
1986	Paul C. Lauterbur	1996	Stanley B. Prusiner	2005	Stuart H. Orkin
1987	Joseph Larner	1997	David M. Livingston	2006	François M. Abboud
1988	Alfred G. Gilman	1998	Mario R. Capecchi	**2007**	**Seymour J. Klebanoff**
1989	Sanford L. Palay		Oliver Smithies		

David E. Rogers Award

The David E. Rogers Award sponsored jointly by the AAMC and the Robert Wood Johnson Foundation was established in 1995. The award is granted annually to a medical school faculty member who has made major contributions to improving the health and health care of the American people. Recipients of this award have been:

1995	Diane M. Becker	2000	Jeremiah Stamler	2004	Michael DeBakey
1996	Robert G. Newman	2001	Barbara Barlow	2005	C. Everett Koop
1997	Julius B. Richmond	2002	David A. Kessler	2006	Eugene Braunwald
1998	Philip R. Lee	2003	Frank E. Speizer;	**2007**	**Robert H. Brook**
1999	William N. Kelley		Walter C. Willett		

Outstanding Community Service Award

The AAMC Award for Outstanding Community Service was first granted in 1993 to recognize the extraordinary contributions that medical schools and teaching hospitals make to their communities. The award recipient must have a broad-based, continuing commitment to community service as reflected in a variety of programs and initiatives that are responsive to community and social needs and show evidence of a true partnership with the community.

1993	University of Miami School of Medicine
1994	University of Medicine and Dentistry of New Jersey New Jersey Medical School
1995	Boston University School of Medicine
1996	Montefiore Medical Center
1997	Wright State University School of Medicine
1998	University of California, Los Angeles, School of Medicine, with Charles R. Drew University of Medicine and Science
1999	Morehouse School of Medicine
2000	University of Colorado School of Medicine
2001	Medical University of South Carolina
2002	University of Washington School of Medicine
2003	Creighton University School of Medicine; University of Nebraska College of Medicine
2004	University of Rochester Medical Center
2005	Medical College of Wisconsin; University of California Davis Health System
2006	West Virginia University School of Medicine
2007	**St. Joseph's Hospital and Medical Center**

Annual Awards and Lectures

Humanism in Medicine Award

The Humanism in Medicine Award recognizes a physician faculty member who exemplifies the qualities of a caring and compassionate mentor in the teaching and advising of medical students and possesses the personal qualities necessary to the practice of patient-centered medicine. The award is sponsored by Pfizer Inc. and Pfizer Medical Humanities Initiative.

1999	Andrew Hsi	2004	Sharad Jain
2000	Richard P. Usatine	2005	Melissa A. Warfield
2001	Coleen H. Kivlahan	2006	Robert J. Paeglow
2002	Edward F. Bell	**2007**	**Yasmin S. Meah**
2003	Samuel LeBaron		

Herbert W. Nickens Award

The Herbert W. Nickens Award was established by the AAMC in 2000 to honor the late Dr. Nickens and his lifelong concerns about the educational, societal, and health care needs of minorities. This award is given to an individual who has made outstanding contributions to promoting justice in medical education and health care. The recipients of this award have been:

2000	Donald E. Wilson	2004	Michael V. Drake
2001	Lee C. Bollinger	2005	Joan Y. Reede
2002	David Satcher	2006	Spero M. Manson
2003	Anna Cherrie Epps	**2007**	**M. Roy Wilson**

Herbert W. Nickens Faculty Fellowship

The Herbert W. Nickens Faculty Fellowship was established by the AAMC in 2000. The award recognizes an outstanding junior faculty member who has demonstrated leadership in the United States in addressing inequities in medical education and health care; demonstrated efforts in addressing educational, societal, and health care needs of minorities; and is committed to a career in academic medicine. The recipients of this award have been:

2000	Charles E. Moore	2004	Katherine J. Mathews
2001	Vanessa B. Sheppard	2005	Ugo A. Ezenkwele
2002	Janice C. Blanchard	2006	Alfredo Quiñones-Hinojosa
2003	Monica J. Mitchell	**2007**	**Thomas D. Sequist**

Herbert W. Nickens Medical Student Scholarships

The Herbert W. Nickens Medical Student Scholarships were established by the AAMC in 2000. These awards consist of five scholarships given to outstanding students entering their third year of medical school who have shown leadership efforts to eliminate inequities in medical education and health care and have demonstrated leadership efforts in addressing educational, societal, and health care needs of minorities in the United States. The recipients of these awards have been:

2000	Opeolu M. Adeoye; Diana I. Bojorquez; Jim F. Hammel; Yolandra Hancock; Sonia Lomeli
2001	Alberto Mendivil; Constance M. Mobley; Chukwuka C. Okafor; Sheneika M. Walker; Melanie M. Watkins
2002	Aimalohi A. Ahonkhai; Lukejohn W. Day; Tarayn A. Grizzard; Alejandrina I. Rincón; David T. Robles
2003	Cedric K. Dark; Francine E. Garrett; David E. Montgomery; Johnnie J. Orozco; Nicholas J. Smith
2004	Nicolas L. Cuttriss; Joy Hsu; Angela Chia-Mei Huang; Risha R. Irby; Richard M. Vidal
2005	Erik S. Cabral; Christopher T. Erb; Harlan B. Harvey; Osita I. Onugha; Sloane L. York
2006	Nehkonti Adams; Dora Cristina Castañeda; Luis Isaac Garcia; AeuMuro Gashaw Lake; Katherine Leila Neuhausen
2007	**Christain A. Corbit; Cheri Cerella Cross; Maria-Esteli Garcia; Marlana M. Li; Danielle Ku`ulei Potter**

Annual Awards and Lectures

Alan Gregg Memorial Lecture

Named in honor of the late Alan Gregg, American physician, educator, and philanthropist, this lecture was presented for the first time at the 1958 annual meeting of the Association of American Medical Colleges. Lectures have been given by:

1958	James B. Conant	1975	William B. Castle	1991	Daniel Callahan
1959	Warren Weaver	1976	William B. Bean	1992	Robert M. Heyssel
1960	Joseph T. Wearn	1977	Donald W. Seldin	1993	Samuel Thier
1961	Wilder G. Penfield	1978	Lewis Thomas	1994	W. French Anderson
1962	C. Sidney Burwell	1979	David E. Rogers	1995	Stanley Chodorow
1963	Willard C. Rappleye	1980	Daniel C. Tosteson	1996	Andrew G. Wallace
1964	Robert S. Morison	1981	David M. Kipnis	1997	David Satcher
1965	Ward Darley	1982	Sherman M.	1998	Richard L. Cruess
1966	James A. Shannon		Mellinkoff	1999	Molly Corbett Broad
1967	Colin M. MacLeod	1983	Robert G. Petersdorf	2000	Donald M. Berwick
1968	John M. Russell	1984	Lloyd H. Smith, Jr.	2001	Steven A. Schroeder
1969	Kingman Brewster, Jr.	1985	Harold T. Shapiro	2002	Deborah Prothrow-Stith
1970	Lincoln Gordon	1986	Thomas F. Eagleton	2003	Harvey V. Fineberg
1971	Alexander Heard	1987	Alvin R. Tarlov	2004	Christine K. Cassell
1972	Clark Kerr	1988	C. Everett Koop	2005	M. Roy Schwarz
1973	John R. Evans	1989	Louis W. Sullivan	2006	Charles L. Rice
1974	Terry Sanford	1990	James D. Watson	**2007**	**Carolyn Clancy**

John A.D. Cooper Lecture

Named in honor of John A.D. Cooper, president of the Association of American Medical Colleges from 1969 to 1986, this lecture was presented for the first time at the 1985 annual meeting of the AAMC. The lecture was originally endowed by the American Hospital Supply Corporation Foundation.

1985	John A. D. Cooper	1995	Sherif S. Abdelhak		Daniel R. Masys,
1986	Paul B. Beeson	1996	Judith Feder		Suzanne S. Stensaas
1987	Uwe E. Reinhardt	1997	David Stern		(panelists)
1988	Henry G. Cisneros	1998	Barbara A. DeBuono	2002	David M. Lawrence
1989	Lauro F. Cavazos	1999	Christopher J.L. Murray	2003	Edward H. Wagner
1990	John F. Sherman	2000	Ruth Rothstein	2004	Clayton Christensen
1991	Margaret Catley-Carlson	2001	Robert L. Marier	2005	David J. Brailer
1992	Leroy Hood		(moderator);	2006	John E. Wenneberg
1993	Bruce M. Alberts		Valerie Florance,	**2007**	**Sara Rosenbaum**
1994	Merwyn R. Greenlick		Edward D. Miller,		

Robert G. Petersdorf Lecture

Named in honor of Robert G. Petersdorf, president of the Association of American Medical Colleges from 1986 to 1994, this lecture was presented for the first time at the 1994 annual meeting of the AAMC.

1994	Christine K. Cassel	2000	Uwe E. Reinhardt	2003	Risa Lavizzo-Mourey
1995	Joseph L. Goldstein	2001	Michael E. Whitcomb;	2004	Julie Gerberding
1996	Francis S. Collins		Donald O. Nutter;	2005	Daniel R. Masys
1997	Judith Rodin		Steven W. Weinberger	2006	Elizabeth G. Nabel
1998	Gilbert S. Omenn		(panelists)	**2007**	**Thomas R. Cech**
1999	David Satcher	2002	Anthony Fauci		

Jordan J. Cohen Leadership in Health Care Lecture

Named in honor of Jordan J. Cohen, president of the Association of American Medical Colleges from 1994 to 2006, this lecture was presented for the first time at the 2006 annual meeting of the AAMC.

2006   William M. Sulivan   **2007   Daniel D. Federman**

Medical School Members

2008–2009

University of Alabama School of Medicine

University of Alabama at Birmingham
1530 3rd Avenue South, FOT 12th Floor
Birmingham, Alabama 35294-3412
205-934-4011 (general information); 934-1111 (dean's office); 934-0333 (fax);
934-2330 (medical student affairs)
Web site: www.uab.edu/uasom

The University of Alabama School of Medicine is a continuation of medical training begun in Mobile more than 100 years ago. The medical school was moved from the Tuscaloosa campus to Birmingham in 1945 and expanded from a two-year to a four-year school. Clinical campuses are located in Tuscaloosa, Huntsville, and Birmingham.

Type: public
2008-2009 total enrollment: 700
Clinical facilities: Chauncey Sparks Center for Developmental and Learning Disorders, University of Alabama Hospitals, Children's Hospital, Spain Rehabilitation Center, the Kirklin Clinic, Veterans Administration Hospital, Center for Psychiatric Medicine, Callahan Eye Foundation Hospital, L. B. Wallace Tumor Institute, Druid City Hospital (Tuscaloosa), Huntsville Hospital, Family Medicine Centers (Birmingham, Huntsville, and Tuscaloosa).

University Officials

Chancellor . . . . Malcolm Portera, Ph.D.
President, University of Alabama at Birmingham. . . . . Carol Z. Garrison, Ph.D.
Provost . . . . Eli I. Capilouto, D.M.D.
Chief Executive Officer, Health System. . . . . Ray L. Watts (Interim)
Associate Vice President for Marketing and Public Relations . . . . Dale G. Turnbough

Medical School Administrative Staff

Senior Vice President and Dean. . . . . Robert R. Rich, M.D.
Senior Associate Dean for Administration and Finance . . . . G. Allen Bolton
Senior Associate Dean for Research . . . . Robert P. Kimberly, M.D.
Senior Associate Dean for Clinical Affairs. . . . . Loring Rue, M.D.
Senior Associate Dean for Academic Affairs . . . . Hughes Evans, M.D.
Senior Associate Dean for Faculty Development . . . . Kathleen G. Nelson, M.D.
Associate Dean, Huntsville Program . . . . Robert M. Centor, M.D.
Associate Dean, Tuscaloosa Program . . . . E. Eugene Marsh III, M.D.
Associate Dean for Student Services . . . . Laura Kezar, M.D.
Associate Dean for Veteran Affairs . . . . Dale A. Freeman, M.D.
Associate Dean for Research Compliance . . . . Sarah W. Morgan, M.D.
Associate Dean for Rural Programs and Primary Care . . . . William A. Curry, M.D.
Associate Dean for Undergraduate Medical Education . . . . Craig J. Hoesley, M.D.
Assistant Dean for Graduate Medical Education . . . . Gustavo Heudebert, M.D.
Assistant Dean for Admissions . . . . Nathan B. Smith, M.D.
Assistant Dean for Faculty and Administration . . . . Margarete A. Roser
Director, Continuing Medical Education. . . . . Jeroan Allison, M.D.
Registrar . . . . Linda P. McCullough

Department and Division or Section Chairs

Basic Sciences

Biochemistry . . . . Tim M. Townes, Ph.D.
Cell Biology. . . . . Etty Benveniste, Ph.D.
Microbiology. . . . . David D. Chaplin, M.D., Ph.D.
Neurobiology. . . . . David Sweatt, Ph.D.
Nutrition Sciences . . . . W. Timothy Garvey, M.D.
Pathology . . . . Jay M. McDonald, M.D.
   Anatomical Pathology. . . . . Gene P. Siegal, M.D.
   Forensic. . . . . Robert M. Brissie, M.D.
   Laboratory Medicine . . . . John A. Smith, M.D., Ph.D.
   Molecular and Cellular Pathology . . . . Thomas Clemens, Ph.D.

Neuropathology . . . . Kevin A. Roth, M.D.
Pharmacology . . . . Dennis Pillion, Ph.D. (Interim)
Physiology and Biophysics . . . . Dale J. Benos, Ph.D.

Clinical Sciences

Anesthesiology. . . . . Keith A. Jones, M.D.
Dermatology . . . . Craig A. Elmets, M.D.
Emergency Medicine . . . . Janyce Sanford, M.D.
Family Medicine . . . . T. Michael Harrington, M.D.
Human Genetics . . . . Bruce R. Korf, M.D.
Medicine. . . . . Edward Abraham, M.D.
    Cardiovascular Disease . . . . Robert C. Bourge, M.D.
    Endocrinology and Metabolism. . . . . Jeffrey E. Kudlow, M.D.
    Gastroenterology and Hepatology . . . . Charles M. Wilcox, M.D.
    General Internal Medicine . . . . Robert M. Centor, M.D.
    Gerontology and Geriatrics. . . . . Richard M. Allman, M.D.
    Hematology and Oncology . . . . Lisle M. Nabell, M.D. (Interim)
    Infectious Diseases . . . . Michael Saag, M.D.
    Nephrology . . . . Anupam Agarwal, M.D.
    Preventive Medicine . . . . Catarina I. Kiefe, M.D.
    Pulmonary and Critical Care. . . . . K. Randall Young, Jr., M.D.
    Rheumatology . . . . Robert Carter, M.D.
Neurology . . . . Ray L. Watts, M.D.
Obstetrics and Gynecology. . . . . John C. Hauth, M.D.
Ophthalmology . . . . Lanning B. Kline, M.D.
Pediatrics . . . . Sergio B. Stagno, M.D.
Physical Medicine and Rehabilitation . . . . Amie B. Jackson, M.D.
Psychiatry . . . . James Meador-Woodruff, M.D.
Radiation Oncology. . . . . James A. Bonner, M.D.
Radiology . . . . Reginald F. Munden, M.D.
    Nuclear Medicine. . . . . Janis P. O'Malley, M.D.
Surgery . . . . Kirby I. Bland, M.D.
    Cardiovascular and Thoracic. . . . . James Kirklan, M.D.
    General Surgery. . . . . Kirby I. Bland, M.D.
    Neurosurgery. . . . . James Markert, M.D.
    Oral Maxillofacial. . . . . Peter Waite, D.D.S., M.D.
    Orthopedic Surgery . . . . Thomas R. Hunt III, M.D.
    Otolaryngology. . . . . Glenn E. Peters, M.D.
    Pediatric Surgery . . . . Keith E. Georgeson, M.D.
    Plastic Surgery . . . . Luis O. Vasconez, M.D.
    Transplantation . . . . Devin E. Eckhoff, M.D.
    Urology . . . . Christopher L. Amling, M.D.

University-wide Interdisciplinary Research Centers

Arthritis and Musculoskeletal Disease Center . . . . Robert P. Kimberly, M.D.
Center for Aging. . . . . Richard M. Allman, M.D.
Center for AIDS Research . . . . Michael S. Saag, M.D.
Center for Clinical and Translational Science . . . . Lisa Guay-Woodford, M.D.
Center for Emerging Infections and Emergency Preparedness. . . . . Richard Whitley, M.D.,
                                                                           and Ziad Kazzi, M.D.
Center for Free Radical Biology . . . . Bruce A. Freeman, Ph.D.
Center for Outcomes and Effectiveness Research and Education . . . . Catarina I. Kiefe, M.D.,
                                                                       and Norman W. Weissman, Ph.D.
Civitan International Research Center . . . . Harald Sontheimer, Ph.D.
Comprehensive Cancer Center. . . . . Edward Partridge, M.D.
Gregory Fleming James Cystic Fibrosis Research Center . . . . Eric J. Sorscher, M.D.
Minority Health and Health Disparities Research Center. . . . . Mona N. Fouad, M.D.

University of South Alabama College of Medicine

307 University Boulevard
Mobile, Alabama 36688
251-460-7176 (admissions); 460-6278 (fax)
Web site: www.southalabama.edu/com

On August 19, 1969, the state legislature passed a resolution that a second medical school should be established in Alabama under the auspices of the University of South Alabama. On January 3, 1973, the charter class entered the University of South Alabama College of Medicine. The Basic Medical Sciences Building is located on the main university campus. Clinical teaching is conducted at the University of South Alabama Hospitals, the Infirmary Health Systems-affiliated hospitals, and numerous ambulatory facilities.

Type: public
2008-2009 total enrollment: 256
Clinical facilities: University of South Alabama Medical Center, University of South Alabama, Children's & Women's Hospital, Infirmary Medical Center, Infirmary West and Thomas Hospital.

University Officials

President. . . . . V. Gordon Moulton
Vice President for Health Sciences . . . . Ronald D. Franks, M.D.

Medical School Administrative Staff

Dean. . . . . Samuel J. Strada, Ph.D.
Associate Dean for Student Affairs and
   Continuing Medical Education . . . . Margaret O'Brien, J.D., M.D.
Assistant Dean for Curriculum . . . . Susan LeDoux, Ph.D.
Assistant Dean, Student Affairs and Educational Enrichment. . . . . Hattie M. Myles, Ph.D.
Assistant Dean, Student Affairs. . . . . John B. Bass Jr., M.D.
Associate Dean for Faculty Practice. . . . . Frederick N. Meyer, M.D.
Associate Dean for Clinical Affairs and Chief of Staff . . . . Richard S. Teplick, M.D.
Assistant Dean for Faculty Development . . . . Mary I. Townsley, Ph.D.
Assistant Dean for Graduate Medical Education . . . . Arnold Luterman, M.D.
Coordinator, Graduate Medical Education . . . . Judy Getty
Assistant Vice President for Medical/Financial Affairs . . . . John Pannelli
Director, Health Sciences Finance and Administration . . . . Susan Sansing
Director, Biomedical Library . . . . Judith F. Burnham
Director of Admissions. . . . . D. Mark Scott
Director, Office of Student Records . . . . Rhonda Smith
Director of Public Relations . . . . Paul Taylor
Chief Executive Officer, Health Services Foundation. . . . . Becky Tate
Vice President for USA Health System . . . . Stanley K. Hammack

University of South Alabama College of Medicine: ALABAMA

Department and Division or Section Chairs

Basic Sciences

Biochemistry and Molecular Biology...................... William T. Gerthoffer, Ph.D.
Comparative Medicine................................. Jonathan G. Scammell, Ph.D.
Microbiology and Immunology................................. David O. Wood, Ph.D.
Pharmacology .... Mark N. Gillespie, Ph.D.
Physiology.. Thomas M. Lincoln, Ph.D.
Cell Biology and Neuroscience................................ Glenn L. Wilson, Ph.D.

Clinical Sciences

Emergency Medicine...................................... Frank S. Pettyjohn, M.D.
Family Medicine .... R. Allen Perkins, M.D.
Internal Medicine .... Errol Crook, M.D.
    Cardiology.. Clara Massey, M.D.
    Gastroenterology/Liver Disease............................. Jack A. DiPalma, M.D.
    Hypertension/Nephrology .... Michael Culpepper, M.D.
    Infectious Diseases..................................... John VandeWaa, Ph.D., D.O.
    Pulmonary.. Ronald C. Allison, M.D.
    Rheumatology .... Errol Crook, M.D.
Medical Genetics.. Wladimir Wertelecki, M.D.
Neurological Surgery..................................... Eugene A. Quindlen, M.D.
Neurology... Bassam Bassam, M.D. (Interim)
Obstetrics and Gynecology.............................. Kathy Porter, M.D.
    Maternal and Fetal Medicine .... Kathy Porter, M.D.
    Reproductive Endocrinology........................... Botros N. Rizk, M.D.
Orthopedic Surgery...................................... Frederick N. Meyer, M.D.
Pathology .... J. Allan Tucker, M.D.
Pediatrics .... Loran T. Clement, M.D.
    Endocrinology .... Kenneth R. Rettig, M.D.
    Gastroenterology and Nutrition .... Karen Crissinger, M.D., Ph.D.
    General Pediatrics .... Ladonna Crews, M.D.
    Hematology and Oncology............................. Felicia Wilson, M.D.
    Infectious Diseases .... Mary C. Mancao, M.D.
    Neonatology... Fabien G. Eyal, M.D.
    Pediatric Critical Care .... Rose Vidal, M.D.
Psychiatry .... Ronald Franks, M.D.
Radiology .... Steven K. Teplick, M.D.
    Radiation Oncology .... Raymond B. Wynn, M.D.
Surgery.. Charles B. Rodning, M.D., Ph.D. (Interim)
    General Surgery...................................... Charles B. Rodning, M.D., Ph.D.
    Otolaryngology/ENT .... Open
    Pediatric Surgery .... Celeste Hollands, M.D.
    Plastic and Reconstructive Surgery .... Curtis N. Harris, M.D.
    Trauma and Critical Care............................. Richard Gonzalez, M.D.
    Urology .... Open

University of Arizona College of Medicine

P.O. Box 245017
Tucson, Arizona 85724-5017
520-626-6214 (Tucson admissions); 520-626-6337 (Tucson dean's office);
602-827-2005 (Phoenix admissions); 602-827-2018 (Phoenix dean's office)
Web site: www.medicine.arizona.edu

In 1961, the board of regents of the Universities and State College of Arizona authorized the University of Arizona to proceed with establishing a full four-year college of medicine on its campus in Tucson. In 1963, the state legislature appropriated funds for planning purposes, and active planning began in 1964. The first class of students was admitted in fall 1967 and graduated in June 1971. The Phoenix campus has trained third- and fourth-year students since 1992. It has been a four-year campus the last two years, matriculating 24 students its first year and 48 students this academic year.

Type: public
2008-2009 total enrollment: 542
Clinical facilities: Phoenix: Barrow Neurological Institute; Carl T. Hayden VA Medical Center; Good Samaritan Hospital and Medical Center; Maricopa Integrated Health System; Mayo Clinic/Scottsdale; Phoenix Baptist Hospital and Medical Center; Phoenix Children's Hospital; Scottsdale Health Care; St. Joseph's Hospital and Medical Center **Tucson:** Tucson Medical Center; Tucson VA Medical Center; University Medical Center; University Physicians Health Care.

University Officials

President. . . . . Robert N. Shelton, Ph.D.
Executive Vice President and Provost . . . . Meredith Hay, Ph.D.
Vice President for Health Sciences . . . . William M. Crist, M.D.
Vice President for Research . . . . Leslie P. Tolbert, Ph.D.

Medical School Administrative Staff

Dean. . . . . Steve Goldschmid, M.D. (Interim)
Dean, Phoenix. . . . . Stuart D. Flynn, M.D. (Interim)
Vice Dean, Academic Affairs . . . . T. Philip Malan, Jr., Ph.D., M.D.
Senior Associate Dean, Admissions and Student Affairs . . . . Christopher A. Leadem, Ph.D.
Senior Associate Dean, Finance and Administration . . . . William R. Elger
Senior Associate Dean, Medical Student Education . . . . Nancy A. Koff, Ph.D.
Associate Dean, Academic Affairs, Phoenix. . . . . Stuart D. Flynn, M.D.
Associate Dean, Administrative Affairs and Chief of Staff. . . . . Sarah M. Hiteman
Associate Dean, Clinical Affairs and CMO. . . . . Bruce M. Coull, M.D. (Interim)
Associate Dean, Clinical Affairs, Phoenix . . . . Jacqueline A. Chadwick, M.D.
Associate Dean, Faculty Affairs . . . . Anne L. Wright, Ph.D.
Associate Dean, Graduate Medical Education . . . . Rebecca L. Potter, M.D.
Associate Dean, Graduate Medical Education, Phoenix . . . . Michael Grossman, M.D.
Associate Dean, Outreach and Multicultural Affairs. . . . . Ana Maria Lopez, M.D.
Associate Dean, Planning and Facilities, Phoenix . . . . Nancy H. Tierney
Assistant Dean, Admissions and Student Affairs, Phoenix. . . . . Alexis G. Hernandez, Ph.D.
Associate Dean, Research. . . . . Anne E. Cress, Ph.D.
Assistant Dean, Finance and Administration, Phoenix . . . . Brenda L. Paulsen (Interim)
Assistant Dean, Clinical Education . . . . Kevin F. Moynahan, M.D.
Assistant Dean, Information Resources, Phoenix. . . . . Howard D. Silverman, M.D.
Assistant Dean, Outreach and Multicultural Affairs . . . . Linda K. Don
Asst. Dean, Outreach and Multicultural Affairs, Phoenix . . . . Doug E. Campos-Outcalt, M.D.
Assistant Dean, Planning and Facilities . . . . Angela M. Souza
Assistant Deans, Student Affairs . . . . John C. Racy, M.D., and Lawrence M. Moher, M.D.
Chief Information Officer . . . . Steven Wormsley, Ph.D.
Senior Director, Development . . . . Brian L. Bateman
Director, Arizona Arthritis Center . . . . Salvatore Albani, M.D., Ph.D.
Director, Arizona Cancer Center . . . . David S. Alberts, M.D.
Director, Arizona Respiratory Center . . . . Fernando D. Martinez, M.D.
Director, AHS Library . . . . Gary A. Freiburger
Director, Sarver Heart Center . . . . Gordon A. Ewy, M.D.
Director, Steele Memorial Children's Research Center . . . . Fayez K. Ghishan, M.D.
Director, Valley Fever Center of Excellence . . . . John N. Galgiani, M.D.

Department Heads and Section Chiefs

Basic Sciences

Basic Medical Sciences, Phoenix. . . . . Mark R. Haussler, Ph.D.
Biochemistry and Molecular Biophysics. . . . . Vicki H. Wysocki, Ph.D.
Cell Biology and Anatomy . . . . Kathleen Dixon, Ph.D.

Immunobiology . . . . Janko Nikolich-Zugich, M.D., Ph.D.
Pharmacology . . . . I. Glenn Sipes, Ph.D.
Physiology . . . . Nicholas A. Delamere, Ph.D.

Clinical Sciences

Anesthesiology . . . . Steven J. Barker, Ph.D., M.D.
Emergency Medicine . . . . Harvey W. Meislin, M.D.
Family and Community Medicine . . . . Tamsen L. Bassford, M.D.
Medicine . . . . Thomas D. Boyer, M.D. (Interim)
 Cardiology . . . . Gordon A. Ewy, M.D.
 Dermatology . . . . James E. Sligh, Jr., Ph.D., M.D.
 Endocrinology . . . . Craig S. Stump, Ph.D., M.D.
 Gastroenterology . . . . Bhaskar Banerjee, M.D. (Interim)
 General Medicine . . . . Jason A. Krupp, M.D.
 Geriatrics . . . . Mindy J. Fain, M.D.
 Hematology and Oncology . . . . Thomas P. Miller, M.D.
 Infectious Diseases . . . . Stephen A. Klotz, M.D.
 Inpatient Medicine . . . . Piyush Tiwari, M.D. (Interim)
 Medical Education . . . . William P. Johnson, M.D.
 Nephrology . . . . Bruce Kaplan, M.D.
 Pulmonary . . . . John W. Bloom, M.D. (Interim)
 Rheumatology . . . . Jeffrey R. Lisse, M.D.
Neurology . . . . David M. Labiner, M.D. (Interim)
Obstetrics and Gynecology . . . . Kathryn L. Reed, M.D.
 Female Pelvic Medicine and Reconstructive Surgery . . . . Kenneth D. Hatch, M.D.
 General Obstetrics and Gynecology . . . . Ilana B. Addis, M.D.
 Gynecologic Oncology . . . . Setsuko K. Chambers, M.D.
 Maternal and Fetal Medicine . . . . Karen B. Lesser, M.D.
Ophthalmology and Vision Science . . . . Joseph M. Miller, M.D.
Orthopaedic Surgery . . . . John T. Ruth, M.D.
Pathology . . . . Achyut S. Bhattacharyya, M.D. (Interim)
Pediatrics . . . . Fayez K. Ghishan, M.D.
 Cardiology . . . . Richard A. Samson, M.D.
 Critical Care . . . . Andreas A. Theodorou, M.D.
 Endocrinology . . . . Mark D. Wheeler, M.D.
 Gastroenterology and Nutrition . . . . Hassan H. Hassan, M.D.
 General Pediatrics and Adolescent Medicine . . . . Conrad Clemens, M.D.
 Hematology and Oncology . . . . Emmanuel Katsanis, M.D.
 Infectious Diseases . . . . Ziad M. Shehab, M.D.
 Medical and Molecular Genetics . . . . Christopher M. Cunniff, M.D.
 Neonatology and Developmental Biology . . . . Alan D. Bedrick, M.D.
 Nephrology . . . . Emmanuel Apostol, M.D.
 Pulmonary . . . . Wayne J. Morgan, M.D.
Psychiatry . . . . John J. Misiaszek, M.D. (Interim)
Radiation Oncology . . . . Baldassarre D. Stea, Ph.D., M.D.
Radiology . . . . Tim B. Hunter, M.D.
 Cross-Sectional Imaging . . . . Eric K. Outwater, M.D.
 GI/GU . . . . Kai Haber, M.D.
 Musculoskeletal . . . . Mihra S. Taljanovic, M.D.
 Neuroradiology . . . . Joachim F. Seeger, M.D.
 Nuclear Medicine . . . . Fabio Almeida, M.D.
 Research . . . . Harrison H. Barrett, M.D.
 Ultrasound . . . . Annemarie Buadu, M.D.
 Vascular and Interventional . . . . Stephen H. Smyth, M.D.
Surgery . . . . Rainer W.G. Gruessner, M.D.
 Cardiovascular and Thoracic . . . . Jack G. Copeland, M.D.
 General Surgery . . . . Amy L. Waer, M.D.
 Neurosurgery . . . . Martin E. Weinand, M.D.
 Research . . . . Ronald L. Heimark, M.D.
 Surgical Oncology . . . . Hugo V. Villar, M.D.
 Trauma and Critical Care . . . . Peter M. Rhee, M.D.
Urology . . . . Mitchell H. Sokoloff, M.D.
Vascular Surgery . . . . Joseph L. Mills, Sr., M.D.

University of Arkansas for Medical Sciences College of Medicine

4301 West Markham Street
Little Rock, Arkansas 72205
501-686-5000; 686-5350 (dean's office); 686-8160 (dean's office fax)
Web site: www.uams.edu

The college of medicine is part of the University of Arkansas for Medical Sciences, one of the 18 campuses of the University system. The college was founded in 1879. Eight area health education centers operate in the larger cities of the state as satellite centers of medical education.

Type: public
2008-2009 total enrollment: 590
Clinical facilities: University Hospital of Arkansas, John L. McClellan Memorial Veterans Administration Hospital, North Little Rock Veterans Administration Hospital, Arkansas State Hospital, Arkansas Children's Hospital, Baptist Rehabilitation Institute of Arkansas, St. Vincent Infirmary Medical Center, Baptist Medical Center, Central Arkansas Radiation Therapy Institute, Sparks Regional Medical Center, St. Edwards Mercy Medical Center, St. Bernards Regional Medical Center, Methodist Hospital of Jonesboro, Jefferson Regional Medical Center, Washington Regional Medical Center Fayetteville City Hospital, Northwest Medical Center, St. Mary-Rogers Memorial Hospital, Veterans Administration Medical Center (Fayetteville), Baxter Regional Medical Center, Medical Center of South Arkansas, Ouachita County Hospital, St. Michael Hospital, Wadley Regional Medical Center, Medical Arts Hospital, White River Medical Center, Stone County Medical Center, Helena Regional Medical Center.

University Officials

President. . . . . B. Alan Sugg, Ph.D.
Chancellor, University of Arkansas for Medical Sciences . . . . I. Dodd Wilson, M.D.
Vice Chancellor for Academic Affairs . . . . Larry D. Milne, Ph.D.
Vice Chancellor for Administration and Fiscal Affairs . . . . Melanie Goodhand
Vice Chancellor for Development and Alumni Relations . . . . John I. Blohm
Executive Director of Clinical Programs . . . . Richard A. Pierson
Director, Library . . . . Mary Ryan
Assistant Hospital Director for CIS . . . . Kari L. Cassel

Medical School Administrative Staff

Dean. . . . . Debra H. Fiser, M.D.
Executive Associate Dean, Finance and Administration . . . . Olan Nugent
Executive Associate Dean, Clinical Affairs . . . . Charles W. Smith, Jr., M.D.
Executive Associate Dean, Academic Affairs . . . . Richard P. Wheeler, M.D.
Associate Dean, AHEC Programs . . . . Mark B. Mengel, M.D.
Associate Dean, Cancer Programs. . . . . Peter Emanuel, M.D.
Associate Dean, Continuing Medical Education
    and Faculty Affairs . . . . Jeannette M. Shorey II, M.D.
Associate Dean, Children's Affairs . . . . Bonnie J. Taylor, M.D.
Executive Associate Dean, Medical Research . . . . Larry Cornett, Ph.D.
Associate Dean for Translational Research . . . . Aubrey J. Hough, Jr., M.D.
Associate Dean, Veterans Administration Affairs . . . . Margie Scott, M.D.
Assistant Dean, Research, Arkansas Children's Research Institute. . . . . Richard Jacobs, M.D.
Associate Dean, Diversity Affairs . . . . Billy R. Thomas, M.D.
Associate Dean, Undergraduate Medical
    Education and Curriculum Development . . . . Bruce W. Newton, Ph.D.
Associate Dean, Graduate Medical Education . . . . James A. Clardy, M.D.
Director, Communications . . . . Leslie Taylor
Chief Operating Officer, Faculty Group Practice. . . . . Olan Nugent
Director, Faculty Group Practice Billing Operations (UAMS) . . . . Beth Wheeler
Director, Faculty Group Practice Billing Operations (ACH). . . . . Gayle Fiser
Director, Lab Animal Medicine . . . . Mildred Randolph
Assistant Dean for Housestaff Affairs and Registrar . . . . Dwana McKay
Executive Director of Alumni Affairs . . . . Judith K. McClain
Assistant Dean for Medical Student Admissions and Financial Aid . . . . Tom G. South
Development Officer for College of Medicine. . . . . Vacant

University of Arkansas for Medical Sciences College of Medicine: ARKANSAS

Department and Division or Section Chairs

Basic Sciences

Neurobiology and Developmental Sciences......................... Gwen V. Childs, Ph.D.
Biochemistry and Molecular Biology............................. Alan D. Elbein, Ph.D.
Biostatistics .... Paula Roberson, Ph.D.
Microbiology and Immunology................................. Richard Morrison, Ph.D.
Pathology .... Bruce R. Smoller, M.D.
Pharmacology and Interdisciplinary Toxicology...................... Nancy Rusch, Ph.D.
Physiology and Biophysics .... Michael Jennings, Ph.D.

Clinical Sciences

Anesthesiology... Carmelita Pablo, M.D.
Dermatology ....John C. Ansel, M.D.
Emergency Medicine .... Marvin Leibovich, M.D.
Family and Preventive Medicine........................... Geoffrey Goldsmith, M.D.
Geriatrics.. Jeanne Wei, M.D. (Interim)
Internal Medicine ....James Marsh, M.D.
   Cardiology.. Open
   Endocrinology and Metabolism.................. Stavros C. Manolagas, M.D., Ph.D.
   Gastroenterology .... Kevin Olden, M.D.
   General Medicine..................................... Susan Beland, M.D.
   Hematology and Oncology........................... Laura Hutchins, M.D.
   Infectious Diseases .... Robert W. Bradsher, Jr., M.D.
   Nephrology .... Sudhir V. Shah, M.D.
   Pulmonary... Larry Johnson, M.D
   Rheumatology .... Hugo E. Jasin, M.D.
Medical Humanities...................................... J. Chrisley Hackler, Ph.D.
Neurology... Sami I. Harik, M.D.
Neurosurgery.. Ossama Al-Mefty, M.D.
Obstetrics and Gynecology................................ Curtis Lowery, M.D.
Ophthalmology .... John P. Shock, M.D.
Orthopaedic Surgery...................................... Richard Nicholas, M.D.
Otolaryngology and Head and Neck Surgery...................James Y. Suen, M.D.
Pediatrics .... Richard F. Jacobs, M.D.
Psychiatry and Behavioral Sciences........................ G. Richard Smith, M.D.
   Child and Adolescent Psychiatry .... J. Lynn Taylor, M.D.
   University Hospital................................ Christopher Cargile, M.D.
   VA Hospitals .... Jeffrey Clothier, M.D.
Radiation Oncology.................................. Vaneerat Ratanatharathorn, M.D.
Radiology .... Ernest J. Ferris, M.D.
Rehabilitation Medicine................................. Kevin Means, M.D.
Surgery .... Michael J. Edwards, M.D.

9

David Geffen School of Medicine at UCLA

10833 Le Conte Avenue
Los Angeles, California 90095
310-825-9111; 825-6373 (dean's office); 206-5046 (fax)
Web site: http://dgsom.healthsciences.ucla.edu/

The UCLA School of Medicine was established in 1951. It is the second oldest of the five medical schools of the University of California (UC). In 1999, it became the David Geffen School of Medicine. The school is on the UCLA campus, part of a complex including the other health science schools of dentistry, nursing, and public health. In 2008, the state-of-the-art Ronald Reagan Medical Center opened. The medical school has two partners jointly admitting 24 students yearly to each program. The Charles Drew University of Medicine and Science is a private, minority-serving medical and health science institution serving California since the 1960s. Its mission is to help society's poorest communities. The UCLA/Drew medical student program was established in 1970. Students do their first two years at UCLA and clinical work through the Drew program. The University of California at Riverside (UCR) is in the Inland Empire region in southern California and has one of the most diverse student bodies of the UC system. In 1966, the UCLA/UCR medical student program was established. Originally, it was an accelerated B.S./M.D. program in seven years but transitioned to a four-year medical program with students doing the first two years of medical school at UCR and transferring to UCLA for the clinical years.

Type: public
2008-2009 total enrollment: 715
Clinical facilities: Ronald Reagan UCLA Medical Center; UCLA Neuropsychiatric Hospital; Brentwood, Sepulveda, and West L.A. VA medical centers; Cedars-Sinai Medical Center; Children's Hospital of L.A.; L.A. County hospitals: Harbor-UCLA Medical Center; Olive View Medical Center; St. Mary Medical Center; Jewish Home for the Aged of Los Angeles (Reseda); Kaiser Foundation hospitals: Panorama City, Sunset Boulevard, West Los Angeles; Woodland Hills; Kern (County) Medical Center; Northridge Hospital Foundation; Rand Corp.; Research and Education Institute; Santa Monica UCLA Medical Center and Orthopaedic Hospital; Shriners Hospitals for Children; Venice Family Clinic; Ventura County General Hospital.

Medical School Administrative Staff

Dean and Vice Chancellor, Medical Sciences . . . . Gerald S. Levey, M.D.
Associate Vice Chancellor, Medical Sciences and
   Executive Associate Dean . . . . Alan G. Robinson, M.D.
Associate Vice Chancellor for Finance and
   Senior Associate Dean, Finance &
   Administration . . . . Judith E. Rothman
Senior Associate Dean, Academic Affairs. . . . . Fawzy Fawzy, M.D.
Senior Associate Dean, Clinical Operations. Jean B. deKernion, M.D.
Senior Associate Dean, Research . . . . Leonard H. Rome, Ph.D.
Associate Dean, Graduate Studies. . . . . Ren Sun, Ph.D.
Senior Associate Dean, Student Affairs and
   Graduate Medical Education . . . . Neil H. Parker, M.D.
Senior Associate Dean, Medical Education . . . . LuAnn Wilkerson, Ed.D.
Associate Dean, Medical Ethics. . . . . Stanley G. Korenman, M.D.
Associate Dean, UCLA, and Dean, Charles R.
   Drew University of Medicine and Science . . . . Richard S. Baker, M.D.
Associate Dean, Harbor-UCLA Medical Center . . . . Gail Anderson, M.D.
Associate Dean, UCR-UCLA Biomedical Sciences Program . . . . Craig Byus, Ph.D.
Associate Dean, Cedars-Sinai Medical Center . . . . Shlomo Melmed, M.D.
Assistant Dean, Biomedical Library. . . . . Judith Consales
Associate Dean, Olive View Medical Center. . . . . William Loos, M.D.
Assistant Deans, Student Affairs . . . . Theodore Hall, Josephine Isabel-Jones, M.D.,
                    Susan Stangl, M.D., Lawrence Bassett, M.D., and Daphne Calmes, M.D.

Department and Division or Section Chairs

Basic Sciences

Biological Chemistry . . . . Michael M. Grunstein, Ph.D.
Biomathematics. . . . . Elliot Landaw, M.D., Ph.D.
Human Genetics . . . . Kenneth Lange, Ph.D.
Microbiology, Immunology, and Molecular Genetics. . . . . Jeffery F. Miller, Ph.D.

Molecular and Medical Pharmacology .... Michael Phelps, Ph.D.
Neurobiology. .... Marie Francoise Chesselet, M.D., Ph.D.
Physiology .... Kenneth Philipson, Ph.D.

Clinical Science

Anesthesiology. .... Patricia A. Kapur, M.D.
   Olive View Medical Center .... Selma Calmes, M.D.
Family Medicine .... Patrick Dowling, M.D.
Medicine. .... Alan Fogelman, M.D.
   Cedars-Sinai Medical Center. .... Glenn Braunstein, M.D.
   Harbor-UCLA Medical Center. .... William Stringer, M.D.
   Kern Medical Center .... Royce Johnson, M.D.
   Olive View Medical Center .... Dennis Cope, M.D.
   Sepulveda VA Medical Center. .... Michael Golub, M.D.
   VA Greater Los Angeles Healthcare System .... Phyllis A. Guze, M.D.
Neurology. .... John Mazziotta, M.D., Ph.D.
   Harbor-UCLA Medical Center. .... Mark A. Goldberg, M.D.
   Olive View Medical Center .... Alan Shewman, M.D.
   Sepulveda VA Medical Center. .... Claude G. Wasterlain, M.D.
Obstetrics and Gynecology. .... Gautam Chaudhuri, M.D., Ph.D.
   Cedars-Sinai Medical Center. .... Richard Azziz, M.D.
   Drew-King Medical Center .... Teiichiro Fukushima, M.D.
   Harbor-UCLA Medical Center. .... Michael Ross, M.D.
   Olive View Medical Center .... Dominic Muzsnai, M.D.
Ophthalmology. .... Bartly Mondino, M.D.
   Drew-King Medical Center .... Richard Casey, M.D.
   Harbor-UCLA Medical Center. .... Sherwin J. Isenberg, M.D.
   Olive View Medical Center .... Robert Engstrom, M.D.
   Sepulveda VA Medical Center. .... John McCann, M.D.
   VA Greater Los Angeles Healthcare System .... Lynn Gordon, M.D.
Orthopaedic Surgery. .... Gerald Finerman, M.D.
Pathology and Laboratory Medicine .... Jonathan Braun, M.D., Ph.D.
   Cedars-Sinai Medical Center. .... Stephen Geller, M.D.
   Harbor-UCLA Medical Center. .... Robert Morin, M.D.
   Olive View Medical Center .... Paul Liu, M.D.
   Wadsworth VA Medical Center .... Joan Howanitz, M.D.
Pediatrics .... Edward McCabe, M.D., Ph.D.
   Cedars-Sinai Medical Center. .... Charles Simmons, Jr., M.D.
   Drew-King Medical Center .... Betti Jo Warren, M.D.
   Harbor-UCLA Medical Center. .... Adam Jonas, M.D.
   Olive View Medical Center .... Mohammed Malekzader, M.D.
Psychiatry and Biobehavioral Sciences. .... Peter C. Whybrow, M.D.
   Cedars-Sinai Medical Center. .... Mark Rapaport, M.D.
   VA Greater Los Angeles Healthcare System .... Andrew Shaner, M.D.
   Drew-King Medical Center .... George Mallory, M.D. (Acting)
   Harbor-UCLA Medical Center. .... Milton H. Miller, M.D.
   Olive View Medical Center .... Albert Ketannis, M.D.
   Sepulveda VA Medical Center. .... Daniel Auerbach, M.D.
Radiation Oncology. .... Michael L. Steinberg, M.D.
Radiological Sciences. .... Dieter Enzmann, M.D.
   Drew-King Medical Center .... Jack Eisenman, M.D.
   Harbor-UCLA Medical Center. .... Mark Mehinger, M.D.
   Olive View Medical Center .... Ramesh Verma, M.D.
   Wadsworth VA Medical Center .... Scott Goodwin, M.D.
Surgery. .... Ronald Busuttil, M.D.
   Cedars-Sinai Medical Center. .... Achilles Demetriou, M.D.
   Drew-King Medical Center .... Nand Dalta, M.D.
   Harbor-UCLA Medical Center. .... Bruce E. Stabile, M.D.
   Olive View Medical Center .... Jessie E. Thompson, M.D.
   VA Greater Los Angeles Healthcare System .... Mathias Stelzner, M.D.
Urology. .... Jean B. deKernion, M.D.
   Harbour-UCLA Medical Center. .... Jacob Rajfer, M.D.
   Olive View Medical Center .... William Aronson, M.D.
   VA Greater Los Angeles Healthcare System .... Carol Bennett, M.D.

Keck School of Medicine of the University of Southern California

1975 Zonal Avenue, KAM 500
Los Angeles, California 90033
323-442-1900 (dean's office); 442-2724 (fax)
E-mail: deanksom@usc.edu
Web site: www.usc.edu/keck

The University of Southern California (USC) was founded in 1880, and its school of medicine was established in 1885 as the region's first medical school. In 1952, the medical school moved to land adjoining the Los Angeles County LAC†USC Medical Center, seven miles from the main university campus. In 1999, the school was renamed the Keck School of Medicine of USC.

Type: private
2008-2009 total enrollment: 677
Clinical facilities: Barlow Hospital, California Hospital Medical Center, Childrens Hospital Los Angeles, Doheny Eye Institute, Queen of Angels/Hollywood Presbyterian Medical Center, Hospital of the Good Samaritan, House Ear Institute, Huntington Memorial Hospital, USC/Norris Comprehensive Cancer Center and Hospital, LAC†USC Medical Center, Presbyterian Intercommunity Hospital, Rancho Los Amigos National Rehabilitation Center, Edward R. Roybal Comprehensive Health Center, El Monte Comprehensive Health Center, H. Claude Hudson Comprehensive Health Center, USC University Hospital, White Memorial Medical Center, Veterans Administration Outpatient Clinic.

University Officials

President. . . . . Steven B. Sample, Ph.D.
Provost and Executive Vice President . . . . C. L. Max Nikias, Ph.D.
Dean. . . . . Carmen A. Puliafito, M.D., M.B.A.

Medical School Administrative Staff

Chief Operating Officer. . . . . Coreen A. Rodgers
Senior Associate Dean for Clinical Affairs. . . . . Vacant
Senior Associate Dean for Faculty Affairs . . . . Judy A. Garner, Ph.D.
Senior Executive Director for Development . . . . William Loadvine
Vice Dean for Educational Affairs . . . . Henri Ford, M.D.
Vice Dean for Research Advancement . . . . M. Elizabeth Fini, Ph.D.
Associate Dean for Curriculum. . . . . Allan V. Abbott, M.D.
Associate Dean for Graduate Medical Education . . . . Lawrence M. Opas, M.D.
Associate Dean for Postgraduate Medical Education . . . . Allan V. Abbott, M.D.
Associate Dean of Undergraduate, Master's, and
    Professional Degree Programs . . . . Elahe Nezame, Ph.D.
Associate Dean for Graduate Programs. . . . . Debbie L. Johnson
Associate Dean for Student Affairs . . . . Donna D. Elliott, M.D., Ed.D.
Associate Dean for Women and Disabled Issues . . . . Raquel Arias, M.D.
Associate Dean for Admissions . . . . Erin Quinn, Ph.D.
Associate Dean for Clinical Research . . . . Thomas A. Buchanan, M.D.
Assistant Dean for Clinical Research Studies . . . . Darcy Spicer, M.D.
Assistant Dean for Minority Affairs . . . . Althea Alexander
Assistant Dean for Basic Science Education and Student Affairs. . . . . . . Joel H. Schechter, Ph.D.
Assistant Dean for Curriculum and Student Affairs (Clinical) . . . . Pamela B. Schaff, M.D.
Associate Vice President, Public Relations. . . . . Jane Brust
Assistant Dean for Faculty Affairs . . . . Frank Sinatra, M.D.
Assistant Dean for Basic Science. . . . . Stanley P. Azen, Ph.D.

Department and Division or Section Chairs

Anesthesiology. . . . . Phillip D. Lumb, M.D.
Biochemistry and Molecular Biology. . . . . Michael R. Stallcup, Ph.D.
Cardiothoracic Surgery . . . . Vaughn A. Starnes, M.D.
Cell and Neurobiology. . . . . Pat R. Levitt, Ph.D.
Colorectal Surgery. . . . . Andreas M. Kaiser, M.D., F.A.C.S.
Dermatology . . . . David T. Woodley, M.D.
Emergency Medicine . . . . Edward J. Newton, M.D.
Family Medicine . . . . Jerry D. Gates, Ph.D. (Interim)
Medicine. . . . . Edward D. Crandall, Ph.D., M.D.

Keck School of Medicine of the University of Southern California: CALIFORNIA

Cancer Medicine and Blood Diseases*............................ Darcy Spicer, M.D.
Cardiovascular Medicine*................................. Leslie A. Saxon, M.D.
Diabetes and Endocrinology* .... Thomas A. Buchanan, M.D.
Gastrointestinal and Liver*............................. Neil Kaplowitz, M.D.
Geriatric, Hospitalist, and General Internal Medicine*............. David Goldstein, M.D.
Infectious Diseases* .... Fred R. Sattler, M.D.
Nephrology* .... Vito M. Campese, M.D.
Pulmonary Diseases*........................... Edward D. Crandall, Ph.D., M.D.
Rheumatology* .... William Stohl, M.D.
Molecular Microbiology and Immunology.................... Jae Jung, Ph.D.
Neurological Surgery............................ Steven L. Giannotta, M.D.
Neurology...................................... Helena Chui, M.D.
Obstetrics and Gynecology....................... Laila I. Muderspach, M.D.
  Gynecology*.................................. Subir Roy, M.D.
    Family Planning* .... Daniel R. Mishell, Jr., M.D.
    Female Pelvic Medicine and Reconstructive Surgery* .... Begum Ozël, M.D.
  Gynecologic Oncology* .... Lynda D. Roman, M.D.
  Maternal and Fetal Medicine*..................... Thomas Goodwin, M.D.
  Reproductive Endocrinology/Infertility* .... Richard Paulson, M.D.
Ophthalmology .... Ronald E. Smith, M.D.
Orthopaedics................................... Michael J. Patzakis, M.D.
Otolaryngology .... Dale H. Rice, M.D.
Pathology .... Michael E. Selsted, M.D., Ph.D.
Pediatrics .... Roberta G. Williams, M.D.
  Adolescent Medicine .... Marvin E. Belzer, M.D.
  Allergy and Clinical Immunology .... Joseph Church, M.D.
  Anesthesiology and Critical Care Medicine .... Randall Wetzel, M.D.
  Bone Marrow Transplant .... Donald B. Kohn, M.D.
  Cardiology.................................. Michael Silka, M.D.
  Emergency Medicine .... Alan Nager, M.D.
  Endocrinology and Metabolism.................... Francine R. Kaufman, M.D.
  Gastroenterology .... Danny Thomas, M.D.
  General Pediatrics/UAP........................ Robert Jacobs, M.D.
  Hematology and Oncology...................... Stuart Siegel, M.D.
  Infectious Diseases .... Wilbert H. Mason, Jr., M.D.
  Medical Genetics .... Linda M. Randolph, M.D. (Interim)
  Neonatology................................. Istvan Seri, M.D., Ph.D.
  Nephrology .... Carl Grushkin, M.D.
  Neurology .... Wendy G. Mitchell, M.D.
  Pediatric Pulmonary........................... Sally Davidson Ward, M.D.
  Psychiatry.................................. Susan Turkel, M.D.
  Rehabilitation............................... Kevin Craig, M.D.
  Research on Children, Youth, and Families.............. Michele Kipke, Ph.D.
  Rheumatology .... Andreas Reiff, M.D.
Physiology and Biophysics .... Richard N. Bergman, Ph.D.
Preventive Medicine............................ Jonathan M. Samet, M.D.
Psychiatry and the Behavioral Sciences.............. Carlos N. Pato, M.D.
Radiation Oncology............................ Parvesh Kumar, M.D.
Radiology .... Edward G. Grant, M.D.
Surgery...................................... Tom R. DeMeester, M.D.
  General Surgery*............................. Tom R. DeMeester, M.D.
    Pediatric Surgery*........................... Henri Ford, M.D.
    Plastic and Reconstructive Surgery*................... Vacant
    Colorectal and Pelvic Floor Surgery .... Howard Kaufman, M.D.
    Emergency Surgery Services.................... Rodney Mason, M.D.
    Hepato/Pancreas and Abdominal Organ Transplant Surgery.......... Rick Selby, M.D.
    Thoracic and Foregut Surgery .... Tom R. DeMeester, M.D.
    Trauma and Critical Care Surgery .... Demetrios Demetriades, M.D.
    Tumor and Endocrine Surgery.................. Dilip Parekh, M.D.
    Vascular Surgery .... Fred Weaver, M.D.
Urology...................................... Inderbir Gil, M.D.

*Specialty without organizational autonomy.

Loma Linda University School of Medicine

11175 Campus Street, Suite A1108
Loma Linda, California 92350
909-558-4462 (general information); 558-4481 (dean's office); 558-0292 (fax)
E-mail: awongworawat@llu.edu
Web site: www.llu.edu/llu/medicine/

The medical school was founded in 1909 and was known as the College of Medical Evangelists until 1961, when it was renamed Loma Linda University. It is owned and operated by the Seventh-Day Adventist Church. From 1909 to 1966, medical students received their first two years of medical education on the Loma Linda campus, and the clinical years were spent on the Los Angeles campus at the White Memorial Medical Center and the Los Angeles County Hospital. After completion of Loma Linda University Medical Center in 1967, the medical school campuses consolidated at Loma Linda. The school has graduated more than 9,000 students, many of whom have served worldwide.

Type: private
2008-2009 total enrollment: 727
Clinical facilities: Loma Linda University Medical Center, Loma Linda University Children's Hospital, Loma Linda University Behavioral Medicine Center, Jerry L. Pettis Veterans Medical Center, Riverside County Regional Medical Center, White Memorial Medical Center, Arrowhead Regional Medical Center, Glendale Adventist Medical Center.

University Officials

President. . . . . Richard H. Hart, M.D., D.P.H.
Chancellor and Chief Executive Officer . . . . Richard H. Hart, M.D., D.P.H.
Vice President and Chief Financial Officer . . . . Kevin J. Lang
Senior Vice Chancellor, Financial Affairs . . . . Verlon W. Strauss
Vice Chancellor, Academic Affairs . . . . Ronald L. Carter, Ph.D.
Vice Chancellor, Information Systems. . . . . David P. Harris, Ph.D.
Vice Chancellor, Public Affairs. . . . . Open
Associate Vice Chancellor, Research Affairs. . . . . Anthony J. Zuccarelli, Ph.D.

Medical School Administrative Staff

Dean. . . . . H. Roger Hadley, M.D.
Associate Dean, Basic Science Faculty. . . . . Lawrence C. Sowers, Ph.D.
Associate Dean, Clinical Faculty . . . . Ricardo L. Peverini, M.D.
Senior Associate Dean, Medical Student Education . . . . Leonard S. Werner, M.D.
Associate Dean, Admissions and Recruitment . . . . Stephen A. Nyirady, Ph.D.
Associate Dean, Finance and Administration. . . . . Rodney D. Neal
Associate Dean, Clinical Education. . . . . Tamara M. Shankel, M.D.
Associate Dean, Graduate Medical Education . . . . Daniel W. Giang, M.D.
Associate Dean, Los Angeles Programs . . . . Leroy A. Reese, M.D.
Associate Dean, Faculty Development. . . . . Tamara L. Thomas, M.D.
Associate Dean, Student Affairs . . . . Henry H. Lamberton, Psy.D.
Assistant Dean, Continuing Medical Education . . . . Open
Assistant Dean, Admissions. . . . . Lenoa Edwards
Assistant Dean, Clinical Site Recruitment . . . . Lynda Daniel-Underwood, M.D.
Assistant Dean, Development . . . . Treva C. Webster
Assistant Dean, Graduate Student Affairs . . . . Penelope J. Duerksen-Hughes, Ph.D.
Assistant Dean, Jerry L. Pettis VA Hospital . . . . Dwight C. Evans, M.D.
Assistant Dean, Program Development and Education. . . . . Loretta B. Johns, Ph.D.
Assistant to the Dean for Basic Science Education. . . . . Resa L. Chase, M.D.
Assistant to the Dean for Diversity . . . . Daisy D. DeLeon, Ph.D.
Assistant to the Dean for Medical Staff Affairs. . . . . Linda J. Mason, M.D.
Director, Records and Student Services. . . . . Marvalee J. Hoffman
Director, University Libraries . . . . Carlene M. Drake

Department and Division or Section Chairs

Basic Sciences

Pathology and Human Anatomy. . . . . Brian S. Bull, M.D.
  Human Anatomy . . . . P. Ben Nava, Ph.D.
  Pathology. . . . . Darryl G. Heustis, M.D.
Basic Sciences . . . . Lawrence C. Sowers, Ph.D.
  Biochemistry . . . . Penelope J. Duerksen-Hughes, Ph.D.

Microbiology . . . . Hansel M. Fletcher, Ph.D.
Pharmacology. . . . . John N. Buchholz, Ph.D.
Physiology . . . . John H. Zhang, M.D., Ph.D.

Centers

Center for Health Disparities and Molecular Medicine . . . . Marino A. DeLeon, Ph.D.
Center for Perinatal Biology. . . . . Lawrence D. Longo, M.D.
Neurosurgery Center for Research, Training, and Education. . . . . Wolff M. Kirsch, M.D.

Clinical Sciences

Anesthesia. . . . . Robert D. Martin, M.D.
    Critical Care*. . . . . Gary R. Stier, M.D.
Cardiovascular and Thoracic Surgery . . . . Anees J. Razzouk, M.D.
Emergency Medicine . . . . Kathleen J. Clem, M.D.
    Pediatric Emergency Medicine* . . . . Lance A. Brown, M.D.
Family Medicine . . . . John K. Testerman, M.D., Ph.D.
General and Trauma Surgery. . . . . Antonio E. Robles, M.D. (Interim)
    General . . . . Antonio E. Robles, M.D.
    Oral Surgery . . . . Alan S. Herford, D.D.S., M.D.
    Pediatric . . . . Donald C. Moores, M.D.
    Surgical Oncology . . . . Jan H. Wong, M.D.
    Transplant. . . . . H. Roger Hadley, M.D. (Interim)
    Trauma . . . . Richard D. Catalano, M.D.
Gynecology and Obstetrics. . . . . William C. Patton, M.D.
Medicine. . . . . Philip M. Gold, M.D. (Interim)
    Cardiology. . . . . Kenneth R. Jutzy, M.D.
    Dermatology . . . . Abel Torres, M.D.
    Endocrinology* . . . . J. Lamont Murdoch, M.D.
    Gastroenterology* . . . . Terence D. Lewis, M.B.B.S.
    General Internal Medicine and Geriatric Medicine . . . . Raymond Wong, M.D.
    Hematology and Oncology* . . . . Chien-Shing Chen, M.D., Ph.D.
    Infectious Disease*. . . . . James J. Couperus, M.D.
    Nephrology* . . . . Siegmund Teichman, M.D.
    Pulmonary* . . . . Philip M. Gold, M.D.
    Rheumatology* . . . . Keith K. Colburn, M.D.
Neurology. . . . . Bryan E. Tsao, M.D.
Neurosurgery. . . . . Austin R. T. Colohan, M.D.
Ophthalmology . . . . Howard V. Gimbel, M.D.
Orthopedic Surgery. . . . . Christopher M. Jobe, M.D.
Otolaryngology: Head and Neck Surgery . . . . Alfred A. Simental, M.D.
Pediatrics . . . . Richard E. Chinnock, M.D.
    Allergy and Immunology*. . . . . Yvonne F. Fanous, M.D.
    Cardiology* . . . . Ranae L. Larsen, M.D.
    Endocrinology* . . . . Eba H. Hathout, M.B.B.S.
    Gastroenterology* . . . . Manoj C. Shah, M.B.B.S.
    General Pediatrics*. . . . . Ravindra Rao, M.B.B.S.
        Adolescent Medicine* . . . . Pushpa Nowrangi, M.B.B.S.
        Forensic Pediatrics*. Clare M. Sheridan-Matney, M.D.
    Genetics*. . . . . Robin D. Clark, M.D.
    Hematology and Oncology* . . . . Antranik A. Bedros, M.D.
    Infectious Disease*. . . . . Jane N. Bork, M.D.
    Neonatology* . . . . Ricardo L. Peverini, M.D.
    Nephrology* . . . . Shobha Sahney, M.B.B.S.
    Neurology* . . . . Stephen Ashwal, M.D.
    Pediatric Critical Care Medicine* . . . . Shamel A. Abd-Allah, M.D.
    Pulmonary* . . . . Yvonne F. Fanous, M.D.
    Rheumatology* . . . . Wendy L. De la Pena, M.D.
Physical Medicine and Rehabilitation . . . . Murray E. Brandstater, M.B.B.S., Ph.D.
Plastic and Reconstructive Surgery . . . . Subhas C. Gupta, M.D., Ph.D.
Preventive Medicine. . . . . Wayne S. Dysinger, M.D.
Psychiatry . . . . William G. Murdoch, M.D. (Interim)
Radiation Medicine . . . . Jerry D. Slater, M.D.
Radiology . . . . David B. Hinshaw, Jr., M.D.
Urology. . . . . Herbert C. Ruckle, M.D.

*Specialty without organizational autonomy.

15

Stanford University School of Medicine

300 Pasteur Drive, Alway Building, Room M121
Stanford, California 94305-5119
650-725-3900 (dean's office); 725-7368 (dean's office fax)
Web site: www.med.stanford.edu

The school of medicine was established in 1908 when the properties and equipment of Cooper Medical College were transferred to Stanford. The medical school is part of the Stanford University Medical Center.

Type: private
2008-2009 total enrollment: 462
Clinical facilities: Stanford University Hospital and Clinics (SHC); Lucile Salter Packard Children's Hospital at Stanford (LPCH); Palo Alto Veterans Administration Medical Center; Santa Clara Valley Medical Center.

University Officials

President. . . . . John L. Hennessy, Ph.D.
Provost . . . . John W. Etchemendy, Ph.D.

Medical School Administrative Staff

Dean, School of Medicine . . . . Philip A. Pizzo, M.D.
Vice Dean and Senior Associate Dean for Academic Affairs. . . . . David K. Stevenson, M.D.
Senior Associate Dean for Adult Clinical Affairs . . . . Norman W. Rizk, M.D.
Senior Associate Dean for Pediatric and Obstetric Clinical Affairs . . . . Kenneth L. Cox, M.D.
Associate Dean for Clinical Affairs . . . . Geoffrey D. Rubin, M.D.
Senior Associate Dean for Diversity and Leadership . . . . . . Hannah A. Valantine, M.D., M.R.C.P.
Senior Associate Dean for Finance and Administration . . . . Marcia Cohen
Senior Associate Dean for Information Resources and Technology . . . . Henry J. Lowe, M.D.
Director of Lane Library . . . . Heidi Heileman (Acting)
Senior Associate Deans for Research and Training . . . . Daria Mochly-Rosen, Ph.D.,
and Harry B. Greenberg, M.D.
Associate Vice President for Medical Development and Alumni Affairs. . . . . . Douglas G. Stewart
Senior Associate Dean for Medical Student Education. . . . . Charles Prober, M.D.
Associate Dean for Medical Admissions. . . . . Gabriel Garcia, M.D.
Associate Dean for Alumni Affairs . . . . Ross D. Bright, M.D.
Associate Dean for Graduate Student Affairs. . . . . Ellen Porzig, Ph.D.
Senior Associate Dean for Graduate Medical Education . . . . Myriam Curet, M.D.
Senior Associate Dean for Graduate Education
and Postdoctoral Affairs. . . . . John Pringle, Ph.D.
Associate Dean for Minority Advising and Programs . . . . Fernando S. Mendoza, M.D.
Assistant Dean for Postdoctoral Affairs . . . . Chequeta Allen
Associate Dean for Pre-Clinical Advising and Research . . . . Patricia C. Cross, Ph.D.
Assistant Dean for Graduate Education. . . . . Anika Green
Assistant Dean for Minority Affairs . . . . Ronald D. Garcia, Ph.D.
Assistant Dean for Student Affairs. . . . . Charlene C. Hamada
Associate Dean for Medical Student Advising . . . . Neil Gesundheit, M.D.
Associate Dean for Veterans Affairs . . . . Lawrence Leung, M.D.
Executive Director, Office of Communication and Public Affairs. . . . . Paul Costello

Department and Division or Section Chairs

Basic Sciences

Biochemistry . . . . Mark Krasnow, Ph.D.
Developmental Biology . . . . Roeland Nusse, Ph.D.
Genetics . . . . Open
Health Research and Policy . . . . Philip W. Lavori, Ph.D.
Microbiology and Immunology. . . . . Karla A. Kirkegaard, Ph.D.
Molecular and Cellular Physiology . . . . Richard S. Lewis, Ph.D.
Molecular Pharmacology . . . . James Ferrell, Ph.D.

16

Neurobiology. . . . . William T. Newsome, Ph.D.
Structural Biology . . . . Joseph D. Puglisi, Ph.D.

Clinical Sciences

Anesthesia. . . . . Ronald G. Pearl, M.D.
Cardiothoracic Surgery . . . . Robert C. Robbins, M.D.
Comparative Medicine. . . . . Linda C. Cork, D.V.M., Ph.D.
Dermatology. . . . . Alfred T. Lane, M.D.
Medicine. . . . . Ralph I. Horwitz, M.D.
  Bone Marrow Transplant . . . . Robert Negrin, M.D.
  Cardiovascular Medicine. Thomas Quertermous, M.D. (Co-Chief),
                                                           and Alan C. Yeung, M.D. (Co-Chief)
  Endocrinology, Gerontology, and Metabolism . . . . Frederic B. Kraemer, M.D.
  Gastroenterology and Hepatology. . . . . Jay Pasricha, M.D.
  General Internal Medicine and Family Community Medicine. . . . . Peter Rudd, M.D.
  Hematology . . . . Linda M. Boxer, M.D.
  Immunology and Rheumatology. . . . . C. Garrison Fathman, M.D.
  Infectious Diseases . . . . Lucy Tompkins, M.D., Ph.D.
  Nephrology . . . . Glenn Chertow, M.D.
  Oncology. . . . . Ronald Levy, M.D.
  Primary Care and Outcomes Research. . . . . Alan M. Garber, M.D., Ph.D.
  Pulmonary and Critical Care Medicine . . . . Glenn D. Rosen, M.D., and Steve Ruoss, M.D.
  Stanford Prevention Research Center . . . . Stephen P. Fortmann, M.D.
  Stanford Medical Informatics . . . . Mark A. Musen, M.D., Ph.D.
Neurology and Neurological Sciences. . . . . Frank M. Longo, M.D, Ph.D.
Neurosurgery. . . . . Gary K. Steinberg, M.D., Ph.D.
Obstetrics and Gynecology. . . . . Jonathan Berek, M.D.
Opthalmology . . . . Mark S. Blumenkranz, M.D.
Orthopedic Surgery. . . . . William J. Maloney, M.D.
  Sports Medicine. . . . . Gordon O. Matheson, M.D.
Otolaryngology . . . . Robert K. Jackler, M.D.
Pathology . . . . Stephen J. Galli, M.D.
Pediatrics . . . . Hugh O'Brodovich, M.D.
  Adolescent Medicine . . . . Neville Golden, M.D.
  Cancer Biology. . . . . Michael Cleary, M.D.
  Cardiology. . . . . Daniel Bernstein, M.D.
  Endocrinology . . . . Darrell M. Wilson, M.D.
  Gastroenterology . . . . Kenneth L. Cox, M.D.
  General Pediatrics . . . . Fernando S. Mendoza, M.D.
  Genetics. . . . . Louanne Hudgins, M.D.
  Hematology and Oncology. . . . . Michael P. Link, M.D.
  Immunology. . . . . Open
  Infectious Diseases . . . . Yvonne Maldonado, M.D. (Acting)
  Neonatology. . . . . William Benitz, M.D. (Acting)
  Nephrology . . . . Steven R. Alexander, M.D.
  Pulmonary, Allergy, and Critical Care . . . . David Cornfield, M.D.
  Rheumatology . . . . Christy L. Sandborg, M.D.
  Stem Cell Transplantation (BMT). . . . . Kenneth Weinberg, M.D.
Psychiatry and Behavioral Sciences. . . . . Alan F. Schatzberg, M.D.
Radiation Oncology. . . . . Richard T. Hoppe, M.D.
Radiology . . . . Gary M. Glazer, M.D.
Surgery. . . . . Thomas M. Krummel, M.D.
  Anatomy . . . . John Gosling, M.D., and Ian Whitmore, M.D.
  Emergency Medicine . . . . Robert L. Norris, M.D.
  General Surgery. . . . . Jeff Norton, M.D.
  Pediatric Surgery . . . . Craig T. Albanese, M.D.
  Plastic and Reconstructive Surgery . . . . Jim Chang, M.D.
  Vascular Surgery. . . . . Ronald L. Dalman, M.D.
  Multi-Organ Transplantation. Carlos O. Esquivel, M.D., Ph.D.
Urology. . . . . Linda Shortliffe, M.D.

17

University of California, Davis, School of Medicine

4610 X Street, Suite 3101
Saramento, California 95817
916-734-7131 (dean's office); 734-7055 (fax)
Web site: www.ucdmc.ucdavis.edu/medschool

The Regents of the University of California authorized the development of a medical school on the Davis campus near Sacramento in 1963, and legislative funds were made available for planning and development in 1966. The school admitted an entering class of 48 students in 1968. By fall 1971, the size of the entering class had more than doubled. Currently, the school admits a first-year class of 105 students who train at the Sacramento and Davis campuses of University of California, Davis, and at affiliated sites.

Type: public
2008-2009 total enrollment: 416
Clinical facilities: University of California, Davis, Medical Center (Sacramento); Veterans' Affairs Northern California System of Clinics (Mather); David Grant Medical Center (Travis Air Force Base); Kaiser Permanente Medical Centers (Sacramento); Mercy Healthcare (Sacramento); Sutter Community Hospitals (Sacramento); San Joaquin General Hospital (Stockton); Merced Community Medical Center; Contra Costa Medical Services (Martinez); Stanislaus Medical Center (Modesto); Mercy General Hospital (Redding); Shriners Children Hospital (Sacramento).

University Officials

President	Mark G. Yudof, L.L.B.
Chancellor, Davis Campus	Larry N. Vanderhoef, Ph.D.
Provost and Executive Vice Chancellor, Davis Campus	Enrique J. Lavernia, Ph.D.
Vice Chancellor, Human Health Sciences	Claire Pomeroy, M.D.

Medical School Administrative Staff

Dean	Claire Pomeroy, M.D.
Executive Associate Dean, Academic Affairs	Ann Bonham, Ph.D.
Executive Associate Dean, Clinical and Administrative Affairs	Thomas Nesbitt, M.D.
Associate Dean, Academic Personnel	Edward Callahan, Ph.D.
Associate Dean, Admissions	Mark Henderson, M.D.
Associate Dean, Basic and Translational Research	Fitz-Roy E. Curry, Ph.D.
Associate Dean, Cancer Programs	Ralph deVere White, M.D.
Director, Practice Group, and Associate Dean, Clinical Affairs	James Goodnight, M.D., Ph.D.
Associate Dean, Clinical and Translational Research	Lars Berglund, M.D., Ph.D.
Associate Dean, Continuing Medical Education	Gibbe Parsons, M.D.
Associate Dean, External, Academic, and Clinical Programs	Timothy Albertson, M.D.
Associate Dean, Faculty Life and Diversity	Jesse Joad, M.D.
Associate Dean, Humanities and Bioethics	Faith T. Fitzgerald, M.D.
Associate Dean, Medical Education	Vacant
Associate Dean, Student Affairs and Graduate Medical Education	James Nuovo, M.D.
Associate Dean, Veterans' Administration Affairs	William Cahill, M.D.
Assistant Dean, Administration	Michael Condrin
Assistant Dean and Executive Director, Facilities Planning and Construction	Michael W. Boyd
Assistant Dean, Finances/Controller	Katherine Wesnousky
Assistant Dean, Health Sciences Advancement	Stephanie Bray
Assistant Dean and Executive Director, Human Resources	Gloria Alvarado
Assistant Dean, Interprofessional Programs	Jana Katz-Bell, M.P.H.
Chief Medical Officer	Allan D. Siefkin, M.D.
Chief Financial Officer	William McGowan
Chief Executive Officer, Hospital and Clinics	Ann Madden Rice
Chief Patient Care Services Officer	Carol Robinson
Chief Information Officer	Michael Minear
Chief Administration and Professional Services Officer	Shelton Duruisseau, Ph.D.
Assistant Director, Public Affairs	Bonnie Hyatt
Coordinator, Alumni Association	Beth Abad

University of California, Davis, School of Medicine: CALIFORNIA

Department and Division or Section Chairs

Basic Sciences

Biochemistry and Molecular Medicine . . . . George Kaysen, M.D. (Acting)
Cell Biology and Human Anatomy . . . . Paul Fitzgerald, Ph.D. (Acting)
Medical Microbiology and Immunology . . . . Satya Dandekar, Ph.D.
Medical Pharmacology and Toxicology . . . . Donald M. Bers, Ph.D.
Physiology and Membrane Biology . . . . Peter M. Cala, Ph.D.

Clinical Sciences

Anesthesiology and Pain Medicine . . . . Peter Moore, M.D.
  Pain Medicine . . . . Scott Fishman, M.D.
Dermatology . . . . Fu-Tong Liu, M.D., Ph.D.
Emergency Medicine . . . . Nathan Kupperman, M.D., Ph.D.
Family and Community Medicine . . . . Klea D. Bertakis, M.D.
Internal Medicine . . . . Frederick J. Meyers, M.D.
  Cardiovascular Medicine . . . . Reginald Low, M.D.
  Endocrinology, Clinical Nutrition, and Vascular Biology . . . . John Rutledge, M.D.
  Gastroenterology . . . . Lorenzo Rossaro, M.D.
  General Medicine . . . . Richard White, M.D.
  Hematology and Oncology . . . . Kit Lam, M.D., Ph.D.
  Infectious Diseases . . . . Richard Pollard, M.D.
  Nephrology . . . . George A. Kaysen, M.D., Ph.D.
  Pulmonary and Critical Care Medicine . . . . Timothy E. Albertson, M.D., Ph.D.
  Rheumatology, Allergy, and Clinical Immunology . . . . M. Eric Gershwin, M.D.
Medical Pathology and Laboratory Medicine . . . . Ralph Green, M.D.
Neurological Surgery . . . . J. Paul Muizelaar, M.D.
Neurology . . . . Michael Rogawski, M.D., Ph.D.
Obstetrics and Gynecology . . . . Lloyd H. Smith, M.D., Ph.D.
Ophthalmology . . . . Mark Mannis, M.D.
Orthopaedic Surgery . . . . Paul DiCesare, M.D.
Otolaryngology . . . . Hilary Brodie, M.D., Ph.D.
Pediatrics . . . . Anthony Philipps, M.D.
  Neonatology . . . . Richard Cooke, M.D.
Physical Medicine and Rehabilitation . . . . David Kilmer, M.D.
Psychiatry and Behavioral Sciences . . . . Robert E. Hales, M.D.
  Child, Adolescent, and Family Psychiatry . . . . Robert Hendren, D.O.
Public Health Sciences . . . . Ellen Gold, Ph.D.
Radiation Oncology . . . . Ralph de Vere White, M.D. (Acting)
Radiology . . . . Raymond Dougherty, M.D. (Acting)
  Nuclear Medicine . . . . David K. Shelton, M.D.
Surgery . . . . David Wisner, M.D. (Acting)
  Burn Surgery . . . . David Greenhalgh, M.D.
  Cardiothoracic Surgery . . . . Nilas Young, M.D.
  Gastrointestinal Surgery . . . . Hung Ho, M.D.
  Plastic Surgery . . . . Thomas R. Stevenson, M.D.
  Surgical Oncology . . . . Philip Schneider, M.D.
  Transplant Surgery . . . . Richard Perez, M.D.
  Trauma Surgery . . . . Lynette Scherer, M.D.
  Vascular Surgery . . . . William Pevec, M.D.
Urology . . . . Chris Evans, M.D.

University of California, Irvine, School of Medicine

Irvine, California 92697-3950
949-824-6119; 824-5926 (dean's office); 824-2676 (fax)
Web site: www.ucihs.uci.edu

Founded in 1898, the California College of Medicine became part of the University of California, Irvine (UCI), one of nine campuses in the University of California System, in 1965. The college officially moved from Los Angeles to a 122-acre site on the Irvine campus in 1968. Today, the UCI School of Medicine provides teaching, research, and patient care facilities at the health sciences complex on the Irvine campus and at UCI Medical Center, the school's principal clinical facility, located in Orange.

Type: public
2008-2009 total enrollment: 428
Clinical facilities: University of California, Irvine, Medical Center (Orange); Veterans Administration Medical Center (Long Beach); Memorial Hospital Medical Center (Long Beach); Family Health Care Center (Santa Ana); Family Health Center (Anaheim); Gottschalk Medical Plaza (Irvine).

University Officials

Chancellor . . . . Michael Drake, M.D.
Executive Vice Chancellor and Provost . . . . Michael Gottfredson, Ph.D.

Medical School Administrative Staff

Vice Chancellor for Health Affairs and Dean, School of Medicine . . . . David N. Bailey, M.D.
Chief Executive Officer, Medical Center . . . . Maureen Zehntner
Chief of Staff, School of Medicine . . . . Ann Briggs Addo
Senior Associate Dean, Academic Affairs . . . . F. Allan Hubbell, M.D.
Senior Associate Dean, Educational Affairs . . . . Gerald Maguire, M.D.
Senior Associate Dean, Clinical Affairs/FPO . . . . John Heydt, M.D.
Senior Associate Dean, Faculty Affairs and Development . . . . Sue P. Duckles, Ph.D.
Senior Associate Dean, Research . . . . William Bunney, M.D.
Chief Financial Officer . . . . Ron King
Corporate Compliance and Privacy Officer . . . . Jim Herron
Associate Vice Chancellor for Administration . . . . Jim Herron
Associate Vice Chancellor, College of Health Sciences . . . . Frank L. Meyskens, M.D.
Associate Dean, Clinical Neurosciences . . . . Ira Lott, M.D.
Associate Dean, Program Development . . . . John Longhurst, M.D., Ph.D.
Associate Dean, Clinical Policy and Health Sciences Research . . . . Sherrie Kaplan, Ph.D.
Associate Dean, Student Affairs . . . . Michael D. Prislin, M.D.
Associate Dean, Curricular Affairs, Clinical . . . . E. M. McDougall, M.D.
Associate Dean, Curricular Affairs, Preclinical . . . . Harry Haigler, M.D.
Associate Dean, Admissions . . . . Ellena Peterson, Ph.D.
Associate Dean, Graduate Medical Education . . . . Russell Williams, M.D.
Assistant Dean, Continuing Medical Education . . . . Scott Rudkin, M.D.
Chief of Staff, VA Medical Center, Long Beach . . . . Sandor Szabo, M.D.
Director, Office of Clinical Research and Trials . . . . Randall F. Holcombe, M.D.
Director, Nursing Sciences . . . . Ellen Olshansky, R.N.
Director, Pharmaceutical Sciences . . . . Mahtab Jafari, Pharm.D.
Director, Public Health Preparedness . . . . Kristi L. Koenig, M.D.

Department and Division or Section Chairs

Basic Sciences

Anatomy and Neurobiology . . . . Ivan Soltesz, Ph.D.
Biological Chemistry . . . . Wen-Hwa Lee, Ph.D.
Microbiology and Molecular Genetics . . . . Rozanne Sandri-Goldin, Ph.D.
Pharmacology . . . . Paolo Sassone-Corsi, Ph.D.
Physiology and Biophysics . . . . Michael Cahalan, Ph.D.

Clinical Sciences

Anesthesiology and Perioperative Care . . . . Zeev N. Kain, M.D.
Dermatology . . . . Christopher Zachary, M.D.

Emergency Medicine . . . . Mark Langdorf, M.D.
Epidemiology . . . . Hoda Anton-Culver, Ph.D.
Family Medicine . . . . Kathryn Larsen, M.D.
Medicine . . . . Alpesh N. Amin, M.D.
  Basic and Clinical Immunology . . . . Sudhir Gupta, M.D.
  Cardiology . . . . Jagat Narula, M.D.
  Endocrinology . . . . Ellis Levin, M.D.
  Gastroenterology . . . . Andrzej Tarnawski, M.D.
  General Internal Medicine . . . . Alpesh Amin, M.D.
  Hematology and Oncology . . . . Randall Holcombe, M.D.
  Infectious Diseases . . . . Donald Forthal, M.D.
  Nephrology . . . . Nosratola D. Vaziri, M.D.
  Occupational Medicine . . . . Dean Baker, M.D.
  Pulmonary Diseases and Critical Care Medicine . . . . Matthew Brenner, M.D.
  Rheumatology and Clinical Immunology . . . . Brian Andrews, M.D.
Neurological Surgery . . . . Mark Linskey, M.D.
Neurology . . . . Steven Schreiber, M.D.
Obstetrics and Gynecology . . . . Manual Porto, M.D.
Ophthalmology . . . . George Baerveldt, M.D.
Orthopedic Surgery . . . . Ranjan Gupta, M.D.
Otolaryngology . . . . William Armstrong, M.D.
Pathology . . . . Michael Sclsted, M.D., Ph.D.
Pediatrics . . . . Feizal Waffain, M.D.
  Cardiology . . . . Nafiz Kiciman, M.D.
  Child Development . . . . James Swanson, Ph.D.
  Critical Care . . . . Mehrdad Jalili, M.D.
  Endocrinology . . . . Floyd Culler, M.D.
  General Pediatrics . . . . Marc Lerner, M.D.
  Hematology and Oncology . . . . Leonard Sender, M.D.
  Human Genetics . . . . Virginia Kimonis, M.D.
  Infectious Disease . . . . Behnoosh Afghani, M.D.
  Neonatal and Perinatal Medicine . . . . Houchang Modanlou, M.D.
  Nephrology . . . . Deepak Rajpoot, M.D.
  Neurology . . . . Ira Lott, M.D.
  Pulmonary . . . . Dan Cooper, M.D.
Physical Medicine and Rehabilitation . . . . Jen Yu, M.D., Ph.D.
Psychiatry and Human Behavior . . . . Barry Chaitin, M.D.
Radiation Oncology . . . . Nilam Ramsinghani, M.D.
Radiological Sciences . . . . Scott Goodwin, M.D.
  Cardiothoracic Radiology . . . . Farhood Saremi, M.D.
  ER Radiology . . . . Duane Vajgrt, M.D.
  General Imaging and CT . . . . Allen Cohen, M.D., Ph.D.
  Magnetic Resonance Imaging . . . . Fred Girensite, M.D.
  Mammography . . . . Stephen Feig, M.D.
  Musculoskeletal . . . . Jamshid Tehranzadeh, M.D.
  Molecular Imaging . . . . Paul Lizotte, D.O.
  Neuro Endovascular Radiology . . . . Varoujan Kostanian, M.D.
  Neuroradiology . . . . Anton Hasso, M.D.
  Pediatric Radiology . . . . Michelle Chandler, M.D.
  Ultrasound . . . . Monica Rivera, M.D.
  Vascular and Interventional . . . . Open
  Women's Imaging . . . . Joan Marshall, M.D.
Surgery . . . . David Hoyt, M.D.
  Colorectal Surgery . . . . Michael Stamos, M.D.
  Gastrointestinal . . . . Ninh Nguyen, M.D.
  Hepatobiliary . . . . David Imagawa, M.D.
  Oncology . . . . John Butler, M.D.
  Pediatric Surgery . . . . Sherif Emil, M.D.
  Plastic Surgery . . . . Gregory Evans, M.D.
  Thoracic Surgery . . . . Jeffrey Milliken, M.D.
  Transplantation . . . . Clarence Foster, M.D.
  Trauma and Critical Care . . . . Michael Lekawa, M.D.
  Vascular Surgery . . . . Roy Fujitani, M.D.
Urology . . . . Ralph Clayman, M.D.

University of California, San Diego, School of Medicine
La Jolla, California 92093
858-534-0830; 534-1501 (dean's office); 534-6573 (fax)
Web site: http://som.ucsd.edu

The University of California Regents voted to establish a school of medicine on the University of California, San Diego (UCSD), campus in 1962. The first medical school class matriculated in fall 1968. Today, the entering class size is 122 new students, including 8-10 M.D./Ph.D. students each year. The school's La Jolla campus complex has grown to encompass the Biomedical Sciences Building, Stein Clinical Research Building, Leichtag Biomedical Research Building, Cellular and Molecular Medicine buildings, and the Center for Molecular Genetics. UCSD's Skaggs School of Pharmacy facility is also located on this complex, and pharmacy students join medical students in several common classes. The primary teaching hospital is located 13 miles south of the campus in Hillcrest. A newer medical center complex with a hospital and specialty centers is located on UCSD campus property east of the school of medicine. Both complexes also have ambulatory care facilities.

Type: public
2008-2009 total enrollment: 508
Clinical facilities: UCSD Medical Center, Hillcrest (complex includes three ambulatory care centers); UCSD Thornton Hospital, Rebecca and John Moores Cancer Center, Donald and Darlene Shiley Eye Center, Perlman Ambulatory Care Center on UCSD's east campus in La Jolla. **Partner Institutions:** Veterans Affairs Medical Center, Children's Hospital and Health Center. Joint Bone Marrow Program with Sharp Hospital. Teaching and service agreements with Scripps Hospitals, Sharp Hospitals, Kaiser Foundation Hospital, Community Clinics.

University Officials

President. . . . . Mark G. Yudof, L.L.B.
Chancellor, San Diego Campus . . . . Marye Anne Fox, Ph.D.

Medical School Administrative Staff

Vice Chancellor and Dean, School of Medicine . . . . David A. Brenner, M.D.
Associate Dean, Academic Affairs . . . . Andy Ries, M.D.
Dean, Clinical Affairs. . . . . Thomas McAfee, M.D.
Dean, Scientific Affairs. . . . . Gordon Gill, M.D.
Associate Dean, Scientific Affairs . . . . Jerrold M. Olefsky, M.D.
Associate Vice Chancellor and Chief Financial Officer. . . . . Thomas E. Jackiewicz
Associate Dean, Admissions and Student Life . . . . Carolyn Kelly, M.D.
Associate Dean, Continuing Education . . . . Terence M. Davidson, M.D.
Associate Dean . . . . Ruth M. Covell, M.D.
Vice Dean for Medical Education. . . . . Maria C. Savoia, M.D.
Assistant Dean, Diversity and Community Outreach . . . . Sandra P. Daley, M.D.
Associate Dean, Veterans Affairs. . . . . Jacqueline G. Parthemore, M.D.
Chief Executive Officer UCSD Medical Center . . . . Richard J. Liekweg
Director, Animal Care Program . . . . Phillip Richter, D.V.M., Ph.D.
Director, Health Sciences Communication . . . . Leslie J. Franz
Associate Dean, Business and Fiscal Affairs . . . . Ron Espiritu

Department Chairs and Division or Section Heads

Anesthesiology. . . . . Gerard Manecke, M.D.
Cellular and Molecular Medicine . . . . Marilyn Farquhar, Ph.D.
Family and Preventive Medicine. . . . . Ted Ganiats, M.D. (Interim)
    Division of Biostatistics and Bioinformatics . . . . Ronald G. Thomas, Ph.D.
    Division of International Health and Cross
        Cultural Medicine . . . . Steffanie A. Strathdee, Ph.D.
    Epidemiology. . . . . Elizabeth Barrett-Connor, M.D.
    Family Medicine. . . . . Gene (Rusty) Kallenberg, M.D.
    Health Care Sciences . . . . Richard G. Kronick, Ph.D.
Medicine. . . . . Kenneth Kaushansky, M.D.
    Allergy, Rheumatology, and Immunology . . . . Gary Firestein, M.D.
    Cardiology. . . . . Kirk Knowlton, M.D.
    Dermatology . . . . Richard Gallo, M.D., Ph.D.
    Endocrinology and Metabolism. . . . . Jerrold M. Olefsky, M.D.
    General Internal Medicine . . . . Joe W. Ramsdell, M.D.
    Genetics. . . . . Maria Dell'Aquilla, Ph.D.

Gastroenterology . . . . John Carethers, M.D.
Hematology and Oncology . . . . Sanford Shattil, M.D.
Infectious Disease . . . . Robert Schooley, M.D.
Nephrology . . . . Roland C. Blantz, M.D.
Physiology . . . . Peter D. Wagner, M.D.
Pulmonary . . . . Patricio Finn, M.D.
Neurosciences . . . . Doris A. Trauner, M.D. (Interim)
Neurology-UCMC . . . . Patrick Lyden, M.D.
Neurology-VAMC . . . . Douglas R. Galasko, M.D.
Neurosciences Graduate Program . . . . Anirvan Ghosh, Ph.D.
Pediatric Neurology . . . . Doris A. Trauner, M.D.
Ophthalmology . . . . Stuart I. Brown, M.D.
Orthopaedics . . . . Steven R. Garfin, M.D.
Pathology . . . . Steve Gonias, M.D.
Laboratory Medicine . . . . Sharon Reed, M.D.
Molecular Pathology Graduate Program . . . . Mark Kamps, Ph.D.
Pediatrics . . . . Gabriel Haddad, M.D.
Cardiology . . . . Stanley Kirkpatrick, M.D. (Acting)
Community Pediatrics . . . . Howard Taras, M.D.
Dermatology . . . . Larry Eichenfield, M.D.
Dysmorphology . . . . Kenneth Lyons Jones, M.D.
Endocrinology . . . . Michael E. Gottschalk, M.D., Ph.D.
Gastroenterology . . . . Joel Lavine, M.D.
Genetics . . . . Tony Wynshaw-Boris, M.D.
Hematology and Oncology . . . . Open
Infectious Diseases . . . . Stephen A. Spector, M.D.
Neonatology and Perinatology . . . . Neil Finer, M.D.
Nephrology and Renal Medicine . . . . Paul Grimm, M.D. (Acting)
Neurology . . . . Doris A. Trauner, M.D.
Primary Care and Adolescent Medicine . . . . Lawrence Friedman, M.D.
Pulmonary Medicine . . . . Mark S. Pian, M.D.
Pharmacology . . . . Joan Heller Brown, Ph.D.
Biomedical Sciences Graduate Program . . . . Jeffrey D. Esko, Ph.D.
Psychiatry . . . . Lewis L. Judd, M.D.
Child Psychiatry . . . . Saul Levine, M.D.
Clinical Psychology Doctoral Program . . . . Robert K. Heaton, Ph.D.
Geropsychiatry . . . . Dilip Jeste, M.D.
Radiology . . . . William Bradley, M.D., Ph.D.
Diagnostic Radiology . . . . John R. Hesselink, M.D.
Nuclear Medicine . . . . Carl K. Hoh, M.D.
Vascular and Interventional . . . . Anne C. Roberts, M.D.
Radiation Oncology . . . . Stephen Seagren, M.D.
Radiological Physics . . . . Michael P. André, Ph.D.
Reproductive Medicine . . . . Thomas R. Moore, M.D.
Gynecologic Oncology . . . . Steven Plaxe, M.D.
Maternal-Fetal (Perinatal) Medicine . . . . Thomas R. Moore, M.D.
Reproductive Endocrinology . . . . R. Jeffrey Chang, M.D.
Surgery . . . . Mark Talamini, M.D.
Anatomy . . . . Mark C. Whitehead, Ph.D.
Cardiothoracic Surgery . . . . Stuart W. Jamieson, M.D.
General Surgery . . . . Mark Talamini, M.D.
Neurosurgery . . . . Lawrence Marshall, M.D.
Otolaryngology-Head and Neck Surgery . . . . Jeffrey P. Harris, M.D., Ph.D.
Plastic Surgery . . . . Marek Dobke, M.D.
Trauma-Burn . . . . Raul Colmbra, M.D.
Urology . . . . Christopher Kane, M.D.

Organized Research Units

Cancer Center . . . . Dennis Carson, M.D.
Institute for Research on Aging . . . . Dilip Jeste, M.D.
AIDS Research Institute . . . . Douglas Richman, M.D.
Institute of Molecular Medicine . . . . Gary S. Firestein, M.D.
Glycobiology Research and Training Center . . . . Ajit Varki, M.D.

University of California, San Francisco, School of Medicine

513 Parnassus Avenue
Room S-224
San Francisco, California 94143-0410
415-476-1000; 476-2342 (dean's office); 476-0689 (fax)
Web site: www.medschool.ucsf.edu

The school of medicine at the University of California, San Francisco, dates from 1864 when it was founded as the Toland Medical College. In 1873, it was formally transferred to the Regents of the University of California.

Type: public
2008-2009 total enrollment: 600
Clinical facilities: UCSF Medical Center; Langley Porter Psychiatric Institute; San Francisco General Hospital Medical Center; San Francisco Veterans Affairs Medical Center; and major teaching hospitals associated with the UCSF/Fresno Medical Education Program.

University Officials

President . . . . Mark G. Yudof
Vice President, Health Sciences and Services . . . . Wyatt R. (Rory) Hume, D.D.S., Ph.D. (Acting)
Chancellor, San Francisco Campus . . . . J. Michael Bishop, M.D.

Medical School Administrative Staff

Dean . . . . Samuel Hawgood, M.B.B.S. (Interim)
Associate Dean, Cancer Center . . . . Frank McCormick, Ph.D.
Associate Dean, Mount Zion Medical Center . . . . Jeffrey M. Pearl, M.D.
Associate Dean, San Francisco General Hospital . . . . Amanda S. Carlisle, M.D., Ph.D.
Associate Dean, San Francisco Veterans Affairs
Medical Center . . . . C. Diana Nicoll, M.D., Ph.D.
Senior Associate Dean, Clinical and
Translational Research . . . . Joseph M. McCune, M.D., Ph.D.
Associate Deans, Clinical and Translational Research . . . . Deborah Grady, M.D., M.P.H.,
Daniel H. Lowenstein, M.D., and Joel M. Palefsky, M.D.
Vice Dean, Academic Affairs . . . . Donna M. Ferriero, M.D.
Associate Deans, Academic Affairs . . . . Renee L. Binder, M.D.,
and J. Renee Navarro, Pharm.D., M.D.
Vice Dean, Administration, Finance, and Clinical Programs . . . . Michael Hindery
Vice Dean, Education . . . . David M. Irby, Ph.D.
Associate Dean, Admissions . . . . David Wofsy, M.D.
Associate Dean, Curricular Affairs . . . . Helen Loeser, M.D.
Associate Dean, Student Affairs . . . . Maxine A. Papadakis, M.D.
Associate Dean, Graduate Medical Education,
and Associate Dean, Continuing Medical
Education . . . . Robert B. Baron, M.D.
Associate Dean, Fresno Medical Education Program . . . . Joan L. Voris, M.D.
Associate Dean, School of Medicine . . . . Peter R. Carroll, M.D., M.P.H.
Executive Vice Dean . . . . Keith R. Yamamoto, Ph.D.
Associate Dean, Research and Special Projects . . . . Dina Gould Halme, Ph.D.
Vice Deans, School of Medicine . . . . Neal H. Cohen, M.D., Nancy Milliken, M.D.,
and Bruce U. Wintroub, M.D.

Department and Division or Section Chairs

Basic Sciences

Anatomy . . . . Allan I. Basbaum, Ph.D.
Anthropology, History, and Social Medicine . . . . Dorothy E. Porter, Ph.D.
Biochemistry and Biophysics . . . . K. Peter Walter, Ph.D.
Cellular and Molecular Pharmacology . . . . Ronald D. Vale, Ph.D.
Epidemiology and Biostatistics . . . . Robert A. Hiatt, M.D., Ph.D., and Neil J. Risch, Ph.D.
Microbiology and Immunology . . . . Anthony L. DeFranco, Ph.D.
Pathology . . . . Abul K. Abbas, M.D.
Physiology . . . . David J. Julius, Ph.D.

University of California, San Francisco, School of Medicine: CALIFORNIA

Clinical Sciences

Anesthesia and Perioperative Care . . . . Ronald D. Miller, M.D.
Dermatology . . . . Bruce U. Wintroub, M.D.
Family and Community Medicine . . . . Kevin Grumbach, M.D.
Laboratory Medicine . . . . Clifford A. Lowell, M.D., Ph.D.
Medicine . . . . Talmadge E. King, Jr., M.D.
Neurological Surgery . . . . Mitchel S. Berger, M.D.
Neurology . . . . Stephen L. Hauser, M.D.
Obstetrics, Gynecology, and Reproductive Sciences . . . . Linda C. Giudice, M.D., Ph.D.
Ophthalmology . . . . Stephen D. McLeod, M.D.
Orthopaedic Surgery . . . . Thomas P. Vail, M.D.
Otolaryngology . . . . David W. Eisele, M.D.
Pediatrics . . . . Samuel Hawgood, M.B.B.S.
Physical Therapy and Rehabilitation Sciences . . . . Kimberly S. Topp, Ph.D. (Interim)
Psychiatry . . . . Renee L. Binder, M.D.
Radiation Oncology . . . . Mack Roach III, M.D.
Radiology and Biomedical Imaging . . . . Ronald L. Arenson, M.D.
Surgery . . . . Nancy L. Ascher, M.D., Ph.D.
Urology . . . . Peter R. Carroll, M.D.

University of Colorado Denver School of Medicine

4200 East Ninth Avenue
Campus Box C290
Denver, Colorado 80262
720-848-0000 (general information); 303-724-8025 (admissions);
303-724-0882 (dean's office); 303-724-6070 (fax)
E-mail: SOMdean@uchsc.edu
Web site: www.uchsc.edu/som

The University of Colorado Denver School of Medicine was opened on the main campus in Boulder in 1883. The school was moved to downtown Denver in 1911 to be merged with the Denver and Gross College of Medicine. In 1922, a facility was built on a 17-acre site in a residential section of east Denver, and the school of medicine was moved there in 1925. The campus has outgrown the present 45-acre site and is in the process of moving six miles east to the Anschutz Medical Campus, site of the former Fitzsimons Army Medical Center in Aurora. The 227-acre Anschutz Medical Campus is adjacent to a 160-acre bioscience park.

Type: public
2008-2009 total enrollment: 620
Clinical facilities: The Children's Hospital, University of Colorado Hospital, Denver Health, National Jewish Medical and Research Center and the nearby Veterans Affairs Medical Center, which is a dean's committee VA center.

University Officials

President. . . . . Bruce Benson
Chancellor, University of Colorado at Denver and Health Sciences . . . . M. Roy Wilson, M.D.
Provost and Vice Chancellor for Academic and Student Affairs . . . . Roderick Nairn, Ph.D.
Vice Chancellor for Administration and Finance. . . . . Teresa Berryman
Vice Chancellor for Advancement and Chief of Staff. . . . . Andy A. Jhanji
Vice Chancellor for External Affairs . . . . Jay Gershen, D.D.S., Ph.D.
Vice Chancellor for Health Affairs and Dean,
    School of Medicine . . . . Richard D. Krugman, M.D.
Vice Chancellor for Research Affairs. . . . . Richard Traystman, Ph.D.

Medical School Administrative Staff

Dean. . . . . Richard D. Krugman, M.D.
Senior Associate Dean for Academic Affairs . . . . E. Chester Ridgway, M.D.
Senior Associate Dean for Administration and Finance . . . . Lilly Marks
Senior Associate Dean for Clinical Affairs. . . . . Joel S. Levine, M.D.
Senior Associate Dean for Education . . . . Robert E. Feinstein, M.D.
Associate Dean . . . . Regina A. Kilkenny, M.D.
Associate Dean for Admissions . . . . Norma Wagoner, Ph.D.
Assistant Dean for Business Affairs . . . . Robert Fries
Associate Dean for Clinical Core Curriculum . . . . Robin R. Deterding, M.D.
Associate Dean for Continuing Medical Education . . . . Ronald S. Gibbs, M.D.
Associate Dean for Curriculum Evaluation . . . . Carol S. Hodgson, Ph.D.
Associate Dean for Essentials Core Curriculum. . . . . Bruce Wallace, Ph.D.
Associate Dean for Faculty Affairs. . . . . Steven R. Lowenstein, M.D.
Associate Dean for Graduate Medical Education . . . . Carol M. Rumack, M.D.
Associate Dean for Research Affairs . . . . John W. Moorhead, M.D.
Associate Dean for Research Development . . . . Richard B. Johnston, Jr., M.D.
Associate Dean for Rural Affairs. . . . . John M. Westfall, M.D.
Associate Dean for Student Advocacy . . . . John E. Repine, M.D.
Associate Dean for Student Affairs . . . . Maureen Garrity, Ph.D.
Associate Dean for Western Slope Branch Planning . . . . David West, M.D.
Assistant Dean for Allied Health. . . . . Margaret L. Schenkman, Ph.D., P.T.
Associate Dean for Research Education . . . . Nancy R. Zahniser, Ph.D.

Department and Division or Section Chairs

Basic Sciences

Biochemistry and Molecular Genetics. . . . . Robert A. Sclafani, Ph.D. (Interim)
Cell and Developmental Biology. . . . . Claude Selitrennikoff, Ph.D. (Interim)
Immunology . . . . John C. Cambier, Ph.D.

Microbiology . . . . Randall K. Holmes, M.D., Ph.D.
Pathology . . . . Ann D. Thor, M.D.
Pharmacology . . . . Boris Tabakoff, Ph.D.
Physiology and Biophysics . . . . William Betz, Ph.D.

Clinical Sciences

Anesthesiology. . . . . Thomas K. Henthorn, M.D.
Dermatology . . . . David A. Norris, M.D.
Family Medicine . . . . Frank deGruy, M.D.
Medicine. . . . . Robert J. Anderson, M.D.
    Allergy and Clinical Immunology . Andrew Fontenot, M.D., and Rafeul Alam, M.D. (Co-Head)
    Cardiology . . . . Peter Buttrick, M.D.
    Clinical Pharmacology and Toxicology . . . . Curt Freed, M.D.
    Endocrinology, Metabolism, and Diabetes . . . . Bryan Haugen, M.D.
    Gastroenterology . . . . Hugo Rosen, M.D.
    General Internal Medicine . . . . Jean Kutner, M.D.
    Geriatrics. . . . . Robert S. Schwartz, M.D.
    Health Care Policy and Research . . . . Andrew Kramer, M.D.
    Hematology . . . . Robert H. Allen, M.D., and Sally P. Stabler, M.D. (Co-Head)
    Infectious Diseases . . . . Thomas Campbell, M.D. (Interim)
    Medical Oncology . . . . Gail S. Eckhardt, M.D.
    Pulmonary Sciences and Critical Care Medicine . . . . Mark Geraci, M.D.
    Renal Diseases and Hypertension . . . . Richard Johnson, M.D.
    Rheumatology . . . . V. Michael Holers, M.D.
Neurology . . . . Donald H. Gilden, M.D.
Neurosurgery. . . . . Kevin Lillehei, M.D.
Obstetrics and Gynecology. . . . . Ronald S. Gibbs, M.D.
Ophthalmology . . . . Naresh Mandava, M.D.
Orthopaedics. . . . . Robert D. D'Ambrosia, M.D.
Otolaryngology . . . . Herman A. Jenkins, M.D.
Pediatrics . . . . Stephen R. Daniels, M.D., Ph.D.
Physical Medicine and Rehabilitation . . . . Dennis Matthews, M.D.
Psychiatry . . . . Robert Freedman, M.D.
    American Indian and Alaska Native Programs . . . . Spero Manson, Ph.D.
    Behavioral Immunology Research Group. . . . . Mark Laudenslager, Ph.D.
    Child Psychiatry . . . . Marianne Z. Wamboldt, M.D.
    Early Developmental Studies. . . . . Robert Emde, M.D.
    Medical Student Education. . . . . Michael Weissberg, M.D.
    Neuro Behavioral Disorders . . . . David Arciniegas, M.D.
    Residency Education. . . . . Alexis Giese, M.D.
    Schizophrenia Research Center. . . . . Robert Freedman, M.D.
    Substance Dependence. . . . . Thomas Crowley, M.D.
Radiation Oncology. . . . . Laurie Gaspar, M.D.
Radiology . . . . Gerald D. Dodd, M.D.
    Abdominal Imaging . . . . Kirsten E. McKinney, M.D.
    Diagnostic Radiology . . . . James Davidson, M.D.
    Interventional Radiology. . . . . Janette D. Durham, M.D.
    Mammography* . . . . Lara Hardesty, M.D.
    Neuroradiology . . . . Robert Bert, M.D.
    Nuclear Medicine*. . . . . Adrienne Gage-El, M.D.
    Radiological Research. . . . . Charles E. Ray, M.D., and Jody L. Tanabe, M.D. (Co-Head)
    Radiological Sciences . . . . Ann Scherzinger, Ph.D.
    Thoracic Radiology*. . . . . James Borgstede, M.D.
Surgery . . . . Frederick L. Grover, M.D.
    Cardiothoracic Surgery. . . . . David Fullerton, M.D.
    Emergency Medicine . . . . Benjamin Honigman, M.D.
    Gastrointestinal, Tumor, and Endocrine Surgery . . . . Gregory Van Stiegmann, M.D.
    Pediatric Surgery* . . . . Frederick Karrer, M.D.
    Plastic and Reconstructive Surgery . . . . Michael Gordon, M.D.
    Transplant Surgery. . . . . Igal Kam, M.D.
    Trauma . . . . Ernest E. Moore, M.D.
    Urology . . . . Randall B. Meacham, M.D.
    Vascular Surgery and Podiatry. . . . . Mark R. Nehler, M.D.

*Specialty without organizational autonomy.

University of Connecticut School of Medicine

263 Farmington Avenue
Farmington, Connecticut 06030
860-679-2000; 679-2594 (dean's office); 679-1255 (fax)
Web site: http://medicine.uchc.edu/

The University of Connecticut School of Medicine appointed its first faculty members in 1963 and admitted its first class in 1968. The University of Connecticut Health Center, 35 miles from the main university campus, includes the school of medicine, school of dental medicine, ambulatory services, and John Dempsey Hospital.

Type: public
2008-2009 total enrollment: 337
Clinical facilities: John Dempsey Hospital, Connecticut Children's Medical Center, Veterans Administration Medical Center (Newington). Bristol Hospital, Hartford Hospital, the Institute of Living, Middlesex Memorial Hospital, Mount Sinai Hospital, New Britain General Hospital, Hospital for Special Care, Saint Francis Hospital and Medical Center, the Hebrew Home and Hospital.

University Officials

President. . . . . Michael J. Hogan
Vice President, Health Affairs. . . . . Cato T. Laurencin, M.D., Ph.D.
Chief Financial Officer. . . . . Daniel L. Upton
Chief Information Officer . . . . Sandra Armstrong
Associate Vice President, Facilities Management . . . . Daniel Penney
Associate Vice President, Research Administration and Finance. . . . . Jeff Small
Associate Vice President, Human Resources . . . . Brian Eaton
Associate Vice President, Communications . . . . James Walter
Associate Vice President, Budget . . . . Lisa Danville
Director, John Dempsey Hospital. . . . . James Thornton
Medical Director, UConn Medical Group. Peter Albertsen, M.D.

Medical School Administrative Staff

Dean. . . . . Cato T. Laurencin, M.D., Ph.D.
Dean for Academic Affairs. . . . . Bruce M. Koeppen, M.D., Ph.D.
Associate Dean, Administration and Finance. . . . . David C. Gillon
Associate Dean, Clinical Affairs. . . . . Peter C. Albertsen, M.D.
Associate Dean, Clinical Research Planning and Coordination. . . . . Peter C. Albertsen, M.D.
Associate Dean for Continuing Education. . . . . Charles Huntington, M.P.H.
Associate Dean, Faculty Affairs . . . . Mary Casey Jacob, Ph.D.
Associate Dean of the Graduate School . . . . Lawrence A. Klobutcher, Ph.D.
Associate Dean, Graduate Medical Education . . . . Jacqueline Nissen, M.D.
Associate Dean, Health Career Opportunity Program . . . . Marja Hurley, M.D.
Associate Dean for Health Informatics . . . . Renee Drabier, Ph.D.
Associate Dean for Postdoctoral and External Affairs. . . . . Gerald D. Maxwell, Ph.D.
Associate Dean, Primary Care. . . . . Bruce Gould, M.D.
Associate Dean, Research Planning and Coordination. . . . . Marc E. Lalande, Ph.D.
Associate Dean, Student Affairs . . . . Anthony J. Ardolino, M.D.
Assistant Dean, Clinical Affairs . . . . Jane Grant-Kels, M.D.
Assistant Dean, Health Career Opportunity Program. . . . . Open
Assistant Dean, Student Affairs. . . . . Keat Sanford, Ph.D.

Department and Division or Section Chairs

Basic Sciences

Cell Biology. . . . . Laurinda A. Jaffe, Ph.D. (Interim)
Community Medicine and Health Care. . . . . Thomas Babor, Ph.D.
Genetics and Developmental Biology . . . . Marc Lalande, Ph.D.
  Division of Genetics . . . . Robert M. Greenstein, M.D.
Immunology . . . . Pramod Srivastava, Ph.D.
Molecular, Microbial, and Structural Biology . . . . Sandra K. Weller, Ph.D.
Neuroscience. . . . . Richard Mains, Ph.D.

Clinical Sciences

Anesthesiology. . . . . Jeffrey B. Gross, M.D.
Dermatology . . . . Jane Grant-Kels, M.D.
Diagnostic Imaging and Therapeutics. . . . . Douglas Fellows, M.D.
  Radiation Oncology . . . . Robert Dowsett, M.D.

Radiology. . . . . Douglas Fellows, M.D.
Nuclear Medicine. . . . . Mozafareddin Karimeddini, M.D.
Family Medicine . . . . Robert A. Cushman, M.D.
Medicine . . . . Joseph Palmisano, M.D. (Interim)
   Cardiology. . . . . Bruce T. Liang, M.D.
   Endocrinology . . . . Andrew Arnold, M.D.
   Gastroenterology . . . . John Birk, M.D.
   General Medicine. . . . . Adam Silverman, M.D.
   Geriatrics. . . . . George Kuchel, M.D.
   Hematology and Oncology . . . . Robert Bona, M.D.
   Hypertension . . . . William B. White, M.D.
   Infectious Diseases . . . . Kevin Dieckhaus, M.D.
   Nephrology . . . . Nancy Adams, M.D.
   Public Health and Population Sciences. . . . . Robert Trestman, M.D., Ph.D.
   Pulmonary and Critical Care Medicine . . . . Daniel McNally, M.D. (Interim)
   Rheumatology . . . . Micha Abeles, M.D. (Interim)
Neurology. . . . . Leslie Wolfson, M.D.
Obstetrics and Gynecology. . . . . James F. X. Egan, M.D.
   Gynecological Oncology* . . . . Molly A. Brewer, M.D.
   Maternal Fetal Medicine*. . . . . Winston A. Campbell, M.D.
   Reproductive Endocrinology and Infertility* . . . . John C. Nulsen, M.D.
   Urogynecology. . . . . Open
   Generalist . . . . Joseph Walsh, M.D.
Orthopaedic Surgery. . . . . Jay Lieberman, M.D.
Pathology and Laboratory Medicine . . . . M. Melinda Sanders, M.D.
Pediatrics . . . . Paul Dworkin, M.D.
   Adolescent Medicine*. . . . . Aric Schichor, M.D.
   Ambulatory and Community Affairs . . . . Open
   Behavioral and Development*. . . . . Neil L. Schechter, M.D.
   Cardiology* . . . . Harry Leopold, M.D.
   Child and Family Studies* . . . . Mary Beth Bruder, Ph.D.
   Community Pediatrics*. . . . . Douglas MacGilpin, M.D., and Larry Scherzer, M.D.
   Critical Care*. . . . . Aaron Zucker, M.D.
   Endocrinology* . . . . Karen R. Rubin, M.D.
   Education and Residency Program* . . . . Edwin L. Zalneraitis, M.D.
   Gastroenterology* . . . . Jeffrey S. Hyams, M.D.
   General Pediatrics*. . . . . Richard C. Antonelli, M.D., and Lee M. Pachter, D.O.
   Hematology and Oncology* . . . . Nathan Hagstrom, M.D.
   Hospitalist Care . . . . Robert Englander, M.D.
   Infectious Diseases* . . . . Peter Krause, M.D.
   Neonatology and Perinatal Medicine. . . . . Victor C. Herson, M.D. (Interim)
   Nephrology* . . . . Majid Rasoulpour, M.D.
   Neurology* . . . . Francis Di Mario, M.D.
   Pediatric Allergy and Immunology*. . . . . Louis Mendelson, M.D.
   Pediatric Emergency Medicine . . . . M. C. Culbertson, M.D.
   Pediatric Dermatology . . . . Mary Chang, M.D.
   Pediatric Pathology*. . . . . Vijay Joshi, M.D.
   Pediatric Psychiatry*. . . . . Robert Sahl, M.D.
   Pediatric Radiology*. . . . . Timothy Brown, M.D.
   Pediatric Rehabilitative Medicine*. . . . . Open
   Pediatric Research* . . . . Georgine S. Burke, Ph.D.
   Pediatric Rheumatology* . . . . Lawrence Zemel, M.D.
   Pulmonary Medicine*. . . . . Craig Schramm, M.D.
Psychiatry . . . . Leighton Huey, M.D.
Surgery . . . . Robert A. Kozol, M.D.
   Cardiothoracic Surgery. . . . . Paul L. Preissler, M.D.
   General Surgery. . . . . Robert A. Kozol, M.D.
   Neurosurgery. . . . . Hilary Onyiuke, M.D.
   Ophthalmology and Clinical. . . . . Jeanine Suchecki, M.D.
   Otorhinolaryngology. . . . . Denis Lafreniere, M.D.
   Plastic Surgery . . . . Rajiv Y. Chandawarkar, M.D.
   Surgery Research . . . . Open
   Urology. . . . . Peter Albertsen, M.D.
Traumatology and Emergency Medicine. . . . . Lenworth Jacobs, M.D.

*Specialty without organizational autonomy.

Yale University School of Medicine

333 Cedar Street; P.O. Box 208055
New Haven, Connecticut 06520-8055
203-785-4672 (dean's office); 785-7437 (fax)
Web site: http://info.med.yale.edu/

The Medical Institution of Yale College was chartered in 1810, opened in 1813, and has been in continuous operation since that date. Yale College became Yale University in 1887; the current designation of the school was adopted in 1918.

Type: private
2008-2009 total enrollment: 805
Clinical facilities: Yale-New Haven Hospital, Veterans Administration Hospital (West Haven), Connecticut Mental Health Center, Hill Health Center, Yale Child Study Center, Bridgeport Hospital, Danbury Hospital, Greenwich Hospital, Griffin Hospital, Lawrence and Memorial Hospitals, Norwalk Hospital, St. Mary's Hospital, Hospital of St. Raphael, Waterbury Hospital, Yale Health Center.

University Officials

President. . . . . Richard C. Levin, Ph.D.
Provost . . . . Andrew D. Hamilton, Ph.D.
Deputy Provost for Biomedical and Health Affairs. . . . . Stephanie S. Spangler, M.D.

Medical School Administrative Staff

Dean. . . . . Robert J. Alpern, M.D.
Dean for Public Health . . . . Paul D. Cleary, Ph.D.
Deputy Dean for Academic and Scientific Affairs . . . . Carolyn W. Slayman, Ph.D.
Deputy Dean for Education . . . . Richard Belitsky, M.D.
Deputy Dean for Finance and Administration. . . . . Cynthia Walker
Deputy Dean for Clinical Affairs. . . . . David J. Leffell, M.D.
Special Advisor to the Dean . . . . Linda C. Mayes, M.D.
Dean's Special Advisor for Research . . . . Richard Lifton, M.D., Ph.D.
Associate Dean for Student Affairs . . . . Nancy Angoff, M.D.
Associate Dean for Student Programs. . . . . James P. Comer, M.D.
Associate Dean for Academic and Faculty Affairs. . . . . Carolyn M. Mazure, Ph.D.
Associate Dean for Graduate Medical Education . . . . Rosemarie L. Fisher, M.D.
Associate Dean for Admissions . . . . Laura Ment, M.D.
Associate Dean for Student Affairs for EPH . . . . Anne F. Pistell
Associate Dean . . . . Merle Waxman
Associate Dean for Veteran Affairs . . . . Michael E. Ebert, M.D.
Associate Dean, Office of Scientific Affairs . . . . Sara Rockwell, Ph.D.
Assistant Dean and Program Director for Physician Associate Program. . . . . Mary Warner
Assistant Dean for Multicultural Affairs. . . . . Forrester A. Lee, M.D.
Director, Division of Animal Care. . . . . James D. Macy, D.V.M.
Director, Medical Library. . . . . Regina K. Marone
Director, Program in Biological and Biomedical Sciences . . . . Lynn Cooley, Ph.D.
Director, Office of Student Research . . . . John N. Forrest, Jr., M.D.
Director, Office of Faculty Development and Equity . . . . Linda Bockenstedt, M.D.

Department, Section, or Center Chairs

Basic Sciences

Cell Biology. . . . . James E. Rothman, M.D., Ph.D.
Cellular and Molecular Physiology . . . . Michael J. Caplan, M.D. (Acting)
Center for Molecular Medicine . . . . Vincent T. Marchesi, M.D., Ph.D.
Comparative Medicine* . . . . Tamas Horvath, D.V.M., Ph.D.
History of Medicine. . . . . John H. Warner, Ph.D.
Immunobiology. . . . . Richard A. Flavell, Ph.D.
Microbial Pathogenesis. . . . . Jorge E. Galan, Ph.D.
Molecular Biophysics and Biochemistry. . . . . Scott Strobel, Ph.D.
Neurobiology*. . . . . Pasko Rakic, M.D., Sc.D.
Pharmacology . . . . Joseph Schlessinger, Ph.D.

Clinical Sciences

Anesthesiology. . . . . Roberta L. Hines, M.D.
Child Study Center† . . . . Fred Volkmar, M.D.

Comprehensive Cancer Center . . . . Richard L. Edelson, M.D.
Dermatology . . . . Richard L. Edelson, M.D.
Diagnostic Radiology . . . . James A. Brink, M.D.
Epidemiology and Public Health . . . . Paul D. Cleary, Ph.D.
   Biostatistics . . . . Theodore R. Holford, Ph.D.
   Chronic Disease Epidemiology . . . . Stanislav V. Kasl, Ph.D.
   Environmental Health Sciences. . . . . Tongzhang Zheng, Ph.D.
   Epidemiology of Microbial Diseases. . . . . Serap Aksoy, Ph.D.
   Health Policy and Administration . . . . Jody Sindelar, Ph.D.
Genetics . . . . Richard Lifton, M.D., Ph.D.
Internal Medicine . . . . Jack A. Elias, M.D.
   Allergy and Immunology . . . . Philip W. Askenase, M.D.
   Cardiology. . . . . Michael Simons, M.D.
   Digestive Diseases. . . . . Michael Nathanson, M.D.
   Endocrine and Metabolism. . . . . Robert Sherwin, M.D. (Interim)
   General Medicine. . . . . Patrick O'Connor, M.D.
   Geriatric Medicine . . . . Leo M. Cooney, M.D.
   Hematology. . . . . Madhav V. Dhodapkar, M.D.
   Infectious Diseases . . . . Erol Fikrig, M.D.
   Nephrology . . . . Stefan Somlo, M.D.
   Oncology. . . . . Edward Chu, M.D.
   Pulmonary and Critical Care. . . . . Lynn T. Tanoue, M.D. (Interim)
   Rheumatology . . . . Joseph E. Craft, M.D.
Laboratory Medicine . . . . Brian R. Smith, M.D.
Neurology . . . . Stephen G. Waxman, M.D., Ph.D.
Neurosurgery. . . . . Dennis D. Spencer, M.D.
Obstetrics and Gynecology. . . . . Charles J. Lockwood, M.D.
Ophthalmology and Visual Sciences . . . . James C. Tsai, M.D.
Orthopedics and Rehabilitation . . . . Gary E. Friedlaender, M.D.
Pathology . . . . Jon S. Morrow, M.D., Ph.D.
Pediatrics . . . . Margaret K. Hostetter, M.D.
   Adolescent Medicine . . . . Sheryl Ryan, M.D.
   Cardiology. . . . . Alan Friedman, M.D. (Acting)
   Critical Care. . . . . Clifford Bogue, M.D.
   Development Biology and Biophysics . . . . Scott Rivkees, M.D.
   Emergency Medicine . . . . Karen Santucci, M.D. (Acting)
   Endocrinology . . . . William Tamborlane, M.D.
   Gastroenterology . . . . Pramod Mistry, M.D.
   General Pediatrics . . . . Paul L. McCarthy, M.D.
   Hematology. . . . . Gary Kupfer, M.D.
   Immunology. . . . . Margaret K. Hostetter, M.D.
   Infectious Diseases . . . . I. George Miller, M.D.
   Nephrology . . . . Alda Tufro, M.D.
   Neurology . . . . Bennett A. Shaywitz, M.D.
   Perinatal Medicine. . . . . Ian Gross, M.D.
   Respiratory Medicine . . . . Alia Buzzy Assad, M.D.
Psychiatry . . . . William Sledge, M.D. (Acting)
Surgery. . . . . Robert Udelsman, M.D.
   Anatomy and Experimental Surgery . . . . William B. Stewart, Ph.D.
   Cardiology. . . . . John Elefteriades, M.D.
   Dentistry* . . . . Suher Baker, D.M.D. (Acting)
   Endocrine Surgery . . . . Sanziana Roman, M.D.
   Emergency Medicine . . . . Gail D'Onofrio, M.D.
   Gross Anatomy. . . . . William B. Stewart, Ph.D.
   Organ Transplantation and Immunology. . . . . Sukru H. Emre, M.D., F.A.C.S.
   Neuropathology. . . . . Laura Manuelidis, M.D.
   Otolaryngology. . . . . Clarence T. Sasaki, M.D.
   Pediatric . . . . R. Lawrence Moss, M.D.
   Plastic and Reconstructive. . . . . John A. Persing, M.D.
   Surgical Gastroenterology . . . . Walter E. Longo, M.D.
   Surgical Oncology . . . . Ronald Salem, M.D.
   Thoracic Surgery . . . . Frank Detterbeck, M.D.
   Trauma and Surgical Critical Care . . . . Kimberly Davis, M.D.
   Urology . . . . Robert M. Weiss, M.D.
   Vascular. . . . . Bauer Sumpio, M.D.
Therapeutic Radiology. . . . . Peter M. Glazer, M.D.

*Autonomous section.
†Autonomous study center.

The George Washington University
School of Medicine and Health Sciences

2300 Eye Street, N.W.
Washington, D.C. 20037
202-994-1000 (university operator); 994-2987 (dean's office); 994-0926 (fax)
Web site: www.gwumc.edu/smhs/

The school of medicine was founded in 1821 as the Medical Department of the Columbian College. In 1974, the name was changed to the school of medicine and health sciences. The Walter G. Ross Hall of Health Sciences, Paul Himmelfarb Health Sciences Library, University Hospital, Burns Memorial Building and Ambulatory Care Center (Medical Faculty Associates, Inc.), and Warwick Building are situated on the main campus and constitute the George Washington University Medical Center.

Type: private
2008-2009 total enrollment: 700
Clinical facilities: Virginia Hospital Center, The George Washington University Hospital, Children's National Medical Center, Fairfax Hospital, Holy Cross Hospital, National Institutes of Health, National Naval Medical Center, National Rehabilitation Hospital, Northern Virginia Mental Health Institute, Psychiatric Institute of Washington, Providence Hospital, Suburban Hospital, Sibley Memorial Hospital, U.S. Soldiers and Airmen Home, Veterans Administration Hospitals (Washington, D.C., and Martinsburg, West Virginia), Walter Reed Army Medical Center, Washington Hospital Center.

University Officials

President. . . . . Steven Knapp, Ph.D.
Vice President for Health Affairs and Provost . . . . John F. Williams, Jr., M.D., Ed.D.

Medical School Administrative Staff

Dean. . . . . James L. Scott, M.D.
Senior Associate Dean for Academic Affairs . . . . W. Scott Schroth, M.D.
Senior Associate Dean for Health Sciences . . . . Jean E. Johnson, Ph.D.
Associate Dean for Academic Affairs at CNMC . . . . Mark L. Batshaw, M.D.
Associate Dean for Administration and Graduate Medical Education . . . . Nancy Gaba, M.D.
Associate Dean for Graduate Studies . . . . Linda Werling, Ph.D.
Associate Dean for Clinical and Translational Research. . . . . Jill Joseph, M.D., Ph.D.
Associate Deans for Health Sciences . . . . Keith Holtermann, D.Ph., and Sylvia Silver, D.A.
Associate Dean for Student Affairs and Education. . . . . Rhonda M. Goldberg
Assistant Dean for Admissions . . . . Diane P. McQuail
Assistant Dean for Community-based Partnerships. . . . . Lisa Alexander, Ed.D.
Assistant Dean for Student and Curricular Affairs . . . . Yolanda C. Haywood, M.D.
Associate Vice President for Faculty and Educational Resources. . . . . Brian J. McGrath, M.D.
Associate Vice President for Health Research . . . . Anne N. Hirshfield, Ph.D.

Department and Division or Section Chairs

Basic Sciences

Anatomy . . . . Robert G. Hawley, Ph.D.
Biochemistry and Molecular Biology. . . . . Allan L. Goldstein, Ph.D.
Microbiology, Immunology, and Tropical Medicine. . . . . Peter J. Hotez, M.D.
Pathology . . . . Donald S. Karcher, M.D.
   Anatomical Pathology. . . . . Sana O. Tabbara, M.D.
   Clinical Pathology . . . . Louis A. DePalma, M.D.
   Surgical Pathology . . . . Arnold M. Schwartz, M.D.
Pharmacology and Physiology. . . . . Vincent A. Chiappinelli, Ph.D.

Clinical Sciences

Anesthesiology. . . . . Michael J. Berrigan, M.D., Ph.D.
   Intensive Care Medicine . . . . Michael G. Seneff, M.D.
Emergency Medicine . . . . Robert F. Shesser, M.D.
Medicine. . . . . Alan G. Wasserman, M.D.
   Cardiology . . . . Richard J. Katz, M.D.

Dermatology . . . . Gary L. Simon, M.D. (Acting)
Endocrinology . . . . Kenneth L. Becker, M.D., Ph.D.
Gastroenterology . . . . Marie Borum, M.D.
Hematology and Oncology . . . . Robert S. Siegel, M.D.
Hospitalist Medicine . . . . Kate Goodrich, M.D.
Infectious Diseases . . . . Gary L. Simon, M.D., Ph.D.
Internal Medicine . . . . Ryan Bosch, M.D. (Interim)
Occupational and Environmental Medicine . . . . Tee Guidotti, M.D.
Pulmonary Diseases and Allergy . . . . Guillermo Gutierrez, M.D., Ph.D.
Renal Diseases . . . . Susie Q. Lew, M.D.
Rheumatology . . . . James Katz, M.D.
Neurological Surgery . . . . Anthony Caputy, M.D.
Neurology . . . . John J. Kelly, M.D.
Obstetrics and Gynecology . . . . John W. Larsen, M.D.
Ophthalmology . . . . Craig E. Geist, M.D.
Orthopaedic Surgery . . . . Robert N. Neviaser, M.D.
Pediatrics . . . . Mark L. Batshaw, M.D.
Adolescent Medicine . . . . Lawrence D'Angelo, M.D.
Allergy, Pulmonary, and Sleep Medicine . . . . Glenna Winnie, M.D.
Anesthesiology . . . . Raafat Hannallah, M.D.
Cardiology . . . . Gerard Martin, M.D.
Cardiovascular Surgery . . . . Richard Jonas, M.D.
Critical Care Medicine . . . . David Wessel, M.D.
Dermatology . . . . Roselyn Epps, M.D.
Diagnostic Imaging and Radiology . . . . Raymond Sze, M.D.
Emergency Medicine . . . . Jim Chamberlain, M.D.
Endocrinology . . . . Paul Kaplowitz, M.D.
Gastroenterology . . . . Benny Kerzner, M.D.
General and Community Pediatrics . . . . Denice Cora-Bramble, M.D.
Hearing and Speech . . . . Sheela Stuart, Ph.D.
Hematology and Oncology . . . . Max Coppes, M.D.
Infectious Disease . . . . Nalini Singh, M.D.
Laboratory Medicine . . . . Naomi Luban, M.D.
Medical Genetics and Metabolism . . . . Cynthia Tifft, M.D.
Neonatology . . . . Billie Lou Short, M.D.
Nephrology . . . . Kanwal Kher, M.D.
Neurology . . . . Roger Packer, M.D.
Neurosurgery . . . . Robert Keating, M.D.
Ophthalmology . . . . Mohamad Jaafar, M.D.
Orthopedics . . . . Laurel Blakemore, M.D.
Otolaryngology . . . . George Zalzal, M.D.
Pathology . . . . Ronald Przygodzsky, M.D.
Pediatric Dentistry . . . . Anupana Pate, D.M.D.
Pediatric Surgery . . . . Anthony Sandler, M.D.
Physical Medicine and Rehabilitation . . . . Sally Evans, M.D.
Psychiatry . . . . Paramjit Joshi, M.D.
Urology . . . . H. Gil Rushton, M.D.
Psychiatry and Behavioral Sciences . . . . Jeffrey S. Akman, M.D.
Radiology . . . . Robert K. Zeman, M.D.
Breast Imaging and Intervention . . . . Rachel F. Brem, M.D.
Diagnostic Radiology . . . . Robert K. Zeman, M.D.
Nuclear Medicine . . . . Esma A. Akin, M.D.
Radiation Oncology and Biophysics . . . . Howard Griffith, Ph.D.
Surgery . . . . Joseph M. Giordano, M.D.
Breast Care Center . . . . Christine B. Teal, M.D.
Colon and Rectal . . . . Bruce A. Orkin, M.D.
General . . . . Paul Lin, M.D.
Otolaryngology . . . . Steven Bielamowicz, M.D.
Plastic . . . . Michael Olding, M.D.
Vascular . . . . Subodh Arora, M.D.
Urology . . . . Thomas Jarrett, M.D.

Georgetown University School of Medicine

3900 Reservoir Road, N.W.
Washington, D.C. 20007
202-687-3922 (dean's office); 687-2792 (fax); 697-5055 (general information)
Web site: http://som.georgetown.edu/

Georgetown University was founded in 1789, and its school of medicine was established in 1851. The school of medicine is part of the Georgetown University Medical Center and is one of four operational units, including the school of nursing and health studies, the Lombardi Comprehensive Cancer Center, and the Biomedical Practice Network, its General Clinical Research Center (one of 37 in the country) and the Integrated Clinical Research Facility are all managed through a partnership with MedStar Health, a not-for-profit organization of seven hospitals in the Baltimore-Washington region. In 2004, the school of medicine opened its Integrated Learning Center, which supports the school of medicine's emphasis on a patient-centered, competence-based curriculum and provides the latest methods of clinical teaching and evaluation. In 2007, medical center research and teaching projects brought in $200 million in sponsored research funding.

Type: private
2008-2009 total enrollment: 725
Clinical facilities: Georgetown University Hospital, Virginia Hospital Center-Arlington, Washington Hospital Center, Fairfax Hospital, Veterans Administration Hospital, Walter Reed Army Medical Center, Providence Hospital, Naval Hospital (Bethesda, Maryland).

University Officials

President. . . . . John J. DeGioia, Ph.D.
Executive Vice President for Health Sciences,
    Director of the Medical Center, and Executive
    Dean . . . . Howard J. Federoff, M.D., Ph.D.

Medical School Administrative Staff

Dean for Medical Education. . . . . Stephen Ray Mitchell, M.D.
Associate Dean for Medical Education and
    Medical Director of Georgetown University
    Hospital . . . . Richard L. Goldberg, M.D.
Associate Vice President Regulatory Affairs . . . . Sheila Zimmet, J.D.
Senior Associate Dean for Faculty Affairs . . . . Herbert Herscowitz, Ph.D.
Senior Associate Dean for Students . . . . Princy Kumar, M.D.
Associate Dean for Educational Planning . . . . F. Daniel Davis, Ph.D. (sabbatical)
Associate Dean for Curriculum. . . . . Shyrl Sistrunk, M.D.
Assistant Dean for Clinical Curriculum . . . . John R. Siberski, M.D., S.J.
Associate Dean for Students and Special Programs . . . . Joy Williams
Associate Dean for Admissions and Student Services . . . . Russell Wall, M.D.
Associate Dean for Graduate Education . . . . Ronald Cihlar, Ph.D.
Assistant Dean of Admissions . . . . Brandon C. Schneider
Assistant Dean of Financial Planning . . . . David Pollock
Assistant Dean of Knowledge Management and Librarian . . . . Jett McCann
Senior Associate Dean for Resource Management and Registrar . . . . Jeanne V. Walther
Associate Dean for International Programs . . . . Irma Frank, D.D.S.
Assistant Dean for Medical Education, INOVA Fairfax. . . . . Craig Cheifetz, M.D.
Assistant Dean for Medical Education, VA
    Hospital Center, Arlington . . . . Robert Holman, M.D.
Assistant Dean for Medical Education, Washington Hospital Center. . . . . . . Deborah Topol, M.D.

Department and Division or Section Chairs

Basic Sciences

Biostatistics, Bioinformatics, and Biomathematics . . . . Françoise Seillier-Moiselwitsch, Ph.D.
Biochemistry and Molecular and Cell Biology. . . . . Elliott Crooke, Ph.D.
Clinical Pathology . . . . Norio Azumi, M.D.
Microbiology and Immunology. . . . . Richard A. Calderone, Ph.D. (Interim)

Neuroscience.. Barbara M. Bayer, Ph.D.
Oncology... Louis M. Weiner, M.D.
Pathology .... Richard Schlegel, M.D., Ph.D. (Acting)
Pharmacology .... Kenneth L. Dretchen, Ph.D.
Physiology and Biophysics .... Zofia Zukowska, M.D., Ph.D.

Clinical Sciences

Anesthesia... Young D. Kim, M.D.
Emergency Medicine .... Mark Smith, M.D.
Family Medicine .... James C. Welsh, M.D. (Interim)
Medicine.. Peter G. Shields, M.D. (Interim)
    Cardiology... David L. Pearle, M.D.
    Dermatology .... Kevin P. Hogan, M.D.
    Endocrinology and Metabolic Diseases .... Joseph Verbalis, M.D.
    Gastroenterology .... Stanley B. Benjamin, M.D.
    Hematology and Oncology.............................. John L. Marshall, M.D.
    Infectious Diseases .... Princy Kumar, M.D.
    Internal Medicine................................... Dennis R. Murphy, M.D.
    Lombardi Cancer Center .... Louis M. Weiner, M.D.
    Nephrology .... Christopher S. Wilcox, M.D., Ph.D.
    Pulmonary Disease .... Anne O'Donnell, M.D.
    Rheumatology, Immunology, and Allergy .... Thomas R. Cupps, M.D.
Neurology.. Edward Healton, M.D.
Neurosurgery.. Kevin McGrail, M.D.
Obstetrics and Gynecology............................. Helain Dicker Landy, M.D.
Ophthalmology .... Howard P. Cupples, M.D.
Orthopedics .... Sam W. Wiesel, M.D.
Otolaryngology and Head and Neck Surgery................... Bruce Davidson, M.D.
Pediatrics .... David B. Nelson, M.D.
Physical Medicine and Rehabilitation .... Edward B. Healton, M.D.
Psychiatry .... Steven A. Epstein, M.D.
Radiation Medicine .... Anatoly Dritschilo, M.D.
Radiology .... James B. Spies, M.D.
    Nuclear Medicine................................... Giuseppe Esposito, M.D.
Surgery... Steven R. T. Evans, M.D.
    Thoracic Surgery .... Blair Marshall, M.D.
Plastic Surgery.. Scott Spear, M.D.
    Transplantation and Hepatobiliary Surgery .... Lynt B. Johnson, M.D.
Urology... John H. Lynch, M.D.

Howard University College of Medicine

520 W Street, N.W.
Washington, D.C. 20059
202-806-6270 (dean's office); 806-7934 (fax)
Web site: http://medicine.howard.edu

The college of medicine had its beginning as the medical department of Howard University when it was chartered by the Congress of the United States on March 2, 1867. Instruction in the department began on November 9, 1868. In 1882, instruction in dentistry and pharmacy was sufficiently formalized to warrant the division of the medical department into the medical, dental, and pharmaceutical colleges. The name of the department was changed to the school of medicine in 1907, and its component parts were named the college of medicine, college of dentistry, and college of pharmacy. The colleges of medicine and dentistry are now autonomous units within the Howard University Center for the Health Sciences, which also encompasses the college of pharmacy, nursing, and allied health sciences, Howard University Hospital, the Louis Stokes Health Sciences Library, and the student health center.

Type: private
2008-2009 total enrollment: 485
Clinical facilities: Howard University Hospital, Inova Fairfax Hospital, Providence Hospital, St. Elizabeth's Hospital, Washington Veterans Affairs Medical Center, Prince George's Hospital Center, Washington Hospital Center, Children's National Medical Center.

University Officials

President. . . . . Sidney A. Ribeau, Ph.D.
Provost and Chief Academic Officer. . . . . Vacant
Senior Vice President for External Affairs and Strategic Planning . . . . . Hassan Minor, Jr., Ph.D.
Senior Vice President for Health Sciences. . . . . Donald E. Wilson, M.D.
Associate Senior Vice President for Health
   Sciences and Director of Graduate Medical
   Education . . . . Robin C. Newton, M.D.
Assistant Vice President for Health Sciences . . . . Celia J. Maxwell, M.D.
Senior Vice President and Secretary of the University . . . . Artis G. Hampshire-Cowan
Senior Vice President and Chief Financial Officer. . . . . Sidney H. Evans, Jr.
General Counsel . . . . Norma B. Leftwich
Vice President for Research and Compliance . . . . Oliver G. McGee III, Ph.D.
Vice Provost for Student Affairs . . . . Franklin D. Chambers, Ph.D.
Vice President for University Advancement. . . . . Virgil E. Ecton
Director, Student Health Center. . . . . Lynette E. Mundey, M.D.
Chief Executive Officer, Howard University Hospital. Larry Warren
Director, Louis Stokes Health Sciences Library . . . . Ellis B. Beteck, Ph.D. (Interim)

Medical School Administrative Staff

Dean. . . . . Robert E. Taylor, M.D., Ph.D.
Associate Dean for Academic Affairs. . . . . Sheik N. Hassan, M.D.
Associate Dean for Administration and Planning. . . . . Sterling M. Lloyd, Jr.
Associate Dean for Clinical Affairs and Chief
   Medical Officer, Howard University Hospital . . . . Thomas E. Gaiter, M.D.
Associate Dean for Research. . . . . Warren K. Ashe, Ph.D. (Acting)
Associate Dean for Student Affairs and Admissions . . . . Dawn L. Cannon, M.D.
Assistant Dean for Medical Education. . . . . Walter P. Bland, M.D.
Director, Curriculum Office. . . . . Scott M. Satterlund, Ph.D.
Director of Development . . . . Karine A. Sewell
Director, Veterinary Services . . . . Doris E. Hughes, D.V.M.
Budget Officer. . . . . Clarence W. Matthews
Director, Office of Continuing Medical Education . . . . Debra White-Coleman, M.D.
Financial Aid Manager. . . . . Rozanna J. Aitcheson
Director, Office of Public Relations . . . . Audrey L. Vaughan
Director of Admissions. . . . . Judith M. Walk

Howard University College of Medicine: DISTRICT OF COLUMBIA

Department and Division or Section Chairs

Basic Sciences

Anatomy . . . . James H. Baker, Ph.D.
Biochemistry and Molecular Biology . . . . Matthew George, Jr., Ph.D.
Microbiology . . . . Agnes A. Day, Ph.D.
Pathology . . . . Edward L. Lee, M.D.
Pharmacology . . . . Yousef Tizabi, Ph.D. (Interim)
Physiology and Biophysics . . . . Werner M. Graf, M.D., Ph.D.

Clinical Sciences

Anesthesiology . . . . Baffour K. Osei, M.D. (Interim)
Cancer Center . . . . Lucile L. Adams-Campbell, Ph.D.
Community and Family Medicine . . . . Charles P. Mouton, M.D.
Dermatology . . . . Rebat M. Halder, M.D.
Medicine . . . . Duane T. Smoot, M.D.
   Allergy/Immunology . . . . Elena R. G. Reece, M.D.
   Cardiology . . . . Steven N. Singh, M.D.
   Clinical Pharmacology . . . . Clifford L. Ferguson, M.D.
   Critical Care and Medical Intensive Care Unit . . . . R. George Adams, M.D.
   Endocrinology . . . . Gail L. Nunlee-Bland, M.D.
   Gastroenterology . . . . Duane T. Smoot, M.D.
   General Internal Medicine . . . . Shelly R. McDonald-Pinkett, M.D.
   Geriatrics . . . . Thomas O. Obesisan, M.D.
   Hematology and Medical Oncology . . . . Victor R. Gordeuk, M.D.
   Infectious Diseases . . . . Vinod R. Mody, M.D.
   Nephrology . . . . Vacant
   Pulmonary Diseases . . . . Alvin V. Thomas, Jr., M.D.
   Rheumatology . . . . Gail S. Kerr, M.D.
Neurology . . . . Annapurni Jayam-Trouth, M.D.
Obstetrics and Gynecology . . . . Kerry M. Lewis, M.D. (Interim)
Ophthalmology . . . . Robert A. Copeland, Jr., M.D.
Orthopaedic Surgery . . . . Terry L. Thompson, M.D.
Pediatrics and Child Health . . . . Michal A. Young, M.D. (Interim)
   Adolescent Medicine . . . . Esther E. Forrester, M.D.
   Allergy and Immunology . . . . Elena R. G. Reece, M.D.
   Ambulatory Pediatrics . . . . Habiballah Shariat, M.D.
   Cardiology . . . . Vacant
   Child Development . . . . Vacant
   Endocrinology . . . . Gail L. Nunlee-Bland, M.D.
   Genetics . . . . Robert F. Murray, Jr., M.D.
   Hematology . . . . Sohail R. Rana, M.D.
   Neonatology . . . . Michal A. Young, M.D.
Physical Medicine and Rehabilitation . . . . Janaki Kalyanam, M.D.
Psychiatry and Behavioral Sciences . . . . William B. Lawson, M.D, Ph.D.
Radiation Oncology . . . . Vacant
Radiology . . . . Roma V. Gumbs, M.D. (Interim)
Sickle Cell Disease Center . . . . Victor R. Gordeuk, M.D.
Surgery . . . . Edward E. Cornwell III, M.D.
   Critical Care . . . . Suryanarayana M. Siram, M.D.
   General Surgery . . . . Wayne A.I. Frederick, M.D.
   Neurosurgery . . . . Vacant
   Otolaryngology . . . . Ernest M. Myers, M.D.
   Plastic and Reconstructive Surgery . . . . Henry Paul, M.D.
   Thoracic and Cardiovascular . . . . Vacant
   Transplant . . . . Clive O. Callender, M.D.
   Urology . . . . Chiledum A. Ahaghotu, M.D.
   Podiatry . . . . Kirk Geter, D.P.M.

Florida State University College of Medicine

1115 West Call Street
Tallahassee, Florida 32306-4300
850-644-1855 (general information); 644-1346 (dean's office); 645-1420 (fax)
E-mail: medinformation@med.fsu.edu
Web site: www.med.fsu.edu

The first new allopathic medical school in over 20 years, the Florida State University (FSU) College of Medicine was established in June 2000 by the Florida legislature for the purpose of training physicians, with special emphasis on the needs of rural, underserved, minority, and elderly populations. The college's educational program uses cutting-edge information technology and focuses on producing compassionate physicians who will practice patient-centered medicine in a rapidly changing health care environment. As a community-based medical school, the FSU College of Medicine partners with existing community medical facilities and practitioners throughout the state rather than operating a teaching hospital. Students have the opportunity to learn on the front lines of the health care delivery system. Community campuses have been developed in Daytona Beach, Fort Pierce, Tallahassee, Pensacola, Orlando, and Sarasota. The college of medicine occupies a newly constructed, state-of-the-art building that houses student communities, classrooms, auditoria, research labs, a simulated clinic, and administrative and faculty offices.

Type: public
2008-2009 total enrollment: 358
Clinical facilities: Act Corp., Daytona Beach; Apalachee Center, Inc., Tallahassee; Baptist Health Care, Pensacola; Bayfront Medical Center, St. Petersburg; Big Bend Hospice, Tallahassee; Bond Community Health Center, Inc., Tallahassee; Capital Health Plan, Tallahassee; Capital Regional Medical Center, Tallahassee; Cleveland Clinic Florida, Weston; Collier Health Services, Inc., Immokalee; Doctors Hospital of Sarasota, Sarasota; Doctors' Memorial Hospital, Perry; Florida Community Health Center, Inc., Fort Pierce; Florida Department of Health, Children's Medical Services, Fort Pierce; Florida Health Care Plans, Inc., Holly Hill; Florida Hospital DeLand, DeLand; Florida Hospital, Orlando; Florida Hospital Ormond Memorial, Ormond Beach; Florida State Hospital, Chattahoochee; Fort Walton Beach Medical Center, Fort Walton; Grove Place Surgery Center, Vero Beach; GulfCoast Surgery Center, Inc., Sarasota; Halifax Medical Center, Daytona Beach; HealthSouth Physicians' Surgical Care Center, Winter Park; HealthSouth Corp., Tallahassee; HealthSouth Treasure Coast Rehabilitation Hospital, Vero Beach; Indian River Memorial Hospital, Vero Beach; Jackson Hospital, Marianna; Lakeview Center, Inc., Pensacola; Lawnwood Regional Medical Center, Fort Pierce; Martin Memorial Health Systems, Stuart; Mayo Clinic, Jacksonville; Morton Plant Hospital, Clearwater; Naval Hospital of Pensacola, Pensacola; Neighborhood Health Services, Tallahassee; Nemours Children's Clinic, Orlando; Nemours Children's Clinic, Pensacola; Orlando Health, Orlando; Raulerson Hospital, Okeechobee; Sacred Heart Health System, Pensacola; Santa Rosa Medical Center, Milton; Sarasota County Health Department, Sarasota; Sarasota Memorial Healthcare System, Sarasota; St. Lucie Medical Center, Port St. Lucie; St. Lucie Surgery Center, Port St. Lucie; St. Vincent's Medical Center, Inc., Jacksonville; Surgery Center of Fort Pierce, Fort Pierce; Surgery Center of Volusia County, Daytona Beach; Surgical Center of the Treasure Coast, Port St. Lucie; Tallahassee Memorial Healthcare, Tallahassee; Tallahassee Outpatient Surgery Center, Tallahassee; Tallahassee Single Day Surgery, Tallahassee; Tallahassee VA Clinic, Tallahassee; Twin Lakes Surgical Center, Daytona Beach; Venice Regional Medical Center, Venice; West Florida Hospital, Pensacola; Westminster Oaks, Tallahassee. Archbold Medical Center, Thomasville, Georgia.

University Officials

President, Florida State University . . . . T.K. Wetherell, Ph.D.
Provost . . . . Lawrence G. Abele, Ph.D.
Senior Vice President for Finance and Administration. . . . . John R. Carnaghi
Vice President for Research . . . . Kirby Kemper, Ph.D.

College of Medicine Administrative Staff

Dean. . . . . John P. Fogarty, M.D.
Senior Associate Dean for Academic Affairs . . . . Alma Littles, M.D.
Associate Dean for Student Affairs, Admissions,
   and Outreach . . . . Elena Reyes, Ph.D. (Interim)
Associate Dean for Research and Graduate Programs . . . . Myra Hurt, Ph.D.
Associate Dean for Health Affairs . . . . Robert G. Brooks, M.D.

Florida State University College of Medicine: FLORIDA

Associate Dean for Curriculum and Evaluation . . . . Lynn Romrell, Ph.D.
Associate Dean for Medical Education . . . . Sebastian Alston, M.D.
Assistant Dean for Admissions . . . . Graham Patrick, Ph.D.
Assistant Dean for Faculty Development . . . . Dennis Baker, Ph.D.
Assistant Dean for Diversity and Outreach . . . . Eugene Trowers, M.D.
Assistant Dean, Daytona Beach . . . . Luckey Dunn, M.D.
Assistant Dean, Fort Pierce . . . . Randall Bertolette, M.D.
Assistant Dean, Orlando Campus . . . . Michael Muszynski, M.D.
Assistant Dean, Pensacola Campus . . . . Paul McLeod, M.D.
Assistant Dean, Sarasota Campus . . . . Bruce Berg, M.D.
Assistant Dean, Tallahassee Campus . . . . Mel Hartsfield, M.D.

Department Chairs

Biomedical Sciences . . . . David Balkwill, Ph.D.
Clinical Sciences . . . . Eugene Ryerson, M.D.
Family Medicine and Rural Health . . . . Daniel Van Durme, M.D.
Geriatrics . . . . Kenneth Brummel-Smith, M.D.
Medical Humanities and Social Sciences . . . . Suzanne Bennett Johnson, Ph.D.

University of Florida College of Medicine

Box 100215, JHMHC
Gainesville, Florida 32610-0215
352-273-7500 (dean's office); 846-3299 (fax)
Web site: www.med.ufl.edu

The college of medicine accepted its first class in September 1956. It is an integral part of the University of Florida and is located on the university campus. The medical school is part of the J. Hillis Miller Health Center.

Type: public
2008-2009 total enrollment: 525
Clinical facilities: Shands at the University of Florida, Shands at Alachua General Hospital, Malcom Randall Veterans Affairs Medical Center, Shands Jacksonville.

University Officials

President. . . . . J. Bernard Machen, D.D.S., Ph.D.
Provost . . . . Joseph Glover, Ph.D.
Senior Vice President for Health Affairs . . . . Douglas J. Barrett, M.D.

Medical School Administrative Staff

Dean. . . . . Michael L. Good, M.D. (Interim)
Senior Associate Dean for Clinical Affairs . . . . TBA
Senior Associate Dean for Educational Affairs. . . . . Kyle E. Rarey, Ph.D. (Interim)
Senior Associate Dean for Faculty Group Practice . . . . Jane T. Schumaker
Dean, Regional Campus in Jacksonville. . . . . Robert C. Nuss, M.D.
Senior Associate Dean for Research Affairs . . . . M. Peter Pevonka, R.Ph.
Director, Research Development . . . . Elaine Young, Ph.D. (Interim)
Associate Dean for Administrative Affairs . . . . Tom V. Harris
Associate Dean for Student and Alumni Affairs. . . . . W. Patrick Duff, M.D.
Associate Dean for Continuing Medical Education . . . . Marvin A. Dewar, M.D.
Associate Dean for Clinical Research & Training. . . . . Peter W. Stacpoole, M.D., Ph.D.
Associate Dean for Graduate Education . . . . Wayne T. McCormack, Ph.D.
Associate Dean for Information Technology . . . . Richard J. Rathe, M.D.
Associate Dean for Education. . . . . Maureen A. Novak, M.D.
Associate Dean for Graduate Medical Education . . . . Timothy C. Flynn, M.D.
Associate Dean for VA Medical Center Relations. . . . . Bradley S. Bender, M.D.
Associate Dean for Financial Services . . . . W. Wayne Tharp
Assistant Dean for Minority Relations . . . . Donna M. Parker, M.D.
Assistant Dean for Minority Relations . . . . Kendall Campbell, M.D.
Assistant Dean for Program Evaluation and Development . . . . Kyle E. Rarey, Ph.D.
Chairman, Medical Selection Committee . . . . Ira H. Gessner, M.D.
Vivarium Director . . . . August H. Battles, D.V.M., Ph.D.
Librarian. . . . . W. Wallace McLendon, M.S.L.S.
Deputy Registrar . . . . Amy Jaworski

Department and Division or Section Chairs

Basic Sciences

Anatomy and Cell Biology . . . . Stephen P. Sugrue, Ph.D.
Biochemistry and Molecular Biology. . . . . James B. Flanegan, Ph.D.
Health Policy and Epidemiology. . . . . Elizabeth Shenkman, Ph.D.
Molecular Genetics and Microbiology. . . . . Henry V. Baker II, Ph.D. (Interim)
Neuroscience. . . . . David R. Borchelt, Ph.D. (Interim)
Pharmacology and Therapeutics. . . . . Stephen P. Baker, Ph.D.
Physiology and Functional Genomics . . . . Charles E. Wood, Ph.D.

Clinical Sciences

Aging and Geriatric Research.................................. Marco Pahor, M.D.
Anesthesiology.. F. Kayser Enneking, M.D.
Community Health and Family Medicine .... R. Whit Curry, Jr., M.D.
Emergency Medicine.................................. Joseph Adrian Tyndall, M.D.
Medicine.. Edward R. Block, M.D.
    Cardiology................................... Jamie B. Conti, M.D. (Interim)
    Dermatology .... Franklin P. Flowers, M.D.
    Endocrinology and Metabolism..................... A. Laurence Kennedy, M.D.
    Gastroenterology, Hepatology, and Nutrition.............. Christopher E. Forsmark, M.D.
    Hematology and Oncology................................ Carmen J. Allegra, M.D.
    Infectious Diseases .... Frederick S. Southwick, M.D.
    Internal Medicine... Aida Vega, M.D.
    Nephrology .... Richard J. Johnson, M.D.
    Physician Assistant Program .... Wayne D. Bottom
    Pulmonary Diseases .... Veena B. Antony, M.D.
    Rheumatology and Clinical Immunology....................... Westley H. Reeves, M.D.
Neurological Surgery....................................... William A. Friedman, M.D.
Neurology.. Edward Valenstein, M.D.
Obstetrics and Gynecology......................... R. Stan Williams, M.D. (Interim)
Ophthalmology... William T. Driebe, M.D.
Orthopaedic Surgery.................................... Peter F. Gearen, M.D.
Otolaryngology .... Patrick J. Antonelli, M.D.
Pathology, Immunology, and Laboratory Medicine .... James M. Crawford, M.D., Ph.D.
    Clinical Pathology .... Kenneth M. Rand, M.D.
Pediatrics .... Richard L. Bucciarelli, M.D.
    Cardiology.................................... Frederick J. Fricker, M.D.
    Cellular and Molecular Therapy .... Arun Srivastava, Ph.D.
    Critical Care................................. Tara Smith, M.D. (Interim)
    Endocrinology .... Janet H. Silverstein, M.D.
    Gastroenterology .... Christopher D. Jolley, M.D.
    General Pediatrics .... John A. Nackashi, M.D.
    Genetics..................................... Roberto T. Zori, M.D.
    Hematology and Oncology.................... William B. Slayton, M.D. (Interim)
    Immunology and Infectious Diseases...................... Melissa E. Elder, M.D.
    Neonatology.................................. David J. Burchfield, M.D.
    Nephrology .... Vikas R. Dharnidharka, M.D.
    Neurology .... Paul R. Carney, M.D.
    Pulmonary Diseases and Cystic Fibrosis .... Sarah E. Chesrown, M.D. (Interim)
Psychiatry .... Mark S. Gold, M.D.
    Child and Adolescent Psychiatry...................... Regina Bussing, M.D. (Interim)
Radiation Oncology.................................... Robert Amdur, M.D. (Interim)
Radiology .... Anthony A. Mancuso, M.D.
Surgery................. Kevin Behrns, M.D. (Interim), and Matt Nguyen, M.D. (Interim)
    Burn and Trauma .... David W. Mozingo, M.D.
    General .... Kevin Behrns, M.D.
    Pediatric .... David Kays, M.D.
    Plastic and Reconstructive.......................... Brent Seagle, M.D.
    Surgical Oncology .... Steven Hochwald, M.D.
    Thoracic and Cardiovascular........................ Curtis G. Tribble, M.D.
    Transplantation .... Alan Hemming, M.D.
    Vascular...................................... James M. Seeger, M.D.
Urology.. Johannes Vieweg, M.D.

University of Miami Miller School of Medicine

1600 N.W. 10th Avenue
P.O. Box 016099 (R699)
Miami, Florida 33101
305-243-6545 (dean's office); 243-4888 (fax)
E-mail: pgoldschmidt@med.miami.edu
Web site: www.miami.edu

The University of Miami School of Medicine was founded in 1952 and is located in the University of Miami-Jackson Memorial Hospital Medical Center, approximately eight miles from the University of Miami Coral Gables campus. The Rosenstiel Medical Sciences Building, which serves as the center of the school's educational activities, opened in 1969.

Type: private
2008-2009 total enrollment: 606
Clinical facilities: Anne Bates Leach Eye Hospital/Bascom Palmer Eye Institute/Jackson Memorial Hospital, Mailman Center for Child Development, University of Miami Hospital and Clinics/ Sylvester Comprehensive Cancer Center, William L. McKnight Vision Research Center, Mount Sinai Hospital, Veterans Administration Medical Center, Gautier Medical Science Building, Papanicolaou Cancer Research Building, General Clinical Research Center, Diabetes Research Institute, University of Miami Hospital.

University Officials

President. . . . . Donna E. Shalala, Ph.D.
Provost and Executive Vice President . . . . Thomas Leblanc, Ph.D.
Senior Vice President for Business and Finance . . . . Joe Natoli
Senior Vice President for Medical Affairs . . . . Pascal J. Goldschmidt, M.D.
Vice President for Governmental Relations. . . . . Rudy Fernandez
Vice President and General Counsel. . . . . Aileen M. Ugalde, J.D.
Vice President for Student Affairs. . . . . Patricia A. Whitley, Ph.D.
Vice President for Development. . . . . Sergio Gonzalez
Vice President for Medical Administration and
    Chief Operating and Strategy Officer . . . . William Donelan
Assistant Vice President for Business Services . . . . Alan Fish
Vice President and Treasurer. . . . . Diane M. Cook
Senior Executive Advisor to the Senior Vice
    President for Medical Affairs and Dean . . . . Bart Chernow, M.D.
Executive Dean for Clinical Affairs. . . . . William O'Neill, M.D.
Executive Dean for Education and Policy . . . . Laurence B. Gardner, M.D.
Executive Dean for Research and Research Training. . . . . Richard J. Bookman, Ph.D.
Executive Dean of Clinical Affairs at FAU. . . . . Steven Falcone, M.D.
Regional Dean, University of Miami Miller
    School of Medicine at FAU . . . . Michael Friedland, M.D.
Secretary of the University . . . . Aileen M. Ugalde, J.D.
Controller . . . . Aida Diaz-Piedra

Medical School Administrative Staff

Senior Vice President for Medical Affairs and Dean . . . . Pascal J. Goldschmidt, M.D.
Associate Vice President for Medical Affairs and
    Medical Director . . . . Alan S. Livingstone, M.D., and Leo B. Twiggs, M.D.
Associate Vice President for Medical Affairs and
    Managing Director of Group Practice . . . . TBA
Associate Vice President and Director for Hospital Operations . . . . Michelle Chulick
Associate Vice President for Financial Affairs . . . . Thomas Fitzpatrick
Associate Vice President for Human Resources. . . . . Paul C. Hudgins
Associate Vice President for Medical Communications . . . . Christine Morris
Associate Vice President for Medical Development and Alumni Relations . . . . Marsha Kegley
Assistant Vice President for Health Program Development . . . . Richard Iacino
Senior Associate Dean for Clinical Affairs. . . . . Gerard A. Kaiser, M.D.
Senior Associate Dean for Faculty Affairs . . . . Richard Thurer, M.D.
Associate Dean for Faculty Diversity and Development . . . . Sheri Keitz, M.D., Ph.D.
Senior Associate Dean for Medical Education . . . . Mark O'Connell, M.D.
Senior Associate Dean for Medical Student Administration . . . . Robert Hernandez, M.D.

Senior Associate Dean for Graduate Medical Education . . . . Jeanette Mladenovic, M.D.
Associate Regional Dean for Medical Education
at University of Miami FAU . . . . Daniel Lichtstein, M.D.
Senior Associate Dean for Quality, Safety, and Risk Prevention . . . . David Lubarsky, M.D.
Associate Executive Dean for Pediatric Health . . . . Steven E. Lipshultz, M.D.
Associate Dean for Research. . . . . Camillo Ricordi, M.D.
Associate Dean for Graduate Studies . . . . John Bixby, Ph.D.
Associate Dean for Medical Admissions. . . . . Richard S. Weisman, Pharm.D.
Associate Dean for Undergraduate Medical Education . . . . Alex J. Mechaber, M.D.
Associate Dean for Community Affairs . . . . Arthur M. Fournier, M.D.
Associate Dean for Minority Affairs. . . . . Ana Campo, M.D. (Interim)

Department and Division or Section Chairs

Basic Sciences

Anatomy and Cell Biology . . . . Robert H. Warren, Ph.D. (Interim)
Biochemistry and Molecular Biology. Louis J. Elsas II, M.D. (Interim)
Microbiology and Immunology. . . . . Eckhard Podack, Ph.D.
Molecular and Cellular Pharmacology . . . . Charles W. Luetje, Ph.D. (Interim)
Pathology . . . . Mehrdad Nadji, M.D. (Interim)
Physiology and Biophysics . . . . Karl L. Magleby, Ph.D.

Clinical Sciences

Anesthesiology. . . . . David A. Lubarsky, M.D.
Dermatology and Cutaneous Surgery . . . . Lawrence Schachner, M.D.
Epidemiology and Public Health . . . . José Szapocznik, Ph.D.
Family Medicine . . . . E. Robert Schwartz, M.D.
Medicine. . . . . Marc Lippman, M.D.
    Arthritis. . . . . Robert Hoffman, M.D.
    Cardiology . . . . Joshua Hare, M.D.
    Endocrinology, Diabetes, and Metabolism . . . . Anthony Bianco, M.D.
    Gastroenterology . . . . Maria T. Abreu, M.D.
    General Medicine. . . . . Marco L. Gonzalez, M.D.
    Genetic Medicine. . . . . Karl H. Muench, M.D.
    Gerontology and Geriatrics. . . . . Bernard Roos, M.D.
    Hematology and Oncology. . . . . Joseph Rosenblatt, M.D.
    Hepatology . . . . Paul Martin, M.D.
    Infectious Disease. . . . . Gordon Dickinson, Jr., M.D.
    Nephrology . . . . Jochen Reiser, M.D.
    Pulmonary Diseases . . . . Matthias Salathe, M.D.
Neurological Surgery. . . . . Barth A. Green, M.D.
Neurology. . . . . Ralph Sacco, M.D.
Obstetrics and Gynecology. . . . . Leo B. Twiggs, M.D.
Ophthalmology . . . . Eduardo Alfonso, M.D. (Interim)
Orthopaedics and Rehabilitation . . . . Frank J. Eismont, M.D.
Otolaryngology . . . . Thomas J. Balkany, M.D.
Pediatrics . . . . Steven Lipshultz, M.D.
Physical Therapy . . . . Sherrill H. Hayes, Ph.D.
Psychiatry . . . . Ewald Horwath, M.D.
Radiation Oncology. . . . . Alan Pollack, M.D., Ph.D., and Arnold M. Markoe, M.D.
Radiology . . . . Robert Quencer, M.D.
Rehabilitation Medicine. . . . . Diana Cardenas, M.D.
Surgery . . . . Alan S. Livingstone, M.D.
    Oncology. . . . . Alan S. Livingstone, M.D.
    Oral. . . . . Robert E. Marx, D.D.S.
    Pediatric . . . . Raleigh Thompson, M.D.
    Plastic . . . . Seth Thaller, M.D.
    Thoracic and Cardiovascular. . . . . Thomas Salerno, M.D.
    Kidney and Pancreas Transplantation . . . . George Burke, M.D.
    Liver and G.I. Transplantation . . . . Andreas Tzakis, M.D.
    Trauma . . . . Mark G. McKenney, M.D.
Urology. . . . . Mark Soloway, M.D.

University of South Florida College of Medicine

12901 Bruce B. Downs Boulevard
MDC 2
Tampa, Florida 33612-4742
813-974-2196 (USF Health/dean's office); 974-3886 (fax)
Web site: http://health.usf.edu/medicine/home.html

The college of medicine was open for the instruction of students in 1971. It is an integral part of the University of South Florida (USF) and is located on the campus. The medical school is part of USF Health.

Type: public
2008-2009 total enrollment: 480
Clinical facilities: USF Health South Tampa Center for Advanced Health Care, Carol and Frank Morsani Center for Advanced Health Care, USF Medical Clinic, Harbourside Medical Tower, USF Eye Institute, USF ENT Center, USF Health Orthopedic Surgery and Sports Medicine, USF Children's Medical Services, USF Health Physical Therapy Center, Suncoast Alzheimer's and Gerontology Center, Tampa General Hospital, James A. Haley Veterans Affairs Hospital, All Children's Hospital, Shriners Hospital for Children, USF Health Psychiatry Center, H. Lee Moffitt Cancer Center and Research Institute, Bay Pines Veterans Affairs Medical Center, University Community Hospital.

University Officials

President. . . . . Judy Lynn Genshaft, Ph.D.
Vice President, USF Health . . . . Stephen K. Klasko, M.D.
Chief Administrative Liaison . . . . John C. Ekarius
Senior Associate Vice President for Research . . . . Abdul S. Rao, M.B.B.S., D.Phil.
Associate Vice President for Administration, Finance, and Technology. . . . . . . Joann M. Strobbe
Associate Vice President for Clinical Affairs and
    Venture Development . . . . William G. Marshall, Jr., M.D.
Associate Vice President for Clinical Quality Improvement . . . . Michael T. Parsons, M.D.
Associate Vice President for Communications and Marketing . . . . Michael J. Hoad
Associate Vice President for Continuing
    Professional Development . . . . Deborah Sutherland, Ph.D.
Associate Vice President of Development/USF Health. Steve Blair
Associate Vice President for Faculty and Academic Affairs. . . . . John S. Curran, M.D.
Associate Vice President for Health Law, Policy, and Safety. . . . . Jay Wolfson, Dr.PH.
Associate Vice President for International Programs . . . . Ann DeBaldo, Ph.D.
Associate Vice President for Strategic
    Partnership and Governmental Affairs . . . . Phillip J. Marty, Ph.D.
Associate Vice President for Strategic Planning and Policy. . . . . Patricia C. Haynie, Ph.D.
Assistant Vice President for Budget and Policy Analysis. . . . . Karen M. Burdash
Assistant Vice President, Information
    Technology, and Chief Information Officer . . . . James McKenzie

Medical School Administrative Staff

Dean. . . . . Stephen K. Klasko, M.D.
Vice Dean, Administration, Finance, and Technology . . . . Joann M. Strobbe
Vice Dean, Clinical Affairs . . . . Robert J. Belsole, M.D.
Vice Dean, Educational Affairs. . . . . Alicia D. H. Monroe, M.D.
Vice Dean for Research, Graduate, and
    Postdoctoral Affairs . . . . Abdul S. Rao, M.B.B.S., D.Phil.
Senior Executive Associate Dean for Faculty and Academic Affairs. . . . . John S. Curran, M.D.
Associate Dean for Clinical Outreach . . . . Richard P. Hoffmann, M.D.
Associate Dean for Clinical Research . . . . Patricia J. Emmanuel, M.D.
Associate Dean for Continuing Professional Development. . . . . Deborah Sutherland, Ph.D.
Associate Dean for Diversity Initiatives . . . . Marvin T. Williams, Ph.D.
Associate Dean for Graduate Medical Education and Veterans Affairs . . . . . . Peter J. Fabri, M.D.
Associate Dean for International Affairs . . . . John Sinnott, M.D.
Associate Dean for Postdoctoral and Graduate Affairs. . . . . Michael J. Barber, D.Phil.
Associate Dean for Research. . . . . Vacant
Associate Dean for Strategic Planning and Policy . . . . Patricia C. Haynie, Ph.D.

Associate Dean for Student Affairs and Admissions . . . . Steven C. Specter, Ph.D.
Assistant Dean for Clinical Outreach . . . . Heidi M. Stephens, M.D.
Assistant Dean for Clinical Finance. . . . . Karen M. Burdash
Director of Admissions. . . . . Gretchen Koehler, Ph.D.
Director of Area Health Education Center . . . . Cynthia S. Selleck, D.S.N.
Director of Business Affairs . . . . Jean G. Nixon
Director of Compliance . . . . Patricia J. Bickel
Director of Professional Relations. . . . . Mathis L. Becker, M.D.
Executive Director of University of South Florida Physicians Group . . . . Rick Green

Department and Division or Section Chairs

Basic Sciences

Molecular Medicine. . . . . Duane C. Eichler, Ph.D. (Interim)
Molecular Pharmacology and Physiology. . . . . Bruce G. Lindsey, Ph.D.
Pathology and Cell Biology . . . . Santo V. Nicosia, M.D.

Clinical Sciences

Dermatology . . . . Neil A. Fenske, M.D.
Family Medicine . . . . H. James Brownlee, M.D.
Internal Medicine . . . . Allan L. Goldman, M.D.
  Allergy and Immunology . . . . Richard F. Lockey, M.D.
  Cardiovascular Services. . . . . Anne B. Curtis, M.D.
  Digestive Diseases and Nutrition . . . . Patrick G. Brady, M.D.
  Emergency Medicine . . . . David J. Orban, M.D.
  Endocrinology and Metabolism. . . . . Anthony D. Morrison, M.D.
  General Internal Medicine/Ambulatory. Elizabeth P. Warner, M.D.
  General Internal Medicine/Inpatient . . . . Charles M. Edwards, M.D.
  Geriatric Medicine . . . . Vincent D. Perron, M.D.
  Infectious Disease and International Medicine. . . . . John T. Sinnott, M.D.
  Ethics, Humanities, and Palliative Medicine. . . . . Robert M. Walker, M.D.
  Nephrology and Hypertension . . . . Jacques A. Durr, M.D.
  Physical Medicine and Rehabilitation . . . . Steven G. Scott, M.D.
  Prevention and Occupational Medicine. . . . . Stuart M. Brooks, M.D.
  Pulmonary, Critical Care, and Sleep Medicine. . . . . David A. Solomon, M.D.
  Rheumatology . . . . John D. Carter, M.D.
Neurology. . . . . Clifton L. Gooch, M.D.
Neurosurgery. . . . . Harry R. van Loveren, M.D.
Obstetrics-Gynecology . . . . David L. Keefe, M.D.
Oncologic Sciences . . . . Lynn C. Moscinski, M.D.
Ophthalmology . . . . Peter R. Pavan, M.D.
Orthopedics . . . . Robert A. Pedowitz, M.D., Ph.D.
SMART Program . . . . Jeff G. Konin, Ph.D.
Otolaryngology . . . . Thomas V. McCaffrey, M.D., Ph.D.
Pathology and Cell Biology . . . . Santo V. Nicosia, M.D.
Pediatrics . . . . Robert M. Nelson, Jr., M.D.
Physical Therapy, School of . . . . W. Sandy Quillen, Ph.D.
Psychiatry and Behavioral Medicine . . . . Francisco Fernandez, M.D.
Radiology . . . . Todd R. Hazelton, M.D.
Surgery . . . . Richard C. Karl, M.D.
  General/Tampa General Hospital. . . . . Vacant
  Plastic Surgery . . . . David J. Smith, Jr., M.D.
  Surgical Oncology . . . . Richard C. Karl, M.D.
  Trauma . . . . David J. Ciesla, M.D.
  Vascular. . . . . Dennis F. Bandyk, M.D.

Emory University School of Medicine

1648 Pierce Drive
Atlanta, Georgia 30322
404-727-5640 (general information); 727-5631 (dean's office); 727-0473 (fax);
727-5655 (medical educ. & stud. aff.); 727-0045 (fax)
Web site: http://med.emory.edu

The history of the school began with the chartering of Atlanta Medical College in 1854. This was the first of a series of institutions that eventually consolidated in 1913 and became the school of medicine of Emory University in 1915. Since 1917, the school has operated and developed both in the downtown area and on the main university campus in Druid Hills. The medical school is part of the Robert W. Woodruff Health Sciences Center.

Type: private
2008-2009 total enrollment: 495
Clinical facilities: Grady Memorial Hospital, Emory University Hospital, Veterans Affairs Medical Center, Wesley Woods Center of Emory University, Emory Adventist Hospital, The Emory Clinic, Children's Healthcare of Atlanta, Crawford Long Hospital of Emory University, Emory Johns Creek Hospital.

University Officials

President. . . . . James W. Wagner, Ph.D.
Executive Vice President for Health Affairs and
  Chief Executive Officer, Woodruff Health
  Sciences Center . . . . Fred Sanfilippo, M.D., Ph.D.

Medical School Administrative Staff

Dean. . . . . Thomas J. Lawley, M.D.
Executive Associate Dean of Administration and
  Faculty Affairs . . . . Claudia R. Adkison, J.D., Ph.D.
Executive Associate Dean for Medical Education and Student Affairs. . . . . . J. William Eley, M.D.
Executive Associate Dean for Research . . . . Raymond J. Dingledine, Ph.D. (Interim)
Executive Associate Dean for Clinical Affairs at Grady Hospital . . . . William J. Casarella, M.D.
Executive Associate Dean for Fiscal Affairs and
  Chief Financial Officer . . . . Barbara V. Schroeder
Associate Dean for Clinical Services, Grady Hospital . . . . William R. Sexson, M.D.
Associate Dean for Admissions . . . . Ira K. Schwartz, M.D.
Associate Dean for Graduate Medical Education . . . . James R. Zaidan, M.D.
Associate Dean for Clinical Education . . . . Joel M. Felner, M.D.
Associate Dean for Multicultural Medical Student Affairs. . . . . Robert Lee, Ph.D.
Associate Dean for Medical Education and Student Affairs . . . . J. Alan Otsuki, M.D.
Associate Dean for Faculty Development. . . . . Sharon W. Weiss, M.D.
Associate Dean for Research. . . . . Carolyn C. Meltzer, M.D.
Associate Dean for Research. . . . . Raymond J. Dingledine, Ph.D.
Associate Dean for Clinical and Translational Research. . . . . Jeff M. Sands, M.D.
Associate Dean for Administration . . . . Brenda J. Seiton, J.D.
Associate Dean for Administration . . . . Joshua Barwick, J.D.
Assistant Dean for Research . . . . Patricia Haugaard
Assistant Dean for Graduate Medical Education . . . . Marilane Bond, Ed.D.
Assistant Dean for Medical Education and Student Affairs. . . . . Sheryl L. Heron, M.D.
Assistant Dean for Postdoctoral Education . . . . Mary J. Delong, Ph.D.
Assistant Dean for Business and Finance. . . . . Sharen B. Olson
Assistant Dean for Business and Finance. . . . . Constance B. Nagle
Assistant Dean for Clinical Trials . . . . Carlton Dampier, M.D.

Department and Division or Section Chairs

Basic Sciences

Biochemistry. . . . . Richard D. Cummings, Ph.D.
Biomedical Engineering. . . . . Larry McIntire, Ph.D.
Cell Biology. . . . . Barry D. Shur, Ph.D.
Human Genetics . . . . Stephen T. Warren, Ph.D.
Microbiology and Immunology. . . . . Charles Moran, Ph.D. (Interim)
Pharmacology . . . . Raymond J. Dingledine, Ph.D.
Physiology. . . . . Douglas Eaton, Ph.D.

Clinical Sciences

Anesthesiology... James R. Zaidan, M.D.
Dermatology.................................... Robert A. Swerlick, M.D. (Interim)
Emergency Medicine............................... Katherine L. Heilpern, M.D.
Family and Preventive Medicine........................... Lawrence J. Lutz, M.D.
Gynecology and Obstetrics................................ Sarah L. Berga, M.D.
Hematology and Medical Oncology......................... Fadlo R. Khuri, M.D.
Medicine..................................... R. Wayne Alexander, M.D., Ph.D.
   Cardiology... David G. Harrison, M.D.
   Digestive Diseases........................... Vincent W. Yang, M.D., Ph.D.
   Endocrinology, Metabolism, and Lipids...................... Roberto Pacifici, M.D.
   General Medicine.............................. William T. Branch, Jr., M.D.
   Geriatric Medicine and Gerontology.................. Theodore Johnson II, M.D.
   Infectious Diseases.............................. David S. Stephens, M.D.
   Pulmonary, Allergy, and Critical Care Medicine............. Jesse Roman-Rodriguez, M.D.
   Renal... Jeff M. Sands, M.D.
   Rheumatology and Human Immunology................... Jorg Goronzy, M.D., Ph.D.
Neurology.................................... Allan J. Levey, M.D., Ph.D.
Neurosurgery..................................... Daniel L. Barrow, M.D.
Ophthalmology...................................... Timothy Olsen, M.D.
Orthopaedics................................... James R. Roberson, M.D.
   Spine Center.. Scott Boden, M.D.
Otolaryngology-Head and Neck Surgery.................. Douglas E. Mattox, M.D.
Pathology and Laboratory Medicine................ Tristram G. Parslow, M.D., Ph.D.
Pediatrics... Barbara J. Stoll, M.D.
   Cardiology.. Robert Campbell, M.D.
   Neonatology and Perinatology...................... David Carlton, M.D.
   Emergency Medicine............................... Naghma Khan, M.D.
   Endocrinology.................................... Andrew Muir, M.D.
   Gastroenterology................................. Benjamin Gold, M.D.
   General Pediatrics............. Corrine Taylor, M.D., and Frank Berkowitz, M.D.
   Hematology, Oncologyy, and BMT.................... William Woods, M.D.
   Infectious Diseases and Immunology................. Paul Spearman, M.D.
   Nephrology.................................... Larry Greenbaum, M.D.
   Neurology....................................... John Sladky, M.D.
   Pulmonology, Allergy, Cystic Fibrosis, and Sleep.......... Arlene Stecenko, M.D.
Psychiatry and Behavioral Sciences.................. Charles B. Nemeroff, M.D., Ph.D.
   Child/Adolescent Psychiatry and Forensic Psychiatry................. Peter Ash, M.D.
   Consultation-Liaison............................. Bernard Frankel, M.D.
   Geriatric Psychiatry......................... William M. McDonald, M.D.
Radiation Oncology................................. Walter Curran, M.D.
Radiology...................................... Carolyn C. Meltzer, M.D.
   Abdominal Imaging......................... William Small, M.D., Ph.D.
   Breast Imaging...................................... Carl D'Orsi, M.D.
   Cardiothoracic Imaging................... Arthur E. Stillman, M.D., Ph.D.
   Community Radiology............................. Martin Sheline, M.D.
   Emergency Radiology.................... William Torres, M.D. (Acting)
   Interventional Radiology............................. Hyun Kim, M.D.
   Musculoskeletal Imaging......................... Michael Terk, M.D.
   Neuro-interventional Radiology.................... Jacques Dion, M.D.
   Neuroradiology............................. A. Jackson Fountain, M.D.
   Nuclear Medicine................................ David Schuster, M.D.
   Pediatric Imaging........................... Stephen Simoneaux, M.D.
Rehabilitation Medicine........................... David T. Burke, M.D.
Surgery.. William C. Wood, M.D.
   CardioThoracic.................................. Robert A. Guyton, M.D.
   General... Collin J. Weber, M.D.
   Oral and Maxillofacial...................... Steven M. Roser, D.M.D., M.D.
   Pediatric.................................. Richard R. Ricketts, M.D.
   Plastic and Reconstructive...................... T. Roderick Hester, M.D.
   Surgical Oncology............................... Charles Staley, M.D.
   Transplantation........................... Christian P. Larsen, M.D., D.Ph.
   Trauma/Surgical Critical Care.................. Grace S. Rozycki, M.D.
   Vascular................................. Elliot Chaikof, M.D., Ph.D.
Urology... Fray F. Marshall, M.D.

Medical College of Georgia School of Medicine

1120 Fifteenth Street
Augusta, Georgia 30912-4750
706-721-0211; 721-2231 (dean's office); 721-7035 (fax)
Web site: www.mcg.edu/som

The Medical College of Georgia (MCG) School of Medicine was originally chartered in 1828 as the Medical Academy of Georgia; the school of medicine was the founding school of what has evolved to become Georgia's health sciences university: the Medical College of Georgia. Now in its 181st year, the MCG School of Medicine is Georgia's only public medical school. Among the health sciences schools of MCG are allied health sciences, dentistry, medicine, nursing, and graduate studies. The university's mission—to improve health and reduce the burden of illness on society—is central to every facet of MCG's educational, research, and clinical initiatives.

Type: public
2008-2009 total enrollment: 739
Clinical facilities: Medical College of Georgia Hospital and Clinics, Augusta, Georgia; Atlanta Medical Center, Atlanta, Georgia; Charlie Norwood Veterans Administration Medical Center, Augusta, Georgia; Dwight David Eisenhower Army Medical Center, Augusta, Georgia; Memorial Health University Medical Center, Savannah, Georgia; Phoebe Putney Memorial Hospital, Albany, Georgia.

Medical College Officials

President. . . . . Daniel W. Rahn, M.D.
Senior Vice President for Academic Affairs and Provost. . . . . Barry D. Goldstein, Ph.D.
Senior Vice President for Health Affairs . . . . D. Douglas Miller, M.D., C.M.
Senior Vice President for Finance and Administration. . . . . William R. Bowes
Vice President for Research . . . . Frank A. Treiber, Ph.D.
Vice President for Enrollment and Student Services . . . . Kevin B. Frazier, D.D.S.
Vice President for Instruction. . . . . Roman M. Cibirka, D.D.S.
Vice President for Administration. . . . . J. Michael Ash, M.D.
Vice President for Information Technology . . . . Beth P. Brigdon
Vice President for Decision Support. . . . . Deborah L. Barshafsky
Vice President for Legal Affairs . . . . Andrew R. H. Newton

Medical School Administrative Staff

Dean. . . . . D. Douglas Miller, M.D., C.M.
Vice Dean for Academic Affairs . . . . Ruth-Marie E. Fincher, M.D.
Campus Dean, Athens . . . . Barbara L. Schuster, M.D.
Associate Dean for Admissions . . . . Geoffrey H. Young, Ph.D.
Associate Dean for Student Affairs . . . . Kathleen M. McKie, M.D.
Assistant Dean for Educational Outreach and Partnerships . . . . Wilma Sykes-Brown
Associate Dean for Curriculum. . . . . T. Andrew Albritton, M.D.
Associate Dean for Evaluation . . . . Andria Thomas, Ph.D.
Associate Dean for Regional Campus Coordination. . . . . Linda Boyd, D.O.
Assistant Dean, Southwest Georgia Clinical Campus . . . . Iqbal Khan, Ph.D.
Assistant Dean, Southeast Georgia Clinical Campus. . . . . Kathryn R. Martin, Ph.D.
Senior Associate Dean for Graduate Medical
   Education and Veterans Administration Affairs . . . . Walter J. Moore, M.D.
Senior Associate Dean for Basic Science Research. . . . . John D. Catravas, Ph.D.
Senior Associate Dean for Clinical Research . . . . Anthony L. Mulloy, D.O., Ph.D.
Senior Associate Dean for Clinical Affairs. . . . . Vacant
Senior Associate Dean for Primary Care and Community Affairs . . . . Joseph Hobbs, M.D.
Associate Dean for Faculty Development. Christopher B. White, M.D.
Associate Dean for Leadership Development. . . . . Peter F. Buckley, M.D.
Executive Associate Dean for Administration. . . . . Michael A. Herbert
Chief Operations Officer . . . . Joel J. Covar
Chief of Staff. . . . . Donna Dauphinais

Medical College of Georgia School of Medicine: GEORGIA

Department and Division or Section Chairs

Basic Sciences

Biochemistry and Molecular Biology. . . . . Vadivel Ganapathy, Ph.D.
Cellular Biology and Anatomy . . . . Sally S. Atherton, Ph.D.
Pharmacology and Toxicology . . . . R. William Caldwell, Ph.D.
Physiology. . . . . R. Clinton Webb, Ph.D.

Clinical Sciences

Anesthesiology and Perioperative Medicine. C. Alvin Head, M.D.
Cardiothoracic and Vascular Surgery . . . . Vijay S. Patel, M.D. (Interim)
Emergency Medicine. . . . . Richard B. Schwartz, M.D.
Family Medicine . . . . Joseph Hobbs, M.D.
Medicine. . . . . Michael P. Madaio, M.D.
   Allergy and Immunology . . . . Dennis R. Ownby, M.D.
   Cardiology. . . . . Robert A. Sorrentino, M.D. (Interim)
   Dermatology . . . . Jack L. Lesher, Jr., M.D.
   Endocrinology, Diabetes, and Metabolism . . . . Anthony L. Mulloy, D.O., Ph.D.
   Gastroenterology and Hepatology. . . . . Robert R. Schade, M.D.
   General Internal Medicine . . . . Reynolds G. Jarvis, M.D. (Interim)
   Hematology and Oncology. . . . . Anand Jillella, M.D.
   Infectious Disease . . . . J. Peter Rissing, M.D.
   Nephrology, Hypertension, and Transplantation Medicine. . . . . Laura L. Mulloy, D.O.
   Pulmonary . . . . William B. Davis, M.D.
   Rheumatology . . . . Walter J. Moore, M.D.
Neurology. . . . . David C. Hess, M.D.
   Child Neurology. . . . . James E. Carroll, M.D.
Obstetrics and Gynecology. . . . . Ana A. Murphy, M.D.
   General Gynecology and Obstetrics. . . . . Vacant
   Gynecologic Oncology . . . . Michael S. MacFee, M.D.
   Maternal-Fetal Medicine. . . . . Andrew W. Helfgott, M.D.
   Reproductive Endocrinology, Infertility, and Genetics . . . . Lawrence C. Layman, M.D.
   Urogynecology and Pelvic Surgery. . . . . Sean L. Francis, M.D. (Interim)
Ophthalmology . . . . Julian J. Nussbaum, M.D.
Orthopaedics. . . . . Norman B. Chutkan, M.D.
Otolaryngology . . . . David J. Terris, M.D.
Pathology . . . . John C. H. Steele, Jr., M.D.
   Anatomic Pathology. . . . . Paul Biddinger, M.D.
   Clinical Pathology . . . . John C. H. Steele, Jr., M.D.
Pediatrics . . . . William P. Kanto, M.D.
   Allergy and Immunology . . . . Dennis R. Ownby, M.D.
   Cardiology. . . . . Henry B. Wiles, M.D.
   Critical Care Medicine. . . . . Anthony L. Pearson-Shaver, M.D.
   Endocrinology, Diabetes, and Metabolism . . . . Christopher Houk, M.D.
   General Pediatrics and Adolescent Medicine. . . . . Reda Bassali, M.D.
   Hematology and Oncology. . . . . Roger A. Vega, M.D.
   Infectious Diseases . . . . Dennis L. Murray, M.D.
   Neonatology. . . . . Jatinder J. S. Bhatia, M.D.
   Nephrology, Hypertension, and Transplantation Medicine. . . . . Luiz A. Ortiz, M.D.
   Rheumatology . . . . Rita S. Jerath, M.D.
Psychiatry and Health Behavior . . . . Peter F. Buckley, M.D.
   Child, Adolescent, and Family Psychiatry. . . . . Sandra B. Sexson, M.D.
Radiology . . . . James V. Rawson, M.D.
   Radiation Oncology . . . . John F. Greskovich, Jr., M.D.
Surgery. . . . . Bruce V. MacFadyen, Jr., M.D.
   General Surgery. . . . . Bruce V. MacFadyen, Jr., M.D.
   Oral and Maxillofacial Surgery . . . . Allen L. Sisk, D.D.S.
   Pediatric Surgery . . . . Charles G. Howell, Jr., M.D.
   Plastic Surgery . . . . Jack Yu, M.D.
   Urology. . . . . Ronald W. Lewis, M.D.

Mercer University School of Medicine

1550 College Street
Macon, Georgia 31207
478-301-2600; 301-5570 (dean's office); 301-2547 (fax)
Web site: www.medicine.mercer.edu

The Mercer University School of Medicine was founded in June 1982 and graduated its charter class in June 1986. Its school of medicine is located on the main campus of Mercer University. A second campus in Savannah opened for new first-year students in August 2008.

Type: private
2008-2009 total enrollment: 278
Clinical facilities: Medical Center of Central Georgia, Memorial Health-University Medical Center, Floyd Medical Center, Atlanta Medical Center, Columbus Medical Center, Phoebe Putney Memorial Hospital.

University Officials

President. . . . . William D. Underwood, J.D.
Senior Vice President for Marketing
  Communications and Chief of Staff . . . . Larry D. Brumley
Provost . . . . Wallace L. Daniel, Ph.D.
Senior Vice President for Administration and Finance. . . . . James S. Netherton, Ph.D.
Senior Vice President and General Counsel . . . . William Solomon, J.D.
Senior Vice President for Enrollment Management. . . . . Brian F. Dalton
Senior Vice President for University
  Advancement and Atlanta campus . . . . Richard Swindle, Ph.D.
Vice President for Health Sciences . . . . Hewitt W. Matthews, Ph.D.
Vice President for Audit and Compliance. . . . . James S. Calhoun
Associate Vice President for Regulatory Compliance . . . . David L. Innes, Ph.D.
Chancellor . . . . R. Kirby Godsey, Ph.D.

Medical School Administrative Staff

Dean. . . . . William F. Bina III, M.D. (Interim)
Senior Associate Dean, Savannah campus . . . . Wayne Glasgow, Ph.D.
Associate Dean for Admissions and Student Affairs . . . . Maurice S. Clifton, M.D.
Associate Dean for Academic Affairs, Macon campus. . . . . Robert S. Donner, M.D.
Associate Dean for Faculty Development. . . . . Dona L. Harris, Ph.D.
Associate Dean for Academic Affairs, Savannah campus. . . . . Tina L. Thompson, Ph.D.
Senior Associate Dean for Medical Center of Central Georgia . . . . James Cunningham, M.D.
Associate Dean for Medical Center of Central
  Georgia Programs . . . . Marcia B. Hutchinson, M.D.
Senior Associate Dean for Clinical Affairs, Savannah campus. . . . . Ramon V. Meguiar, M.D.
Associate Dean for Graduate Medical Education,
  Savannah campus . . . . Edward E. Abrams, D.Ed.
Assistant Dean for Admissions and Student
  Affairs, Savannah campus . . . . Samuel D. Murray, M.D.
Assistant Dean for Faculty Development, Savannah campus. . . . . Marie Dent, Ph.D.
Assistant Dean for Research, Macon campus. . . . . Joseph M. Van De Water, M.D.
Assistant Dean for Research, Savannah campus. Jeffrey Boyd, Ph.D.
Director of Finance . . . . Barbara Moore
Director, Medical Library. . . . . Jan Labeause
Registrar and Director, Financial Aid and Office
  of Practice Opportunities . . . . Youvette Hudson
Director of Information Technology and Media Services. . . . . Shane Milam

Department and Division or Section Chairs

Basic Sciences

Basic Sciences . . . . Wayne Glasgow, Ph.D. (Interim)
Biomedical Sciences, Savannah campus . . . . Wayne Glasgow, Ph.D.

Clinical Sciences

Anesthesiology. . . . . Ken McDonald, M.D.
Community Medicine. . . . . William F. Bina III, M.D., M.P.H.
Emergency Medicine, Macon campus. . . . . Ralph C. Griffin, M.D.
Emergency Medicine, Savannah campus. . . . . Jay Goldstein, M.D.
Family Medicine, Macon campus . . . . Fred Girton, M.D.
Family Medicine, Savannah campus . . . . Robert M. Pallay, M.D. (Interim)
Internal Medicine, Macon campus . . . . David Parish, M.D. (Interim)
Internal Medicine, Savannah campus . . . . Steven Carpenter, M.D.
Obstetrics and Gynecology, Macon campus. . . . . William Butler, M.D.
Obstetrics and Gynecology, Savannah campus. . . . . Donald G. Gallup, M.D.
Pathology . . . . Robert S. Donner, M.D.
Pediatrics, Macon campus . . . . Frank P. Bowyer, M.D.
Pediatrics, Savannah campus . . . . Jean A. Wright, M.D.
Psychiatry and Behavioral Science, Macon campus . . . . Melton Strozier, Ph.D.
Psychiatry and Behavioral Science, Savannah campus . . . . TBA
Radiology, Macon campus . . . . William A. Bootle, M.D.
Radiology, Savannah campus . . . . Charles Brown, M.D.
Surgery, Macon campus. . . . . Don Nakayama, M.D.
Surgery, Savannah campus. . . . . Steven T. Brower, M.D.

Morehouse School of Medicine

720 Westview Drive, S.W.
Atlanta, Georgia 30310
404-752-1500; 752-1720 (dean's office); 752-1594 (fax)
Web site: www.msm.edu

The Morehouse School of Medicine is a historically black institution established to recruit and train minority and other students as physicians, biomedical scientists, and public health professionals committed to the primary health care needs of the underserved. Founded in 1975 as the school of medicine at Morehouse College, the Morehouse School of Medicine became independent from Morehouse College in 1981 and became a member of the Atlanta University Center in 1983. An active biomedical research program tied together by an emphasis on disease processes that disproportionately affect minority communities supports Ph.D., M.D., M.P.H., and M.S.C.R. programs.

Type: private
2008-2009 total enrollment: 279
Clinical facilities: Grady Memorial Hospital, South Fulton Medical Center, Georgia Regional Hospital, Atlanta, Tuskegee Veterans Administration Medical Center.

Medical School Administrative Staff

President. . . . . John E. Maupin, Jr., D.D.S.
Dean and Senior Vice President for Academic Affairs . . . . Eve J. Higginbotham, M.D.
Vice President for Campus Planning and Operations . . . . Walter W. Sullivan, Ph.D.
Vice President for Finance. . . . . Eli H. Phillips
Vice President for Institutional Advancement
   and Marketing and Communications . . . . Sally M. Davis
Vice President and Associate Dean for
   Sponsored Research Administration . . . . Sandra A. Harris-Hooker, Ph.D.
Associate Vice President, Community Relations
   and Development . . . . Willie H. Clemons, Ph.D.
Associate Vice President of Human Resources. . . . . Denise Britt
Vice Dean and Associate Vice President for
   Academic and Student Affairs . . . . Angela L. W. Franklin, Ph.D.
Associate Vice President of Major Gifts. . . . . Juan A. McGruder, Ph.D.
Deputy to the President for Governmental
   Relations and Community Affairs . . . . Terri A. Winston
Chief Information Officer . . . . Cigdem Delano
Senior Associate Dean, Education and Faculty Affairs . . . . Martha L. Elks, M.D., Ph.D.
Associate Dean for Administration . . . . Sandra E. Watson
Associate Dean for Clinical Affairs . . . . Lawrence L. Sanders, Jr., M.D.
Associate Dean for Clinical Research . . . . Elizabeth Ofili, M.D., M.P.H.
Associate Dean for Community Programs . . . . Daniel S. Blumenthal, M.D.
Associate Dean for Veterans Affairs . . . . Samuel M. Aguayo, M.D.
Assistant Director for Admissions and Student
   Affairs . . . . Ngozi Anachebe, M.D., Pharm.D. (Interim)
Assistant Dean for Graduate Studies. . . . . Douglas F. Paulsen, Ph.D.
Director, Admissions . . . . Sterling Roaf, M.D.
Director, Campus Operations and Capital Resources. Tony Collier
Director, Library . . . . Cynthia L. Henderson
Director, Graduate Medical Education Administration. . . . . William E. Booth
Director, Marketing and Communications . . . . Cherie Richardson
Director, Planning and Institutional Research. . . . . Andrea D. Fox, M.B.A.
Director, Risk Management . . . . Marilyn A. Pruitt
Director, Student Information Systems, and Registrar . . . . Derreck Pressley
Controller. . . . . David H. Byrd

Department Chairs

Basic Sciences

Anatomy and Neurobiology . . . . Peter R. MacLeish, Ph.D.

Microbiology, Biochemistry, and Immunology. . . . . Myrtle J. Thierry-Palmer, Ph.D. (Interim)

Pharmacology and Toxicology . . . . Mohamed A. Bayorh, Ph.D. (Interim)

Physiology . . . . David R. Mann, Ph.D. (Interim)

Clinical Sciences

Community Health and Preventive Medicine . . . . Daniel S. Blumenthal, M.D., M.P.H.

Family Medicine . . . . Harry S. Strothers III, M.D. (Interim)

Internal Medicine . . . . Myra E. Rose, M.D. (Interim)

Medical Education. . . . . Martha L. Elks, M.D., Ph.D.

Obstetrics and Gynecology. . . . . Roland Matthews, M.D.

Pathology . . . . Marjorie M. Smith, M.D.

Pediatrics . . . . Frances J. Dunston, M.D., M.P.H.

Psychiatry and Behavioral Science . . . . Gail A. Mattox, M.D.

Surgery . . . . William Lynn Weaver, M.D.

University of Hawaii at Mānoa John A. Burns School of Medicine

651 Ilalo Street, Medical Education Building
Honolulu, Hawaii 96813-5534
808-692-0899 (general information); 692-0881 (dean's office); 692-1247 (fax)
Web site: http://jabsom.hawaii.edu

The school of medicine was established in 1965 and functioned as a two-year school until 1973. At that time, expansion to a full M.D. degree-granting program was approved. The first class graduated in 1975. Since 1989, Problem Based Learning (PBL) has been utilized extensively throughout the curriculum.

Type: public
2008-2009 total enrollment: 260
Clinical facilities: Hawaii State Hospital, Hilo Medical Center, Kaiser Foundation Hospital, Kapiolani Medical Center for Women and Children, Kuakini Medical Center, Leahi Hospital, The Physician Center at Mililani, Queen Emma Clinics, The Queen's Medical Center, Rehabilitation Hospital of the Pacific, Shriner's Hospital for Children, Straub Clinic and Hospital, Straub Hospital for Children, Tripler Army Medical Center, Castle Medical Center, Hawaii Medical Center East, Department of Veterans Affairs Pacific Island Health Care System, Wahiawa General Hospital.

University Officials

President. . . . . David McClain, Ph.D.
Chancellor . . . . Virginia S. Hinshaw, Ph.D.

Medical School Administrative Staff

Dean. . . . . Jerris Hedges, M.D.
Associate Dean for Academic Affairs. . . . . Satoru Izutsu, Ph.D. (Interim)
Assistant Dean for Graduate Student Services . . . . Open
Director of Student Affairs. . . . . Mary Ann Antonelli, M.D.
Director of Medical Education . . . . Richard T. Kasuya, M.D.
Director of Faculty Affairs . . . . Rosanne C. Harrigan, Ed.D.
Director of Clinical Research . . . . David Easa, M.D.
Director of Postgraduate Medical Education . . . . William F. Haning III, M.D.
Director of Telehealth Research. . . . . Lawrence P. A. Burgess, M.D.
Director of Women in Biomedical Science and Minority Affairs. . . . . . Mary Ann Antonelli, M.D.
Director of Admissions. . . . . Satoru Izutsu, Ph.D.
Director of Development, UH Foundation . . . . Jeffrie Jones
Director of Office of Public Health Studies. . . . . Jay Maddock, Ph.D.
Director of Information Technology. . . . . Grant Murata (Acting)
Director of Fiscal and Administrative Affairs . . . . Corinne Seymour
Director of Communications . . . . Tina Shelton
Contracts Officer, Hospital and External Business Affairs . . . . Lauren Kwak, J.D.
Director of Human Resources . . . . Kim Uyehara, M.P.H.
Director of Facilities Management and Planning. . . . . Francis Blanco
Director of Translational Research . . . . David Curb, M.D.

University of Hawaii at Mānoa John A. Burns School of Medicine: HAWAII

Department and Division or Section Chairs

Basic Sciences

Anatomy, Biochemistry, Physiology, and Reproductive Biology . . . . Scott Lozanoff, Ph.D.
Cell and Molecular Biology . . . . Marla J. Berry, Ph.D.
Pathology . . . . Michele Carbone, M.D.
Public Health Sciences and Epidemiology. . . . . Jason E. Maddock, Ph.D.
Tropical Medicine, Medical Microbiology, and Pharmacology . . . . Duane J. Gubler, Ph.D.

Clinical Sciences

Complementary and Alternative Medicine . . . . Rosanne C. Harrigan, Ed.D.
Family Medicine and Community Health . . . . Neal A. Palafox, M.D.
Geriatric Medicine. . . . . Patricia L. Blanchette, M.D.
Medicine. . . . . Elizabeth K. Tam, M.D.
Native Hawaiian Health . . . . Marjorie K. Mau, M.D.
Obstetrics, Gynecology, and Women's Health . . . . Lynnae Millar Sauvage, M.D. (Interim)
Pediatrics . . . . Raul C. Rudoy, M.D.
Psychiatry . . . . Naleen N. Andrade, M.D.
Surgery . . . . Danny M. Takanishi, M.D.

Other Medical Sciences

Allied Medical Sciences . . . . Satoru Izutsu, Ph.D
Medical Technology. . . . . Open
Speech Pathology and Audiology . . . . James T. Yates, Ph.D.

University of Chicago
Division of the Biological Sciences
Pritzker School of Medicine

5841 South Maryland Avenue
Chicago, Illinois 60637
773-702-1939; 702-9000 (dean's office); 702-1897 (fax)
Web site: www.uchicago.edu

The school of medicine of the University of Chicago was established in 1927. In 1968, it was renamed the Pritzker School of Medicine.

Type: private
2008-2009 total enrollment: 428
Clinical facilities: University of Chicago Hospitals, LaRabida Children's Hospital and Research Center, Louis A. Weiss Memorial Hospital, MacNeal Hospital.

University Officials

President. . . . . Robert J. Zimmer, Ph.D.
Provost . . . . Thomas Rosenbaum, Ph.D.

Medical School Administrative Staff

Dean, Division of Biological Sciences, Pritzker School of Medicine . . . . . James L. Madara, M.D.
Dean for Medical Education. . . . . Holly J. Humphrey, M.D.
Executive Vice Dean, Biological Sciences Division. . . . . Vinay Kumar, M.D.
Associate Dean, Admissions . . . . Herbert Abelson, M.D.
Associate Dean, Multicultural Affairs. . . . . William McDade, M.D., Ph.D.
Dean, Graduate Affairs. . . . . Nancy B. Schwartz, Ph.D.
Dean for Clinical Affairs and Chief Medical Officer . . . . Harvey Golomb, M.D.
Associate Dean and Master, Biological Science Collegiate Division. . . . . Jose Quintans, M.D.
Associate Dean for Administration . . . . Ann Schwind
Associate Dean and Vice President for
  Organizational Strategy and Planning . . . . Kenneth J. Sharigian
Associate Dean and Vice President for Medical Center Development. . . . . Michele Schiele
Associate Dean and Vice President, Medical Practice Administration . . . . Carolyn Wilson
Associate Dean for Clinical Research . . . . Walter Stadler, M.D.
Associate Dean, Organismal and Evolutionary Biology. . . . . Neil Shubin, Ph.D.
Faculty Dean, Office of Academic Affairs . . . . Martin Feder, Ph.D.

Department and Division or Section Chairs

Basic Sciences

Ben May Department for Cancer Research. Marsha R. Rosner, Ph.D.
Biochemistry and Molecular Biology. Anthony A. Kossiakoff, Ph.D.
Cancer Biology* . . . . Geoffrey Greene, Ph.D.
Cancer Research Center. . . . . Michelle Le Beau, M.D.
Cell Physiology*. . . . . Eric Beyer, M.D.
Computational Neuroscience, Committee of*. Philip Ulinski, Ph.D.
Committee on Clinical Pharmacology and Pharmacogenomics*. . . . . Mark A. Ratain, M.D.
Developmental Biology*. . . . . Victoria Prince, Ph.D.
Ecology and Evolution. . . . . Joy Bergelson, Ph.D.
Evolutionary Biology* . . . . David Jablonski, Ph.D.
Genetics* . . . . Douglas Bishop, Ph.D.
Human Genetics . . . . T. Conrad Gilliam, Ph.D.
Immunology* . . . . Albert Bendelac, Ph.D.
Institute for Biophysical Dynamics . . . . Stephen Kent, Ph.D.
Institute for Cardiovascular Research* . . . . Elizabeth McNally, M.D., Ph.D.
Institute for Genomics and Systems Biology* . . . . Kevin White, Ph.D.
Ludwig Center for Metastasis Research*. . . . . Ralph Weichselbaum, M.D.
Medical Physics, Committee of* . . . . Maryellen L. Giger, Ph.D.
Microbiology. . . . . Olaf Schneewind, M.D., Ph.D.
Molecular Genetics and Cell Biology . . . . Richard Fehon, Ph.D.
Molecular Medicine, Committee on* . . . . Julian Solway, M.D.
Molecular Metabolism and Nutrition* . . . . Christopher Rhodes, Ph.D.
Neurobiology, Committee on* . . . . Peggy Mason, Ph.D.
Neurobiology. . . . . S. Murray Sherman, Ph.D.

Organismal Biology and Anatomy . . . . Jan-Marino Ramirez, Ph.D.

Clinical Sciences

Anesthesia and Critical Care . . . . Jeffrey L. Apfelbaum, M.D.
Family Medicine . . . . Bernard G. Ewigman, M.D.
Health Studies . . . . Ronald A. Thisted, Ph.D.
Medicine . . . . Joe G.N. Garcia, M.D.
    Cardiology* . . . . Stephen Archer, M.D.
    Dermatology* . . . . Christopher Shea, M.D.
    Emergency Medicine* . . . . James J. Walter, M.D.
    Endocrinology* . . . . Roy Weiss, M.D., Ph.D.
    Gastroenterology* . . . . Stephen Hanauer, M.D.
    Genetic Medicine . . . . Nancy Cox, M.D.
    General Internal Medicine* . . . . Deborah Burnet, M.D.
    Geriatrics, Section of* . . . . Greg Sachs, M.D.
    Hematology and Oncology* . . . . Everett E. Vokes, M.D.
    Infectious Diseases* . . . . David Pitrak, M.D.
    Nephrology* . . . . Richard Quigg, M.D.
    Pulmonary and Critical Care* . . . . Jesse Hall, M.D.
    Rheumatology* . . . . Marcus Clark, M.D.
Neurology . . . . Christopher Gomez, M.D., Ph.D.
Obstetrics and Gynecology . . . . Arthur Haney, M.D.
Ophthalmology and Visual Science . . . . William F. Mieler, M.D.
Pathology . . . . Vinay Kumar, M.D.
Pediatrics . . . . Michael D. Schreiber, Ph.D. (Interim)
    Allergy and Immunology* . . . . Raoul L. Wolf, M.D.
    Cardiac Surgery . . . . TBA
    Cardiology* . . . . Brojendra Agarwala, M.D.
    Chronic Diseases* . . . . Izhar Qamar, M.D.
    Developmental and Behavioral Pediatrics* . . . . Michael Msall, M.D.
    Endocrinology* . . . . TBA
    Gastroenterology, Hepatology, and Nutrition* . . . . Stefano Guandalini, M.D.
    General Pediatrics* . . . . John D. Lantos, M.D.
    Hematology and Oncology* . . . . John Cunningham, M.D.
    Infectious Diseases* . . . . Kenneth Alexander, M.D.
    Neonatology* . . . . Kwang-sun Lee, M.D.
    Nephrology* . . . . Christopher Clardy, M.D.
    Neurology* . . . . TBA
    Neurosurgery* . . . . David M. Frim, M.D., Ph.D.
    Pediatric Emergency Medicine* . . . . Mark A. Hostetler, M.D.
    Pulmonology* . . . . Lucille Lester, M.D.
    Rheumatology* . . . . Charles Spencer, M.D.
    Urology* . . . . Clare Close, M.D.
Psychiatry . . . . Emil Coccaro, Ph.D.
Radiation and Cellular Oncology . . . . Ralph R. Weichselbaum, M.D.
Radiology . . . . Richard Baron, M.D.
Surgery . . . . Jeffrey Matthews, M.D.
    Cardiac and Thoracic Surgery* . . . . Valluvan Jeevanandam, M.D.
    General Dentistry* . . . . Joseph Toljanic, D.D.S., and Chris Smith, D.D.S.
    General Surgery* . . . . Mitchell Posner, M.D.
    Neurosurgery* . . . . Richard Fessler, M.D.
    Orthopaedic Surgery* . . . . Terrance Peabody, M.D.
    Otolaryngology/Head and Neck Surgery* . . . . Robert M. Naclerio, M.D.
    Pediatric Surgery* . . . . Donald Liu, M.D., Ph.D.
    Plastic and Reconstructive* . . . . David Song, M.D.
    Transplantation Surgery* . . . . J. Michael Millis, M.D.
    Urology* . . . . Arieh Shalhav, M.D.
    Vascular* . . . . Hisham Bassiouny, M.D.

*Specialty without organizational autonomy.

Chicago Medical School
At Rosalind Franklin University of Medicine and Science

3333 Green Bay Road
North Chicago, Illinois 60064
847-578-3000; 578-3301 (dean's office); 578-3343 (fax)
Web site: www.rosalindfranklin.edu

The Chicago Medical School was founded in 1912 as the Chicago Hospital College of Medicine. In 1919, the name of the institution was changed to the Chicago Medical School. In 1930, the school moved to the West Side Medical Center and remained there until it completed a move to North Chicago in 1980. In 1967, with the establishment of the University of Health Sciences, the academic programs were broadened to include the school of graduate and postdoctoral studies and the school of related health sciences in addition to the Chicago Medical School. In 1993, the university was renamed Finch University of Health Sciences. In 2004, the university was renamed in honor of Rosalind Franklin. In 2002, the Dr. William M. Scholl College of Podiatric Medicine became a college of the university.

Type: private
2008-2009 total enrollment: 746
Clinical facilities: North Chicago Veterans Affairs Medical Center, Stroger Hospital of Cook County, Mount Sinai Hospital Medical Center, Swedish Covenant Hospital, Lutheran General Hospital, Norwalk Hospital (CT), Illinois Masonic Hospital, Christ Hospital.

University Officials

President and Chief Executive Officer . . . . K. Michael Welch, M.B.,Ch.B, F.R.C.P.
Executive Vice President and Chief Operating Officer. . . . . Margot Surridge
Vice President for Academic Affairs . . . . Timothy R. Hansen, Ph.D.
Vice President for Medical Affairs. . . . . Arthur J. Ross III, M.D., M.B.A.
Vice President for Research . . . . Michael Sarras, Ph.D.

University Deans and Administrative Staff

Dean, Chicago Medical School. . . . . Arthur J. Ross III, M.D., M.B.A.
Dean, School of Graduate and Postdoctoral Studies . . . . Michael Sarras, Ph.D.
Dean, College of Health Professions. . . . . Wendy L. Rheault, Ph.D.
Dean, Dr. William M. Scholl College of Podiatric Medicine . . . . Terence Albright, D.P.M.
Executive Director, Division of Student Affairs . . . . Rebecca Durkin
Associate Vice President of Enrollment Services . . . . Maryann DeCaire
Coordinator, Student Housing . . . . Jennifer Smith

Medical School Administrative Staff

Senior Associate Dean for Clinical Affairs. . . . . Charles P. Barsano, M.D., Ph.D.
Senior Associate Dean for Student Affairs and Medical Eduation. . . . . Cathy Lazarus, M.D.
Associate Dean for Veterans Affairs . . . . Tariq Hassan, M.D.
Associate Dean for Mount Sinai Hospital Medical Center . . . . Robert Parker, M.D.
Associate Dean for Curriculum. . . . . John Tomkowiak, M.D.
Associate Dean for Research. . . . . Kenneth Neet, Ph.D.
Senior Associate Dean for Advocate Health Care . . . . Lee Sacks, M.D.
Associate Dean for Advocate Health Care. . . . . Open
Assistant Dean for Advocate Health Care . . . . Mary Ann Clemens
Assistant Dean for Advocate Lutheran General Hospital . . . . Kris Narasimhan, M.D.
Assistant Dean for Advocate Christ Medical Center . . . . Robert Stein, M.D.
Assistant Dean for Advocate Illinois Masonic Medical Center. . . . . William Werner, M.D.

Department and Division or Section Chairs

Basic Sciences

Biochemistry and Molecular Biology. . . . . Rami Haddad, M.D.
Cell Biology and Anatomy . . . . William N. Frost, Ph.D.
Cellular and Molecular Pharmacology . . . . Gloria E. Meredith, Ph.D.
Microbiology and Immunology. . . . . Bala Chandran, Ph.D.
Neuroscience. . . . . Marina E. Wolf, Ph.D.
Pathology . . . . Arthur S. Schneider, M.D.
Physiology and Biophysics . . . . Robert Bridges, Ph.D.

Clinical Sciences

Anesthesiology. . . . . Open
Emergency Medicine . . . . Leslie Zun, M.D.
Family and Preventive Medicine . . . . Judith Gravdal, M.D.
Medicine. . . . . Eric P. Gall, M.D.
  Allergy
  Cardiology. . . . . Rohit Arora, M.D.
  Critical Care Medicine . . . . Raul Gazmuri, M.D.
  Endocrinology . . . . Sant P. Singh, M.D.
  Epidemiology. . . . . Open
  Gastroenterology . . . . Alex Feller, M.D.
  General Medicine. . . . . Cathy Lazarus, M.D.
  Geriatric Medicine . . . . William Rhoades, D.O.
  Hematology and Oncology . . . . Rami Haddad, M.D.
  Infectious Diseases . . . . Open
  Nephrology . . . . Earl Smith, M.D.
  Pulmonary Diseases . . . . Ashok Fulambarker, M.D.
  Rheumatology/Allergy . . . . Eric Gall, M.D.
Neurology. . . . . Nutan Vaidya, M.D. (Interim)
Obstetrics and Gynecology. . . . . Josef Blankstein, M.D.
  Gynecologic Oncology . . . . Hyung-Shik Kang, M.D.
  Gynecology . . . . Hyung-Shik Kang, M.D.
  Maternal Fetal Medicine. . . . . E. C. Lampley, M.D.
  Reproductive Endocrinology. . . . . Josef Blankstein, M.D.
Ophthalmology . . . . Alan J. Axelrod, M.D.
Pediatrics . . . . Henry H. Mangurten, M.D. (Interim)
  Ambulatory Pediatrics. . . . . Jay Mayefsky, M.D.
  Child Protective Services. . . . . Michelle Lorand, M.D.
  Pediatric Allergy/Immunology . . . . James Moy, M.D.
  Pediatric Cardiology . . . . Zahra Naheed, M.D. (Acting)
  Pediatric Emergency Service . . . . J. Thomas Senko, D.O.
  Pediatric Endocrinology . . . . Kunika Ghai, M.D.
  Pediatric Hematology and Oncology . . . . Lilly Mathew, M.D.
  Pediatric Neonatology. . . . . Suma Pyati, M.D.
Psychiatry and Behavioral Sciences . . . . Nutan Vaidya, M.D.
  Addiction Psychiatry. . . . . Vamsi Garlapati, M.D.
  Child Psychiatry . . . . Balasubramania P. S. Sarma, M.D.
  Community Psychiatry . . . . David Baron, M.D.
  Consultation Liaison Psychiatry. . . . . Viktoria Erhardt, M.D.
  Forensic Psychiatry. . . . . Amin Daghestani, M.D.
  Gertiatric Psychiatry . . . . Zafeer Berki, M.D.
  Hospital Psychiatry. . . . . Chandra Vedak, M.D.
  Neuropsychiatry . . . . Lori Moss, M.D,
  Psychotherapy . . . . Ruth Rosenthal, M.D., and Amanda Weiss, M.D.
Radiology . . . . Ejaz Rahim, M.D. (Interim)
Surgery . . . . Thomas Vargish, M.D. (Interim)
  Critical Care. . . . . Michelle Holevar, M.D.
  General Surgery . . . . Allan Fredland, M.D.
  Neurosurgery . . . . Hernando Torres, M.D.
  Orthopedic Surgery . . . . Prahlad Pyati, M.D.
  Otolaryngology. . . . . Nedra Joyner, M.D.
  Surgical Nutrition. . . . . Stephen R. Wise, M.D.
  Urology . . . . Nejd Alsikafi, M.D.

University of Illinois at Chicago College of Medicine
1853 West Polk Street (M/C 784)
Chicago, Illinois 60612
312-996-3500; 996-9006 (fax)
Web site: www.medicine.uic.edu/departments_programs

Founded in 1881 as the College of Physicians and Surgeons of Chicago, the school affiliated with the University of Illinois in 1897 and became known as the University of Illinois College of Medicine in 1900. The dean's office is located on the campus of the University of Illinois at Chicago, 135 miles from the Urbana-Champaign campus of the university. In 1970, the college was regionalized to include programs of medical education in Chicago, Peoria, Rockford, and Urbana-Champaign.

Type: public
2008-2009 total enrollment: 1,250
Clinical facilities: Chicago area-University of Illinois at Chicago Hospital Medical Center, Jesse Brown VA Medical Center, Advocate Christ Hospital Medical Center, Advocate Illinois Masonic Medical Center, Mercy Hospital Medical Center, St. Francis HospitalGreat Lakes Naval Medical Center, Advocate Lutheran General Hospital, St. Anthony's Hospital Michael Reese Hospital and Medical Center, John H. Stroger Hospital of Cook County; Peoria area-Allied Agencies Center, Institute of Physical Medicine and Rehabilitation, Methodist Medical Center of Illinois, Julia Rackley Perry Memorial Hospital, Pekin Memorial Hospital, Proctor Community Hospital, St. Francis Medical Center, George A. Zeller Mental Health Center, Graham Hospital; Rockford area-Carrie Lynn Children's Center, Wesley Willows, Rockford Memorial Hospital, St. Anthony Hospital, H. Douglas Singer Zone Center, Swedish-American Hospital; Urbana-Champaign area-BroMenn Regional Medical Center, Christie Clinic, Decatur Memorial Hospital, Francis Nelson Health Center, Lake View Memorial Hospital, McKinley Health Center, Planned Parenthood, Veterans Administration Hospital (Danville), Carle Foundation Hospital, Provena Covenant Medical Center, United Samaritans Medical Center.

University Officials

President. . . . . B. Joseph White, Ph.D.

University of Illinois at Chicago Officials

Chancellor . . . . Eric A. Gislason, Ph.D. (Interim)
Provost and Vice Chancellor for Academic Affairs. . . . . R. Michael Tanner, Ph.D.
Vice Chancellor for Student Affairs . . . . Barbara Henley, Ph.D.
Vice Chancellor for Research. . . . . Larry H. Danziger, Ph.D. (Interim)
Associate Vice Chancellor for Health Affairs. . . . . John J. DeNardo
Executive Assistant Vice President for Business
    and Finance . . . . Heather J. Haberaecker, Ph.D.
Dean of the Graduate College . . . . Clark Hulse, Ph.D.
University Librarian. . . . . Mary M. Case

Medical School Administrative Staff

Dean. . . . . Joseph A. Flaherty, M.D.
Vice Dean . . . . Sarah J. Kilpatrick, M.D., Ph.D.
Senior Associate Dean for Educational Affairs. . . . . Leslie J. Sandlow, M.D.
Senior Associate Dean for Research . . . . Larry Tobacman, M.D., Ph.D.
Senior Associate Dean of Students . . . . Kathleen Kashima, Ph.D.
Associate Dean for Fiscal Affairs. . . . . Arnim Dontes
Associate Dean for Veterans Affairs . . . . Subhash C. Kukreja, M.D.
Associate Dean and Director, Admissions . . . . Jorge A. Girotti, Ph.D.
Director for Faculty Affairs. . . . . Gillian Coombs
Assistant Dean for Faculty Development. . . . . Claudia Morrissey
Associate Dean for Medical Center Affairs . . . . William H. Chamberlin, M.D.
Associate Dean for Graduate Research and Education. . . . . Karen Colley, Ph.D.
Assistant Dean for Urban Health Program . . . . Javette Orgain, M.D.
Associate Dean for Advancement . . . . Craig Bazzani (Interim)
Director, Medical Service Plan . . . . William R. Nicholas, Ph.D.
Director, Records and Registration. . . . . Susan Huhndorf
Director, Financial Aid. . . . . Carmelita Gee

Programs of Undergraduate Medical Education

College of Medicine at Chicago
1853 West Polk Street (M/C 784)
Chicago, Illinois 60612
312-996-3500; 996-9006 (fax)

Assistant Dean for Student Affairs. . . . . Kathleen J. Kashima, Ph.D.
Associate Dean for Informational Resources . . . . Robert J. McAuley, Ph.D.
Associate Dean for Curriculum. . . . . David Mayer, M.D.
Associate Dean for Educational Planning . . . . Loreen Troy
Assistant Dean for Informational Resources . . . . Donald R. Atkinson
Senior Associate Dean for Clinical Affairs. . . . . Open
Associate Dean and Director, Special Curricular
  Programs; Director, Medical College
  Admissions . . . . Jorge A. Girotti, M.D.

Basic Sciences

Anatomy and Cell Biology . . . . Scott Brady, Ph.D.
Biochemistry and Molecular Genetics. . . . . Jack H. Kaplan, Ph.D.
Medical Education. . . . . Leslie J. Sandlow, M.D.
Microbiology and Immunology. . . . . Bellur S. Prabhakar, Ph.D.
Pharmacology . . . . Asrar B. Malik, Ph.D.
Physiology and Biophysics . . . . R. John Solaro, Ph.D.

Clinical Sciences

Anesthesiology. . . . . David E. Schwartz, M.D. (Interim)
Dermatology . . . . Lawrence Chan, M.D.
Emergency Medicine . . . . Gary R. Strange, M.D.
Family Medicine . . . . Patrick A. Tranmer, M.D.
Medicine. . . . . Thomas J. Layden, M.D.
  Allergy and Immunology*. . . . . John Latall, M.D.
  Cardiology* . . . . Samuel Dudley, M.D.
  Digestive Disease and Nutrition*. . . . . Gail A. Hecht, M.D.
  Endocrinology* . . . . Theodore Mazzone, M.D.
  General Internal Medicine* . . . . John Tulley, M.D.
  Geriatric Medicine* . . . . Donald Jurivich, D.O.
  Hematology* . . . . Gary Kruh, M.D., Ph.D. (Interim)
  Hepatology*. . . . . Scott Cotler, M.D.
  Infectious Diseases* . . . . James L. Cook, M.D.
  Nephrology* . . . . Jose A. L. Arruda, M.D.
  Oncology*. . . . . Gary Kruh, M.D., Ph.D. (Interim)
  Respiratory and Critical Care* . . . . John Christman, M.D.
  Rheumatology* . . . . William Swedler, M.D. (Interim)
Neurology and Rehabilitation Medicine . . . . Philip B. Gorelick, M.D.
Neurological Surgery. . . . . Fady Charbel, M.D.
Obstetrics and Gynecology. . . . . Sara Kilpatrick, M.D., Ph.D.
Ophthalmology and Visual Sciences . . . . Dimitri T. Azar, M.D.
Orthopaedic Surgery . . . . Mark A. Gonzalez, M.D.
Otolaryngology-Head and Neck Surgery . . . . J. Regan Thomas, M.D.
Pathology . . . . Robert Folberg, M.D.
Pediatrics . . . . Usha Raj, M.D.
Psychiatry . . . . Anand Kumar, M.D.
Radiation Oncology. . . . . Jeffrey Feinstein, M.D.
Radiology . . . . Masoud Hemmati, M.D. (Interim)
Surgery. . . . . Enrico Benedetti, M.D.
  Cardio-Thoracic Surgery* . . . . Malek G. Massad, M.D. (Int. Chief)
  Colorectal Surgery* . . . . Jose Cintron, M.D.
  General Surgery* . . . . Pier Cristoforo Giulianotti, M.D.
  Pediatric Surgery* . . . . Mark Holterman, M.D.
  Plastic Surgery* . . . . Mimis N. Cohen, M.D.
  Transplantation Surgery* . . . . Jose Obherholzer, M.D. (Interim)
  Vascular Surgery*. . . . . Martin Borhani, M.D.
Surgical Oncology . . . . Tapas K. Das Gupta, M.D., Ph.D.

Urology. . . . . Craig Niederberger, M.D.

*Specialty without organizational autonomy.

College of Medicine at Peoria
One Illini Drive
P.O. Box 1649
Peoria, Illinois 61656
309-671-8402 (regional dean's office); 671-8438 (fax)

Regional Dean. . . . . Sara L. Rusch, M.D.
Regional Vice Dean. . . . . Vacant
Associate Dean for Academic Affairs. . . . . Gwen J. Lombard, Ph.D.
Associate Dean for Community Health. . . . . John G. Halvorsen, M.D.
Associate Dean for Fiscal Affairs and Administration. . . . . Vacant
Associate Dean for Graduate Medical Education. . . . . Thomas Santoro, M.D. (Visiting)
Associate Dean for Research and Development. . . . . Vacant
Assistant Dean for Student Services . . . . Linda Rowe, Ed.D.
Assistant Dean for Clinical Curriculum and Evaluation . . . . James Crane, M.D.
Assistant Dean for Education/MMCI . . . . Richard Anderson, M.D.
Assistant Dean for Pre-Clinical Curriculum and Evaluation . . . . Glenn Miller, M.D.
Assistant Dean for Education, SFMC. . . . . Tim Miller, M.D.
Assistant Dean for Medical Education and Evaluation . . . . Lynne Meyer, Ph.D.
Director of Fiscal Services . . . . Lawrence Kloc
Cancer Biology and Pharmacology. . . . . Jasti Rao, Ph.D.
Dermatology . . . . Rodney A. Lorenz, M.D. (Interim)
Family and Community Medicine. . . . . John G. Halvorsen, M.D.
Internal Medicine . . . . Sara L. Rusch, M.D.
Neurology. . . . . Jorge C. Kattah, M.D.
Neurosurgery. . . . . Patrick Tracy, M.D. (Interim)
Obstetrics and Gynecology. . . . . Rida Boulos, M.D. (Interim)
Pathology . . . . Roger Geiss, M.D.
Pediatrics . . . . Pedro de Alarcon, M.D. (Chair)
Psychiatry and Behavioral Medicine . . . . Timothy Bruce, Ph.D. (Int. Chair)
Radiology . . . . Thomas J. Cusack, M.D.
Rehabilitation Medicine. . . . . Rodney Lorenz, M.D.
Surgery. . . . . Norman C. Estes, M.D.

College of Medicine at Rockford
1601 Parkview Avenue
Rockford, Illinois 61107
815-395-5600 (regional dean's office); 395-5887 (fax)

Regional Dean. . . . . Martin S. Lipsky, M.D.
Associate Dean for Academic Affairs. . . . . Mitchell King, M.D.
Associate Dean for Fiscal Affairs and Administration . . . . Rick Hampton
Assistant Dean for Medical Education and Evaluation . . . . Margaret Maynard, M.D.
Assistant Dean for Health Systems Research . . . . Joel B. Cowen
Biomedical Sciences. . . . . K. Ramaswamy, Ph.D.
Family and Community Medicine. . . . . Erick Henley, M.D.
Medicine. . . . . Glenn Netto, M.D. (Interim)
Obstetrics and Gynecology. . . . . Timothy J. Durkee, M.D., Ph.D.
Pathology . . . . Gary L. Anderson, M.D. (Interim)
Pediatrics . . . . David E. Deutsch, M.D.
Psychiatry . . . . Steven Kouris, D.O., M.P.H. (Interim)
Surgery. . . . . Samuel Appavu, M.D.

College of Medicine at Urbana-Champaign
190 Medical Sciences Building
506 South Mathews
Urbana, Illinois 61801
217-333-5465 (regional dean's office); 333-8868 (fax)

Regional Dean. . . . . Bradford S. Schwartz, M.D.
Director of Business and Financial Systems. . . . . Richard J. Schimmel, Ed.D.
Associate Dean for Academic Affairs. . . . . Richard I. Gumport, Ph.D.
Associate Dean for Student Affairs and Medical Scholars Program. . . . . James W. Hall, Ed.D.
Associate Dean for Academic Curriculum Management. . . . . Susan Kies, Ed.D.
Associate Dean for Clinical Affairs . . . . Robert W. Kirby, M.D.
Executive Assistant Dean for Student Affairs and
  Medical Scholars Program . . . . Nora J. Few, Ph.D.
Associate Dean for Administration . . . . Dedra M. Williams
Director of Medical Scholars Program . . . . James Slauch, Ph.D.
Director of Advancement. . . . . Madeleine Jaehne
Director of Computer and Information Science . . . . Tod A. Jebe
Medical Humanities and Social Sciences Program. . . . . Evan M. Melhado, Ph.D.
Biochemistry . . . . Colin A. Wraight, Ph.D.
Cell and Structural Biology . . . . Martha L.U. Gillette, Ph.D.
Family Medicine . . . . Christian Wagner, M.D.
Internal Medicine . . . . Janet Jokela, M.D.
Medical Information Science . . . . Bruce R. Schatz, Ph.D. (Interim)
Microbiology . . . . John E. Cronan, Ph.D.
Molecular and Integrative Physiology . . . . Byron W. Kemper, Ph.D.
Obstetrics and Gynecology. . . . . Ralph J. Kehl, M.D.
Pathology . . . . Gregory G. Freund, M.D.
Pediatrics . . . . M. Kathleen Buetow, M.D., Dr.P.H.
Pharmacology . . . . Byron W. Kemper, Ph.D.
Psychiatry . . . . Sari Gilman Aronson, M.D.
Surgery . . . . Uretz J. Oliphant, M.D.

Loyola University Chicago Stritch School of Medicine

2160 South First Avenue
Maywood, Illinois 60153
708-216-9000; 216-3223 (dean's office); 216-8881 (fax)
Web site: www.stritch.luc.edu

Stritch School of Medicine is part of Loyola University Chicago, an urban Catholic university composed of a culturally and religiously diverse faculty, student body, and administration. Established in 1909, Stritch specifically calls upon its Jesuit tradition of education, which emphasizes the full development of its students, rigorous concern for the quality of its academic programs, and promotion of a broad educational curriculum that encourages leadership in the service of others and advances social justice. The school is located at Loyola's medical center campus in Maywood, Illinois, a suburb 12 miles west of Chicago's lake front. The 200,000 square-foot medical education building includes a variety of contemporary teaching spaces, student life/lounge/study areas, computer facilities, standardized patient center, human simulation center, and administrative offices. A 62,000 square-foot health and fitness center is adjacent to the school. Stritch's curriculum relies on small-group sessions and problem-based learning as much as it does on traditional lectures and labs. Medical students are required to develop particular competencies to the level expected of new physicians entering graduate medical education programs. Students are broadly trained and prepared to undertake advanced training and choose careers in academic medicine, community medicine, and/or research. Faculty members are committed as teachers, mentors, and role models to support the development of these student competencies.

Type: private
2008-2009 total enrollment: 563
Clinical facilities: Loyola University Hospital, Edward Hines Veterans Administration Medical Center, Madden Mental Health Center, Provident Hospital of Cook County, Alexian Brothers Health System, Resurrection Medical Center, MacNeal Hospital, West Suburban Medical Center, Gottlieb Memorial Hospital.

University Officials

President. . . . . Michael J. Garanzini, S.J., Ph.D.
Vice President for the Health Sciences . . . . Paul K. Whelton, M.D.

Medical School Administrative Staff

Dean, Stritch School of Medicine. . . . . John M. Lee, M.D., Ph.D.
Senior Associate Dean, Education Program. . . . . Myles Sheehan, S.J., M.D.
Senior Associate Dean, Research . . . . Richard Kennedy, Ph.D.
Associate Dean, Computers in Education . . . . Arcot J. Chandrasekhar, M.D.
Associate Dean, Educational Affairs . . . . Gregory Gruener, M.D.
Associate Dean, Faculty Administration. . . . . Donna Halinski
Associate Dean, Fiscal Affairs . . . . Cindy Gonya
Associate Dean, Graduate Medical Education . . . . William Cannon, M.D.
Associate Dean, Health Sciences Library. . . . . Logan Ludwig, Ph.D.
Associate Dean, Information Systems . . . . Ron Price, Jr.
Associate Dean, Student Affairs . . . . Teresa Wronski
Associate Dean, Veterans Affairs. . . . . Barbara K. Temeck, M.D.
Assistant Dean, Admissions and Recruitment . . . . Adrian Jones
Assistant Dean, Clinical Education . . . . Paul Hering, M.D.
Assistant Dean, Clinical and Translational Research . . . . Linda Brubaker, M.D.
Assistant Dean, Educational Affairs. . . . . Keith Muccino, S.J., M.D.
Assistant Dean, Comparative Studies. . . . . Lee Cera, D.V.M., Ph.D.
Assistant Dean, Educational Affairs. . . . . Patricia McNally, Ph.D.
Assistant Dean, Student Affairs . . . . Michael Lambesis
Assistant Dean, Student Affairs. . . . . James Mendez
Director, Education Program Administration . . . . Linda Massari
Director, Financial Aid. . . . . Donna Sobie
Director, Registration and Records. . . . . Helene Orloff
Director, Research Services . . . . Jamie Caldwell

Loyola University Chicago Stritch School of Medicine: ILLINOIS

Department and Division or Section Chairs

Basic Sciences

Cell Biology, Neurobiology, and Anatomy . . . . John Clancy, Jr., Ph.D.
Microbiology and Immunology . . . . Katherine Knight, Ph.D.
Pharmacology and Experimental Therapeutics . . . . Tarun Patel, Ph.D.
Physiology . . . . Pieter deTumbe, Ph.D.

Clinical Sciences

Anesthesiology . . . . W. Scott Jellish, M.D., Ph.D.
Family Medicine . . . . Eva Bading, M.D.
Medicine . . . . David Hecht, M.D. (Acting)
    Allergy, Immunology, and Rheumatology . . . . Elaine Adams, M.D.
    Bioethics and Health Policy . . . . Mark Kuczewski, Ph.D.
    Cardiology . . . . David Wilber, M.D.
    Dermatology . . . . James Swan, M.D.
    Endocrinology . . . . Nicholas Emanuele, M.D.
    Gastroenterology . . . . Claus Fimmel, M.D.
    General Internal Medicine . . . . Edward Gurza, M.D.
    Hematology and Oncology . . . . Patrick Stiff, M.D.
    Infectious Disease . . . . David Hecht, M.D.
    Nephrology . . . . Anil Bidani, M.D.
    Pulmonary Disease . . . . Martin Tobin, M.D.
Neurological Surgery . . . . Thomas Origitano, M.D., Ph.D.
Neurology . . . . Jose Biller, M.D.
Obstetrics and Gynecology . . . . John Gianopoulos, M.D.
Ophthalmology . . . . Charles Bouchard, M.D.
Orthopedic Surgery and Rehabilitation . . . . Terry Light, M.D.
Otolaryngology . . . . James Stankiewicz, M.D.
Pathology . . . . Eva Wojcik, M.D.
Pediatrics . . . . Jerold Stirling, M.D.
Preventive Medicine and Epidemiology . . . . Richard Cooper, M.D.
Psychiatry and Behavioral Neurosciences . . . . Angelos Halaris, M.D., Ph.D.
Radiation Oncology . . . . Bahman Emami, M.D.
Radiology . . . . Marc Borge, M.D. (Acting)
Surgery . . . . Richard Gamelli, M.D.
    Emergency Medical Services . . . . Mark Cichon, D.O.
    General Surgery . . . . Steven DeJong, M.D.
    Oral and Maxillofacial Surgery and Dental Medicine . . . . Open
    Peripheral Vascular Surgery . . . . Open
    Plastic and Reconstructive Surgery . . . . Juan Angelats, M.D.
    Surgical Oncology . . . . Margo Shoup, M.D.
    Trauma, Surgical Critical Care, and Burns . . . . Thomas Esposito, M.D.
Thoracic and Cardiovascular Surgery . . . . Mamdouh Bakhos, M.D.
Urology . . . . Robert Flanigan, M.D.

Interdisciplinary Research Institutes and Directors

Burn and Shock Trauma Institute . . . . Richard Gamelli, M.D.
Infectious Disease and Immunology Institute . . David Hecht, M.D., and Katherine Knight, Ph.D.
Leischner Institute for Medical Education . . . . Myles Sheehan, S.J., M.D.
Oncology Institute . . . . Brian Nickoloff, M.D., Ph.D.
Cardiovascular Institute . . . . David Wilber, M.D.
Neiswanger Institute for Bioethics and Health Policy . . . . Mark Kuczewski, Ph.D.
Neuroscience and Aging Institute . . . . Charles Schuster, Ph.D.

Northwestern University
The Feinberg School of Medicine

303 East Chicago Avenue
Chicago, Illinois 60611-3008
312-503-8649 (campus operator); 503-0340 (dean's office);
503-7757 (dean's office fax)
Web site: www.feinberg.northwestern.edu

Northwestern University Feinberg School of Medicine was organized in 1859 as the Medical Department of Lind University. In 1863, it continued under the name of Chicago Medical College. In 1879, the college was affiliated with Northwestern University. Together with the schools of law and continuing education division, the school has been located on the Chicago campus of the university since 1926.

Type: private
2008-2009 total enrollment: 719
Clinical facilities: Children's Memorial Hospital, Evanston Northwestern Healthcare, Northwestern Memorial Hospital, Rehabilitation Institute of Chicago, VA Chicago Health Care System.

University Officials

President. . . . . Henry S. Bienen, Ph.D.
Provost . . . . Daniel H. Linzer, Ph.D.
Senior Vice President, Business and Finance. Eugene S. Sunshine
Vice President for Research and Dean of Graduate Studies . . . . . . Joseph Tonry Walsh, Jr., Ph.D.
Vice President for Medical Affairs. . . . . J. Larry Jameson, M.D., Ph.D.

Medical School Administrative Staff

Dean. . . . . J. Larry Jameson, M.D., Ph.D.
Executive Assistant to the Dean . . . . Kristine Shontz
Vice Dean, Chief Operating Officer . . . . Jeffrey C. Miller
Vice Dean, Chief Academic Officer . . . . Jeffrey L. Glassroth, M.D.
Dean, Clinical Affairs. . . . . Michael Abecassis, M.D.
Dean, Education . . . . Raymond H. Curry, M.D.
Dean, Faculty Affairs . . . . William L. Love, Jr., M.D.
Dean, Research . . . . Rex L. Chisholm, Ph.D.
Senior Associate Dean for Research . . . . Jonathan P. Leis, Ph.D.
Senior Associate Dean for Clinical and Translational Research . . . . Philip Greenland, M.D.
Dean for Medical Development . . . . Katherine Kurtz
Assistant Dean for Education Administration . . . . Heather Winn
Associate Dean, Admissions . . . . Warren H. Wallace, M.D.
Senior Associate Dean for Medical Education . . . . John X. Thomas, Jr., Ph.D.
Senior Associate Dean for Graduate Medical Education . . . . Sharon L. Dooley, M.D.
Associate Dean for Faculty Development. . . . . Linda Van Horn, Ph.D.
Senior Associate Dean, Finance and Budget . . . . Randy J. Wilson
Associate Dean, Minority and Cultural Affairs . . . . John E. Franklin, M.D.
Associate Dean, Research Operations . . . . David Johnson, Ph.D.
Associate Dean, Student Programs and
    Professional Development . . . . Angela Nuzzarello, M.D.
Assistant Dean, Medical Education . . . . Marianne Green, M.D.
Assistant Dean, Alumni Relations . . . . Virginia Darakjian
Director, Finance and Budget . . . . Dieter E. Nevels
Assistant Dean, Management Information Systems. . . . . Jonathan C. Lewis
Director, Continuing Medical Education. . . . . Genevieve Napier
Associate Dean for Strategic Planning and Management . . . . David H. Browdy
Director, Galter Health Sciences Library. . . . . James Shedlock
Assistant Dean, Faculty Affairs . . . . Marcie Weiss
Assistant Dean for Hospital Affairs . . . . Lisa Anastos
Dean for Regulatory Affairs, Chief Compliance Officer . . . . Robert M. Rosa, M.D.
Associate Dean for Faculty Recruitment and
    Professional Development . . . . Rick McGee, Ph.D.
Associate Dean for Clinical Affairs at Jesse
    Brown VA Medical Center . . . . Wendy Weinstock Brown, M.D.
Associate Dean for Clinical Affairs at the RIC . . . . Todd A. Kuiken, M.D., Ph.D.
Associate Dean for Clinical Affairs at CMH. . . . . Edward S. Ogata, M.D.

Associate Dean for Clinical Affairs, Northwestern
  Medical Faculty Foundation .... James L. Schroeder, M.D.
Associate Dean for Clinical Affairs at NMH. .... Charles M. Watts, M.D.
Senior Associate Dean for Administration............................. Rebecca Cooke
Assistant Dean for Clinical Affairs............................. Michael Ruchim, M.D.

Department and Division or Section Chairs

Basic Sciences

Cell and Molecular Biology .... Robert D. Goldman, Ph.D.
Microbiology and Immunology............................. Laimonis Laimins, Ph.D.
Molecular Pharmacology and Biological Chemistry .... Eugene M. Silinsky, Ph.D.
Pathology .... William A. Muller, M.D., Ph.D.
Physiology.. D. James Surmeier, Jr., Ph.D.

Clinical Sciences

Anesthesiology.. M. Christine Stock, M.D.
Dermatology .... Amy Paller, M.D.
Emergency Medicine .... James Adams, M.D.
Family Medicine .... Russell Robertson, M.D.
Medicine... Douglas Vaughan, M.D.
Neurology.. John A. Kessler, M.D.
Neurosurgery... H. Hunt Batjer, M.D.
Obstetrics and Gynecology................................. Sherman Elias, M.D.
Ophthalmology .... Lee M. Jampol, M.D.
Orthopaedic Surgery .... Michael F. Schafer, M.D.
Otolaryngology and Head and Neck Surgery........................ Robert Kern, M.D.
Pediatrics .... Thomas Green, M.D.
Physical Medicine and Rehabilitation .... Elliot J. Roth, M.D.
Physical Therapy and Human Movement Science .... Jules Dewald, Ph.D.
Preventive Medicine........................ Linda Van Horn, Ph.D., R.D. (Interim)
Psychiatry and Behavioral Sciences.......................... John G. Csernansky, M.D.
Radiation Oncology...................................... Bharat B. Mittal, M.D.
Radiology .... Eric J. Russell, M.D.
Surgery .... Nathaniel Soper, M.D.
Urology.. Anthony J. Schaeffer, M.D.

Centers, Institutes, and Special Programs

Buehler Center on Aging, Health, and Society .... Linda Emanuel, M.D., Ph.D.
Center for Bioethics, Science, and Society .... Laurie Zoloth, Ph.D.
Center for Genetic Medicine .... Peter Kopp, Ph.D. (Interim)
Center for the Study of Obesity and Weight Management............. Lewis Landsberg, M.D.
Cognitive Neurology and Alzheimer's Disease Center .... M. Marsel Mesulam, M.D.
Comprehensive AIDS Center .... Steven M. Wolinsky, M.D.
Feinberg Cardiovascular Research Institute.................... Douglas W. Losordo, M.D.
Feinberg Clinical Neurosciences Research Institute.................. John A. Kessler, M.D.
Institute for BioNanotechnology in Medicine .... Sam Stupp, Ph.D.
Institute for Healthcare Studies .... Jane Holl, M.D., M.P.H. (Interim)
Institute for Women's Health Research........................ Teresa K. Woodruff, Ph.D.
Interdepartmental Immunobiology Center .... Stephen D. Miller, Ph.D.
Medical Humanities and Bioethics .... Kathryn K. Montgomery, Ph.D.
Northwestern University Clinical and
  Translational Sciences Institute .... Philip Greenland, M.D.
Northwestern University Interdepartmental
  Neuroscience Program .... John F. Disterhoft, Ph.D.
Robert H. Lurie Comprehensive Cancer Center .... Steven T. Rosen, M.D.

Rush Medical College of Rush University Medical Center

600 South Paulina
Chicago, Illinois 60612
312-942-5000 (general information); 942-6909 (dean's office); 942-2828 (fax)
E-mail: medcol@rush.edu
Web site: www.rush.edu

Rush Medical College was chartered in 1837. The early Rush faculty was involved with other developing institutions in Chicago: St. Luke's Hospital, established in 1864; Presbyterian Hospital, opened at the urging of Rush faculty in 1884; and the University of Chicago, with which Rush Medical College was affiliated and later united from 1898 to 1942. In the early 1940s, Rush discontinued undergraduate education; its faculty continued to teach at the University of Illinois School of Medicine. In 1969, Rush Medical College reactivated its charter and merged with Presbyterian-St. Luke's Hospital, which itself had been formed through merger in 1956, to form Rush-Presbyterian-St. Luke's Medical Center. Rush University, which now includes colleges of medicine, nursing, health sciences, and basic science, was established in 1972. In 2003, the medical center changed its name to Rush University Medical Center.

Type: private
2008-2009 total enrollment: 1,593
Clinical facilities: Rush University Medical Center, including 613-bed hospital serving adults and children and 61-bed rehabilitation and senior care facility; system affiliate Rush Oak Park Hospital with 176 beds. **Other system affiliates:** Rush-Copley Medical Center in Aurora, Rush North Shore Medical Center in Skokie, and Riverside HealthCare in Kankakee. Rush Medical College is the primary medical college for John H. Stroger Jr. Hospital of Cook County.

University Officials

President. . . . . Larry J. Goodman, M.D.
Provost . . . . Thomas A. Deutsch, M.D.
Vice Provost and Vice President of University Affairs. . . . . Lois A. Halstead, R.N., Ph.D.
Associate Provost, Research and Vice President, Research Affairs. . . . . . James L. Mulshine, M.D.
Associate Provost, Student Affairs . . . . Paul Jones, M.D.
Assistant Provost for Community Research . . . . Martha Clare Morris, Sc.D.
Dean, Rush Medical College, and Senior Vice
    President, Medical Affairs . . . . Thomas A. Deutsch, M.D.
College of Nursing. . . . . Melanie C. Dreher, R.N., Ph.D.
Dean, College of Health Sciences. . . . . David C. Shelledy, Ph.D., R.R.T.
Dean, Graduate College. . . . . Paul M. Carvey, Ph.D.
Executive Vice President and Chief Operating Officer. . . . . Peter W. Butler
Senior Vice President, Corporate and Hospital Affairs. . . . . J. Robert Clapp, Jr.
Senior Vice President, Corporate and External Affairs. . . . . Avery Miller
Senior Vice President, Strategic Planning and
    Finance, and Chief Financial Officer and
    Treasurer . . . . Catherine A. Jacobson
Senior Vice President, Information Services, and Chief Information Officer. . . . . . Lac Van Tran
Vice President of Medical Affairs, Clinical
    Practice, and Executive Director, Rush
    University Medical Group . . . . Brian T. Smith
Associate Vice President, Principal Business Officer. . . . . Richard K. Davis
Associate Vice President, University Relations . . . . Mary Katherine Krause

Medical School Administrative Staff

Dean. . . . . Thomas A. Deutsch, M.D.
Associate Dean, Hospital Affairs . . . . David A. Ansell, M.D.
Associate Dean, Medical Sciences and Services . . . . Robert E. Kimura, M.D.
Associate Dean, Surgical Sciences and Services . . . . Keith W. Millikan, M.D.
Associate Dean, Basic Sciences . . . . Paul M. Carvey, Ph.D.
Associate Dean, Medical Student Programs. Susan K. Jacob, Ph.D.
Associate Dean, Postgraduate Education. Harold A. Kessler, M.D.
Associate Dean, Graduate Medical Education . . . . Susan Vanderberg-Dean, M.D.
Associate Dean, Research Development . . . . Joshua J. Jacobs, M.D.

Rush Medical College of Rush University Medical Center: ILLINOIS

Associate Dean, Academic Affiliations . . . . David M. Rothenberg, M.D.
Associate Vice President, Medical Affairs Administration . . . . Richard K. Davis
Director of Admissions . . . . Jill M. Porter, M.S.Ed.
Assistant Dean for Student Development . . . . Mary C. Anderson, M.D.
Assistant Dean for Curricular Innovation . . . . Keith Boyd, M.D.
Assistant Dean, Preclinical Programs . . . . Ada A. Cole, Ph.D.
Assistant Dean for Clinical Curriculum . . . . Robert L. Rosen, M.D.

Department Chairs

Basic Sciences

Anatomy and Cell Biology . . . . R. Dale Sumner, Ph.D.
Behavioral Sciences . . . . Stevan E. Hobfoll, Ph.D.
Biochemistry . . . . Theodore R. Oegema, Jr., Ph.D.
Immunology and Microbiology . . . . Alan L. Landay, Ph.D.
Molecular Biophysics and Physiology . . . . Robert S. Eisenberg, Ph.D.
Pharmacology . . . . Paul M. Carvey, Ph.D.
Preventive Medicine . . . . Lynda H. Powell, Ph.D.

Medical Sciences

Dermatology . . . . Michael D. Tharp, M.D.
Emergency Medicine . . . . Dino Rumoro, D.O. (Acting)
Family Medicine . . . . William A. Schwer, M.D.
Internal Medicine . . . . Stuart Levin, M.D.
Neurological Sciences . . . . Jacob H. Fox, M.D.
Pediatrics . . . . Kenneth M. Boyer, M.D.
Physical Medicine and Rehabilitation . . . . James A. Young, M.D.
Psychiatry . . . . William A. Scheftner, M.D.

Surgical Sciences

Anesthesiology . . . . Kenneth J. Tuman, M.D.
Cardiovascular-Thoracic Surgery . . . . Robert S. D. Higgins, M.D.
Diagnostic Radiology and Nuclear Medicine . . . . David A. Turner, M.D.
General Surgery . . . . Richard A. Prinz, M.D.
Neurosurgery . . . . Richard W. Byrne, M.D.
Obstetrics and Gynecology . . . . Howard T. Strassner, M.D.
Ophthalmology . . . . Kirk H. Packo, M.D.
Orthopedic Surgery . . . . Joshua J. Jacobs, M.D.
Otolaryngology and Bronchoesophagology . . . . David D. Caldarelli, M.D.
Pathology . . . . Robert P. De Cresce, M.D.
Plastic and Reconstructive Surgery . . . . John W. Polley, M.D.
Radiation Oncology . . . . Ross A. Abrams, M.D.
Urology . . . . Charles F. McKiel, Jr., M.D.

Southern Illinois University School of Medicine

801 North Rutledge
P.O. Box 19620
Springfield, Illinois 62794-9620
1-800-342-5748; 217-545-3625 (dean's office); 545-0786 (fax)
Web site: www.siumed.edu

Southern Illinois University School of Medicine was established in 1969. Teaching facilities are located on the campus of Southern Illinois University at Carbondale and Springfield.

Type: public
2008-2009 total enrollment: 288
Clinical facilities: Memorial Medical Center and St. John's Hospital (Springfield), Veterans Affairs Medical Center (Marion).

University Official

Chancellor . . . . Samuel Goldman, Ph.D. (Interim)

Medical School Administrative Staff

Dean and Provost . . . . J. Kevin Dorsey, M.D., Ph.D.
Associate Dean for Graduate Medical Education . . . . Karen Broquet, M.D.
Director of Development . . . . Deborah Case
Director, Cancer Institute . . . . K. Thomas Robbins, M.D.
Associate Dean for Education and Curriculum . . . . Debra Klamen, M.D., M.H.P.E.
Associate Dean for Information Resources . . . . Connie Poole
Associate Dean for Research and Faculty Affairs . . . . Linda Toth, D.V.M., Ph.D.
Associate Dean for Student Affairs . . . . Erik J. Constance, M.D.
Associate Provost for External and Health Affairs . . . . Phillip V. Davis, Ph.D.
Director of Continuing Education . . . . Ann Hamilton
Executive Director for Human Resources . . . . Kay H. Titchenal
Assistant Dean for Institutional Planning and Management Information . . . . Gary Giacomelli
Assistant Dean for Rural and Alumni Affairs . . . . Julie E. Robbs
Assistant Dean for Student Affairs (Minority
    Affairs) and MEDPREP . . . . Harold R. Bardo, Ph.D.
Associate Provost for Finance and Administration . . . . Pamela J. Speer
Comptroller . . . . Robert C. Ross
Director, Laboratory Animal Medicine . . . . Teresa Liberati, Ph.D., D.V.M.
Chief Executive Officer, SIU Physicians and Surgeons . . . . David J. Tkach
Chief Financial Officer and Treasurer, SIU Physicians and Surgeons . . . . Wendy Cox-Largent
Chief Operating Officer, SIU Physicians and Surgeons . . . . Kathryn Mahaffey
Director, Patient Business Services, SIU Physicians and Surgeons . . . . Cheryl McGill
Medical Director, SIU Physicians and Surgeons . . . . Vacant
Executive Director, Capital Planning and Service Operations . . . . Gary Pezall
Assistant Provost, Financial Affairs . . . . Connie Hess
Director, Medical Library . . . . Connie Poole
Director, Communications and Public Relations . . . . Nancy S. Zimmers
Senior Associate Legal Counsels . . . . Virginia Cooper, J.D., and Luke Crater, J.D.

Southern Illinois University School of Medicine: ILLINOIS

Department and Division or Section Chairs

Basic and Clinical Sciences

Center for Alzheimer Disease and Related Disorders . . . . Rodger J. Elble, M.D., Ph.D.
Anatomy . . . . Richard Clough, Ph.D.
Anesthesiology . . . . Reginald Bulkley, M.D.
Family and Community Medicine . . . . Jerry Kruse, M.D.
Information and Communication Sciences . . . . Connie Poole
Internal Medicine . . . . David E. Steward, M.D.
  Cardiology . . . . Frank Aguirre, M.D.
  Dermatology . . . . Jonathan N. Goldfarb, M.D.
  Endocrinology . . . . Romesh Khardori, M.D., Ph.D.
  Gastroenterology . . . . Howard Chodash, M.D.
  General Internal Medicine . . . . Donald Scott, M.D.
  Infectious Diseases . . . . Nancy Khardori, M.D., Ph.D.
  Informatics, Biostatistics, and Research . . . . Vacant
  Medicine and Psychiatry . . . . David S. Resch, M.D.
  Nephrology . . . . Laurence Smith, M.D.
  Oncology . . . . John Godwin, M.D.
  Pulmonary Medicine . . . . Joseph Q. Henkle, M.D.
  Rheumatology . . . . Mark L. Francis, M.D.
Medical Biochemistry . . . . Ramesh Gupta, Ph.D.
Medical Education . . . . Debra L. Klamen, M.D., M.H.P.E.
Medical Humanities . . . . Ross D. Silverman, J.D., M.P.H.
Medical Microbiology and Immunology . . . . Morris D. Cooper, Ph.D.
Neurology . . . . Rodger J. Elble, Jr., M.D., Ph.D.
Obstetrics and Gynecology . . . . J. Ricardo Loret de Mola, M.D.
Pathology . . . . John Murphy, M.D.
Pediatrics . . . . Mark Puczynski, M.D.
Pharmacology . . . . Carl L. Faingold, Ph.D.
Physiology . . . . Richard J. Steger, Ph.D.
Psychiatry . . . . Stephen Soltys, M.D.
  Child Psychiatry . . . . David H. Decker, M.D.
Radiology . . . . Andrew D. Sherrick, M.D.
Surgery . . . . Gary L. Dunnington, M.D.
  Cardiothoracic Surgery . . . . Stephen R. Hazelrigg, M.D.
  General Surgery . . . . Ed Alfrey, M.D.
  Neurosurgery . . . . Jose Espinosa, M.D.
  Orthopedics . . . . D. Gordon Allan, M.D.
  Otolaryngology . . . . Gayle Woodson, M.D.
  Plastic Surgery . . . . Michael Neumeister, M.D.
  Urology . . . . Patrick McKenna, M.D.

Indiana University School of Medicine

340 West 10th Street
Indianapolis, Indiana 46202-3082
317-274-5000 (general information); 274-8157 (dean's office); 274-8439 (fax)
Web site: www.medicine.iu.edu/

The Indiana University School of Medicine was organized in Bloomington in 1903 through a series of mergers of various medical schools. In 1958, the school was consolidated and located at Indianapolis with the exception of a basic medical science program, which remains on the Bloomington campus. In 1971, the school's programs were expanded by the addition of basic medical science programs at Evansville, Fort Wayne, Gary, Lafayette, Muncie, South Bend, and Terre Haute.

Type: public
2008-2009 total enrollment: 1,208
Clinical facilities: Clarian Health Partners, Inc. (Clarian North, Clarian West, Methodist Hospital, Indiana University Hospital, James Whitcomb Riley Hospital for Children), Wishard Health Services, Indianapolis Veterans Affairs Hospital, Larue Carter Memorial Hospital.

University Officials

President. . . . . Michael A. McRobbie, Ph.D.
Vice President and Chancellor (Indianapolis). Charles R. Bantz, Ph.D.

Medical School Administrative Staff

Dean. . . . . D. Craig Brater, M.D.
Executive Associate Dean for Clinical Affairs. John F. Fitzgerald, M.D.
Executive Associate Dean for Educational Affairs . . . . Stephen B. Leapman, M.D.
Executive Associate Dean for Faculty Affairs and
    Professional Development . . . . Stephen P. Bogdewic, Ph.D.
Executive Associate Dean for Research Affairs. . . . . Ora H. Pescovitz, M.D.
Executive Associate Dean for Strategic Planning, Analysis, and Operations. . . . . Open
Associate Dean for Bioethics . . . . Eric M. Meslin, Ph.D.
Associate Dean for Cancer Research. . . . . Stephen D. Williams, M.D.
Associate Dean for Clarian Affairs. . . . . Eric S. Williams, M.D.
Associate Dean for Clinical Research . . . . Rafat Abonour, M.D.
Associate Dean for Continuing Medical Education . . . . Charles M. Clark, Jr., M.D.
Associate Dean for Development . . . . Elizabeth A. Elkas
Associate Dean for Diversity Affairs. . . . . Open
Associate Dean for Graduate Medical Education. . . . . Peter M. Nalin, M.D.
Associate Dean for Graduate Studies . . . . Simon J. Rhodes, Ph.D.
Associate Dean for Health Care Research . . . . Thomas S. Inui, M.D.
Associate Dean for Information Resources and
    Educational Technology . . . . Julie J. McGowan, Ph.D.
Associate Dean for Information Technology . . . . Vincent J. Sheehan
Associate Dean for International Programs . . . . Robert M. Einterz, M.D.
Associate Dean for Medical Education and Curricular Affairs . . . . Debra K. Litzelman, M.D.
Associate Deans for Medical Student Affairs . . . . James J. Brokaw, Ph.D.,
    and Herbert E. Cushing III, M.D.
Associate Dean for Primary Care . . . . John F. Fitzgerald, M.D.
Associate Dean for Research. . . . . Rose S. Fife, M.D.
Associate Dean for Translational Research . . . . Anantha Shekhar, M.B.B.S., Ph.D.
Associate Dean for VA Affairs. . . . . Kenneth E. Klotz, Jr., M.D.
Associate Dean for Wishard Affairs. . . . . Lisa E. Harris, M.D.
Assistant Deans for Faculty Affairs and Professional Development . . . . . Mary E. Dankoski, Ph.D.,
    Lia S. Logio, M.D., and Randy R. Brutkiewicz, Ph.D.
Assistant Dean for Medical Education. . . . . Paula S. Wales, Ed.D.
Assistant Dean for Medical Service-Learning . . . . Open
Assistant Dean and Director, Medical Sciences
    Program (Bloomington) . . . . John B. Watkins III, Ph.D.
Assistant Dean and Director, IUSM–Evansville. . . . . Rex D. Stith, Ph.D.
Assistant Dean and Director, IUSM–Fort Wayne . . . . Fen-Lei F. Chang, M.D., Ph.D.
Assistant Dean and Director, IUSM–Lafayette . . . . Gordon L. Coppoc, Ph.D., D.V.M.
Assistant Dean and Director, IUSM–Muncie . . . . T. Stuart Walker, Ph.D.
Assistant Dean and Director, IUSM–Northwest . . . . Patrick W. Bankston, Ph.D.
Assistant Dean and Director, IUSM–South Bend . . . . Rudolph M. Navari, M.D., Ph.D.
Assistant Dean and Director, IUSM–Terre Haute . . . . Taihung Duong, Ph.D.
Director of Admissions. . . . . Robert M. Stump, Jr.

Director of Graduate Medical Education. . . . . Nancy J. Baxter

Department and Division or Section Chairs

Basic Sciences

Anatomy and Cell Biology . . . . David B. Burr, Ph.D.
Biochemistry and Molecular Biology. . . . . Zhong-Yin Zhang, Ph.D.
Cellular and Integrative Physiology. . . . . Michael S. Sturek, Ph.D.
Microbiology and Immunology. . . . . Hal E. Broxmeyer, Ph.D.
Pharmacology and Toxicology . . . . Michael R. Vasko, Ph.D.

Clinical Sciences

Anesthesia. . . . . John F. Butterworth IV, M.D.
Dermatology . . . . Jeffrey B. Travers, M.D., Ph.D.
Emergency Medicine . . . . Roland B. McGrath, M.D.
Family Medicine . . . . Douglas B. McKeag, M.D.
Medical and Molecular Genetics. . . . . Kenneth G. Cornetta, M.D.
Medicine. . . . . David W. Crabb, M.D.
   Biostatistics . . . . Barry P. Katz, Ph.D.
   Cardiology. . . . . Peng-Sheng Chen, M.D.
   Clinical Pharmacology . . . . David A. Flockhart, M.D., Ph.D.
   Endocrinology and Metabolism. . . . . Michael J. Econs, M.D.
   Gastroenterology and Hepatology. . . . . Naga P. Chalasani, M.B.B.S.
   General Internal Medicine and Geriatrics . . . . Greg A. Sachs, M.D.
   Hematology and Oncology. . . . . Patrick J. Loehrer, M.D.
   Infectious Diseases . . . . Stanley M. Spinola, M.D.
   Nephrology . . . . Bruce A. Molitoris, M.D.
   Pulmonary and Critical Care Medicine . . . . Homer L. Twigg III, M.D.
   Rheumatology . . . . Rafael G. Grau, M.D.
Neurological Surgery. . . . . Paul B. Nelson, M.D.
Neurology . . . . Robert M. Pascuzzi, M.D.
Obstetrics and Gynecology. . . . . Lee A. Learman, M.D., Ph.D.
Ophthalmology . . . . Robert D. Yee, M.D.
Orthopaedic Surgery . . . . Jeffrey O. Anglen, M.D.
Otolaryngology-Head and Neck Surgery . . . . Richard T. Miyamoto, M.D.
Pathology and Laboratory Medicine. . . . . John N. Eble, M.D.
Pediatrics . . . . Richard L. Schreiner, M.D.
   Adolescent Medicine . . . . Donald P. Orr, M.D.
   Cardiology. . . . . Randall L. Caldwell, M.D.
   Child Development . . . . John D. Rau, M.D.
   Developmental Pediatrics . . . . Gregory A. Wilson, M.D.
   Endocrinology and Diabetes. . . . . Erica A. Eugster, M.D.
   Gastroenterology . . . . Jean P. Molleston, M.D.
   General and Community Pediatrics. . . . . Stephen M. Downs, M.D.
   Health Services Research . . . . Stephen M. Downs, M.D.
   Hematology and Oncology. . . . . Robert J. Fallon, M.D., Ph.D.
   Infectious Diseases . . . . John C. Christenson, M.D.
   Neonatal and Perinatal Medicine . . . . James A. Lemons, M.D.
   Nephrology . . . . Sharon P. Andreoli, M.D.
   Pulmonary Disease . . . . Howard Eigen, M.D.
   Rheumatology . . . . Suzanne L. Bowyer, M.D.
Physical Medicine and Rehabilitation . . . . Ralph M. Buschbacher, M.D.
Psychiatry . . . . Christopher J. McDougle, M.D.
Public Health . . . . Gregory A. Wilson, M.D. (Acting)
Radiation Oncology. . . . . Peter A. S. Johnstone, M.D.
Radiology . . . . Valerie P. Jackson, M.D.
Surgery. . . . . Keith D. Lillemoe, M.D.
   Cardiothoracic Surgery. . . . . John W. Brown, M.D.
   General Surgery. . . . . Eric A. Wiebke, M.D.
   Pediatric Surgery . . . . Frederick J. Rescorla, M.D.
   Plastic Surgery . . . . John J. Coleman III, M.D.
   Transplant Surgery. . . . . A. Joseph Tector, M.D., Ph.D.
   Vascular Surgery. . . . . Michael C. Dalsing, M.D.
Urology. . . . . Michael O. Koch, M.D.

University of Iowa Roy J. and Lucille A. Carver College of Medicine

200 Medicine Administration Building
Iowa City, Iowa 52242-1101
319-335-8053 (admissions/student aff.); 319-384-4547 (dean's office);
319-335-8049 (fax-admissions/student aff.); 319-353-5617 (fax-dean's office)
Web site: www.medicine.uiowa.edu

The University of Iowa Roy J. and Lucille A. Carver College of Medicine originated as the Medical Department of the University of Iowa in 1850. In 1870, the medical department was moved from Keokuk to the campus at Iowa City and became known as the University of Iowa College of Medicine. In 2002, the Carver name was adopted in honor of a landmark gift to the college.

Type: public
2008-2009 total enrollment: 476
Clinical facilities: University of Iowa Hospitals and Clinics, Veterans Affairs Medical Center (Iowa City); St. Luke's Hospital, Mercy Medical Center (Cedar Rapids); Genesis Medical Center (Davenport); Broadlawns Medical Center, Iowa Lutheran Hospital, Iowa Methodist Medical Center, Veterans Affairs Medical Center (Des Moines); Mercy Medical Center-North Iowa (Mason City); Mercy Medical Center-Sioux City; St. Luke's Regional Medical Center (Sioux City); Allen Memorial Hospital, Covenant Medical Center (Waterloo).

University Officials

President	Sally Mason
Provost	William D. Loh
Vice President for Finance and University Services	Douglas K. True
Vice President for Research	Jordan L. Cohen, Ph.D. (Interim)
Vice President for Medical Affairs	Jean E. Robillard, M.D.

Medical School Administrative Staff

Dean	Paul B. Rothman, M.D.
Executive Dean	Peter Densen, M.D.
Senior Associate Dean for Scientific Affairs	Michael A. Apicella, M.D.
Associate Dean, Student Affairs and Curriculum	Christopher Cooper, M.D.
Associate Dean, Veterans Affairs	John S. Cowdery, M.D.
Associate Dean, Faculty Affairs	Lois J. Geist, M.D.
Associate Dean for Communications and Advancement	Steven Maravetz
Associate Dean, Finance and Administration	Patrick A. Thompson
Assistant Dean for Facilities Planning and Management	James Henderson
Assistant Dean, Student Affairs and Curriculum	Thomas Schmidt, Ph.D.
Assistant Dean, Student Affairs and Curriculum and Director of Admissions	Catherine Solow
Assistant Dean and Director, Office of Statewide Clinical Education Programs	Roger D. Tracy
Assistant Dean, Research and Graduate Programs	S. Ramaswamy
Assistant Vice President for Health Policy	Stacey T. Cyphert, Ph.D.
Associate Dean for Diversity	Benita D. Wolff

Department and Division or Section Chairs

Basic Sciences

Anatomy and Cell Biology	John F. Engelhardt, Ph.D.
Biochemistry	John E. Donelson, Ph.D.
Microbiology	Michael A. Apicella, M.D.
Molecular Physiology and Biophysics	Kevin P. Campbell, Ph.D.
Pharmacology	Donna Hammond, Ph.D. (Interim)

Clinical Sciences

Anesthesia	Michael M. Todd, M.D.
Cardiothoracic Surgery	Mark D. Iannettoni, M.D.
Dermatology	Janet Fairley, M.D.
Emergency Medicine	Eric W. Dickson, M.D.
Family Medicine	Paul A. James, M.D.
Internal Medicine	Jeffrey Field, M.D.
Allergy and Immunology	Zuhair K. Ballas, M.D.
Cardiovascular Diseases	Mark Anderson, M.D.

University of Iowa Roy J. and Lucille A. Carver College of Medicine: IOWA

Clinical Pharmacology .... William G. Haynes, M.B., Ch.B., M.D.
Endocrinology and Metabolism.............................. William Sivitz, M.D.
Gastroenterology and Hepatology.......................... Bruce Luxon, M.D., Ph.D.
General Medicine, Clinical Epidemiology, and
   Health Services Research .... Gary E. Rosenthal, M.D.
Hematology and Oncology.......................... Steven R. Lentz, M.D., Ph.D.
Infectious Diseases .... Jack T. Stapleton, M.D.
Nephrology .... John B. Stokes III, M.D.
Pulmonary Diseases .... Joseph Zabner, M.D. (Interim)
Rheumatology .... Geordie Lawry, M.D. (Interim)
Neurology.. Robert L. Rodnitzky, M.D.
Neurosurgery.. Matthew A. Howard III, M.D.
Obstetrics and Gynecology............................... Jennifer R. Niebyl, M.D.
Ophthalmology and Visual Sciences......................... Keith Carter, M.D.
Orthopaedics and Rehabilitation .... Joseph A. Buckwalter, M.D.
Otolaryngology-Head and Neck Surgery.................... Bruce J. Gantz, M.D.
Pathology .... Michael B. Cohen, M.D.
Pediatrics .... Michael Artman, M.D.
   Allergy and Pulmonary.......................... Miles M. Weinberger, M.D.
   Cardiology.. Thomas Scholz, M.D.
   Child Psychology .... Lynn C. Richman, Ph.D.
   Critical Care.. Fred S. Lamb, M.D., Ph.D.
   Developmental and Behavioral Medicine...................... Stacy McConkey, M.D.
   Endocrinology and Diabetes............................. Eva Tsalikian, M.D.
   Gastroenterology .... Warren P. Bishop, M.D.
   General Pediatrics and Adolescent Medicine................. Jerold C. Woodhead, M.D.
   Genetics.................................... Val C. Sheffield, M.D., Ph.D.
   Hematology, Oncology, and Rheumatology........... Raymond Tannous, M.D. (Interim)
   Infectious Diseases .... Charles Grose, M.D.
   Neonatology... Jeffrey Segar, M.D.
   Nephrology and Hypertension .... Patrick Brophy, M.D., Ph.D.
   Neurology.. Katherine D. Mathews, M.D.
   Nutrition/Metabolism........................... Michael Artman, M.D. (Interim)
   Specialized Child Health Services .... Brian Wilkes, M.D.
Psychiatry .... Robert G. Robinson, M.D.
Radiation Oncology.................................... John Buatti, M.D.
Radiology .... Laurie L. Fajardo, M.D.
   Nuclear Medicine.................... Michael M. Graham, M.D., Ph.D. (Div. Dir.)
Surgery .... Ronald J. Weigel, M.D.
   Gastrointestinal, Minimally Invasive and Bariatric........................ Open
   Pediatric Surgery .... Joel Shilyansky, M.D.
   Plastic and Reconstructive Surgery .... Open
   Surgical Oncology and Endocrine Surgery.................. James R. Howe, V, M.D.
   Transplant Surgery.................................. Alan Reed, M.D.
   Trauma, Critical Care, and Burn Surgery .... G. Patrick Kealey, M.D.
   Vascular Surgery................................... Jamal J. Hoballah, M.D.
Urology.. Richard D. Williams, M.D.

College of Public Health

Dean.. James A. Merchant, M.D., Dr.P.H.
Associate Dean for Research and Academic Affairs .... Leon F. Burmeister, Ph.D.
Associate Dean for Education and Student Affairs........... Tanya M. Uden-Holman, Ph.D.
Associate Dean for Public Health Practice...................... Christopher G. Atchison
Associate Dean for Diversity................................. Joe D. Coulter, Ph.D.
Assistant Dean and Director of the Master of
   Public Health Program .... Mary L. Aquilino, Ph.D.
Biostatistics .... Kathryn M. Chaloner, Ph.D.
Community and Behavioral Health .... Linda Snetselaar, Ph.D.
Epidemiology.................................... James C. Torner, Ph.D.
Health Management and Policy .... Barry R. Greene, Ph.D.
Occupational and Environmental Health................. Craig S. Zwerling, M.D., Ph.D.

University of Kansas School of Medicine

3901 Rainbow Boulevard
Kansas City, Kansas 66160-7300
913-588-5200 (general information); 588-5287 (executive dean); 588-7222 (fax)
Web site: www.kumc.edu/som/

The University of Kansas established a "preparatory medical course" in 1880, and began to offer a four-year medical curriculum in 1906. The school of medicine is part of the University of Kansas Medical Center, which began to develop its current site in Kansas City, Kansas, in 1924. In 1971, the school of medicine established a campus in Wichita, where a portion of each class receives its clinical training in the last two years.

Type: public
2008-2009 total enrollment: 706
Clinical facilities: University of Kansas Hospital, Research Medical Center, Geary Community Hospital, St. Joseph Hospital, Wesley Hospital, Via Christi Hospital, Veteran Administration Centers (Kansas City, Missouri; Leavenworth; Topeka; Wichita).

University Officials

Chancellor . . . . Robert Hemenway, Ph.D.
Executive Vice Chancellor . . . . Barbara F. Atkinson, M.D.
Chief of Staff. . . . . Shelley Gebar
Senior Vice Chancellor for Academic and Student Affairs . . . . Karen Miller, Ph.D.
Vice Chancellor for Academic Affairs . . . . Allen Rawitch, Ph.D.
Vice Chancellor for Administration . . . . H. Edward Phillips
Vice Chancellor for Research . . . . Paul Terranova, Ph.D.
Vice Chancellor for External Affairs . . . . David Adkins, J.D.

Medical School Administrative Staff

Executive Dean . . . . Barbara F. Atkinson, M.D.
Vice Dean . . . . Vacant
Senior Associate Dean for Clinical Affairs . . . . Douglas A. Girod, M.D.
Senior Associate Dean for Finance . . . . Kimberly A. Meyer, Ph.D.
Senior Associate Dean for Operations and Administration. . . . . Shelly Gebar
Senior Associate Dean for Research and Graduate Studies. . . . . Paul Terranova, Ph.D.
Associate Dean for Graduate Medical Education . . . . Timothy Bennett, M.D.
Associate Dean for Student Affairs . . . . Mark Meyer, M.D.
Associate Dean for Cultural Enhancement and Diversity . . . . Patricia Thomas, M.D.
Associate Dean for Medical Graduate Studies . . . . Jared Grantham, M.D.
Associate Dean for Admissions . . . . Sandra J. McCurdy
Associate Dean for Continuing Medical Education . . . . Joseph L. Kyner, M.D.
Associate Dean for Medical Education . . . . Giulia A. Bonaminio, Ph.D.
Associate Dean for Academic Affairs. . . . . Robert Klein, Ph.D.

Department and Division or Section Chairs

Basic Sciences

Anatomy and Cell Biology . . . . Dale Abrahamson, Ph.D.
Biochemistry and Molecular Biology. . . . . Gerald Carlson, Ph.D.
Cancer Institute. . . . . Roy Jensen, M.D.
Health Policy and Management . . . . Glendon C. Cox, M.D.
History of Medicine. . . . . Christopher Crenner, M.D.
Microbiology, Molecular Genetics, and Immunology . . . . Michael J. Parmely, Ph.D. (Interim)
Molecular and Integrative Physiology . . . . Paul D. Cheney, Ph.D.
Pathology and Laboratory Medicine . . . . Patricia A. Thomas, M.D.
Pharmacology, Toxicology, and Therapeutics . . . . Curtis D. Klaassen, Ph.D.
Preventive Medicine. . . . . Edward F. Ellerbeck, M.D.

Clinical Sciences

Anesthesiology. . . . . James D. Kindscher, M.D.
Family Medicine . . . . Joshua Freeman, M.D.
Medicine. . . . . Steven Stites, M.D.
Neurology. . . . . Richard Barohn, M.D.
Obstetrics and Gynecology. . . . . Carl Weiner, M.D.
Ophthalmology . . . . John Sutphin, M.D.
Otolaryngology . . . . Douglas Girod, M.D.
Pediatrics . . . . Chet Johnson, M.D.
Psychiatry and Behavioral Sciences. . . . . : . . . . William Gabrielli, M.D., Ph.D.
Radiation Oncology. . . . . Eashwer Reddy, M.D. (Interim)
Radiology . . . . Stanton J. Rosenthal, M.D.
Rehabilitation Medicine. . . . . George Varghese, M.D.
Surgery . . . . James Thomas, M.D.
Surgery Neurological. . . . . John Grant, M.D.
Surgery Orthopedic. . . . . Bruce Toby, M.D.
Surgery Urological. . . . . Brantley Thrasher, M.D.

University of Kansas School of Medicine
Wichita Campus
1010 North Kansas
Wichita, Kansas 67214
316-261-2600 (dean's office)

Dean. . . . . S. Edward Dismuke, M.D.
Associate Dean, Academic and Student Affairs . . . . Garold Minns, M.D.
Associate Dean for Administration . . . . Janice Arbuckle
Associate Dean for Graduate Medical Education. . . . . Donald Brada, M.D.
Associate Dean for Faculty Development. . . . . Anne Walling, M.D.
Associate Dean for Research. . . . . David Grainger, M.D.

Department Chairs

Anesthesiology. . . . . Robert McKay, M.D.
Family and Community Medicine. . . . . Rick Kellerman, M.D.
Internal Medicine . . . . Jon P. Schrage, M.D.
Obstetrics and Gynecology. . . . . Douglas Horbelt, M.D.
Pathology . . . . Joe J. Lin, M.D.
Preventive Medicine and Public Health . . . . Douglas D. Bradham, M.D,
Pediatrics . . . . Robert R. Wittler, M.D.
Psychiatry . . . . Russell Scheffer, M.D.
Radiology . . . . David Brake, M.D.
Surgery . . . . Alex Ammar, M.D.

University of Kentucky College of Medicine

138 Leader Avenue
Lexington, Kentucky 40506-9983
859-323-5000; 323-6582 (dean's office); 323-2039 (fax)
Web site: www.mc.uky.edu/medicine

The college of medicine opened in September 1960. It is one of the units of the University of Kentucky A.B. Chandler Medical Center, which also includes the colleges of dentistry, health sciences, public health, nursing, and pharmacy; the University Hospital; Kentucky Clinic, with its off-site facilities; the Medical Center Library; and the University Student Health Service.

Type: public
2008-2009 total enrollment: 430
Clinical facilities: Primary: UK Chandler Hospital, the Kentucky Clinic and its off-site facilities, The Center for Rural Health, The Markey Cancer Center, The Gill Heart Institute, and the Veterans Affairs Medical Center. **Additionally:** Appalachian Regional Medical Center, Central Baptist Hospital, Cardinal Hill Rehabilitiation Hospital, Ridge Behavioral Health System, Eastern State Hospital, Samaritan Hospital, Shriner's Hospital for Crippled Children, St. Claire Regional Medical Center, and Rockcastle Hospital and Respiratory Care Center.

University Officials

President	Lee T. Todd, Jr., Ph.D.
Provost	Kumble Subbaswamy, Ph.D.
Vice President for Research	James W. Tracy, Ph.D.

Medical Center Campus Officials

Executive Vice President for Health Affairs	Michael Karpf, M.D.
Vice President for Clinical Affairs	Jay A. Perman, M.D.
Director of Institutional Affairs	Frank A. Butler
Vice Provost for Budget and Administrative Services	Karen T. Combs
Vice President of Health Care Operations and Chief Clinical Officer	Richard P. Lofgren, M.D.
Senior Vice President for Health Affairs and Chief Financial Officer	Sergio Melgar
Chief Medical Officer	Paul DePriest, M.D.
Associate Vice President for Clinical Network Development	Joseph O. Claypool
Associate Vice President for Information Technology	Zed Day
Associate Vice President for Medical Center Operations	Murray Clark
Director of Strategic Marketing	Bill Gombeski
Chief Development Officer	Vicky Myers
Director, Medical Center Library	Janet Stith
Director, University Student Health Services	Gregory R. Moore, M.D.

Medical School Administrative Staff

Dean	Jay A. Perman, M.D.
Senior Associate Dean for Basic Science Affairs	Louis B. Hersh, Ph.D.
Senior Associate Dean for Medical Education	C. Darrell Jennings, M.D.
Senior Associate Dean for Clinical Affairs	Open
Senior Associate Dean for Research	Open
Associate Dean for AHEC, and Community Outreach	James C. Norton, Ph.D.
Associate Dean for Administration and Finance	Peter N. Gilbert
Associate Dean for Admissions and Institutional Advancement	Carol L. Elam, Ed.D.
Assistant Dean for Student Affairs	Todd R. Cheever, M.D.
Assistant Dean of Curriculum	David W. Rudy, M.D.
Assistant Dean for Student Assessment and Program Evaluation	Terry D. Stratton, Ph.D.
Assistant Dean of Graduate Medical Education	Susan McDowell, M.D.
Assistant Dean for Administration	Sandra Jaros
Senior Assistant Dean for Graduate Education and Administration	Jane Serumgard Harrison, Ph.D.
Manager for Clinical Contracting and Special Projects	Jennifer Collins
Budget Director	Patricia Polly
Director of Development	Richard McKenzie
Associate Director of Alumni and Development	Open

University of Kentucky College of Medicine: KENTUCKY

Chief of Staff. . . . . Julane Hamon

Institute/Center Directors

Lucille P. Markey Cancer Center . . . . Robert Means, M.D. (Interim)
MRI and Spectroscopy Center . . . . Don M. Gash, Ph.D.
Linda and Jack Gill Heart Institute. Victor A. Ferraris, M.D., Ph.D., and David J. Moliterno, M.D.
Center for the Advancement of Women's Health . . . . Leslie Crofford, M.D.
Multidisciplinary Research Center for Drug and Alcohol Abuse. . . . . . Carl G. Leukefeld, D.S.W.
Sanders-Brown Center on Aging. . . . . William R. Markesbery, M.D.
Spinal Cord and Brain Injury Research Center . . . . Edward H. Hall, Ph.D.
University of Kentucky Center on Rural Health. . . . . Baretta Casey, M.D.
Cardiovascular Research Center . . . . Alan Daugherty, M.D.

Department and Division or Section Chairs

Basic Health Sciences

Anatomy and Neurobiology . . . . Don M. Gash, Ph.D.
Behavioral Science. . . . . Carl G. Leukefeld, D.S.W.
Graduate Center for Nutritional Science. . . . . Lisa Cassis, Ph.D.
Graduate Center for Toxicology. . . . . Mary Vore, Ph.D.
Molecular and Cellular Biochemistry . . . . Louis B. Hersh, Ph.D.
Microbiology, Immunology, and Molecular Genetics. . . . . Alan M. Kaplan, Ph.D.
Molecular and Biomedical Pharmacology . . . . Philip S. Landfield, Ph.D.
Physiology and Biophysics . . . . Michael B. Reid, Ph.D.

Clinical Sciences

Anesthesiology. . . . . Edwin A. Bowe, M.D.
Diagnostic Radiology . . . . Open
Emergency Medicine . . . . Roger L. Humphries, M.D.
Family and Community Medicine . . . . Samuel C. Matheny, M.D.
Medicine. . . . . Frederick C. deBeer, M.D.
   Allergy, Immunology, and Rheumatology . . . . Beth Miller, M.D.
   Cardiology. . . . . David Moliterno, M.D.
   Endocrinology . . . . Lisa Tannock, M.D.
   Gastroenterology . . . . Willem de Villiers, M.D.
   General Medicine and Geriatrics. . . . . T. Shawn Caudill, M.D.
   Hematology. . . . . Kevin McDonagh, M.D.
   Infectious Disease. . . . . Beth Miller, M.D. (Interim)
   Molecular Medicine and Endocrinology . . . . Frederick C. deBeer, M.D.
   Nephrology . . . . Hartmut H. Malluche, M.D.
   Pulmonary Disease . . . . James McCormick, M.D.
   Rheumatology and Women's Health . . . . Leslie Crofford, M.D.
Neurology. . . . . Joseph R. Berger, M.D.
Neurosurgery. . . . . A. Byron Young, M.D.
Obstetrics and Gynecology. . . . . James E. Ferguson II, M.D.
Ophthalmology . . . . Andrew Pearson, M.D.
Orthopaedic Surgery . . . . Darren L. Johnson, M.D.
Pathology . . . . Paul Bachner, M.D.
Pediatrics . . . . Timothy Bricker, M.D.
Psychiatry . . . . Lon R. Hays, M.D.
Radiation Medicine . . . . Marcus E. Randall, M.D.
Rehabilitation Medicine. . . . . Gerald V. Klim, M.D.
Surgery. . . . . Joseph B. Zwischenberger, M.D.
   Cardiothoracic Surgery. . . . . Mark Plankett, M.D.
   General Surgery. . . . . Patrick McGrath, M.D.
   Otolaryngology-Head and Neck Surgery . . . . Raleigh O. Jones, M.D.
   Pediatric Surgery . . . . Andrew R. Pulito, M.D.
   Plastic Surgery . . . . Henry C. Vasconez, M.D.
   Transplantation . . . . Dinesh Ranjan, M.D.
   Urology. . . . . Stephen E. Strup, M.D.

*Specialty without organizational autonomy.

University of Louisville School of Medicine

Health Sciences Center
Abell Administration Center, 323 East Chestnut Street
Louisville, Kentucky 40202
502-852-1499 (dean's office); 852-1484 (fax); 852-5555 (general information)
Web site: www.louisville.edu/medschool

Medical education in Louisville began on February 2, 1833, with the granting of a charter for the Louisville Medical Institute. The medical school is part of the health sciences center.

Type: public
2008-2009 total enrollment: 600
Clinical facilities: University of Louisville Hospital, Kosair Children's Hospital, Veterans Administration Medical Center, James Graham Brown Cancer Center. **Other affiliates:** The Bingham Child Guidance Clinic Inc., Central State Hospital, Norton Audubon Hospital, Frazier Rehabilitation Center, Jewish Hospital, Norton Hospital, Portland Family Health Center, Trover Campus (Madisonville).

University Officials

President. . . . . James R. Ramsey, Ph.D.
Executive Vice President for Health Affairs. . . . . Larry N. Cook, M.D.

Medical School Administrative Staff

Dean. . . . . Edward C. Halperin, M.D.
Vice Dean for Academic Affairs and Associate Vice President . . . . David L. Wiegman, Ph.D.
Vice Dean for Clinical Affairs. . . . . Vacant
Vice Dean for Research . . . . Russell A. Prough, Ph.D.
Senior Associate Dean for Student and Academic Affairs. . . . . Toni M. Ganzel, M.D.
Associate Dean for Admissions . . . . Stephen Wheeler, M.D.
Associate Dean for Faculty Affairs. . . . . Tracy D. Eells, Ph.D.
Associate Dean for Graduate Medical Education . . . . John L. Roberts, M.D.
Associate Dean for Medical Education . . . . Ruth Greenberg, Ph.D.
Associate Dean for Research. . . . . Peter Rowell, Ph.D.
Associate Dean for Trover Campus. . . . . William J. Crump, M.D.
Associate Dean for Minority and Rural Affairs. . . . . V. Faye Jones, M.D.
Assistant Dean, Continuing Health Sciences Education . . . . Sharon Whitmer, Ed.D.
Assistant Dean, Liaison, University Hospital . . . . Kristine Krueger, M.D.
Director of Administration and Finance . . . . Terry D. Gossom

Institute/Center Directors

Center for Health Hazard Preparedness . . . Ronald M. Atlas, Ph.D., and Richard D. Clover, M.D.
Center for Genetics and Molecular Medicine . . . . Kenneth S. Ramos, Ph.D.
Gheens Center on Aging . . . . Eugenia Wang, Ph.D.
Institute for Bioethics, Health Policy, and Law . . . . Mark A. Rothstein, J.D.
Institute for Cellular Therapeutics . . . . Suzanne T. Ildstad, M.D.
Institute for Molecular Cardiology . . . . Roberto Bolli, M.D.
James Graham Brown Cancer Center . . . . Donald M. Miller, M.D., Ph.D.
Jewish Hospital Cardiothoracic Surgical Research Institute . . . . Laman A. Gray, Jr., M.D.
Kentucky Spinal Cord Injury Research Center. . . . . Scott R. Whittemore, Ph.D.
Kosair Children's Hospital Research Institute . . . . David Gozal, M.D.
Outcomes Research Institute . . . . Daniel I. Sessler, M.D.
Price Institute for Surgical Research. . . . . Susan Galandiuk, M.D.
University of Louisville Birth Defects Center. . . . . Robert M. Greene, Ph.D.
Center for Cancer Nursing Education and Research . . . . Vacant
Cardiovascular Innovation Institute. . . . . Stuart Williams, Ph.D.

Department and Division or Section Chairs

Basic Sciences

Anatomical Sciences and Neurobiology. . . . . Fred J. Roisen, Ph.D.
Biochemistry and Molecular Biology. . . . . William L. Dean, Ph.D. (Acting)
Microbiology and Immunology. . . . . Robert D. Stout, Ph.D.
Pathology and Laboratory Medicine . . . . Ronald J. Elin, M.D., Ph.D.
Pharmacology and Toxicology . . . . David W. Hein, Ph.D.
Physiology and Biophysics . . . . Irving G. Joshua, Ph.D.

Clinical Sciences

Anesthesiology and Perioperative Medicine. . . . . Gary Loyd, M.D. (Acting)
Emergency Medicine . . . . Daniel F. Danzl, M.D.

Family and Geriatric Medicine . . . . James G. O'Brien, M.D.
Medicine . . . . Richard N. Redinger, M.D.
   Cardiology . . . . Roberto Bolli, M.D.
   Dermatology . . . . Jeffrey P. Callen, M.D.
   Endocrinology and Metabolism . . . . Stephen J. Winters, M.D.
   Gastroenterology and Hepatology . . . . Richard A. Wright, M.D.
   General Internal Medicine, Geriatrics, and Health Policy Research . . . . Monica Shaw, M.D.
   Infectious Diseases . . . . Julio A. Ramirez, M.D.
   Medical Oncology and Hematology . . . . Donald M. Miller, M.D., Ph.D.
   Nephrology . . . . George R. Aronoff, M.D.
   Pulmonary, Critical Care, and Environmental Medicine . . . . Rodney Folz, M.D., Ph.D.
   Rheumatology . . . . Michael J. Edwards, M.D. (Acting)
Neurological Surgery . . . . Christopher B. Shields, M.D.
Neurology . . . . Kerri Remmel, M.D. (Acting)
Obstetrics, Gynecology, and Women's Health . . . . Christine L. Cook, M.D.
   Endocrinology . . . . Steven T. Nakajima, M.D.
   General Gynecology . . . . James Shwayder, M.D.
   Family Planning and Outpatient Clinic Director . . . . Elaine Stauble, M.D.
   Maternal and Fetal Medicine . . . . Vacant
   Pediatric and Adolescent Gynecology . . . . Paige Hertweck, M.D.
   Oncology . . . . Lynn Parker, M.D.
   Urogynecology . . . . Susan B. Tate, M.D.
Ophthalmology and Visual Sciences . . . . Henry J. Kaplan, M.D.
Orthopedic Surgery . . . . John R. Johnson, M.D.
Pediatrics . . . . Gerard P. Rabalais, M.D.
   Adolescent and Rheumatology . . . . Kenneth N. Schikler, M.D.
   Allergy and Immunology . . . . James L. Sublett, M.D.
   Ambulatory and General Pediatrics . . . . Sofia Franco, M.D. (Acting)
   Cardiology . . . . Christopher L. Johnsrude, M.D. (Acting)
   Child Behavior and Evaluation and Genetics . . . . Joseph H. Hersh, M.D.
   Critical Care . . . . Vicki L. Montgomery, M.D.
   Emergency Pediatrics . . . . Ronald I. Paul, M.D.
   Endocrinology . . . . Michael Foster, M.D. (Acting)
   Forensic Medicine . . . . Melissa L. Currie, M.D.
   Gastroenterology . . . . Thomas C. Stephen, M.D.
   Hematology and Oncology . . . . Salvatore J. Bertolone, M.D.
   Infectious Diseases . . . . Gary Marshall, M.D.
   International Pediatrics . . . . George Rodgers, M.D., Ph.D.
   Neonatology . . . . David H. Adamkin, M.D.
   Nephrology . . . . Lawrence R. Shoemaker, M.D.
   Pathology . . . . John J. Buchino, M.D.
   Pulmonary and Cystic Fibrosis . . . . Nemr S. Eid, M.D.
   Sleep Medicine . . . . David Gozal, M.D. (Acting)
Physical Medicine and Rehabilitation . . . . Kenneth Mook, M.D.
Psychiatry and Behavioral Sciences . . . . Allan Tasman, M.D.
   Children and Adolescents . . . . Allan M. Josephson, M.D.
   Adult Psychiatry . . . . Kathy Vincent, M.D.
Radiation Oncology . . . . William J. Spanos, M.D.
Radiology . . . . Gregory C. Postel, M.D.
Surgery . . . . Kelly M. McMasters, M.D., Ph.D.
   Audiology . . . . Ian Windmill, Ph.D.
   Colon-Rectal Surgery . . . . Susan Galandiuk, M.D.
   Endoscopy . . . . Gary C. Vitale, M.D.
   General . . . . Frank B. Miller, M.D.
   Hand Surgery . . . . Joseph Kutz, M.D.
   Oncology . . . . Robert C. Martin, M.D.
   Otolaryngology . . . . Jeffrey M. Bumpous, M.D.
   Pediatric . . . . Mary E. Fallat, M.D.
   Plastic and Reconstructive . . . . Bradon Wilhelmi, M.D.
   Speech Pathology . . . . Barbara Baker, Ph.D.
   Thoracic and Cardiovascular . . . . Mark Slaughter, M.D.
Urology . . . . Anthony Casale, M.D.

Louisiana State University Health Sciences Center
School of Medicine in New Orleans
2020 Gravier Street
New Orleans, Louisiana 70112-2822
504-568-4007 (dean's office); 568-4008 (fax)
Web site: www.medschool.lsuhsc.edu

The Louisiana State University School of Medicine in New Orleans was established on October 1, 1931. The main campus of the parent university, Louisiana State University, is located in Baton Rouge. The school of medicine is one of five professional schools in the Louisiana State University Health Sciences Center.

Type: public
2008-2009 total enrollment: 710
Clinical facilities: LSU Hospitals: Medical Center of Louisiana (Charity and University Hospitals), Earl K. Long Hospital (Baton Rouge), University Medical Center (Lafayette), LSU Clinics; Children's Hospital; Touro Infirmary; Veterans Administration Hospital; Ochsner Foundation Hospital; Kenner Regional Medical Center; and Memorial Medical Center (Baptist and Mercy Hospitals).

University Officials

President of University System and Board Secretary	John V. Lombardi, Ph.D.
Chancellor of LSU Health Science Center	Larry H. Hollier, M.D.
Vice Chancellor for Academic Affairs	Joseph M. Moerschbaecher III, Ph.D.
Vice Chancellor for Administration and Finance	Ronald E. Smith
Director of Information Services	Leslie L. Capo
Vice Chancellor for Administrative and Community Affairs	Ronald Gardner

Medical School Administrative Staff

Dean	Steve Nelson, M.D.
Associate Dean for Academic Affairs	Charles Hilton, M.D.
Associate Dean for Alumni Affairs and Development	Russell C. Klein, M.D.
Associate Dean for Community and Minority Health Education	Edward J. Helm, M.D.
Associate Dean for Faculty and Institutional Affairs	Janis G. Letourneau, M.D.
Associate Dean for Finance	Keith G. Schroth
Associate Dean for Healthcare Quality and Safety	Frank Opelka, M.D.
Associate Dean for Student Affairs and Records	Joseph Delcarpio, Ph.D.
Associate Dean for Clinical Affairs	Frank Opelka, M.D.
Associate Dean for Admissions	Samuel McClugage, Ph.D.
Associate Dean for Research	Wayne Backes, Ph.D.
Assistant Dean for Student Affairs	Fred Lopez, M.D.
Assistant Dean for Undergraduate Education	Richard DiCarlo, M.D.
Director, Library	Wilba Swearingen
Coordinator, Office for Research	Kenneth E. Kratz, Ph.D.
Vivarium Director	Reynaldo R. Gonzalez, D.V.M.
Director of Basic Science Curriculum	Michael G. Levitzky, Ph.D.
Director of Clinical Science Curriculum	Richard DiCarlo, M.D.

Department and Division or Section Chairs

Basic Sciences

Biochemistry and Molecular Biology	Arthur Haas, Ph.D.
Genetics	Wayne V. Vedeckis, Ph.D. (Interim)
Cell Biology and Anatomy	Samuel G. McClugage, Ph.D.
Microbiology, Immunology, and Parasitology	Ronald B. Luftig, Ph.D.
Pharmacology and Experimental Therapeutics	Kurt Varner, Ph.D. (Interim)
Physiology	Patricia E. Molina, M.D., Ph.D.

Clinical Sciences

Anesthesiology	Alan D. Kaye, M.D., Ph.D.
Dermatology	Lee T. Nesbitt, Jr., M.D.
Family Medicine	Kim Edward LeBlanc, M.D., Ph.D.

Medicine . . . . Charles V. Sanders, M.D.
   Allergy and Clinical Immunology . . . . Prem Kumar, M.D.
   Cardiology . . . . Roberto E. Quintal, M.D.
   Comprehensive Medicine . . . . David Borne, M.D. (Interim)
   Emergency Medicine . . . . Keith W. Van Meter, M.D.
   Endocrinology and Metabolism . . . . Frank Svec, M.D., Ph.D.
   Gastroenterology . . . . Luis Balart, M.D.
   Geriatric Medicine . . . . Charles A. Cefalu, M.D.
   Hematology and Oncology . . . . John Cole, M.D.
   Infectious Diseases . . . . David H. Martin, M.D.
   International Medicine . . . . Charles V. Sanders, M.D.
   Nephrology . . . . Efrain Reisin, M.D.
   Nutrition and Metabolism . . . . Alfredo Lopez, M.D.
   Physical Medicine and Rehabilitation . . . . Gary Glynn, M.D.
   Pulmonary and Critical Care Medicine . . . . Steve Nelson, M.D.
   Rheumatology . . . . Luis R. Espinoza, M.D.
   Rural and Community Medicine . . . . Open
Neurology . . . . John D. England, M.D.
Neurosurgery . . . . Frank Culicchia, M.D.
Obstetrics and Gynecology . . . . Thomas E. Nolan, M.D., M.B.A.
   General Obstetrics and Gynecology . . . . Vacant
   Gynecologic Oncology . . . . Danny Barnhill, M.D.
   Maternal and Fetal Medicine . . . . Joseph M. Miller, M.D.
   Reproductive Endocrinology . . . . Richard Dickey, M.D.
   Urogynecology . . . . Ralph Chesson, M.D.
Ophthalmology . . . . Donald R. Bergsma, M.D.
Orthopaedics . . . . Barry Riemer, M.D.
Otolaryngology-Head and Neck Surgery . . . . Daniel Nuss, M.D.
   Kresge Hearing Research Laboratory . . . . Vacant
Pathology . . . . Jack P. Strong, M.D.
   Epidemiology . . . . Vacant
Pediatrics . . . . Ricardo U. Sorensen, M.D.
   Allergy and Immunology . . . . Cleveland Moore, M.D.
   Ambulatory Pediatrics . . . . Suzanne LeFevre, M.D.
   Cardiology . . . . Aluizio Stopa, M.D.
   Clinical Genetics . . . . Yves Lacassie, M.D.
   Critical Care . . . . Bonnie C. Desselle, M.D.
   Developmental and Behavioral Pediatrics . . . . Joy D. Osofsky, Ph.D.
   Emergency Medicine . . . . Raghubir Mangat, M.D.
   Endocrinology, Diabetes, and Metabolic Disorders . . . . Stuart Chalew, M.D.
   Gastroenterology and Nutrition . . . . Eberhard Schmidt-Sommerfeld, M.D.
   Hematology and Oncology . . . . Lolie C. Yu, M.D.
   Infectious Diseases . . . . Rodolfo Begue, M.D.
   Neonatology and Perinatology . . . . Brian Barkemeyer, M.D.
   Nephrology . . . . Matti Vehaskari, M.D.
   Public Health . . . . Susan Berry, M.D.
   Rheumatology . . . . Abraham Gedalia, M.D.
Psychiatry . . . . Howard J. Osofsky, M.D., Ph.D.
   Adult Psychology . . . . James G. Barbee, M.D.
   Child Psychiatry . . . . Martin J. Drell, M.D.
   Psychology . . . . Vacant
   Social Work . . . . Patricia E. Morse, Ph.D.
Radiology . . . . Leonard R. Bok, M.D., M.B.A., J.D.
Surgery . . . . Christopher C. Baker, M.D. (Interim)
   Bariatric . . . . Louis Martin, M.D.
   Pediatric Surgery . . . . Vacant
   Peripheral Vascular Surgery . . . . Robert C. Batson, M.D.
   Plastic Surgery . . . . Charles Dupin, M.D.
   Surgical Oncology . . . . Eugene A. Woltering, M.D.
   Thoracic Surgery . . . . Herman Heck, M.D.
   Transplant . . . . Daniel J. Frey, M.D.
   Trauma . . . . John Hunt, M.D.
Urology . . . . J. Chris Winters, M.D.

Louisiana State University School of Medicine at Shreveport

P.O. Box 33932
Shreveport, Louisiana 71130-3932
318-675-5000; 675-5240 (dean's office); 675-5244 (fax)
Web site: www.sh.lsuhsc.edu

Established in 1965-66 by acts of the Louisiana legislature, the school of medicine in Shreveport graduated its first class of students in 1973. In 1975, the school of medicine complex was completed, and
a class enrollment of 100 students per year was approved. The medical school is part of the Louisiana
State University Health Sciences Center at Shreveport.

Type: public
2008-2009 total enrollment: 439
Clinical facilities: (Shreveport) - Louisiana State University Hospital-Shreveport, E.A. Conway Medi-
cal Center (Monroe), Veterans Administration Medical Center, Schumpert Medical Center, Shriners
Hospitals for Children-Shreveport, Willis-Knighton Health System, Northwest Development Center
(Bossier City), Huey P. Long Medical Center (Pineville).

University Officials

President of the University System and Board Secretary. . . . . John V. Lombardi, Ph.D.
Chancellor . . . . John C. McDonald, M.D.
Vice Chancellor for Business and Reimbursements . . . . Harold W. White
Vice Chancellor for Clinical Affairs and Medical Director . . . . Roy G. Clay, M.D.
Assistant Vice Chancellor for Information Technology . . . . Lee Bairnsfather, Ph.D.
Assistant Vice Chancellor for Graduate Medical Education . . . . Donnie F. Aultman, M.D.

Medical School Administrative Staff

Dean. . . . . , ... John C. McDonald, M.D.
Associate Dean for Academic Affairs. . . . . Andrew L. Chesson, Jr., M.D.
Assistant Dean for Student Admissions . . . . F. Scott Kennedy, Ph.D.
Assistant Dean for Student Affairs. . . . . Mark Platt, Ph.D.
Assistant Dean for E. A. Conway Affairs . . . . Roy G. Clay, M.D.
Assistant Dean for VA Medical Center . . . . Open
Executive Assistant to the Dean . . . . Open
Hospital Administrator. . . . . Joseph M. Miciotto
Director of Public and Governmental Relations . . . . Elaine T. King
Coordinator of Legal Affairs. . . . . Rogers M. Prestridge
Director, Arthritis Center of Excellence . . . . Seth M. Berney, M.D.
Director, Cancer Center of Excellence . . . . Jonathan Glass, M.D.
Assistant Dean for Educational Program Development . . . . Jane M. Eggerstedt, M.D.

Department and Division or Section Chairs

Basic Sciences

Biochemistry and Molecular Biology. . . . . Robert E. Rhoads, Ph.D.
Bioinformatics and Computational Biology. . . . . Lee Bairnsfather, Ph.D.
Cellular Biology and Anatomy . . . . John Beal, Ph.D. (Acting)
Medical Library Science . . . . Marianne L. Comegys
Microbiology and Immunology. . . . . Dennis J. O'Callaghan, Ph.D.
Molecular and Cellular Physiology . . . . D. Neil Granger, Ph.D.
Pharmacology, Toxicology, and Neuroscience. . . . . Nicholas E. Goeders, Ph.D.

Clinical Sciences

Anesthesiology. . . . . Ashok Rao, M.D.
Emergency Medicine . . . . Thomas C. Arnold, M.D.
  Toxicology. . . . . Joseph E. Manno, Ph.D.
Family Medicine and Comprehensive Care . . . . Arthur T. Fort, M.D.
Medicine. . . . . Daniel E. Banks, M.D.
  Cardiology. . . . . Pratap C. Reddy, M.D.

Dermatology . . . . Open
Endocrinology and Metabolic Disease . . . . Steven N. Levine, M.D.
Gastroenterology . . . . Paul Jordan, M.D.
General Medicine. . . . . Deirdre Barfield, M.D.
Hematology . . . . Jonathan Glass, M.D.
Infectious Diseases . . . . Robert L. Penn, M.D.
Nephrology . . . . Kenneth D. Abreo, M.D.
Pulmonary and Critical Care. . . . . D. Keith Payne, M.D.
Rheumatology . . . . Seth M. Berney, M.D.
Neurology . . . . Roger E. Kelley, M.D.
Neurosurgery. . . . . Anil Nanda, M.D.
Obstetrics and Gynecology. . . . . Lynn Groome, M.D.
Ophthalmology . . . . Donald E. Texada, M.D. (Acting)
Orthopaedic Surgery . . . . Richard E. McCall, M.D.
Oral and Maxillofacial Surgery. . . . . G. E. Ghali, M.D., D.D.S.
Otolaryngology and Head and Neck Surgery. . . . . Frederick J. Stucker, Jr., M.D.
Pathology . . . . Stephen M. Bonsib, M.D.
Pediatrics . . . . Joseph A. Bocchini, M.D.
  Allergy and Immunology . . . . Sami L. Bahna, M.D.
  Cardiology. . . . . Ernest Kiel, M.D.
  Clinical Pharmacology . . . . John T. Wilson, M.D.
  Endocrinology . . . . Robert McVie, M.D.
  Gastroenterology . . . . John Herbst, M.D.
  General Pediatrics . . . . Steven Bienvenu, M.D.
  Hematology and Oncology . . . . Majed A. Jeroudi, M.D.
  Infectious Diseases . . . . Joseph A. Bocchini, M.D.
  Neonatology. . . . . Joseph A. Bocchini, M.D.
  Nephrology . . . . Kenneth D. Abreo, M.D.
  Neurology . . . . Arun Kalra, M.D.
  Pulmonary . . . . Kimberly L. Jones, M.D.
Psychiatry . . . . Paul D. Ware, M.D.
Radiology . . . . Horacio R. D'Agostino, M.D.
Surgery . . . . Richard H. Turnage, M.D.
  Burn* . . . . Kevin M. Sittig, M.D.
  Cardiothoracic* . . . . Richard H. Turnage, M.D. (Acting)
  Oncology* . . . . Benjamin D. L. Li, M.D.
  Pediatric*. . . . . Kevin Boykin, M.D. (Acting)
  Plastic* . . . . Open
  Transplantation* . . . . Gazi B. Zibari, M.D.
  Trauma* . . . . Cuthbert O. Simpkins, M.D.
  Vascular* . . . . Charles A. West, M.D.
Urology. . . . . Dennis D. Venable, M.D.

*Specialty without organizational autonomy.

Tulane University School of Medicine

1430 Tulane Avenue
New Orleans, Louisiana 70112
504-988-5462 (dean's office); 988-2945 (fax)
Web site: www.som.tulane.edu

Founded in 1834 as the Medical College of Louisiana, the school of medicine was incorporated into the University of Louisiana at its establishment in 1847. It has been called Tulane University since 1884. The medical school is part of the Tulane Health Sciences Center.

Type: private
2008-2009 total enrollment: 667
Clinical facilities: Tulane University Hospital and Clinic; Tulane Lakeside Hospital; Baton Rouge General Hospital; Children's Hospital; Dermatopathology Association; East Jefferson General Hospital; East Louisiana Mental Health System; Huey P. Long Regional Medical Center Hospital; Jefferson Parish Health Service Authority; Kindred Hospital; Louisiana Heart Hospital; Lady of the Lake Hospital; Lakeview Regional Medical Center; Medical Center of Louisiana at New Orleans; MD Anderson; Methodist Hospital, Houston; Ochsner Hospital; OSHA; Southeast Louisiana; Texas Heart; Touro Infirmary; University of North Carolina; Veterans Administration at Alexandria, Biloxi, Baton Rouge, Houston (Baylor); West Jefferson Medical Center.

University Officials

President. . . . . Scott S. Cowen, D.B.A.
Senior Vice President. . . . . Benjamin P. Sachs, M.D., B.S., D.P.H.
Director of Continuing Education for Health Sciences . . . . Melinda A. Epperson
Librarian for Health Sciences. . . . . Millie Moore (Interim)

Medical School Administrative Staff

Dean. . . . . Benjamin P. Sachs, M.D., B.S., D.P.H.
Vice President for Health Services Systems . . . . Mary W. Brown
Executive Vice Dean . . . . L. Lee Hamm, M.D.
Vice Dean for Academic Affairs . . . . N. Kevin Krane, M.D.
Vice Dean for Community Affairs and Health Care Policy. . . . . Karen B. DeSalvo
Vice Dean for Research . . . . John D. Clements, Ph.D.
Senior Associate Dean for Admissions and Student Affairs. . . . . Marc J. Kahn, M.D.
Associate Dean for Clinical Research . . . . Roy Weiner, M.D.
Associate Dean for Graduate Medical Education. Jeffrey Wiese, M.D.
Assistant Dean for Admissions . . . . Barbara S. Beckman, Ph.D.
Assistant Dean for Graduate Studies in Biomedical Sciences . . . . Robert F. Garry, Jr., Ph.D.
Assistant Dean for Lakeside Affairs. . . . . Gabriella Pridjian, M.D.
Assistant Dean, Medical Center of Louisiana-New
   Orleans Affairs . . . . Michele M. Zembo, M.D.
Assistant Dean, M.D./M.P.H. Combined Degree Program . . . . Marie A. Krousel-Wood, M.D.
Assistant Dean for Program Review and Strategic Analysis . . . . Susan K. Pollack
Assistant Dean for Student Affairs. . . . . Ernest Sneed, M.D.
Assistant Dean for Veterans Affairs. . . . . Paul S. Rosenfeld, M.D.

Department and Division or Section Chairs

Basic Sciences

Biochemistry . . . . Jim D. Karam, Ph.D.
Microbiology and Immunology. . . . . John D. Clements, Ph.D.
Pharmacology . . . . Krishna C. Agrawal, Ph.D.
Physiology. . . . . Luis Gabriel Navar, Ph.D.
Structural and Cellular Biology. . . . . Steven M. Hill, Ph.D.

Clinical Sciences

Anesthesiology. . . . . Frank Rosinia, M.D.
Dermatology . . . . Erin Boh, M.D., Ph.D.
Family and Community Medicine. . . . . Richard H. Streiffer, M.D.
Medicine. . . . . L. Lee Hamm, M.D.
   Clinical Immunology, Allergy, and Rheumatology . . . . Laurianne G. Wild, M.D. (Interim)
   Endocrinology . . . . Vivian A. Fonseca, M.D.
   Gastroenterology and Hepatology. . . . . Luisa Balart, M.D.
   General Internal Medicine and Geriatrics . . . . Karen B. DeSalvo, M.D.
   Heart and Vascular Institute . . . . Patrice Delafontaine, M.D.
   Hematology and Medical Oncology. . . . . Cindy A. Leissinger, M.D. (Interim)
   Infectious Diseases . . . . David M. Mushatt, M.D.
   Nephrology . . . . Eric Simon, M.D. (Interim)
   Pulmonary Diseases, Critical Care, and Environmental Medicine . . . . . . Joseph A. Lasky, M.D.
Neurosurgery. . . . . Miguel A. Melgar, M.D., Ph.D. (Interim)
Obstetrics and Gynecology. . . . . Gabriella Pridjian, M.D.
Ophthalmology. . . . . Delmar R. Caldwell, M.D.
Orthopedics . . . . Raoul P. Rodriguez, M.D.
Otolaryngology . . . . Paul Friedlander, M.D.
Pathology . . . . John R. Krause, M.D.
Pediatrics . . . . Samir El-Dahr, M.D.
   Adolescent Medicine . . . . Sue Ellen Abdalian, M.D.
   Pediatric Allergy, Immunology, and Rheumatology . . . . Jane El-Dahr, M.D.
   Pediatric Cardiology. . . . . Mitch Recto, M.D.
   Pediatric Critical Care . . . . Edwin Frieberg, M.D.
   Pediatric Emergency Medicine . . . . Carla Alcid, M.D.
   Pediatric Endocrinology . . . . Meera Ramayya, M.D.
   Pediatric Gastroenterology . . . . Ilana Fortgang, M.D.
   General Academic Pediatrics. . . . . Hosea Doucet, M.D., M.P.H.
   Pediatric Hematology and Oncology. . . . . Charles Scher, M.D.
   Pediatric Infectious Diseases . . . . Russell Van Dyke, M.D.
   Neonatology. . . . . William Gill, M.D.
   Pediatric Nephrology . . . . Samir El-Dahr, M.D.
   Pediatric Pulmonary. . . . . Robert Hopkins, M.D.
Psychiatry and Neurology. . . . . Daniel K. Winstead, M.D.
Radiology . . . . Harold R. Neitzschman, M.D.
Surgery . . . . Douglas P. Slakey, M.D.
   Plastic Surgery . . . . Ralph E. Newsome, M.D.
Urology. . . . . Raju Thomas, M.D.

Johns Hopkins University School of Medicine

733 North Broadway
Baltimore, Maryland 21205
410-955-5000; 955-3180 (dean's office); 955-0889 (fax)
Web site: www.hopkinsmedicine.org

The school of medicine was opened for the instruction of students in October 1893, four years after the opening of the Johns Hopkins Hospital.

Type: private
2008-2009 total enrollment: 475
Clinical facilities: Johns Hopkins Hospital, Johns Hopkins Bayview Medical Center, Kennedy Kreiger Institute, Good Samaritan Hospital, Sinai Hospital of Baltimore, Greater Baltimore Medical Center.

University Officials

Chair, University Board of Trustees . . . . Pamela Flaherty
Chair, Medicine Board of Trustees . . . . C. Michael Armstrong
President . . . . William R. Brody, M.D., Ph.D.
Provost and Vice President for Academic Affairs . . . . Kristina Johnson, Ph.D.
Senior Vice President for Administration . . . . James McGill, Ph.D.
Secretary . . . . Jerome Schnydman
Vice President for Development and Alumni . . . . Michael C. Eicher

Medical School Administrative Staff

Dean of the Medical Faculty and Chief Executive
   Officer, Johns Hopkins Medicine . . . . Edward D. Miller, M.D.
Vice Dean for Faculty Affairs . . . . Janice E. Clements, Ph.D.
Vice Dean for Education . . . . David G. Nichols, M.D.
Senior Vice President for Johns Hopkins Medicine . . . . Steven J. Thompson
Chief Financial Officer, Johns Hopkins Medicine . . . . Richard A. Grossi
Vice Dean for Clinical Affairs . . . . William A. Baumgartner, M.D.
Vice Dean for Clinical Investigation . . . . Daniel E. Ford, M.D.
Vice Dean for Research . . . . Chi Van Dang, M.D., Ph.D.
Vice Dean for Bayview . . . . David B. Hellmann, M.D.
Associate Dean for Admissions . . . . James Weiss, M.D.
Associate Dean for Student Affairs . . . . Thomas W. Koenig, M.D.
Associate Dean for Graduate Students . . . . Peter C. Maloney, Ph.D.
Associate Dean for Postdoctoral Affairs . . . . Levi Watkins, Jr., M.D.
Associate Dean for Graduate Medical Education . . . . Julia McMillan, M.D.
Associate Dean for Curriculum . . . . Patricia Thomas, M.D.
Associate Dean and Registrar . . . . Mary E. Foy
Associate Dean for Research Administration . . . . Michael B. Amey
Associate Dean for Continuing Medical Education . . . . Todd Dorman, M.D.
Associate Dean for Emerging Technologies . . . . Peter S. Greene, M.D.
Associate Dean, Executive Director, Clinical Practice Association . . . . Kenneth P. Wilczek
Assistant Dean for Admissions and Financial Aid . . . . Hermione Hicks
Assistant Dean for Medicine . . . . Christine H. White
Assistant Dean for Policy Coordination . . . . Julie Gottlieb
Assistant Dean and Director, Office of Academic Computing . . . . Harry Goldberg, Ph.D.
Assistant Dean for Student Affairs . . . . Redonda Miller, M.D.
Assistant Dean for Faculty, Development, and Equity . . . . Lisa Heiser
Assistant Dean for Student Affairs . . . . Vacant
Assistant Dean for Student Affairs . . . . Michael Barone, M.D.
Assistant Dean for Human Subject Research Compliance . . . . Barbara Starklauf
Assistant Dean and Compliance Officer for
   Graduate Medical Education . . . . John Rybock, M.D.

Department and Division or Section Chairs

Basic Sciences

Biological Chemistry . . . . Gerald W. Hart, Ph.D.
Biomedical Engineering . . . . Elliot R. McVeigh, Ph.D.
Biophysics . . . . L. Mario Amzel, Ph.D.
Cell Biology . . . . Peter M. Devreotes, Ph.D.
Comparative Medicine . . . . M. Christine Zink, D.V.M., Ph.D. (Interim)
Health Sciences Informatics* . . . . Nancy K. Roderer

88

History of Medicine.. Randall Packard, Ph.D.
Institute for Basic Biomedical Sciences.................... Stephen Desiderio, M.D., Ph.D.
Molecular Biology and Genetics................................. Carol Greider, Ph.D.
Neuroscience... Richard L. Huganir, Ph.D.
Pharmacology and Molecular Sciences .... Philip A. Cole, M.D., Ph.D.
Physiology... William B. Guggino, Ph.D.

Clinical Sciences

Anesthesiology and Critical Care Medicine......................... John Ulatowski, M.D.
Dermatology .... Charles W. Cummings, M.D. (Interim)
Emergency Medicine.. Gabor D. Kelen, M.D.
Medicine... Myron L. Weisfeldt, M.D.
    Allergy and Clinical Immunology* .... Bruce Bochner, M.D.
    Cardiology* .... Gordon Tomaselli, M.D.
    Clinical Pharmacology* .... Theresa B. Shapiro, M.D., Ph.D.
    Endocrine and Metabolic*...................................... Paul W. Ladenson, M.D.
    Gastroenterology* .... Anthony Kalloo, M.D.
    Geriatric Medicine and Gerontology*........................ Samuel C. Durso, M.D.
    Hematology* .... Robert Brodsky, M.D.
    Infectious Diseases* .... David Thomas, M.D.
    Internal Medicine*... Frederick Brancati, M.D.
    Molecular Medicine* .... Andrew Feinberg, M.D.
    Nephrology* .... Paul Scheel, M.D.
    Pulmonary and Critical Care Medicine* .... Landon King, M.D.
    Rheumatology* .... Antony Rosen, M.D.
Neurological Surgery... Henry Brem, M.D.
Neurology.. Justin McArthur, M.B.B.S. (Interim)
Neuroscience.. Richard L. Huganir, Ph.D.
Obstetrics-Gynecology .... Harold Fox, M.D.
Oncology... Martin D. Abeloff, M.D.
Ophthalmology.. Peter McDonnell, M.D.
Orthopedic Surgery.. Frank J. Frassica, M.D.
Otolaryngology-Head and Neck Surgery........................... Lloyd Minor, M.D.
    Oral*.. James Christian, D.D.S.
Pathology .... J. Brooks Jackson, M.D.
Pediatrics .... George Dover, M.D.
Psychiatry and Behavioral Science .... Raymond DePaulo, M.D.
    Child Psychiatry .... Mark A. Riddle, M.D.
Radiation Oncology.. Theodore L. DeWeese, M.D.
Radiology .... Jonathan Lewin, M.D.
    Nuclear Medicine*... Richard Wahl, M.D.
Physical Medicine and Rehabilitation .... Jeffrey Palmer, M.D.
Surgery.. Julie Freischlag, M.D.
    Acute Care Surgery: Trauma, Critical Care,
      Emergency, and General Surgery .... David Efron, M.D.
    Cardiac Surgery .... William A. Baumgartner, M.D.
    General Surgery .... Frederic Eckhauser, M.D.
    Pediatric Surgery* .... Paul M. Colombani, M.D.
    Plastic Surgery* .... Paul N. Manson, M.D.
    Surgical Critical Care .... Pamela Lipsett, M.D.
    Surgical Oncology .... Michael Choti, M.D., and Richard Schulick, M.D.
    Thoracic Surgery .... Stephen C. Yang, M.D.
    Transplantation .... Robert Montgomery, M.D.
    Vascular Surgery... Bruce Perler, M.D.
Urology... Alan W. Partin, M.D., Ph.D.

*Specialty without organizational autonomy.

University of Maryland School of Medicine

655 West Baltimore Street
Baltimore, Maryland 21201
410-706-3100 (campus); 706-7410 (dean's office); 706-0235 (fax)
E-mail: deanmed@som.umaryland.edu
Web site: http://medschool.umaryland.edu

The University of Maryland School of Medicine was founded in 1807 as the College of Medicine of Maryland. Davidge Hall, its first building, was constructed in 1812 and is the oldest building in North America used continuously for medical education. The school of medicine is one of six professional schools that comprise the university's campus in downtown Baltimore.

Type: public
2008-2009 total enrollment: 617
Clinical facilities: University of Maryland Medical Center (UM Marlene and Stewart Greenebaum Cancer Center and the R Adams Cowley Shock Trauma Center); Mercy Medical Center; VA Maryland Health Care System, Baltimore; Eastern Shore and Western Maryland AHEC.

University Officials

Chancellor, University System of Maryland . . . . William E. Kirwan, Ph.D.
President, University of Maryland Baltimore . . . . David J. Ramsay, D.M., D.Phil.
Vice President for Academic Affairs and Dean of
   the Graduate School . . . . Malinda B. Orlin, Ph.D.
Vice President for Medical Affairs. . . . . E. Albert Reece, M.D., Ph.D.

Medical School Administrative Staff

Dean. . . . . E. Albert Reece, M.D., Ph.D.
Executive Vice Dean . . . . Bruce E. Jarrell, M.D.
Vice Dean for Clinical Affairs. . . . . Robert A. Barish, M.D.
Senior Associate Dean for Finance and Resource Management . . . . Gregory F. Handlir
Associate Dean, Business Affairs, and Senior Advisor to the Dean . . . . Jerry D. Carr, J.D.
Associate Dean for Admissions . . . . Milford M. Foxwell, Jr., M.D.
Associate Dean for Faculty Affairs and
   Professional Development . . . . Nancy Ryan Lowitt, M.D.
Associate Dean for Development . . . . Dennis J. Narango (Acting)
Associate Dean for Medical Education . . . . David B. Mallott, M.D.
Associate Dean for Information Services . . . . James E. McNamee, Ph.D.
Associate Dean for Policy and Planning . . . . Claudia R. Baquet, M.D.
Associate Dean for Research. . . . . Vacant
Associate Dean for Student Affairs . . . . Donna Parker, M.D.
Associate Dean for Veterans Affairs . . . . Dorothy A. Snow, M.D.
Assistant Dean for Public Affairs. . . . . Jennifer Litchman
Assistant Dean for Programs and Planning . . . . Jeanette K. Balotin

Department and Division or Section Chairs

Basic Sciences and Allied Health Chairs

Anatomy and Neurobiology . . . . Michael T. Shipley, Ph.D.
Biochemistry and Molecular Biology. . . . . Richard L. Eckert, Ph.D.
Epidemiology and Preventive Medicine. . . . . Jay S. Magaziner, Ph.D.
Medical and Research Technology . . . . Sanford A. Stass, M.D. (Interim)
Microbiology and Immunology. . . . . James B. Kaper, Ph.D.
Pharmacology and Experimental Therapeutics . . . . Edson X. Albuquerque, M.D., Ph.D.
Physical Therapy and Rehabilitation Science. . . . . Mary M. Rodgers, Ph.D.
Physiology . . . . Meredith Bond, Ph.D.

Clinical Sciences Chairs and Program Directors

Anesthesiology. . . . . Peter Rock, M.D.
Dermatology . . . . Anthony A. Gaspari, M.D.
Diagnostic Radiology and Nuclear Medicine . . . . Reuben Mezrich, M.D., Ph.D.
Emergency Medicine . . . . Brian J. Browne, M.D., F.A.C.E.P. (Acting)
Family and Community Medicine. . . . . David L. Stewart, M.D.
Medicine. . . . . Frank M. Calia, M.D., M.A.C.P.
   Cardiology . . . . Mandeep Mehra, M.D.

Endocrinology, Diabetes, and Nutrition. . . . . Alan R. Shuldiner, M.D.
Gastroenterology and Hepatology . . . . Jean-Pierre Raufman, M.D.
General Internal Medicine . . . . Louis J. Domenici, M.D.
Geographic Medicine . . . . Myron M. Levine, M.D., D.T.P.H.
Gerontology. . . . . Andrew P. Goldberg, M.D.
Hematology and Oncology . . . . Barry R. Meisenberg, M.D.
Infectious Diseases . . . . Robert R. Redfield, M.D.
Nephrology . . . . Matthew R. Weir, M.D.
Pulmonary and Critical Care Medicine . . . . Jeffrey D. Hasday, M.D.
Rheumatology and Clinical Immunology. . . . . Marc C. Hochberg, M.D.
Neurology. . . . . William J. Weiner, M.D.
Neurosurgery. . . . . Howard M. Eisenberg, M.D.
Obstetrics, Gynecology, and Reproductive Sciences . . . . Hugh E. Mighty, M.D.
General Obstetrics and Gynecology. . . . . May Blanchard, M.D.
Gynecologic Oncology . . . . Neil Rosenshein, M.D.
Maternal-Fetal Medicine . . . . Christopher R. Harman, M.D.
Reproductive Endocrinology. . . . . Howard D. McClamrock, M.D.
Urogynecology and Pelvic Reconstruction . . . . Harry W. Johnson, M.D.
Oncology Program, UM Cancer Center . . . . Kevin J. Cullen, M.D.
Ophthalmology and Visual Sciences . . . . Ramzi K. Hemady, M.D. (Acting)
Orthopaedics. . . . . Vincent D. Pellegrini, M.D.
Otorhinolaryngology-Head and Neck Surgery. . . . . Scott E. Strome, M.D.
Pathology . . . . Sanford A. Stass, M.D.
Pediatrics . . . . Steven J. Czinn, M.D.
Adolescent Medicine . . . . Ligia Peralta, M.D.
Cardiology . . . . Mubadda Salim, M.D.
Critical Care. . . . . John Straumanis, M.D.
Emergency Medicine . . . . Keyvan Rafei, M.D.
Gastroenterology and Nutrition . . . . Samra Blanchard, M.D.
General Pediatrics . . . . James King, M.D.
Infectious Diseases and Tropical Pediatrics . . . . James Nataro, M.D., Ph.D.
Neonatology. . . . . Ronald Gutberlet, M.D. (Interim)
Nephrology . . . . Susan Mendley, M.D.
Pulmonary and Allergy. . . . . Mary Bollinger, D.O.
Psychiatry . . . . Anthony F. Lehman, M.D.
Adult Psychiatry . . . . Angela O. Onwuanibe, M.D. (Acting)
Alcohol and Drug Abuse. . . . . Eric Weintraub, M.D.
Child and Adolescent Psychiatry . . . . David B. Pruitt, M.D.
Community Psychiatry . . . . Jill RachBeisel, M.D.
Consultation/Liaison Psychiatry . . . . Mark Ehrenreich, M.D.
Division of Services Research . . . . Lisa B. Dixon, M.D.
Geriatric Psychiatry. . . . . William T. Regenold, M.D.
Maryland Psychiatric Research Center. . . . . William T. Carpenter, Jr., M.D.
Walter P. Carter Center Clinical Director . . . . Louis Cohen, M.D.
Radiation Oncology. . . . . William F. Regine, M.D.
Surgery. . . . . Stephen T. Bartlett, M.D.
Cardiac Surgery . . . . Bartley P. Griffith, M.D.
General Surgery. . . . . Adrian Park, M.D.
Pediatric Surgery . . . . Roger Voigt, M.B.B.S., F.R.C.S.
Plastic and Reconstructive Surgery . . . . Ronald Silverman, M.D.
Surgical Critical Care . . . . Steven Johnson, M.D.
Thoracic Surgery . . . . Richard J. Battafarano, M.D., Ph.D.
Transplant Surgery. . . . . Benjamin Philosphe, M.D.
Urology . . . . Michael J. Naslund, M.D. (Acting)
Vascular Surgery. . . . . Marshall Benjamin, M.D. (Acting)
Trauma Program-Shock Trauma Center . . . . Thomas M. Scalea, M.D.

Institute and Center Directors

Institute of Human Virology. . . . . Robert C. Gallo, M.D.
University of Maryland Institute for Genome Sciences. . . . . Claire M. Fraser-Liggett, Ph.D.
Health Policy and Health Services Research . . . . Claudia R. Baquet, M.D.
Integrative Medicine . . . . Brian M. Berman, M.D.
Mucosal Biology. . . . . Alessio Fasano, M.D.
Vascular and Inflammatory Diseases . . . . Dudley K. Strickland, Ph.D.
Research on Aging. . . . . Andrew P. Goldberg, M.D., and Jay S. Magaziner, Ph.D.
Trauma and Anesthesiology Research. . . . . Thomas M. Scalea, M.D., and Peter Rock, M.D.
Vaccine Development . . . . Myron M. Levine, M.D., D.T.P.H.

Uniformed Services University of the Health Sciences
F. Edward Hébert School of Medicine
4301 Jones Bridge Road
Bethesda, Maryland 20814-4799
301-295-3016 (dean's office); 295-3542 (fax)
Web site: www.usuhs.mil

Upon enactment in 1972 of the Uniformed Services Health Professions Revitalization Act (PL 92-426), Congress authorized establishment of the Uniformed Services University of the Health Sciences. The governing board of regents planned and developed the school of medicine as the initial academic component within the university. The first class of 32 medical officer candidates enrolled on October 12, 1976; the present first-year enrollment is 171.

Type: public
2008-2009 total enrollment: 670
Clinical facilities: Naval Hospital (Bethesda), Walter Reed Army Medical Center, Malcolm Grow U.S. Air Force Medical Center, Wilford Hall U.S. Air Force Medical Center.

University Officials

Chair, Board of Regents. . . . . Everett Alvarez, Jr., J.D.
Executive Secretary, Board of Regents . . . . Carol Scheman
President. . . . . Charles L. Rice, M.D.
Senior Vice President. . . . . Dale C. Smith, Ph.D.
Vice President for Research . . . . Steven Kaminsky, Ph.D.
Vice President for Recruitment and Diversity
    Affairs . . . . Cynthia Macri, M.D. (CAPT, MC, USN)
Vice President, External Affairs . . . . Carol Scheman
Vice President, Finance and Administration . . . . Stephen C. Rice
Chief of Staff. . . . . Stephen J. Henske
General Counsel . . . . John E. Baker, J.D.
Director, Continuing Education for Health
    Professionals . . . . Jaime A. Luke (CAPT, NC, USN)
Brigade Commander . . . . John W. Wempe (COL, MC, USA)

Medical School Administrative Staff

Dean, School of Medicine . . . . Larry W. Laughlin, M.D., Ph.D.
Vice Dean, School of Medicine. . . . . John E. McManigle, M.D.
Commandant . . . . Kenneth M. Tashiro, M.D. (COL, USAF, MC)
Associate Dean, Clinical Affairs. . . . . Emmanuel G. Cassimatis, M.D.
Associate Dean, Faculty Affairs . . . . Eric S. Marks, M.D.
Associate Dean, Faculty Development . . . . William H. J. Haffner, M.D. (Acting)
Associate Dean, Graduate Education. . . . . Eleanor S. Metcalf, Ph.D.
Associate Dean, Graduate Medical Education . . . . Howard E. Fauver, Jr., M.D.
Associate Dean, Medical Education. . . . . Donna M. Waechter, Ph.D.
Associate Dean, Recruitment and Admissions . . . . Margaret Calloway, M.D. (CDR, MC, USN)
                                                                                                 (Acting)
Associate Dean, Simulation Education . . . . Joseph O. Lopreiato, M.D. (CAPT, MC, USN)
Associate Dean, Student Affairs . . . . Richard M. MacDonald, M.D.
Assistant Dean, Clinical Sciences. . . . . Lisa Moores (COL, MC, USA)

Uniformed Services University of the Health Sciences
F.Edward Hébert School of Medicine: MARYLAND

Department Chairs

Basic Sciences

Anatomy, Physiology, and Genetics . . . . Harvey B. Pollard, M.D., Ph.D.
Biochemistry . . . . Teresa Dunn, Ph.D.
Biomedical Informatics . . . . A. Leon Moore, Ph.D. (Interim)
Medical and Clinical Psychology . . . . David S. Krantz, Ph.D.
Medical History . . . . Trueman W. Sharp, M.D. (CAPT, MC, USN) (Acting)
Microbiology and Immunology . . . . Alison D. O'Brien, Ph.D.
Military and Emergency Medicine . . . . Trueman W. Sharp, M.D. (CAPT, MC, USN)
Pathology . . . . Robert M. Friedman, M.D.
Pharmacology . . . . Jeffrey M. Harmon, Ph.D.
Preventive Medicine and Biometrics . . . . Gerald V. Quinnan, Jr., M.D. (CAPT, USPHS)
Radiation Biology . . . . Terry C. Pellmar, Ph.D.

Clinical Sciences

Anesthesiology . . . . Cynthia Shields, M.D. (COL, MC, USA) (Acting)
Dermatology . . . . Leonard B. Sperling, M.D.
Family Medicine . . . . Brian V. Reamy, M.D. (COL, USAF, MC)
Medicine . . . . Louis Pangaro, M.D.
Neurology . . . . William W. Campbell, Jr., M.D. (COL, MC, USA)
Obstetrics and Gynecology . . . . Christopher M. Zahn, M.D. (COL, USAF, MC)
Pediatrics . . . . Ildy M. Katona, M.D.
Psychiatry . . . . Robert J. Ursano, M.D.
Radiology and Nuclear Medicine . . . . James G. Smirniotopoulos, M.D.
Surgery . . . . David G. Burris, M.D. (COL, MC, USA)

Boston University School of Medicine

72 East Concord Street
Boston, Massachusetts 02118
617-638-5300 (dean's office); 638-5258 (fax)
E-mail: busmdean@bu.edu
Web site: www.bumc.bu.edu

In 1873, Boston University established its school of medicine by merging with the New England Female Medical College, which had been founded in 1848 as the first medical college for women in the world. In 1962, the school of medicine became a constituent member of Boston University Medical Center. It is located approximately two miles from the Charles River campus of Boston University, the parent university.

Type: private
2008-2009 total enrollment: 628
Clinical facilities: Bay Ridge Hospital, Baystate Medical Center, Beverly Hospital, Boston Medical Center, Bournewood Medical Center, Cape Cod Hospital, Carney Hospital, Solomon Carter Fuller Mental Health Center, Franciscan Children's Hospital, Human Resources Institute, Jewish Memorial Hospital, Lahey Clinic Medical Center, Columbia MetroWest Medical Center Framingham Union Campus, North Shore Childrens Hospital, Norwood Hospital, Shriners Hospital for Crippled Children, Veterans Administration hospitals (Boston, Bedford), Waltham Deaconess Hospital, Westwood Lodge Hospital, Roger Williams Hospital (Providence, Rhode Island), Central Maine Medical Center (Lewiston, Maine), Quincy Medical Center.

University Officials

President. . . . . Robert A. Brown, Ph.D.
Provost, Medical Campus. . . . . Karen H. Antman, M.D., Ph.D.
Associate Provost. . . . . Thomas J. Moore, M.D.
Associate Provost, Research . . . . Mark S. Klempner, M.D.
Associate Provost for Global Health . . . . Gerald T. Keusch, M.D.
Assistant Provost for Translational Research . . . . David M. Center, M.D.
Assistant Provost for Compliance . . . . Susan Frey, J.D.

Medical School Administrative Staff

Dean. . . . . Karen H. Antman, M.D.
Associate Dean for Academic Affairs. . . . . Sharon A. Levine, M.D.
Associate Dean for Admissions . . . . Robert A. Witzburg, M.D.
Associate Dean for Student Affairs . . . . Phyllis L. Carr, M.D.
Associate Dean for Clinical Affairs . . . . Ravin Davidoff, M.D.
Associate Dean for Continuing Medical Education . . . . Barry M. Manuel, M.D.
Associate Dean for Graduate Medical Sciences . . . . Carl Franzblau, Ph.D.
Associate Dean for Students and Office of
    Diversity and Multicultural Affairs . . . . Jonathan Woodson, M.D.
Assistant Dean for Admissions . . . . Gary J. Balady, M.D.
Assistant Dean for Admissions . . . . Selwyn A. Broitman, Ph.D.
Assistant Dean for Admissions . . . . Deborah Vaughan, Ph.D.
Assistant Dean for Enrichment Programs . . . . Suzanne Sarfaty, M.D.
Assistant Dean for Student Affairs. . . . . Paul O'Bryan, Ph.D.
Assistant Dean for VA Affairs . . . . Michael Charness, M.D.
Assistant Dean for Continuing Medical
    Education and Alumni Affairs . . . . Howard Bauchner, M.D.
Assistant Dean for Alumni Affairs. . . . . Jean Ramsey, M.D.
Assistant Dean for Student Affairs. . . . . Kenneth M. Grundfast, M.D.
Assistant Dean for Student Affairs. . . . . John Polk, M.D.
Registrar and Coordinator for Advanced Standing Admissions. . . . . Ellen J. DiFiore
Librarian. . . . . David S. Ginn, Ph.D.

Boston University School of Medicine: MASSACHUSETTS

Department and Division or Section Chairs

Basic Sciences

Anatomy and Neurobiology . . . . Mark B. Moss, Ph.D.
Biochemistry . . . . Carl Franzblau, Ph.D.
Microbiology . . . . Ronald B. Corley, Ph.D.
Pathology and Laboratory Medicine . . . . Daniel G. Remick, M.D.
Pharmacology and Experimental Therapeutics . . . . David H. Farb, Ph.D.
Physiology and Biophysics . . . . David Atkinson, Ph.D.
Socio-Medical Sciences and Community Medicine . . . . Robert F. Meenan, M.D.

Clinical Sciences

Anesthesiology . . . . Keith Lewis, M.D.
Dermatology . . . . Barbara A. Gilchrest, M.D.
Emergency Medicine . . . . Jonathan S. Olshaker, M.D.
Family Medicine . . . . Larry Culpepper, M.D.
Medicine . . . . David L. Coleman, M.D.
Neurology . . . . Carlos Kase, M.D.
Obstetrics and Gynecology . . . . Linda J. Heffner, M.D., Ph.D.
Ophthalmology . . . . Edward Feinberg, M.D.
Pediatrics . . . . Barry S. Zuckerman, M.D.
Psychiatry . . . . Domenic A. Ciraulo, M.D.
Radiology . . . . Alexander M. Norbash, M.D.
Rehabilitation Medicine . . . . Steve R. Williams, M.D.
Surgery . . . . James M. Becker, M.D.
   Cardiothoracic Surgery* . . . . Benedict D. T. Daly, M.D.
   Neurosurgery* . . . . Lawrence Chin, M.D.
   Orthopedic Surgery* . . . . Thomas A. Einhorn, M.D.
   Otolaryngology* . . . . Kenneth M. Grundfast, M.D.
   Urology* . . . . Richard K. Babayan, M.D.

*Specialty without organizational autonomy.

Harvard Medical School

25 Shattuck Street
Boston, Massachusetts 02115
617-432-1000; 432-1501 (dean's office); 432-3907 (fax)
Web site: www.hms.harvard.edu

On September 19, 1782, the President and Fellows of Harvard College officially adopted a plan for instituting medical instruction. The school's present buildings opened in 1906 and are located in Boston across the Charles River from the university in Cambridge.

Type: private
2008-2009 total enrollment: 739
Clinical facilities: Beth Israel Deaconess Medical Center, Brigham and Women's Hospital, VA Boston Healthcare System, Cambridge Health Alliance, The Center for Blood Research, Children's Hospital, Dana Farber Cancer Institute, Harvard Pilgrim Health Care, Joslin Diabetes Center, Judge Baker Children's Center, McLean Hospital, Massachusetts Eye and Ear Infirmary, Massachusetts General Hospital, Massachusetts Mental Health Center, Mount Auburn Hospital, Schepens Eye Research Institute, Spaulding Rehabilitation Hospital.

University Official

President. . . . . Drew G. Faust

Medical School Administrative Staff

Dean. . . . . Jeffrey S. Flier, M.D.
Executive Dean for Administration and Finance . . . . Daniel G. Ennis, M.B.A., M.P.A.
Dean for Academic and Clinical Affairs . . . . Nancy Tarbell, M.D.
Dean for Faculty Affairs . . . . Ellice Lieberman, M.D., D.P.H.
Dean for Faculty and Research Integrity. . . . . Gretchen Brodnicki, J.D.
Dean for Education . . . . Thomas Michel, M.D., Ph.D.
Dean for Medical Education. . . . . Jules L. Dienstag, M.D.
Dean for Students . . . . Nancy E. Oriol, M.D.
Dean for Diversity and Community Partnership . . . . Joan Reede, M.D.
Dean for Operations and Business Affairs. . . . . Richard Mills
Dean for Resource Development . . . . Susan Rapp
Dean for International Programs . . . . Richard Mills
Associate Dean for Faculty Affairs. . . . . Maureen Connelly, M.D.
Associate Dean for Finance . . . . Okey Agba
Associate Dean for Human Resources. Beth Marshall (Acting)
Associate Dean for Public Affairs . . . . Robert H. Neal (Acting)
Associate Dean for Basic Graduate Studies . . . . David L. Cardozo, Ph.D.
Associate Dean for Graduate Education . . . . Thomas O. Fox, Ph.D.
Faculty Dean for Continuing Medical Education. . . . . Sanjiv Chopra, M.D.
Faculty Dean for Graduate Education. Thomas M. Roberts, Ph.D.
Faculty Associate Dean for Admissions . . . . Robert Mayer, M.D.
Faculty Associate Dean for Student Affairs . . . . Alvin F. Poussaint, M.D.
Faculty Assistant Dean for Admissions. . . . . Darrell Smith, M.D.
Chief Information Officer . . . . John D. Halamka, M.D.
Director of the Academy Center for Teaching and Learning . . . . Charles Hatem, M.D.
Registrar . . . . Terese Galuszka
Director of the Countway Library. . . . . Issac S. Kohane, M.D., Ph.D.

Department and Division or Section Chairs

Basic Sciences

Biological Chemistry and Molecular Pharmacology . . . . Edward E. Harlow, Ph.D.
Cell Biology. . . . . Joan S. Brugge, Ph.D.
Genetics . . . . Cliff Tabin, Ph.D.
Health Care Policy. . . . . Barbara J. McNeil, M.D., Ph.D.
Microbiology and Molecular Genetics. . . . . John J. Mekalanos, Ph.D.
Neurobiology. . . . . Michael E. Greenberg, Ph.D.
Pathology . . . . Peter M. Howley, M.D.
Social Medicine and Global Health . . . . Jim Yong Kim, M.D., Ph.D.
Systems Biology. . . . . Marc Kirschner, Ph.D.

Clinical Science Departments

Ambulatory Care and Prevention .... Richard Platt, M.D.
Anaesthesia .... Charles A. Vacanti, M.D. (Chair, Exec. Committee)
   Beth Israel Deaconess Medical Center.................... Alan Lisbon, M.D. (Acting)
   Brigham and Women's Hospital .... Charles A. Vacanti, M.D.
   Children's Hospital .... Paul R. Hickey, M.D.
   Massachusetts General Hospital.................. Jeanine P. Weiner-Kronish, M.D.
Dermatology .... David Fisher, M.D., Ph.D.
Medicine...................... Mark L. Zeidel, M.D. (Chair, Exec. Committee)
   Beth Israel Deaconess Medical Center.................... Mark L. Zeidel, M.D.
   Brigham and Women's Hospital .... Joseph Loscalzo, M.D., Ph.D.
   Massachusetts General Hospital.................... Dennis A. Ausiello, M.D.
Neurology .... Scott Pomeroy, M.D., Ph.D, (Chair, Exec. Committee)
   Beth Israel Deaconess Medical Center.................. Clifford B. Saper, M.D., Ph.D.
   Brigham and Women's Hospital .... Martin A. Samuels, M.D.
   Children's Hospital .... Scott Pomeroy, M.D.
   Massachusetts General Hospital.................... Anne B. Young, M.D., Ph.D.
Obstetrics, Gynecology, and Reproductive
   Biology .... Isaac Schiff, M.D. (Chair, Exec. Committee)
   Beth Israel Deaconess Medical Center............. DeWayne M. Pursley, M.D., M.P.H.
   Brigham and Women's Hospital .... Robert L. Barbieri, M.D.
   Massachusetts General Hospital.......................... Isaac Schiff, M.D.
Ophthalmology .... Joan Miller, M.D.
Orthopedic Surgery................. Thomas S. Thornhill, M.D. (Chair, Exec. Committee)
   Beth Israel Deaconess Medical Center........................ Marc Gebhardt, M.D.
   Brigham and Women's Hospital .... Thomas S. Thornhill, M.D.
   Children's Hospital .... James R. Kasser, M.D.
   Massachusetts General Hospital..................... Harry E. Rubash, M.D.
Otology and Laryngology...................... Joseph B. Nadol, Jr., M.D.
Pathology .... Peter M. Howley, M.D. (Chair, Exec. Committee)
   Beth Israel Deaconess Medical Center..................... Jeffrey Saffitz, M.D., Ph.D.
   Brigham and Women's Hospital .... Michael A. Gimbrone, Jr., M.D.
   Children's Hospital .... Mark Fleming, M.D., D.Phil. (Acting)
   Massachusetts General Hospital....................... David N. Louis, M.D.
Pediatrics .... Frederick H. Lovejoy, M.D. (Chair, Exec. Committee)
   Children's Hospital .... Gary Fleisher, M.D.
   Massachusetts General Hospital..................... Ronald E. Kleinman, M.D.
Physical Medicine and Rehabilitation .... Ross D. Zafonte, D.O.
Psychiatry .... Jerrold F. Rosenbaum, M.D. (Chair, Exec. Committee)
   Beth Israel Deaconess Medical Center.................... Mary Anne Badaracco, M.D.
   Brigham and Women's Hospital .... Jonathan F. Borus, M.D.
   VA Boston Healthcare System...................... Robert W. McCarley, M.D.
   Cambridge Health Alliance.............................. Jack D. Burke, M.D.
   Children's Hospital .... David R. Demaso, M.D.
   McLean Hospital .... Scott L. Rauch, M.D.
   Massachusetts General Hospital.................... Jerrold F. Rosenbaum, M.D.
   Massachusetts Mental Health Center...................... Mary Anne Badaracco, M.D.
Radiation Oncology...................... Jay S. Loeffler, M.D. (Chair, Exec. Committee)
   Brigham and Women's Hospital/Children's
   Hospital/Dana Farber Cancer Institute .... Jay R. Harris, M.D.
   Beth Israel Deaconess Medical Center............... Mary Ann Stevenson, M.D., Ph.D.
   Massachusetts General Hospital....................... Jay S. Loeffler, M.D.
Radiology .... Steven E. Seltzer, M.D. (Chair, Exec. Committee)
   Beth Israel Deaconess Medical Center................... Vassilios Raptopoulos, M.D.
   Brigham and Women's Hospital .... Steven E. Seltzer, M.D.
   Children's Hospital .... George A. Taylor, M.D.
   Massachusetts General Hospital....................... James H. Thrall, M.D.
Surgery .... Robert C. Shamberger, M.D. (Chair, Exec. Committee)
   Beth Israel Deaconess Medical Center........................ Josef Fischer, M.D.
   Brigham and Women's Hospital .... Michael J. Zinner, M.D.
   Children's Hospital .... Robert C. Shamberger, M.D.
   Massachusetts General Hospital..................... Andrew L. Warshaw, M.D.

University of Massachusetts Medical School

55 Lake Avenue North
Worcester, Massachusetts 01655
508-856-8000 (dean's office); 856-8181 (fax)
E-mail: terry.flotte@umassmed.edu
Web site: www.umassmed.edu

The Medical School was established by an act of the General Court in 1962. The teaching hospital is UMass Memorial Medical Center. The first freshman class was admitted in fall 1970.

Type: public
2008-2009 total enrollment:
Clinical facilities: UMass Memorial-University and Memorial Campuses, Berkshire Medical Center, St. Vincent Hospital, St. Elizabeth's Medical Center, Milford-Whitinsville Regional Hospital.

University Officials

President. . . . . Jack Wilson, Ph.D.
Senior Vice President for Health Sciences and
    Chancellor . . . . Michael F. Collins, M.D. (Interim)
Vice Chancellor for Commonwealth Medicine
    and Strategic Facilities Planning . . . . Thomas D. Manning
Vice Chancellor for University Relations. . . . . Albert Sherman
Vice Chancellor for Administration and Finance. . . . . Robert Jenal
Vice Chancellor for Development. . . . . Charles Pagnam
Vice Provost for School Services . . . . Deborah Harmon Hines, Ph.D.
Associate Vice Chancellor for Diversity and Equal Opportunity . . . . Marian V. Wilson, Ph.D.
Associate Vice Chancellor for Human Resources. . . . . Joanne Derr
Associate Vice Chancellor for University Relations. . . . . Mark L. Shelton

Medical School Administrative Staff

Dean, Provost, and Executive Deputy Chancellor . . . . Terence R. Flotte, M.D.
Vice Provost for Research. . . . . John Sullivan, M.D.
Vice Provost for Faculty Affairs. . . . . Judith K. Ockene, Ph.D. (Interim)
Senior Associate Dean for Educational Affairs. . . . . Michele P. Pugnaire, M.D.
Associate Vice Provost for Clinical and Population Health Research. . . . . . . Walter Ettinger, M.D.
Associate Vice Provost for Research . . . . Thoru Pederson, Ph.D.
Associate Dean for Admissions . . . . John Paraskos, M.D.
Associate Dean for Student Affairs . . . . Mai-Lan Rogoff, M.D.
Associate Dean for Graduate Medical Education . . . . Deborah M. DeMarco, M.D.
Associate Dean for Continuing Education. . . . . Richard V. Aghababian, M.D.
Associate Dean and Director of Medical
    Education, Berkshire Medical Center . . . . Robert Cella, M.D.
Associate Dean, Worcester Medical Center . . . . David A. Kaufman, M.D.
Associate Dean for Community Programs. . . . . Michael Huppert
Assistant Dean of Student Affairs/Diversity and Minority Affairs . . . . Danna Peterson, M.D.
Assistant Dean, Academic Achievement. . . . . Mark E. Quirk, M.D.
Assistant Dean, Academic Advising . . . . Michael C. Ennis, M.D.
Director of Animal Medicine . . . . Gerald Silverman, D.V.M.

Department and Division or Section Chairs

Basic Sciences

Biochemistry and Molecular Pharmacology................... C. Robert Matthews, Ph.D.
Cancer Biology .... Dario Altieri, M.D.
Cell Biology... Gary S. Stein, Ph.D.
Molecular Genetics and Microbiology......................... Allan S. Jacobson, Ph.D.
Molecular Medicine.. Michael P. Czech, Ph.D.
Neurobiology.. Steven M. Reppert, M.D.
Physiology.. James G. Dobson, Ph.D. (Interim)
Program in Gene Function and Expression................... Michael Green, M.D., Ph.D.

Clinical Sciences

Anesthesiology.. Stephen O. Heard, M.D.
Emergency Medicine .... Greg Volturo, M.D.
Family and Community Medicine........................... Daniel H. Lasser, M.D.
Medicine... Robert W. Finberg, M.D.
Neurology.. Robert Brown, M.D.
Obstetrics and Gynecology........................ Harrison Ball, M.D. (Interim)
Orthopedics and Physical Rehabilitation......................... David Ayers, M.D.
Otolaryngology .... William G. Lavelle, M.D.
Pathology .... Kenneth L. Rock, M.D.
Pediatrics .... Marianne E. Felice, M.D.
Psychiatry .... Douglas M. Ziedonis, M.D.
Radiation Oncology....................................... Thomas Fitzgerald, M.D.
Radiology .... Joseph Ferrucci, M.D.
Surgery... Demetrius Litwin, M.D.

Tufts University School of Medicine

136 Harrison Avenue
Boston, Massachusetts 02111
617-636-7000; 636-6565 (dean's office); 636-0375 (fax)
Web site: www.tufts.edu/med

Tufts University School of Medicine is located in downtown Boston, two blocks south and east of the historic Boston Common. Established in 1893 as one of the component schools of Tufts College, its name was changed from Tufts College Medical School to its present title in 1955 when the original Tufts College, founded in 1852, changed to its university status. The medical and dental schools, the USDA Human Nutrition Research Center on Aging, the Gerald J. and Dorothy R. Friedman School of Nutrition Science and Policy, and the Sackler School of Graduate Biomedical Sciences are located in Boston. The Cummings School of Veterinary Medicine at Tufts University is located in Grafton, just west of Boston. The university's undergraduate campus is in Medford, just north of Boston.

Type: private
2008-2009 total enrollment: 698
Clinical facilities: Tufts-New England Medical Center and the Floating Hospital for Children, Baystate Medical Center; Cambridge Hospital; Caritas Carney Hospital, Caritas St. Elizabeth's Medical Center; Eastern Maine Medical Center; Faulkner Hospital; Lahey Clinic; Lemuel Shattuck Hospital; Maine Medical Center; MetroWest Medical Center; Newton-Wellesley Hospital; North Shore Medical Center-Salem Hospital; St. Anne's Hospital; Winchester Hospital.

University Officials

President. . . . . Lawrence S. Bacow
Senior Vice President and Provost . . . . Jamshed Bharucha
Vice Provost. . . . . Margaret S. Newell
Executive Vice President . . . . Steven S. Manos
Associate Provost . . . . Mary Y. Lee
Associate Provost . . . . Vincent Manno

Medical School Administrative Staff

Dean. . . . . Michael Rosenblatt, M.D.
Vice Dean . . . . Harris A. Berman, M.D.
Dean for Educational Affairs . . . . Scott Epstein, M.D.
Dean for Information Technology . . . . David A. Damassa, Ph.D.
Dean for Student Affairs . . . . Amy Kuhlik, M.D.
Dean for Baystate Medical Center. . . . . Hal B. Jenson, M.D.
Dean for Admissions . . . . David A. Neumeyer, M.D.
Dean for International Affairs . . . . Adel Abu-moustafa, Ph.D.
Associate Dean for Administration and Finance . . . . Joseph M. Carroll
Associate Dean for Educational Affairs . . . . Carolyn C. McVoy
Associate Dean for Students. . . . . Janet Kerle
Associate Dean for Admissions and Enrollment Services . . . . John A. Matias
Assistant Dean for Faculty Development . . . . Maria Blanco, Ed.D.
Assistant Dean for Public Health and Professional Degree Programs . . . . Robin Glover
Executive Administrative Dean . . . . Marsha Semuels
Senior Director of Development and Alumni Relations-Medicine. . . . . Leslie Kolterman
Director of Interschool Affairs . . . . Norman S. Stearns, M.D.
Director of Continuing Medical Education . . . . Rosalie Phillips
Director of Student Programs and Minority Affairs . . . . Colleen Romain
Director of Financial Aid . . . . Tara Olsen
Director of Admissions. . . . . Thomas Slavin
Director of the Hirsh Health Sciences Library. Eric D. Albright
Registrar . . . . Carol A. Duffey
Budget and Fiscal Officer. . . . . Patrice Ambrosia
Academic Dean at Lahey Clinic . . . . David J. Schoetz, M.D.
Director of Evaluation . . . . Keith White, Ph.D.

Tufts University School of Medicine: MASSACHUSETTS

Department and Division or Section Chairs

Basic Sciences

Anatomy and Cellular Biology . . . . James E. Schwob, M.D., Ph.D.
Biochemistry . . . . Brian S. Schaffhausen, Ph.D.
Molecular Biology and Microbiology. . . . . Abraham L. Sonenshein, Ph.D. (Acting)
Neuroscience. . . . . Philip G. Haydon, Ph.D.
Pathology . . . . Henry H. Wortis, M.D.
Pharmacology and Experimental Therapeutics . . . . David Greenblatt, M.D.
Physiology . . . . Eric Frank, M.D.

Clinical Sciences

Anesthesiology. . . . . Michael H. Entrup, M.D.
Dermatology . . . . Alice B. Gottlieb, M.D., Ph.D.
Emergency Medicine . . . . Niels K. Rathlev, M.D.
Medicine . . . . Deeb N. Salem, M.D.
Neurology . . . . Thomas D. Sabin, M.D. (Acting)
Neurosurgery. . . . . Carl Heilman, M.D.
Obstetrics and Gynecology . . . . Kenneth L. Noller, M.D.
Ophthalmology . . . . Jay S. Duker, M.D.
Orthopaedic Surgery . . . . Charles Cassidy, M.D.
Otolaryngology-Head and Neck Surgery . . . . Elie Rebeiz, M.D.
Pediatrics . . . . John Schreiber, M.D., Ph.D.
Physical Medicine and Rehabilitation . . . . Harry C. Webster, M.D. (Acting)
Psychiatry . . . . Paul Summergard, M.D.
Public Health and Family Medicine . . . . Aviva Must, Ph.D.
Radiation Oncology. . . . . David E. Wazer, M.D.
Radiology . . . . E. Kent Yucel, M.D.
Surgery. . . . . William C. Mackey, M.D.
Urology. . . . . Gennaro A. Carpinito, M.D.

Michigan State University College of Human Medicine
A-110 East Fee Hall
East Lansing, Michigan 48824
517-353-1730 (dean's office); 353-9969 (fax)
Web site: www.humanmedicine.msu.edu

In 1960, there was a societal demand for more physicians, nationally and within the state. The college of human medicine thus began in 1964 with expectations that the college would make the maximum use of community health care facilities for clinical training and would place strong emphasis on training primary care physicians. Issues of minority admissions, affirmative action, educational supports for disadvantaged students, and medical care for the poor are preeminent in the fabric of the college.

Type: public
2008-2009 total enrollment: 475
Clinical facilities: Michigan State University Clinical Center; Flint Area Medical Education (Hurley Medical Center, McLaren Regional Medical Center, Genesys Regional Medical Center); Grand Rapids Area Medical Education Center (Spectrum Health System, Pine Rest Christian Hospital, St. Mary's Mercy Medical Center); Kalamazoo Center for Medical Studies (Bronson Methodist Hospital, Borgess Medical Center), Lansing Campus (Sparrow Health System, Ingham Regional Medical Center); Synergy Medical Education Alliance (Covenant Health System, St. Mary's Medical Center); Upper Peninsula Health Education Corporation (Marquette General Hospital).

University Officials

President. . . . . Lou Anna Kimsey Simon, Ph.D.
Provost . . . . Kim A. Wilcox, Ph.D.

Medical School Administrative Staff

Dean. . . . . Marsha D. Rappley, M.D.
Executive Dean for East Lansing . . . . Kevin McMahon
Executive Dean for Grand Rapids. . . . . Rosemary Martino
Senior Associate Dean for Academic Affairs . . . . Aron Sousa, M.D.
Associate Dean for Graduate Medical Education . . . . Peter Coggan, M.D.
Associate Dean for Government Relations and Outreach. . . . . Denise Holmes
Associate Dean for College Wide Assessment . . . . Dianne Wagner, M.D.
Associate Dean for Research and Graduate Programs . . . . Jeffrey Dwyer, Ph.D.
Associate Dean for Faculty Development. . . . . William Wadland, M.D.
Assistant Dean for Capital and Strategic Planning . . . . Elizabeth Lawrence
Assistant Dean for Flint . . . . John B. Molidor, Ph.D.
Assistant Dean for Grand Rapids . . . . Margaret Thompson, M.D.
Assistant Dean for Kalamazoo. . . . . Elizabeth Burns, M.D.
Assistant Dean for Lansing. . . . . Renuka Gera, M.D.
Assistant Dean for Saginaw. . . . . Rae Schnuth, Ph.D.
Assistant Dean for Upper Peninsula . . . . David M. Luoma, M.D.
Assistant Dean for Student Affairs, Diversity, and Outreach . . . . Wanda D. Lipscomb, Ph.D.
Assistant Dean for Admissions . . . . Christine L. Shafer, M.D.
Assistant Dean for Preclinical Curriculum. . . . . Janet Osuch, M.D.

Michigan State University College of Human Medicine: MICHIGAN

Department and Division or Section Chairs

Basic Sciences

Anatomy . . . . E. James Potchen, M.D.
Biochemistry . . . . Thomas D. Sharkey, Ph.D.
Epidemiology . . . . James Anthony, Ph.D.
Microbiology . . . . Walter Esselman, Ph.D.
Pharmacology . . . . J. R. Haywood, Ph.D.
Physiology . . . . William S. Spielman, Ph.D.

Clinical Sciences

Dermatology . . . . Animesh A. Sinha, M.D.
Family Medicine . . . . William Wadland, M.D.
Medical Humanities . . . . Tom Tomlinson, Ph.D.
Medicine . . . . Mary D. Nettleman, M.D.
Neurology and Ophthalmology . . . . David Kaufman, D.O.
Obstetrics and Gynecology . . . . Richard E. Leach, M.D.
Office of Medical Education Research and Development . . . . Brian Mavis, Ph.D.
Pathology Teaching Unit . . . . William S. Spielman, Ph.D.
Pediatrics and Human Development . . . . H. Dele Davies, M.D., M.Sc.
Psychiatry . . . . Jed Magen, D.O.
Radiology . . . . E. James Potchen, M.D.
Surgery . . . . Richard E. Leach, M.D.

University of Michigan Medical School

1301 Catherine Street
4101 Medical Science Building I
Ann Arbor, Michigan 48109-5624
734-763-9600; 764-8175 (dean's office); 763-4936
Web site: www.med.umich.edu/medschool

The University of Michigan Medical School admitted its first class of 91 entering students in 1850. Women were admitted as early as 1870. In 1880, the course was lengthened to three years, and in 1890 it was lengthened to four years.

Type: public
2008-2009 total enrollment: 693
Clinical facilities: The University of Michigan Hospitals and Health Centers, including C. S. Mott Children's Hospital, Holden Perinatal Hospital, University Hospital, W. K. Kellogg Eye Center, Cancer Center and Geriatrics Center, Maternal Child Health Center; Catherine McAuley Health Center (St. Joseph Mercy Hospital); Veterans Administration Medical Center (Ann Arbor).

University Officials

President. . . . . Mary Sue Coleman, Ph.D.
Chancellor, University of Michigan-Dearborn . . . . Daniel Little, Ph.D.
Chancellor, University of Michigan-Flint. . . . . Jack Kay, Ph.D. (Acting)
Executive Vice President for Academic Affairs and Provost . . . . Teresa Sullivan, Ph.D.
Executive Vice President and Chief Financial Officer . . . . Timothy P. Slottow
Executive Vice President for Medical Affairs . . . . Robert Kelch, M.D.
Vice President for Development. . . . . Jerry A. May
Vice President for Research . . . . Stephen R. Forrest, Ph.D.
Vice President for Government Relations . . . . Cynthia H. Wilbanks
Vice President for Student Affairs. . . . . E. Royster Harper
Vice President and Secretary of the University . . . . Sally Churchhill

Medical School Administrative Staff

Dean. . . . . James O. Woolliscroft, M.D.
Senior Associate Dean for Clinical Affairs . . . . David A. Spahlinger, M.D.
Senior Associate Dean for Research . . . . Steven L. Kunkel, Ph.D.
Associate Dean for Student Programs . . . . Elizabeth M. Petty, M.D., Ph.D.
Associate Dean for Clinical Affairs . . . . John E. Billi, M.D.
Associate Dean for Faculty Affairs. . . . . Margaret R. Gyetko, M.D.
Associate Dean for Graduate Medical Education . . . . Lisa Colletti, M.D.
Associate Dean for Medical Education . . . . Joseph C. Fantone III, M.D.
Associate Dean for Diversity and Career Development. . . . . David Gordon, M.D.
Associate Dean for Regulatory Affairs . . . . Raymond J. Hutchinson, M.D.
Associate Dean for Clinical and Translational Research . . . . Daniel J. Clauw, M.D.
Assistant Dean for Admissions . . . . Steven E. Gay, M.D.
Assistant Dean for Graduate Medical Education . . . . Monica Lypson, M.D.
Assistant Dean for Clinical Faculty . . . . Elisabeth Quint, M.D.
Assistant Dean for Instructional Faculty . . . . James Albers, M.D.
Assistant Dean for Clinical Affairs. . . . . Darrell A. Campbell, Jr., M.D.
Assistant Dean for Faculty Affairs . . . . Jayne A. Thorson, Ph.D.
Assistant Dean for Medical Education . . . . Casey B. White, Ph.D.
Assistant Dean for Graduate and Postdoctoral Studies. . . . . Victor J. DiRita, Ph.D.
Assistant Dean for Research . . . . Samuel M. Silver, M.D., Ph.D.
Assistant Dean for Student Programs . . . . James F. Peggs, M.D.
Assistant Dean-VA Medical Center . . . . Eric W. Young, M.D.
Director, Medical Center Alumni and Development Office . . . . James S. Thomas
Director, Laboratory Animal Medicine . . . . Howard G. Rush, D.V.M.

Department and Division or Section Chairs

Basic Sciences

Cell and Developmental Biology. . . . . J. Douglas Engel, Ph.D.
Biological Chemistry . . . . William L. Smith, Ph.D.
Human Genetics . . . . Sally Camper, Ph.D.
Medical Education. . . . . Larry D. Gruppen, Ph.D.
Microbiology and Immunology. . . . . Harry L. T. Mobley, Ph.D.
Molecular and Integrative Physiology . . . . M. Bishr Omary, M.D., Ph.D.
Pharmacology . . . . Paul F. Hollenberg, Ph.D.

Clinical Sciences

Anesthesiology. . . . . Kevin K. Tremper, M.D., Ph.D.
Dermatology . . . . John J. Voorhees, M.D.
Emergency Medicine . . . . William G. Barsan, M.D.
Family Medicine . . . . Thomas L. Schwenk, M.D.
Internal Medicine . . . . Robert F. Todd III, M.D., Ph.D. (Interim)
Neurology . . . . David J. Fink, M.D.
Neurosurgery. . . . . Karin M. Muraszko, M.D.
Obstetrics and Gynecology. . . . . Timothy R. B. Johnson, M.D.
Ophthalmology and Visual Sciences . . . . Paul R. Lichter, M.D.
Orthopaedic Surgery . . . . James E. Carpenter, M.D.
Otolaryngology . . . . Gregory T. Wolf, M.D.
Pathology . . . . Jay Hess, M.D., Ph.D.
Pediatrics and Communicable Diseases. . . . . Valerie P. Castle, M.D.
Physical Medicine and Rehabilitation . . . . Edward A. Hurvitz, M.D
Psychiatry . . . . Gregory W. Dalack, M.D. (Interim)
Radiation Oncology. . . . . Theodore S. Lawrence, M.D., Ph.D.
Radiology . . . . N. Reed Dunnick, M.D.
Surgery. . . . . Michael W. Mulholland, M.D., Ph.D.
Urology. . . . . David A. Bloom, M.D.

Institutes, Centers, and Program Directors

A. Alfred Taubman Medical Research Institute . . . . Eva L. Feldman, M.D., Ph.D.
Cardiovascular Center . . . . Kim A. Eagle, M.D., Richard L. Prager, M.D., David Pinsky, M.D.,
and James Stanley, M.D. (co-dir.)
Comprehensive Cancer Center. . . . . Max S. Wicha, M.D.
Depression Center. . . . . John F. Greden, M.D.
Institute of Gerontology. . . . . Jeffrey B. Halter, M.D.
Kresge Hearing Research Institute . . . . Jochen H. Schacht, Ph.D.
Medical Scientist Training Program . . . . Ronald J. Koenig, M.D., Ph.D.
Michigan Center for Translational Pathology . . . . Arul M. Chinnaiyan, M.D.
Michigan Comprehensive Diabetes Center . . . . Peter R. Arvan, M.D., Ph.D.
Michigan Institute for Clinical and Health Research . . . . Daniel J. Clauw, M.D.
Michigan Metabolical and Obesity Center. . . . . Charles Burant, M.D., Ph.D.
Michigan Nanotechnology Institute for Medicine
and Biological Sciences . . . . James R. Baker, Jr., M.D.
Molecular and Behavioral Neuroscience Institute . . . . Stanley J. Watson, M.D., Ph.D.,
and Huda Akil, Ph.D. (co-dir.)

Wayne State University School of Medicine

540 East Canfield
Detroit, Michigan 48201
313-577-1335 (dean's office); 577-8777 (fax)
Web site: www.med.wayne.edu

The school of medicine was founded in 1868 as the Detroit Medical College. It was the first established school of what was to become, in 1956, Wayne State University. It is one of the largest single-campus medical schools in the country.

Type: public
2008-2009 total enrollment: 1,065
Clinical facilities: Barbara Ann Karmanos Cancer Institute, Detroit Receiving Hospital and University Health Center, Children's Hospital of Michigan, Harper University Hospital, Hutzel Womens Hospital, Sinai-Grace Hospital, Veterans Administration Medical Center, Rehabilitation Institute of Michigan, Kresge Eye Institute, Michigan Orthopaedic Specialty Hospital, William Beaumont Hospital, Huron Valley Sinai Hospital, Providence Hospital, North Oakland Medical Center, St. John Hospital and Medical Center, Oakwood Healthcare System, Bon Secours Hospital, St. Joseph Hospital (Pontiac), St. Joseph Hospital (Ann Arbor), Henry Ford Health System.

University Officials

President. . . . . Jay Noren, M.D., M.P.H.
Provost and Senior Vice President for Academic Affairs. . . . . Nancy S. Barrett, Ph.D.
Senior Advisor to the President for Medical Affairs. . . . . Robert M. Mentzer, Jr., M.D.
Vice President for Research . . . . Hilary Ratner, Ph.D.

Medical School Administrative Staff

Dean. . . . . Robert M. Mentzer, Jr., M.D.
Executive Vice Dean . . . . Robert R. Frank, M.D.
Associate Dean for Administration and Chief Administrative Officer . . . . Kenneth Lee
Assistant Dean for Admissions . . . . Silas Norman, M.D.
Assistant Dean for Student Affairs. . . . . Kertia Black, M.D.
Assistant Dean for Basic Science Curriculum. Matthew Jackson, Ph.D.
Assistant Dean for Undergraduate Medical Education. . . . . Thomas Roe, M.D.
Assistant Dean for Medical Evaluation and Education Research. . . . . Patrick Bridge, Ph.D.
Associate Dean for Graduate Medical Education . . . . Mark Juzych, M.D.
Assistant Dean for Continuing Medical Education. . . . . David Pieper, Ph.D.
Assistant Dean for Veterans Administration Affairs . . . . Basim Dubaybo, M.D.
Associate Dean for Research. . . . . Daniel Walz, Ph.D.
Assistant Dean for Clinical Research. . . . . Michael Diamond, M.D.
Assistant Dean for Affiliate Research Programs . . . . Margot LaPointe, M.D.
Associate Dean for Graduate Programs. . . . . Kenneth Palmer, Ph.D.
Vice Dean for Hospital Relations and Clinical Affairs . . . . Valerie Parisi, M.D.
Associate Dean for Faculty Affairs. . . . . Stephen Lerner, M.D.
Assistant Dean for Community Outreach and Urban Health . . . . Herbert Smitherman, M.D.
Associate Dean for Affiliate Programs. . . . . Henry Lim, M.D.
Executive Director of Advancement . . . . Douglas Czajkowski
Manager of Public Affairs. . . . . Philip Van Hulle
Assistant Director of Financial Aid . . . . Deidre Moore
Registrar . . . . JaEsta Jones

Department Chairs and Division Heads

Basic Sciences

Anatomy and Cell Biology . . . . Linda Hazlett, Ph.D.
Biochemistry and Molecular Biology. . . . . Barry P. Rosen, Ph.D.
Immunology and Microbiology. . . . . Paul C. Montgomery, Ph.D.
Center for Molecular Medicine and Genetics . . . . Larry Grossman, Ph.D.
Pathology . . . . Wael Sakr, M.D.
Pharmacology . . . . Bonnie Sloane, Ph.D.

Physiology . . . . David Lawson, Ph.D. (Interim)

Department and Division or Section Chairs

Clinical Sciences

Anesthesiology. . . . . H. Michael Marsh, M.B.B.S.
Cancer Institute. . . . . John C. Ruckdeschel, M.D.
Dermatology . . . . Darius Mehregan, M.D.
Emergency Medicine . . . . Suzanne White, M.D.
Family Medicine . . . . Maryjean Schenk, M.D.
   Behavioral Science and Mental Health . . . . John Porcerelli, Ph.D.
   Occupational and Environmental Medicine. . . . . Bengt Arnetz, M.D., Ph.D.
Internal Medicine . . . . John M. Flack, M.D. (Interim)
   Cardiology. . . . . Peter Vaitkevicius, M.D.
   Critical Care and Pulmonary. . . . . Safwan Badr, M.D.
   Endocrinology . . . . Abdul B. Abou-Samra, M.D., Ph.D.
   Gastroenterology . . . . Milton Mutchnick, M.D.
   General Medicine. . . . . Donald Levine, M.D.
   Hematology and Oncology . . . . Joseph P. Uberti, M.D., Ph.D.
   Infectious Diseases . . . . Jack D. Sobel, M.D.
   Nephrology . . . . Stephen Migdal, M.D.
   Rheumatology . . . . Donald Levine, M.D. (Interim)
Neurology. . . . . Robert P. Lisak, M.D.
Neurosurgery. . . . . Murali Guthikonda, M.D.
Obstetrics and Gynecology. . . . . Theodore Jones, M.D. (Interim)
Ophthalmology . . . . Gary Abrams, M.D.
Orthopedic Surgery. . . . . Lawrence Morawa, M.D.
Otolaryngology . . . . Robert H. Mathog, M.D.
Pediatrics . . . . Bonita F. Stanton, M.D.
   Allergy, Immunology, and Rheumatology . . . . Ellen Moore, M.D.
   Cardiology . . . . Richard Humes, M.D. (Interim)
   Critical Care Medicine . . . . Mary Lieh-Lai, M.D., and Ashok Sarnaik, M.D.
   Emergency Medicine . . . . Stephen Knazik, D.O.
   Endocrinology . . . . Chandra Edwin, M.D.
   Gastroenterology . . . . Mohammed El-Baba, M.D.
   General Pediatrics . . . . Howard Fischer, M.D.
   Genetics and Metabolism . . . . Erawati Bawle, M.D.
   Hematology and Oncology . . . . . . Jeanne Lusher, M.D., and Yaddanapudi Ravindranath, M.D.
   Infectious Diseases . . . . Basim Asmar, M.D.
   Neonatology. . . . . Seetha Shankaran, M.D.
   Nephrology . . . . Tej Mattoo, M.D.
   Neurology . . . . Henry Chugani, M.D.
   Pharmacology and Toxicology . . . . Jacob Aranda, M.D., Ph.D.
   PM&R . . . . Edward Dabrowski, M.D.
   Prevention . . . . Xiaoming Li, Ph.D.
   Pulmonary Diseases . . . . Ibrahim A. Abdulhamid, M.D.
Physical Medicine and Rehabilitation . . . . Jay Meythaler, M.D., J.D.
Psychiatry and Behavioral Neurosciences . . . . Manuel Tancer, M.D.
Radiation Oncology. . . . . Maria Vlachaki, M.D. (Interim)
Radiology . . . . Wilbur Smith, M.D.
Surgery. . . . . Donald Weaver, M.D.
   Breast . . . . David Bouwman, M.D.
   Cardiothoracic. . . . . Larry Stephenson, M.D.
   General Surgery. . . . . Donald Weaver, M.D.
   Pediatric Surgery . . . . Michael Klein, M.D.
   Plastic and Reconstructive. . . . . Eti Gursel, M.D.
   Transplantation . . . . Scott Gruber, M.D.
   Trauma . . . . James Tyburski, M.D.
   Vascular . . . . O.W. Brown, M.D., Ph.D.
   Veteran Affairs. . . . . Marc Basson, M.D.
Urology. . . . . Michael Cher, M.D.

Mayo Medical School
200 First Street, S.W.
Rochester, Minnesota 55905
507-538-4897; 266-5299 (dean's office); 284-2634 (fax)
E-mail: lindor.keith@mayo.edu
Web site: www.mayo.edu

Mayo Medical School, founded in 1972, is part of the Mayo Clinic. Other schools at the Mayo Clinic are the Mayo School of Graduate Medical Education, founded in 1915; the Mayo Graduate School, formalized in 1989; the Mayo School of Health Sciences, formalized in 1972; and the Mayo School of Continuing Medical Education, established in 1996.

Type: private
2008-2009 total enrollment: 168
Clinical facilities: Mayo Clinic, Saint Marys Hospital, Methodist Hospital (Rochester, Minnesota); Mayo Clinic Jacksonville, St. Luke's Hospital (Jacksonville, Florida); Mayo Clinic Scottsdale (Arizona), Mayo Clinic Hospital and regional affiliates.

Mayo Clinic Officials

Chair, Board of Trustees . . . . James A. Barksdale
President and Chief Executive Officer . . . . Denis A. Cortese, M.D.
Vice President and Chief Administrative Officer . . . . Shirley A. Weis
Vice President . . . . Nina M. Schwenk, M.D.
Vice President and Chief Executive Officer, Mayo Clinic, Florida . . . . George B. Bartley, M.D.
Vice President and Chief Executive Officer,
    Mayo Clinic, Rochester . . . . Glenn S. Forbes, M.D.
Vice President and Chief Executive Officer, Mayo Clinic, Arizona . . . . Victor F. Trastek, M.D.
Executive Dean for Education . . . . Terrence Cascino, M.D.
Director for Research, Jacksonville . . . . Thomas G. Brott, M.D.
Executive Dean for Research, Rochester . . . . Robert A. Rizza, M.D.
Director for Research, Arizona . . . . Laurence J. Miller, M.D.
Chair, Clinical Practice Committee, Florida . . . . Stephen M. Lange, M.D.
Chair, Clinical Practice Committee, Rochester . . . . C. Michael Harper, M.D.
Chair, Clinical Practice Committee, Arizona . . . . Richard Helmers, M.D.

Department of Education Services Officials

Chair, Department of Education Administration . . . . Paula Menkosky
Dean, Mayo Medical School . . . . Keith D. Lindor, M.D.
Associate Dean for Academic Affairs, Mayo Medical School . . . . Joseph Grande, M.D., Ph.D.
Associate Dean for Faculty Affairs, Mayo Medical School . . . . Thomas R. Viggiano, M.D.
Associate Dean for Student Affairs, Mayo Medical School . . . . Patricia A. Barrier, M.D.
Associate Dean for Undergraduate Education, Jacksonville . . . . Gerardo Colon-Otero, M.D.
Associate Dean for Undergraduate Education, Arizona . . . . Lois Krahn, M.D.
Division Chair, Jacksonville . . . . Mary R. Anderson
Division Chair, Arizona . . . . Sheila A. Collins
Dean, Mayo School of Graduate Medical Education . . . . Mark Warner, M.D.
Vice Dean . . . . Steve Rose, M.D.
Associate Dean, Internal Medicine and Medical Subspecialties . . . . Joseph C. Farmer, M.D.
Associate Dean, Medical and Laboratory Specialties . . . . Lisa A. Drage, M.D.
Associate Dean, Surgery and Surgical Specialties . . . . Steven H. Rose, M.D.
Associate Dean for Internal Medicine and
    Medical Subspecialties, Jacksonville . . . . Kenneth G. Nix, Jr., M.D.
Associate Dean for Medical and Laboratory
    Specialties, Jacksonville . . . . David Capobianco, M.D.
Associate Dean for Surgery and Surgical Specialties, Jacksonville . . . . Steven Petrou, M.D.
Associate Dean for Internal Medicine and
    Medical Specialties, Arizona . . . . Keith Cannon, M.D.
Associate Dean for Medical and Laboratory Specialties, Arizona . . . . James A. Yiannias, M.D.
Associate Dean for Surgery and Surgical Specialties, Arizona . . . . Renee E. Caswell, M.D.
Dean, Mayo Graduate School . . . . Diane F. Jelinek, Ph.D.
Associate Dean for Academic Affairs, Mayo Graduate School . . . . L. James Maher III, Ph.D.
Associate Dean for Student Affairs, Mayo Graduate School . . . . Bruce F. Horazdovsky, Ph.D.
Dean, Mayo School of Health Sciences . . . . Claire E. Bender, M.D.
Associate Dean for Student Affairs, Mayo School of Health Sciences . . . . David Agerter, M.D.
Associate Dean for Academic Affairs . . . . Michael Silber, M.D.
Associate Dean, Jacksonville . . . . Galen Perdikis, M.D.

Associate Dean, Arizona. . . . . Catherine Roberts, M.D.
Dean, Mayo School of Continuing Medical Education. . . . . Richard A. Berger, M.D.
Associate Dean, Rochester . . . . Darryl S. Chutka, M.D.
Associate Dean, Jacksonville . . . . James S. Scolapio, M.D.
Associate Dean, Arizona. . . . . Russell I. Heigh, M.D.
Library Director, Mayo Foundation. . . . . J. Michael Homan
Public Information Director. . . . . John La Forgia

Department and Division or Section Chairs

Basic Sciences

Anatomy . . . . Wojciech Pawlina, M.D.
Biochemistry and Molecular Biology. . . . . Mark A. McNiven, Ph.D.
Health Sciences Research. . . . . Veronique Roger, M.D.
Immunology . . . . Larry R. Pease, Ph.D.
Laboratory Medicine and Pathology . . . . Paula Santrach, M.D.
Pharmacology . . . . Matthew M. Ames, Ph.D.
Physiology and Biomedical Engineering . . . . Gary C. Sieck, Ph.D.

Clinical Sciences

Anesthesiology. . . . . Bradley Narr, M.D.
Dentistry . . . . Kevin I. Reid, D.M.D.
Dermatology . . . . Randall K. Roenigk, M.D.
Diagnostic Radiology . . . . Bernard King, M.D.
Emergency Medical Services. . . . . Wyatt W. Decker, M.D.
Family Medicine . . . . Steve Adamson, M.D.
Internal Medicine . . . . Morie A. Gertz, M.D.
    Allergic Diseases. . . . . James T. C. Li, M.D.
    Cardiovascular Diseases. . . . . David L. Hayes, M.D.
    Community Internal Medicine . . . . Eric G. Tangalos, M.D.
    Endocrinology and Metabolism. . . . . John C. Morris, M.D.
    Gastroenterology . . . . Gregory J. Gores, M.D.
    General Internal Medicine . . . . J. Taylor Hays, M.D.
    Hematology . . . . Dennis Gastineau, M.D.
    Hypertension . . . . Gary L. Schwartz, M.D.
    Infectious Diseases . . . . James M. Steckelberg, M.D.
    Nephrology . . . . Vincente Torres, M.D.
    Preventive Medicine . . . . Donald Hensrud, M.D.
    Pulmonary and Critical Care Medicine . . . . Andrew H. Limper, M.D.
    Rheumatology . . . . Eric Matteson, M.D.
Medical Genetics . . . . Dusica Babovic-Vuksanovic, M.D.
Neurologic Surgery . . . . Fredric B. Meyer, M.D.
Neurology . . . . Robert Brown, M.D.
Obstetrics and Gynecology. . . . . C. Robert Stanhope, M.D.
Oncology. . . . . Charles Erlichman, M.D.
    Developmental Oncology Research . . . . Scott H. Kaufmann, M.D., Ph.D.
    Medical Oncology . . . . Jan C. Buckner, M.D.
    Radiation Oncology . . . . Paula J. Schomberg, M.D.
Ophthalmology . . . . Jonathan M. Holmes, M.D.
Orthopedics . . . . Daniel J. Berry, M.D.
Otorhinolaryngology . . . . Charles W. Beatty, M.D.
Pediatrics . . . . Robert M. Jacobson, M.D.
Physical Medicine and Rehabilitation . . . . Kathryn A. Stolp, M.D.
Psychiatry and Psychology . . . . David A. Mrazek, M.D.
Surgery . . . . Claude Deschamps, M.D.
    Cardiovascular . . . . Hartzell V. Schaff, M.D.
    Colon and Rectal . . . . Bruce Wolff, M.D.
    Gastroenterologic. . . . . Michael B. Farnell, M.D.
    Plastic and Reconstructive. . . . . Craig H. Johnson, M.D.
    Pediatric Surgery . . . . Michael Ishitani, M.D.
    Thoracic and Cardiovascular. . . . . Mark S. Allen, M.D.
    Transplantation . . . . Mark D. Stegall, M.D.
    Vascular. . . . . Peter Gloviczki, M.D.
Urology. . . . . Douglas Husmann, M.D.

University of Minnesota Medical School

Mayo Mail Code 293
420 Delaware Street, S.E.
Minneapolis, Minnesota 55455
612-624-1188 (admissions/student affairs); 625-3622 (curriculum affairs);
626-4949 (dean's office)
Web site: www.med.umn.edu

The medical school, founded in 1888, is a major unit of the academic health center of the University of Minnesota. The buildings of the medical school, the University of Minnesota Medical Center, and the other units of the academic health center are located on the east bank portion of the Twin Cities campus of the University of Minnesota in Minneapolis and on the Duluth campus. The mission of the Duluth campus is educating future rural family physicians.

Type: public
2008-2009 total enrollment: 929
Clinical facilities: University of Minnesota Medical Center, Fairview; Hennepin County Medical Center; Regions Hospital; Veterans Affairs Medical Center (Minneapolis); Children's Health Care; and several other community hospitals. Duluth Family Practice Center, Miller-Dwan Hospital and Medical Center, St. Luke's Hospital, St. Mary's Medical Center.

University Officials

President. . . . . Robert H. Bruininks, Ph.D.
Senior Vice President, Health Sciences. . . . . Frank B. Cerra, M.D.

Medical School Administrative Staff

Dean of the Medical School. . . . . Deborah E. Powell, M.D.
Vice Dean, Clinical Affairs . . . . Roby C. Thompson, M.D.
Vice Dean, Education . . . . Lindsey C. Henson, M.D., Ph.D.
Vice Dean, Research and Operations . . . . Charles F. Moldow, M.D.
Senior Associate Dean, Duluth Campus . . . . Gary L. Davis, Ph.D.
Associate Dean, Academic Administration. . . . . Patricia A. Mulcahy
Associate Dean, Clinical Research. . . . . Jasjit S. Ahluwalia, M.D.
Associate Dean, Curriculum and Evaluation . . . . Linda J. Perkowski, Ph.D.
Associate Dean, Faculty Affairs . . . . Roberta E. Sonnino, M.D.
Associate Dean, Finance and Administration. . . . . Peter J. Mitsch
Associate Dean, Graduate Medical Education . . . . Louis J. Ling, M.D.
Associate Dean, Primary Care. . . . . Kathleen D. Brooks, M.D.
Associate Dean, Social Medicine and Medical Humanities . . . . Mary Faith Marshall, Ph.D.
Associate Dean, Student Affairs . . . . Helene M. Horwitz, Ph.D.
Associate Dean, Students and Student Learning . . . . Kathleen V. Watson, M.D.
Special Advisor, Basic Sciences. . . . . Harry T. Orr, Ph.D.
Assistant Dean, Admissions. . . . . Paul T. White, J.D.
Assistant Dean, Faculty Development . . . . Carole J. Bland, Ph.D.
Director, International Medical Education . . . . Phillip K. Peterson, M.D.

Department and Division or Section Chairs

Basic Sciences

Biochemistry, Molecular Biology, and Biophysics. . . . . David A. Bernlohr, Ph.D.
Genetics, Cell Biology, and Development . . . . Brian G. Van Ness, Ph.D.
Integrative Biology and Physiology . . . . Joseph M. Metzger, M.D.
Laboratory Medicine and Pathology . . . . Leo T. Furcht, M.D.
Microbiology . . . . Ashley T. Haase, M.D.
Neuroscience. . . . . Timothy J. Ebner, M.D., Ph.D.
Pharmacology . . . . Horace H. Loh, Ph.D.

Clinical Sciences

Anesthesiology. . . . . Richard C. Prielipp, M.D.
Dermatology . . . . Maria D. Hordinsky, M.D.
Emergency Medicine . . . . Joseph E. Clinton, M.D.
Family Medicine and Community Health . . . . Macaran A. Baird, M.D.
Medicine. . . . . Wesley J. Miller, M.D. (Interim)
Neurology . . . . David C. Anderson, M.D.
Neurosurgery. . . . . Stephen J. Haines, M.D., Ph.D.
Obstetrics, Gynecology, and Women's Health . . . . Linda F. Carson, M.D.
Ophthalmology . . . . Jay H. Krachmer, M.D.
Orthopaedic Surgery . . . . Denis R. Clohisy, M.D.
Otolaryngology . . . . Bevan Yueh, M.D.
Pediatrics . . . . Aaron L. Friedman, M.D.
Physical Medicine and Rehabilitation . . . . Dennis D. Dykstra, M.D., Ph.D.
Psychiatry . . . . S. Charles Schulz, M.D.
Radiology . . . . Charles A. Dietz, M.D.
Surgery . . . . Selwyn M. Vickers, M.D.
Therapeutic Radiology and Radiation Oncology . . . . Kathryn E. Dusenbery, M.D.
Urologic Surgery . . . . Eduardo T. Fernandes, M.D. (Interim)

Other Programs

Engineering in Medicine, Institute for . . . . Jeffrey McCullough, M.D.
Center for Developmental Biology . . . . Scott B. Selleck, M.D.
Clinical Outcomes Research Center . . . . Marc F. Swiontkowski, M.D.
General Clinical Research Center. . . . . Elizabeth R. Seaquist, M.D.
History of Medicine. . . . . Jennifer Gunn, Ph.D. (Interim)
Immunology Center. . . . . Matthew F. Mescher, Ph.D.
Institute for Human Genetics. . . . . Harry T. Orr, Ph.D.
Lillehei Heart Institute. . . . . Daniel J. Garry, M.D.
Lung Science and Health, Center for . . . . Marshall I. Hertz, M.D.
M.D.-Ph.D. Program. . . . . W. Tucker LeBien, Ph.D.
Deborah E. Powell Center for Women's Health . . . . Nancy C. Raymond, M.D.
Rural Physician Associate Program . . . . TBD
Stem Cell Institute. . . . . Jonathan M.W. Slack, M.D.

*School of Public Health.

University of Mississippi School of Medicine

2500 North State Street
Jackson, Mississippi 39216-4505
601-984-1000; 984-1010 (dean's office); 984-1011 (fax)
Web site: www.umc.edu

The University of Mississippi School of Medicine was established at Oxford in 1903 as a two-year school. In 1955, it was moved to the University of Mississippi Medical Center in Jackson and expanded to a four-year program. The first degrees were awarded in 1957.

Type: public
2008-2009 total enrollment: 407
Clinical facilities: University Hospital, Blair E. Batson Hospital for Children, Winfred L. Wiser Hospital for Women and Infants, Wallace Conerly Hospital for Critical Care, University Rehabilitation Center, Mississippi Children's Cancer Clinic, G.V. "Sonny" Montgomery Department of Veterans Affairs Medical Center (Jackson), University Hospital and Clinics-Holmes County.

University Officials

Chancellor . . . . Robert C. Khayat
Vice Chancellor for Health Affairs, Medical Center. . . . . Daniel W. Jones, M.D.
Associate Vice Chancellor for Academic Affairs. . . . . Helen R. Turner, M.D., Ph.D.
Associate Vice Chancellor for Financial Affairs, Medical Center. . . . . J. Michael Lightsey
Associate Vice Chancellor for Health Systems
  and Chief Executive Officer, University
  Hospitals and Clinics . . . . William Ferniany, Ph.D.
Associate Vice Chancellor for Administrative Affairs, Medical Center. . . . . . David L. Powe, Ed.D.
Associate Vice Chancellor for Strategic Research
  Alliances, Medical Center . . . . David Dzielak, Ph.D.
Associate Vice Chancellor for Research, Medical Center . . . . John Hall, Ph.D.
Associate Vice Chancellor, Multicultural Affairs, Medical Center . . . . Jasmine Taylor, M.D.
Associate Vice Chancellor for Nursing, Medical Center. . . . . Kaye Bender, Ph.D.
Associate Vice Chancellor, Clinical Affairs, Medical Center . . . . Scott P. Stringer, M.D.
Dean, School of Graduate Studies in the Health Sciences . . . . Joey Granger, Ph.D.
Assistant Vice Chancellor for VA Affairs, Medical Center. . . . . Kent A. Kirchner, M.D.
Director, Student Records and Registrar, Medical Center . . . . Barbara Westerfield
Director, Public Affairs, Medical Center . . . . Tena McKenzie (Interim)
Director, Continuing Health Professional
  Education, Medical Center . . . . Shirley Schlessinger, M.D.
Director, Rowland Medical Library, Medical Center . . . . Susan B. Clark, M.L.S. (Interim)

Medical School Administrative Staff

Dean. . . . . Daniel W. Jones, M.D.
Associate Dean, Student Affairs . . . . Jerry F. Clark, Ph.D.
Associate Dean, Admissions . . . . Steven T. Case, Ph.D.
Associate Dean, Graduate Medical Education . . . . Shirley Schlessinger, M.D.
Associate Dean, Academic Affairs. . . . . LouAnn Woodward, M.D.
Associate Dean for Coordination of Education at VA . . . . Sharon P. Douglas, M.D.
Assistant Dean, Academic Affairs . . . . Loretta Jackson-Williams, M.D., Ph.D.
Director, Laboratory Animal Facilities. . . . . Andrew W. Grady, D.V.M.

University of Mississippi School of Medicine: MISSISSIPPI

Department and Division or Section Chairs

Basic Sciences

Anatomy . . . . Duane E. Haines, Ph.D.
Biochemistry . . . . Donald B. Sittman, Jr., Ph.D. (Interim)
Microbiology . . . . Richard J. O'Callaghan, Ph.D.
Pathology . . . . Steven A. Bigler, M.D.
Pharmacology and Toxicology . . . . Jerry M. Farley, Ph.D. (Interim)
Physiology and Biophysics . . . . John E. Hall, Ph.D.
Preventive Medicine. . . . . Vacant

Clinical Sciences

Anesthesiology. . . . . Claude D. Brunson, M.D.
Emergency Medicine . . . . Robert L. Galli, M.D.
Family Medicine . . . . Diane K. Beebe, M.D.
Medicine. . . . . Richard D. deShazo, M.D.
Neurology. . . . . Hartmut Uschmann, M.D. (Interim)
Neurosurgery. . . . . H. Louis Harkey, M.D. (Interim)
Obstetrics and Gynecology. . . . . Bryan D. Cowan, M.D.
Ophthalmology . . . . Ching J. Chen, M.D.
Orthopedic Surgery. . . . . Robert A. McGuire, Jr., M.D.
Otolaryngology and Communication Sciences. . . . . Scott P. Stringer, M.D.
Pediatrics . . . . Owen B. Evans, M.D.
Psychiatry . . . . Grayson Norquist, M.D.
Radiation Oncology. . . . . Srinivasan Vijayakumar, M.B.B.S
Radiology . . . . Timothy McCowan, M.D.
Surgery . . . . Marc E. Mitchell, M.D.

University of Missouri—Columbia School of Medicine

MA202 Medical Sciences Building, DC018.00
One Hospital Drive
Columbia, Missouri 65212
573-882-2923 (medical education); 882-1566 (dean's office); 882-9219 (curriculum);
884-4808 (fax)
Web site: http://som.missouri.edu

Founded in 1841, the University of Missouri School of Medicine offered only a two-year basic sciences program for much of its early existence. The present four-year program dates from 1956 when the University Hospital opened. Partnering with the University of Missouri Health Care, the school of medicine is located on the Columbia campus.

Type: public
2008-2009 total enrollment: 384
Clinical facilities: University Hospital; Children's Hospital; Columbia Regional Hospital; Ellis Fischel Cancer Center; Harry S Truman Veterans Affairs Hospital; Howard A. Rusk Rehabilitation Center; Mid-Missouri Mental Health Center; Missouri Rehabilitation Center at Mt. Vernon, Missouri; Capital Region Medical Center, Jefferson City, Missouri; and Cooper County Memorial Hospital, Boonville, Missouri.

University Officials

President. . . . . Gary D. Forsee
Vice President for Academic Affairs . . . . Steven Graham, Ph.D. (Interim)
Vice President for Finance and Administration . . . . Nikki Krawitz, Ph.D.
Chancellor, Columbia campus . . . . Brady Deaton, Ph.D.
Vice Chancellor for Health Sciences. . . . . Harold A. Williamson, Jr., M.D. (Interim)
Provost, Columbia campus . . . . Brian L. Foster, Ph.D.

Medical School Administrative Staff

Dean. . . . . Robert Churchill, M.D. (Interim)
Senior Associate Dean for Administration and Finance and Executive Director, UP . . . . . . Open
Associate Dean for Administration and Finance . . . . Kenneth Hammann
Senior Associate Dean for Research . . . . Jamal A. Ibdah, M.D., Ph.D.
Senior Associate Dean for Education and Faculty Development. . . . . Linda Headrick, M.D.
Associate Dean for Alumni Affairs . . . . Ted D. Groshong, M.D.
Associate Dean for Curriculum. . . . . Open
Associate Dean for Education Evaluation and Improvement . . . . Kimberly Hoffman, Ph.D.
Associate Dean for Graduate Medical Education . . . . John W. Gay, M.D.
Associate Dean for Research. . . . . Jerry Parker, Ph.D.
Associate Dean for Student Programs . . . . Rachel Brown, M.B.B.S.
Director, Center for Health Care Quality . . . . Douglas Wakefield, Ph.D.
Director, Health Sciences Library. . . . . Deborah H. Ward
Director, International Psychosocial Trauma Center . . . . Arshad Husain, M.D.
Director, Missouri Institute of Mental Health . . . . Danny Wedding, Ph.D.
Director, Diabetes and Cardiovascular Research . . . . James R. Sowers, M.D.
Director, Ellis Fischel Cancer Center . . . . Charles W. Caldwell, M.D., Ph.D.
Director, National Center for Gender Physiology . . . . Virginia Huxley, Ph.D.

Department and Division or Section Chairs

Basic Sciences

Biochemistry . . . . Gerald L. Hazelbauer, Ph.D.
Molecular Microbiology and Immunology. . . . . Mark McIntosh, Ph.D.
Medical Pharmacology and Physiology . . . . Ronald Korthuis, Ph.D.

Clinical Sciences

Anesthesiology and Perioperative Medicine. . . . . Joel Johnson, M.D., Ph.D.
Child Health . . . . Open

Cardiology . . . . Zuhdi Lababidi, M.D.
Developmental Pediatrics . . . . Tracy Stroud, D.O.
Diabetes and Endocrinology . . . . Bert Bachrach, M.D.
Gastroenterology . . . . Alejandro Ramirez, M.D.
General Pediatrics . . . . Thomas Selva, M.D.
Genetics. . . . . Jerome Gorski, M.D.
Hematology and Oncology . . . . Barbara Gruner, M.D. (Interim)
Infectious Disease, Immunology, and Rheumatology . . . . Michael Cooperstock, M.D.
Neonatology. . . . . John A. Pardalos, M.D.
Nephrology . . . . Ted D. Groshong, M.D.
Neurology . . . . Nitin Patel, M.D.
Pediatric Intensive Care . . . . Patricia Wankum, M.D.
Pulmonary Medicine and Allergy . . . . Peter Konig, M.D.
Dermatology . . . . Karen Edison, M.D.
Emergency Medicine . . . . John Yanos, M.D.
Family and Community Medicine . . . . Steven C. Zweig, M.D.
Internal Medicine . . . . Kevin C. Dellsperger, M.D., Ph.D.
Cardiovascular Medicine. . . . . William Fay, M.D., Ph.D.
Endocrinology, Diabetes, and Metabolism . . . . James R. Sowers, M.D.
Gastroenterology and Hepatology . . . . Jamal A. Ibdah, M.D., Ph.D.
General Internal Medicine . . . . William C. Steinmann, M.D.
Hematology and Medical Oncology. Carl Freter, M.D., Ph.D.
Immunology and Rheumatology . . . . William C. Steinmann, M.D. (Interim)
Infectious Disease. . . . . William Salzer, M.D. (Interim)
Nephrology . . . . Ramesh Khanna, M.D.
Pulmonary, Critical Care, and Environmental Medicine . . . . Rajiv Dhand, M.D.
Neurology . . . . Pradeep Sahota, M.D.
Obstetrics, Gynecology, and Women's Health . . . . Hung Winn, M.D., J.D.
Gynecologic Oncology . . . . Mark I. Hunter, M.D.
Maternal Fetal Medicine. . . . . Randall C. Floyd, M.D.
Obstetrics and Gynecology Generalist . . . . James R. Green, M.D.
Obstetrics and Gynecology Research . . . . Kathy Timms, Ph.D.
Reproductive Endocrinology and Infertility . . . . Danny J. Schust, M.D.
Urogynecology . . . . Raymond Foster, M.D.
Ophthalmology . . . . John W. Cowden, M.D.
Orthopaedic Surgery . . . . Jason Calhoun, M.D.
Otolaryngology-Head and Neck Surgery . . . . Karen Calhoun, M.D.
Pathology and Anatomical Sciences . . . . Douglas Anthony, M.D., Ph.D.
Physical Medicine and Rehabilitation . . . . Greg Worsowicz, M.D.
Psychiatry . . . . Open
Radiology . . . . Robert Churchill, M.D.
Diagnostic Radiology . . . . Robert Churchill, M.D.
Nuclear . . . . Amolak Singh, M.D.
Radiation Oncology . . . . Stephen Westgate, M.D.
Surgery . . . . Steve Eubanks, M.D.
Cardiothoracic . . . . John Markley, M.D. (Interim)
General Surgery and Critical Care. . . . . Bruce Ramshaw, M.D.
Neurosurgery . . . . N. Scott Litofsky, M.D.
Plastic and Reconstructive Surgery . . . . Charles L. Puckett, M.D.
Surgical Oncology . . . . Paul S. Dale, M.D.
Urology . . . . Durwood E. Neal, M.D.
Vascular Surgery. . . . . W. Kirt Nichols, M.D.

Other

Health Management and Informatics . . . . Grant T. Savage, Ph.D.
Nutrition and Health Sciences . . . . Christopher D. Hardin, Ph.D.

University of Missouri—Kansas City School of Medicine

2411 Holmes Street
Kansas City, Missouri 64108-2792
816-235-1808 (dean's office); 235-5277 (fax)
Web site: www.med.umkc.edu

The school of medicine is part of a four-campus university system in Missouri that includes Kansas City, Columbia, St. Louis, and Rolla. It is one of four health science schools in Kansas City. The medical school offers a six-year combined B.A.-M.D. program. The first class enrolled in fall 1971.

Type: public
2008-2009 total enrollment: 630
Clinical facilities: Children's Mercy Hospital, Truman Medical Center-West, Truman Medical Center-Lakewood, Western Missouri Mental Health Center, St. Luke's Hospital, Research Hospital and Medical Center, Menorah Medical Center, Veterans Administration Hospital.

University Officials

President. . . . . Gary D. Forsee, Ph.D.
Chancellor . . . . Guy H. Bailey, Ph.D.
Provost and Vice Chancellor for Academic Affairs. . . . . Gail Hackett, Ph.D.
Provost for Health Sciences Emeritus . . . . E. Grey Dimond, M.D.

Medical School Administrative Staff

Dean. . . . . Betty M. Drees, M.D.
Senior Associate Dean . . . . Paul G. Cuddy, Pharm.D.
Chief Financial Officer. . . . . Chuck Henning
Associate Dean for Student Affairs . . . . Brenda Rogers, M.D.
Associate Dean and Chair, Graduate Medical Education . . . . Open
Assistant Dean for Graduate Medical Education . . . . Open
Assistant Dean for Student Affairs. . . . . Open
Associate Dean for Medical Education . . . . Louise M. Arnold, Ph.D.
Assistant Dean for Medical Education. . . . . Steven Go, M.D.
Director, Health Sciences Library. . . . . Margaret P. Mullaly-Quijas
Associate Dean for St. Luke's Programs . . . . Diana Dark, M.D.
Assistant Dean for St. Luke's Programs. . . . . Open
Associate Dean for Children's Mercy Programs. . . . . Kevin J. Kelly, M.D.
Chair, Council of Docents . . . . David Wooldridge, M.D.
Chair, Faculty Council . . . . John Foxworth, Pharm.D.
Director, Internal Medicine Residency Program . . . . Brent Beasley, M.D.
Director, Office of Educational Resources. . . . . Open
Associate Dean, Office of Minority Affairs. . . . . Susan Wilson, Ph.D.
Director, Office of Student Affairs . . . . Marilyn K. McGuyre
Director, Computer and Evaluation Resource Center . . . . Open
Associate Dean for Western Missouri Mental
  Health Center Programs . . . . Rob K. Hornstra, M.D.
Associate Dean for Truman Medical Center Programs. . . . . Mark T. Steele, M.D.
Assistant Dean, Council on Evaluation . . . . Daryl A. Lynch, M.D.
Associate Dean of Clinical Research . . . . Christopher J. Papasian, Ph.D. (Interim)
Assistant Dean for Truman Medical Center, Lakewood Programs. . . . . Rose J. Zwerenz, M.D.
Assistant to the Dean. . . . . Melvin Davis
Assistant Dean, Council on Selection . . . . Christine Sullivan (Interim)

Department and Division or Section Chairs

Basic Medical Science

Chair. . . . . Christopher J. Papasian, Ph.D.

Clinical Sciences

Anesthesia. . . . . Eugene E. Fibuch, M.D.
Community and Family Medicine. . . . . Open

Geriatrics... Jon F. Dedon, M.D.
Emergency Health Services .... Matthew Gratton, M.D.
Medicine... George R. Reisz, M.D.
    Cardiology... Mukesh Garg, M.D.
    Dermatology and Rheumatology........................... Lynn I. DeMarco, M.D.
    Endocrinology..................................... Lamont Weide, M.D., Ph.D.
    Gastroenterology .... Stuart Chen, M.D.
    General Internal Medicine .... Eyad Al-Hihi, M.D.
    Hematology and Oncology............................... Jill Moormeier, M.D.
    Infectious Disease..................................... David Bamberger, M.D.
    Neurology .... Daryl W. Thompson, M.D.
    Pharmacology and Therapeutics......................... Paul G. Cuddy, Pharm.D.
    Respiratory Diseases and Critical Care................. Gary A. Salzman, M.D.
Obstetrics and Gynecology.............................. Dev Maulik, M.D., Ph.D.
    Adolescent Gynecology................................. Julie Strickland, M.D.
    Eurogynecology .... Richard F. C. Hill, M.D.
    Gynecologic Oncology .... Darryl L. Wallace, M.D.
    Gynecology .... D. Mark Schnee, D.O. (Interim)
    Neonatology.. P. Gary Pettett, M.D.
    Perinatology (Maternal and Fetal Medicine) .... David C. Mundy, M.D.
    Reproductive Endocrinology............................ Gregory Starks, M.D.
Ophthalmology .... Nelson R. Sabates, M.D.
    Contact Lens .... Dawn Birch, D.O.
    Cornea/Ureitis.. David Gritz, M.D.
    Glaucoma .... Rohit Krishna, M.D.
    Neuro-Ophthalmology .... Billi S. Wallace, M.D.
    Ophthalmologic Pathology............................. Mahendra K. Rupani, M.D.
    Ophthalmologic Plastic Surgery .... David B. Lyon, M.D.
    Retina .... Nelson R. Sabates, M.D.
    Refractive... Jean Hausheer, M.D.
Orthopaedic Surgery .... James J. Hamilton, M.D.
Pathology .... Russell M. Fiorella, M.D.
Pediatrics .... Kevin J. Kelly, M.D.
    Adolescent Medicine .... Daryl Lynch, M.D.
    Allergy and Immunology .... Jay M. Portnoy, M.D.
    Cardiology.. R. Gowdamarajan, M.D.
    Development and Behavioral Sciences.................. Michele G. Kilo, M.D.
    Emergency Medicine .... Laura Fitzmaurice, M.D.
    Endocrinology.. Wayne Moore, M.D.
    Gastroenterology .... Charles C. Roberts, M.D.
    General Pediatrics .... Kenneth L. Wible, M.D.
    Genetics.. Wayne Moore, M.D.
    Hematology and Oncology .... Gerald M. Woods, M.D.
    Infectious Disease..................................... Mary Anne Jackson, M.D.
    Neonatology.. Howard W. Kilbride, M.D.
    Nephrology .... Bradley A. Warady, M.D. (Interim)
    Orthopaedic Surgery .... Brad Olney, M.D.
    Pulmonology .... Terrence Carver, M.D.
    Rheumatology .... Andrew Lasky, M.D.
    Surgery .... George Holcomb III, M.D.
Psychiatry .... J. Stuart Munro, M.D.
Forensic Psychiatry.................................... David Vlach, M.D.
Radiology .... David Dixon, M.D. (Interim)
Surgery .... Glenn Talboy, M.D. (Interim)
    Laparoscopy Surgery................................... Open
    Thoracic .... Charles Van Way III, M.D.
    Neurosurgery... John Gianino, M.D.
    Otolaryngology....................................... Open
    Trauma .... Doug Geehan, M.D.
    Urology .... Narendra K. Khare, M.D.
    Vascular.. Open

Saint Louis University School of Medicine

1402 South Grand Boulevard
Saint Louis, Missouri 63104
314-577-8000 (medical center); 977-9801 (dean's office); 977-9899 (fax)
Web site: http://medschool.slu.edu

The first faculty in medicine of the university was appointed in 1836. The present school of medicine dates from 1903 when the Marion Sims-Beaumont College of Medicine came under the direction of the university. The medical school is part of the St. Louis University Medical Center, which is located one mile from the university proper.

Type: private
2008-2009 total enrollment: 625
Clinical facilities: Saint Louis University Hospital, Cardinal Glennon Children's Medical Center, St. Mary's Health Center, the Anheuser Busch Institute, St. John's Mercy Medical Center, St. Louis Veterans Affairs Medical Center (John Cochran and Jefferson Barracks Divisions), St. Elizabeth's Hospital.

University Officials

President. . . . . Lawrence Biondi, Ph.D., S.J.
Provost . . . . Joseph Weixlmann, Ph.D.
Vice President for Business and Finance. . . . . Robert Woodruff

Medical School Administrative Staff

Dean. . . . . Philip D. Anderson, M.D.
Associate Dean for Graduate Medical Education . . . . Robert M. Heaney, M.D.
Associate Dean for Admissions and Student Affairs . . . . L. James Willmore, M.D.
Associate Dean for Curricular Affairs . . . . Stuart J. Slavin, M.D.
Associate Dean for Finance and Administration . . . . Michael J. Meyer
Associate Dean for Multicultural Affairs . . . . George H. Rausch, Ed.D.
Associate Dean for Research. . . . . Jennifer Lodge, Ph.D.
Assistant Dean for Curricular Affairs. . . . . William C. Mootz, M.D.
Assistant Dean for Student Affairs. . . . . James E. Swierkosz, Ph.D.
Chief Executive Officer, University Medical Group . . . . Michael J. Meyer (Interim)

Department and Division or Section Chairs

Basic Sciences

Biochemistry and Molecular Biology. . . . . William S. Sly, M.D.
Comparative Medicine. . . . . Richard E. Doyle, D.V.M.
Institute for Molecular Virology . . . . Maurice Green, Ph.D.
Molecular Microbiology and Immunology. William S. M. Wold, Ph.D.
Pathology . . . . Carole A. Vogler, M.D. (Interim)
Pharmacological and Physiological Science. Thomas C. Westfall, Ph.D.

Clinical Sciences

Anesthesiology. . . . . Gary R. Haynes, M.D.
Community and Family Medicine. . . . . Richard O. Schamp, M.D. (Interim)
Dermatology . . . . Scott W. Fosko, M.D.
Internal Medicine . . . . Adrian M. Di Bisceglie, M.D. (Interim)
  Allergy and Immunology . . . . Raymond G. Slavin, M.D.
  Bone Marrow Transplantation, Oncology, and Hematology . . . . Paul J. Petruska, M.D.
  Cardiology. . . . . Arthur J. Labovitz, M.D.
  Endocrinology and Metabolism. . . . . John E. Morley, M.D. (Interim)
  Gastroenterology and Hepatology. . . . . Bruce R. Bacon, M.D.
  General Internal Medicine . . . . Thomas J. Olsen, M.D. (Interim)
  Geriatric Medicine . . . . John E. Morley, M.D.
  Immunobiology . . . . Daniel M. Hoft, M.D., Ph.D.
  Infectious Diseases and Immunology. . . . . Robert B. Belshe, M.D.

Nephrology . . . . Kevin J. Martin, M.D.
Pulmonary, Critical Care, and Sleep Medicine . . . . George M. Matuschak, M.D.
Rheumatology . . . . Terry L. Moore, M.D.
Neurology and Psychiatry . . . . Henry J. Kaminski, M.D.
Geriatric Psychiatry . . . . George T. Grossberg, M.D.
Obstetrics, Gynecology, and Women's Health . . . . Raul Artal, M.D.
Ophthalmology . . . . Oscar A. Cruz, M.D.
Orthopaedic Surgery . . . . Berton R. Moed, M.D.
Otolaryngology-Head and Neck Surgery . . . . Mark A. Varvares, M.D.
Pediatrics . . . . Robert W. Wilmott, M.D.
Adolescent Medicine . . . . M. Susan Heaney, M.D., M.P.H. (Interim)
Allergy and Immunology . . . . Raymond G. Slavin, M.D., and Alan P. Knutsen, M.D.
Cardiology . . . . Kenneth Schowengerdt, M.D.
Child Protection . . . . Timothy J. Kutz, M.D.
Critical Care . . . . Robert S. Ream, M.D. (Interim)
Developmental Pediatrics . . . . Timothy J. Fete, M.D., M.P.H. (Interim)
Emergency Medicine . . . . Robert G. Flood, M.D.
Endocrinology . . . . Sherida E. Tollefson, M.D.
Gastroenterology . . . . Jeffrey H. Teckman, M.D.
General Academic Pediatrics . . . . Timothy J. Fete, M.D.
Hematology and Oncology . . . . William S. Ferguson, M.D.
Infectious Diseases . . . . Stephen J. Barenkamp, M.D.
Medical Genetics . . . . Akihiko Noguchi, M.D., M.P.H. (Interim)
Neonatology . . . . William J. Keenan, M.D.
Nephrology . . . . Ellen G. Wood, M.D.
Pulmonology . . . . Blakeslee E. Noyes, M.D.
Rheumatology . . . . Terry L. Moore, M.D.
Toxicology . . . . Anthony J. Scalzo, M.D.
Radiation Oncology . . . . Bruce J. Walz, M.D.
Radiology . . . . Michael K. Wolverson, M.D.
Nuclear Medicine . . . . Medhat M. Osman, M.D.
Surgery . . . . Robert G. Johnson, M.D.
Cardiothoracic Surgery . . . . Keith S. Naunheim, M.D.
Emergency Services . . . . Laurie E. Byrne, M.D.
General Surgery . . . . Eddy C. Hsueh, M.D.
Kidney, Liver, and Pancreas Transplantation . . . . Paul J. Garvin, M.D.
Neurosurgery . . . . Richard D. Bucholz, M.D.
Pediatric Surgery . . . . Charles H. Andrus, M.D.
Plastic Surgery . . . . Christian E. Paletta, M.D.
Trauma Service . . . . Aaron M. Scifres, M.D.
Urology . . . . James M. Cummings, M.D.
Vascular Surgery . . . . Gary J. Peterson, M.D.

Washington University in St. Louis School of Medicine

660 South Euclid Avenue, Box 8106
Saint Louis, Missouri 63110
314-362-5000; 362-6827 (dean's office); 367-6666 (fax)
Web site: http://medinfo.wustl.edu

Medical education began at Washington University in 1891 by affiliation between the university and the St. Louis Medical College. Today, the medical school is part of the Washington University Medical Center.

Type: private
2008-2009 total enrollment: 591
Clinical facilities: Washington University Medical Center: Alvin J. Siteman Cancer Center, Barnard Free Skin and Cancer Hospital, Barnes-Jewish Hospital, Central Institute for the Deaf, St. Louis Children's Hospital. **Other facilities:** Metropolitan Psychiatric Center, St. Louis Shriner's Hospital for Crippled Children, St. Louis Veterans Administration (John Cochran) Hospital.

University Officials

Chancellor	Mark S. Wrighton, Ph.D.
Executive Vice Chancellor for Medical Affairs	Larry J. Shapiro, M.D.

Medical School Administrative Staff

Dean. . . . . Larry J. Shapiro, M.D.
Associate Dean and Associate Vice Chancellor,
  Administration and Finance . . . . Richard J. Stanton
Associate Vice Chancellor, Clinical Affairs. . . . . James P. Crane, M.D.
Associate Dean and Associate Vice Chancellor, Animal Affairs . . . . . . Samuel L. Stanley, Jr., M.D.
Associate Vice Chancellor, Medical Public Affairs . . . . Donald E. Clayton
Associate Vice Chancellor, Medical Alumni and Development Programs . . . . Pamela Buell
Associate Dean and Associate Vice Chancellor,
  Admissions and Continuing Medical
  Education . . . . W. Edwin Dodson, M.D.
Associate Dean, Student Affairs . . . . Leslie E. Kahl, M.D.
Associate Dean, Graduate Medical Education . . . . Rebecca P. McAlister, M.D.
Associate Dean, Medical Student Education . . . . Alison J. Whelan, M.D.
Associate Dean and Director, Medical Library. . . . . Paul Schoening
Associate Dean, Human Studies . . . . Philip A. Ludbrook, M.D.
Associate Dean and Director, Diversity Programs. . . . . Will R. Ross, M.D.
Associate Dean, Clinical Studies Research . . . . Vacant
Assistant Dean, Admissions and Student Affairs. . . . . Koong-Nah Chung, Ph.D.
Assistant Dean, Career Counseling . . . . Kathryn Diemer, M.D.
Assistant Dean and Chief Information Officer. . . . . Michael P. Caputo
Assistant Dean and Director, Center for Clinical Studies . . . . James A. Moran, J.D.
Assistant Vice Chancellor and Assistant Dean,
  Facilities and Chief Facilities Officer . . . . Walter W. Davis, Jr.
Assistant Vice Chancellor and Assistant Dean, Finance . . . . George E. Andersson
Assistant Dean and Director, Program in Medicine . . . . Stephen S. Lefrak, M.D.
Assistant Dean, Academic Affairs and Registrar . . . . Deborah A. Monolo
Assistant Dean and Assistant Vice Chancellor, Special Programs . . . . Glenda Wiman
Assistant Dean, Student Affairs, and Director, Student Financial Aid . . . . Robert McCormack
Assistant Vice Chancellor, Veterinary Affairs . . . . Steven L. Leary, D.V.M.
Associate Vice Chancellor and Chief Counsel . . . . William F. Howard
Director of the Student and Employee Health
  Services, Medical Campus . . . . Karen Winters, M.D.

Department and Division or Section Chairs
Basic Sciences

Division of Biology and Biomedical Sciences. . . . . Philip D. Stahl, Ph.D.
Anatomy and Neurobiology . . . . David C. Van Essen, Ph.D.
Biochemistry and Molecular Biophysics. . . . . Thomas Ellenberger, D.V.M., Ph.D.
Cell Biology and Physiology . . . . Philip D. Stahl, Ph.D.
Genetics . . . . Susan K. Dutcher, Ph.D. (Interim)
Developmental Biology . . . . David M. Ornitz, Ph.D. (Interim)
Molecular Microbiology. . . . . Stephen M. Beverley, Ph.D.
Pathology and Immunology . . . . Herbert W. Virgin IV, M.D., Ph.D.
Division of Biostatistics. . . . . D. C. Rao, Ph.D.
Medical Scientist Training Program . . . . Daniel E. Goldberg, M.D.

Clinical Sciences

Anesthesiology. . . . . Alex S. Evers, M.D.
Internal Medicine . . . . Kenneth S. Polonsky, M.D.
   Allergy and Immunology . . . . H. James Wedner, M.D.
   Bone and Mineral Diseases. . . . . Dwight A. Towler, M.D.,Ph.D.
   Bioorganic Chemistry and Molecular Pharmacology. . . . . Richard W. Gross, M.D., Ph.D.
   Cardiology and Cardiovascular Diseases. . . . . Kenneth S. Polonsky, M.D. (Interim)
   Dermatology . . . . Lynn A. Cornelius, M.D.
   Health Behavior Research. . . . . Mario Schootman, Ph.D.
   Emergency Medicine . . . . Brent E. Ruoff, M.D.
   Endocrinology, Metabolism, and Lipid Research . . . . Clay F. Semenkovich, M.D.
   Gastroenterology . . . . Nicholas O. Davidson, M.D.
   General Medical Sciences. . . . . Bradley A. Evanoff, M.D.
   Geriatrics and Nutritional Science. . . . . Samuel Klein, M.D.
   Hematology. . . . . Stuart A. Kornfeld, M.D., and Phillip W. Majerus, M.D.
   Infectious Diseases . . . . Victoria Fraser, M.D., and Daniel Goldberg, M.D.
   Medical Education . . . . Melvin S. Blanchard, M.D.
   Oncology. . . . . John F. DiPersio, M.D., Ph.D.
   Pulmonary and Critical Care Medicine . . . . Michael J. Holtzman, M.D.
   Renal Diseases . . . . Marc R. Hammerman, M.D.
   Rheumatology . . . . John P. Atkinson, M.D. (Interim)
   VA Medical Service. . . . . Scott G. Hickman, M.D.
Neurology. . . . . David M. Holtzman, M.D.
Neurological Surgery. . . . . Ralph G. Dacey, Jr., M.D.
Obstetrics and Gynecology. . . . . George A. Macones, M.D.
   Gynecology . . . . Jeffrey Peipert, M.D.
   Gynecologic Oncology . . . . David G. Mutch, M.D.
   Maternal-Fetal Medicine. . . . . David Stamilio, M.D.
   Reproductive Endocrinology. . . . . Randall R. Odem, M.D.
   Research . . . . D. Michael Nelson, M.D., Ph.D.
Ophthalmology and Visual Sciences . . . . Michael Kass, M.D.
Orthopaedic Surgery. . . . . Richard H. Gelberman, M.D.
Otolaryngology . . . . Richard A. Chole, M.D., Ph.D.
Pediatrics . . . . Alan L. Schwartz, M.D., Ph.D.
   Allergy and Pulmonary. . . . . Thomas W. Ferkol, M.D.
   Cardiology . . . . George Van Hare, M.D.
   Critical Care Medicine . . . . Allan Doctor, M.D.
   Diagnostic Medicine. . . . . James Keating, M.D.
   Emergency Medicine . . . . David M. Jaffe, M.D.
   Endocrinology and Diabetes . . . . Louis J. Muglia, M.D., Ph.D.
   Gastroenterology . . . . Phillip I. Tarr, M.D.
   Genetics. . . . . Dorothy Grange, M.D.
   Hematology and Oncology. . . . . Robert Hayashi, M.D.
   Immunology and Rheumatology. . . . . Andrew J. White, M.D.
   Infectious Diseases . . . . Gregory A. Storch, M.D.
   Laboratory Medicine . . . . Gregory A. Storch, M.D.
   Nephrology . . . . Keith A. Hruska, M.D.
   Newborn Medicine. . . . . F. Sessions Cole, M.D.
Psychiatry . . . . Charles F. Zorumski, M.D.
Radiology . . . . R. Gilbert Jost, M.D.
   Diagnostic Radiology . . . . Daniel D. Picus, M.D.
   Nuclear Medicine. . . . . Barry A. Siegel, M.D.
   Radiological Sciences . . . . Marcus E. Raichle, M.D.
Radiation Oncology. . . . . Jeff M. Michalski, M.D. (Interim)
Surgery. . . . . Timothy J. Eberlein, M.D.
   Cardiothoracic Surgery. . . . . G. Alexander Patterson, M.D.
   Chief of Surgery at the VA . . . . Jeffrey F. Moley, M.D.
   General Surgery. . . . . Gregorio A. Sicard, M.D.
   Pediatric Surgery . . . . Brad W. Warner, M.D.
   Reconstructive Plastic Surgery. . . . . Susan E. Mackinnon, M.D.
   Urologic Surgery . . . . Gerald L. Andriole, M.D.
   Clinical . . . . Jeff M. Michalski, M.D.
   Medical Physics . . . . David A. Low, M.D.
   Radiation and Cancer Biology. . . . . Joseph L. Roti Roti, Ph.D.
   Bioinformatics and Outcomes Research. . . . . Joseph O. Deasy, Ph.D.

Creighton University School of Medicine

2500 California Plaza
Omaha, Nebraska 68178
402-280-2900; 280-2600 (dean's office); 280-4027 (fax)
Web site: http://medicine.creighton.edu

Creighton University was founded on September 2, 1878, in accordance with the wishes of Edward and Mary Creighton, under the name of Creighton College. On August 14, 1879, the trust created was surrendered to a new corporation, the Creighton University. The Creighton University School of Medicine was opened on October 1, 1892, and became the first professional school of the university. The Creighton University Medical Center includes the schools of medicine, dentistry, nursing, pharmacy, and allied health professions. Creighton University Medical Center and the Boys Town National Research Hospital are located on a single campus with the remainder of the university community.

Type: private
2008-2009 total enrollment: 460
Clinical facilities: Creighton University Medical Center, Boys Town National Research Hospital, Archbishop Bergan Mercy Hospital, Children's Hospital, Ehrling Bergquist USAF Strategic Hospital, Lincoln Regional Center, Veterans Administration Hospital (Omaha), Immanuel Medical Center.

University Officials

President	Father John P. Schlegel, S.J.
Vice President, Health Sciences	Cam E. Enarson, M.D.
Associate Vice President, Health Sciences	Fred H. Salzinger
Associate Vice President, Health Sciences	Sade Kosoko-Lasaki, M.D.
Assistant Vice President, Health Sciences, and Director, Health Sciences Library	James Bothmer
Coordinator, Health Sciences, Public Relations	N. Kathryn Clark
Vice President, University Ministry	Father Andy Alexander, S.J.
Vice President for Academic Affairs	Patrick Borchers, J.D.
Vice President for Administration and Financial Affairs	Daniel E. Burkey
Vice President for Student Services	John C. Cernech, Ph.D.
Vice President for University Relations	Lisa Calvert
Vice President, Information Systems	Brian A. Young
Registrar	John Krecek
Director, Media Services	Charles Lenosky
Assistant Vice President for Marketing and Public Relations	Kim Manning
Assistant Vice President for Research and Compliance	Kathleen Taggart
Director, Grants Administration	Beth Herr
Director of Development, School of Medicine	Matt Gerard

Medical School Administrative Staff

Dean	Cam E. Enarson, M.D.
Senior Associate Dean, Academic and Clinical Affairs	Stephen J. Lanspa, M.D.
Senior Associate Dean, Administration and Finance	Stanette Kennebrew, J.D.
Associate Dean, Academic and Faculty Affairs	Roberta E. Sonnino, M.D.
Chief Executive Officer, Creighton Medical Associates	Open
Associate Dean, Clinical Affairs	Stephen J. Lanspa, M.D.
Associate Dean, Continuing Medical Education	Sally C. O'Neill, Ph.D.
Associate Dean, Hospital Affairs	Linda N. Ollis
Associate Dean, Medical Education	William B. Jeffries, Ph.D.
Associate Dean for Research	Thomas F. Murray, Ph.D.
Associate Dean, Graduate Medical Education	Cecile M. Zielinski, M.D.
Associate Dean, Student Affairs	Michael J. Kavan, Ph.D.
Associate Dean, Veterans Affairs	Rowen K. Zetterman, M.D.
Assistant Dean for Admissions	Henry C. Nipper, Ph.D.
Assistant Dean, Clinical Affairs	Robert W. Dunlay, M.D.
Assistant Dean, Faculty Affairs	Archana Chatterjee, M.D.
Assistant Dean, Medical Education (Clinical)	Alfred D. Fleming, M.D.
Assistant Dean, Graduate Medical Education	Robin E. Graham, M.D.

Creighton University School of Medicine: NEBRASKA

Department and Division or Section Chairs

Basic Sciences

Biomedical Sciences . . . . Richard F. Murphy, Ph.D.
Health Policy and Ethics . . . . Amy Haddad, Ph.D.
Medical Microbiology and Immunology . . . . Richard V. Goering, Ph.D.
Pathology . . . . Roger A. Brumback, M.D.
Pharmacology . . . . Thomas F. Murray, Ph.D.

Clinical Sciences

Anesthesiology . . . . Nahel Saied, M.D.
Emergency Medicine . . . . Wesley S. Grigsby, M.D.
Family Practice . . . . Donald R. Frey, M.D.
Medicine . . . . Syed M. Mohiuddin, M.D.
    Allergy . . . . Thomas B. Casale, M.D.
    Cardiology . . . . Dennis J. Esterbrooks, M.D.
    Dermatology . . . . Christopher J. Huerter, M.D.
    Endocrinology . . . . Robert R. Recker, M.D.
    Gastroenterology . . . . Syed Bin-Saghccr, M.D.
    General Medicine . . . . Anna Maio, M.D.
    Hematology and Oncology . . . . Peter Silberstein, M.D.
    Infectious Diseases . . . . Gary L. Gorby, M.D.
    Nephrology . . . . Robert W. Dunlay, M.D.
    Pulmonary Medicine . . . . Dan Schuller, M.D.
    Rheumatology . . . . John A. Hurley, M.D., and Jay G. Kenik, M.D.
Neurology . . . . John M. Bertoni, M.D., Ph.D.
Obstetrics and Gynecology . . . . Alfred D. Fleming, M.D.
Pediatrics . . . . Terence L. Zach, M.D.
    Allergy and Immunology* . . . . Russell J. Hopp, D.O.
    Developmental Pediatrics* . . . . Andrea J. Steenson, M.D.
    Endocrinology and Adolescent Medicine* . . . . Open
    Gastroenterology* . . . . Open
    General Ambulatory* . . . . Open
    Infectious Disease* . . . . Archana Chatterjee, M.D.
    Metabolism . . . . William B. Rizzo, M.D.
    Newborn Medicine . . . . Terence L. Zach, M.D.
    Pediatric Cardiology* . . . . John Kugler, M.D.
    Pediatric Intensive Care . . . . Javed Akhtar, M.D.
    Rheumatology . . . . Open
Preventive Medicine and Public Health . . . . Henry T. Lynch, M.D.
Psychiatry . . . . Daniel R. Wilson, M.D., Ph.D.
Radiology . . . . Martin L. Goldman, M.D.
Surgery . . . . Jeffrey T. Sugimoto, M.D.
    Cardiothoracic Surgery . . . . Jeffrey T. Sugimoto, M.D.
    General Surgery . . . . Robert J. Fitzgibbons, Jr., M.D.
    Neurosurgery . . . . Charles Taylon, M.D.
    Ophthalmology . . . . Open
    Orthopedic Surgery . . . . Michael H. McGuire, M.D.
    Plastic and Reconstructive Surgery . . . . Open
    Urology . . . . Rei K. Chiou, M.D., Ph.D.
    Vascular Surgery . . . . Open

*Specialty without organizational autonomy.

University of Nebraska College of Medicine

986545 Nebraska Medical Center
Omaha, Nebraska 68198-6545
402-559-4000 (general information); 559-4204 (dean's office);
559-4148 (dean's office fax)
Web site: www.unmc.edu

The Omaha Medical College was incorporated in 1881. When it became part of the University of Nebraska in 1902, the basic sciences years were taught in Lincoln and the clinical years were taught in Omaha. In 1913, a new campus was established in Omaha for all medical education. The medical school is part of the University of Nebraska Medical Center.

Type: public
2008-2009 total enrollment: 486
Clinical facilities: The Nebraska Medical Center (composed of the University of Nebraska Hospital and Bishop Clarkson Memorial Hospital), Methodist Hospital, Children's Hospital, Immanuel Medical Center, Bergan Mercy Hospital, Omaha VA Hospital, Creighton University Medical Center, Boys Town National Research Hospital, Bryan LGH, St. Elizabeth's Hospital, Jennie Edmundson Hospital, Mercy Hospital, Mary Lanning Hospital, Good Samaritan Hospital, West Nebraska General Hospital, Columbus Community Hospital, Faith Regional Health Center, Fremont Area Medical Center, Great Plains Regional Medical Center, Regional West Medical Center, St. Francis Medical Center.

University Officials

President. . . . . James B. Milliken, J.D.
Chancellor and Vice President . . . . Harold M. Maurer, M.D.
Vice Chancellor for Academic Affairs . . . . Rubens J. Pamies, M.D.
Vice Chancellor for Business and Finance . . . . Donald S. Leuenberger
Associate Vice Chancellor, Student Services . . . . John W. McClain, Ph.D.
Director, Library . . . . Nancy N. Woelfl, Ph.D.
Director, Public Affairs. . . . . Renee A. Fry

Medical School Administrative Staff

Dean. . . . . John L. Gollan, M.D., Ph.D.
Executive Assistant to the Dean . . . . Delmer D. Lee
Assistant to the Dean for Special Projects . . . . John A. Benson, Jr., M.D.
Senior Associate Dean for Academic Affairs . . . . Gerald F. Moore, M.D.
Senior Associate Dean for Administration and Director of Finance . . . . Michael R. McGlade
Senior Associate Dean for Clinical Affairs. . . . . Rodney S. Markin, M.D., Ph.D.
Senior Associate Dean for the Health System . . . . Glenn A. Fosdick
Senior Associate Dean for Research Development. . . . . Steven H. Hinrichs, M.D.
Associate Dean for Admissions and Student Affairs . . . . Jeffrey W. Hill, M.D.
Associate Dean for Clinical Research . . . . Jennifer L. Larsen, M.D.
Associate Dean for Curriculum. . . . . Open
Associate Dean for Graduate Medical Education . . . . Robert S. Wigton, M.D.
Associate Dean for Hospital Services. . . . . Stephen B. Smith, M.D.
Associate Dean, School of Allied Health Professions . . . . Kyle P. Meyer, Ph.D.
Associate Dean for Veterans Affairs . . . . Rowen K. Zetterman, M.D.
Assistant Dean for Admissions . . . . Open
Assistant Dean for Graduate Medical Education . . . . James H. Stageman, M.D.
Assistant Dean for Operations . . . . Cory D. Shaw
Assistant Dean for Student and Multicultural Affairs . . . . Kristie D. Hayes, M.D.
Director, Dean's Business Office. . . . . Galen L. Kathol
Director, Comparative Medicine. . . . . Robert S. Dixon, D.V.M.

Department and Division or Section Chairs

Basic Sciences

Biochemistry and Molecular Biology. . . . . Judith K. Christman, Ph.D.
Cellular and Integrative Physiology. . . . . Irving H. Zucker, Ph.D.
Genetics, Cell Biology, and Anatomy . . . . James D. Shull, Ph.D.

Pathology and Microbiology.................................. Steven H. Hinrichs, M.D.
Pharmacology and Experimental Neuroscience................. Howard E. Gendelman, M.D.

Clinical Sciences

Anesthesiology.. Sheila J. Ellis, M.D. (Interim)
Emergency Medicine..................................... Robert L. Muelleman, M.D.
Family Practice .... Michael A. Sitorius, M.D.
Internal Medicine .... Lynell W. Klassen, M.D.
   Cardiology... John R. Windle, M.D.
   Dermatology .... Kristie D. Hayes, M.D.
   Diabetes, Endocrinology, and Metabolism .... Jennifer L. Larsen, M.D.
   Gastroenterology and Hepatology.......................... Mark E. Mailliard, M.D.
   General Internal Medicine .... Thomas G. Tape, M.D.
   Geriatrics and Gerontology............................. Jane F. Potter, M.D.
   Infectious Diseases .... Philip W. Smith, M.D.
   Nephrology .... Gerald C. Groggel, M.D.
   Oncology and Hematology.............................. Julie M. Vose, M.D.
   Pulmonary, Critical Care, Sleep, and Allergy .... Joseph H. Sisson, M.D.
   Rheumatology .... James R. O'Dell, M.D.
Neurological Sciences .... Pierre Fayad, M.D.
Obstetrics and Gynecology................................ Carl V. Smith, M.D.
Ophthalmology and Visual Sciences........................ Carl B. Camras, M.D.
Orthopedic Surgery and Rehabilitation...................... Kevin L. Garvin, M.D.
Otolaryngology-Head and Neck Surgery .... Donald A. Leopold, M.D.
Pediatrics .... John W. Sparks, M.D.
   Cardiology... John D. Kugler, M.D.
   Child Health Policy and City MatCH........................ Magda G. Peck, Sc.D.
   Cytogenetics....................................... Warren G. Sanger, Ph.D.
   Developmental Medicine .... Cynthia R. Ellis, M.D.
   Endocrinology and Diabetes............................. Kevin P. Corley, M.D.
   Gastroenterology and Nutrition .... Open
   General Pediatrics .... John N. Walburn, M.D.
   Genetics.. Open
   Hematology and Oncology.............................. Peter F. Coccia, M.D.
   Infectious Disease.................................... Open
   Inherited Metabolic Diseases............................. William B. Rizzo, M.D.
   Molecular Genetics................................... Shelley D. Smith, Ph.D.
   Nephrology .... Helen B. Lovell, M.D.
   Neurology .... Paul D. Larsen, M.D.
   Newborn Medicine .... Terrence L. Zach, M.D.
   Psychology... Joseph H. Evans, Ph.D.
   Pulmonary Medicine and Cystic Fibrosis .... John L. Colombo, M.D.
   Rehabilitation Medicine .... J. Michael Leibowitz, M.D.
Psychiatry .... Steven P. Wengel, M.D.
Radiation Oncology..................................... Charles A. Enke, M.D.
Radiology .... Craig W. Walker, M.D.
Surgery .... Byers W. Shaw, Jr., M.D.
   Cardiothoracic Surgery................................. Kim F. Duncan, M.D.
   General Surgery...................................... Jon S. Thompson, M.D.
   Neurosurgery....................................... Kenneth A. Follett, M.D.
   Oral and Maxillofacial Surgery .... Leon F. Davis, D.D.S., M.D. (Interim)
   Plastic and Reconstructive Surgery .... Ronald R. Hollins, M.D., D.M.D.
   Surgical Oncology .... James A. Edney, M.D.
   Transplantation Surgery................................ Alan N. Langnas, D.O.
   Urologic Surgery .... George P. Hemstreet III, M.D., Ph.D.

University of Nevada School of Medicine

Pennington Medical Education Building/332
Reno, Nevada 89557-0071
775-784-6001 (general information); 784-6096 (fax)
Web site: www.unr.edu/med

The school of medicine was originally approved in 1969 as a two-year school of basic sciences. In 1977, the university's board of regents and the Nevada state legislature approved the school's conversion to a four-year degree granting school. The first doctor of medicine degrees were awarded in 1980. The school of medicine is a university-based, community-integrated medical school with the basic science campus located on the University of Nevada, Reno, campus and clinical campuses in Reno and Las Vegas. Present enrollment at the school of medicine is 52 students per class.

Type: public
2008-2009 total enrollment: 206
Clinical facilities: VA Medical Center, Washoe Medical Center (Reno), University Medical Center of Southern Nevada (Las Vegas).

University Officials

Chancellor, Nevada Systems of Higher Education . . . . James Rogers
President, University of Nevada, Reno . . . . Milton D. Glick, Ph.D.

Medical School Administrative Staff

Dean. . . . . Ole J. Thienhaus, M.D., M.B.A.
Senior Associate Dean for Basic Science and Research . . . . David M. Lupan, Ph.D.
Associate Dean for Admissions and Student Affairs . . . . Cheryl Hug-English, M.D.
Assistant Dean for Graduate Medical Education . . . . Miriam Bar-on, M.D.
Associate Dean for Medical Education . . . . Jennifer Kimmel, M.D.
Assistant Dean for Education and Health Services Outreach . . . . Caroline J. Ford
Chief Financial Officer. . . . . Jean Regan
Personnel Officer . . . . Feride McAlpine
Director of Continuing Medical Education . . . . Stanley R. Shane, M.D.
Medical Library Director . . . . James Curtis

University of Nevada School of Medicine: NEVADA

Department and Division or Section Chairs

Basic Sciences

Biochemistry . . . . Gary Blomquist, Ph.D.
Microbiology . . . . William Murphy, Ph.D.
Pathology and Laboratory Medicine . . . . Anton P. Sohn, M.D.
Pharmacology . . . . Joseph Hume, Ph.D.
Physiology and Cell Biology . . . . Kenton M. Sanders, Ph.D.

Clinical Sciences

Family and Community Medicine, Las Vegas. . . . . Elissa Palmer, M.D.
Family and Community Medicine, Reno . . . . Daniel Spogen, M.D.
Internal Medicine, Las Vegas . . . . Daniel Goodenberger, M.D.
Internal Medicine, Reno . . . . Catherine Goring, M.D.
Nutrition Education and Research Program . . . . Sachiko St. Jeor, Ph.D.
Obstetrics and Gynecology. . . . . Paul G. Stumpf, M.D.
Pediatrics . . . . David Gremse, M.D.
Psychiatry and Behavioral Sciences, Reno . . . . Michael Daines, M.D.
Psychiatry and Behavioral Sciences, Las Vegas. . . . . Gregory P. Brown, M.D.
Radiology Program . . . . Thomas C. Barcia, M.D.
Speech Pathology and Audiology . . . . Tom Watterson, Ph.D.
Surgery . . . . William Zamboni, M.D.

Dartmouth Medical School

Hanover, New Hampshire 03755-3833
877-367-1797 (general information); 603-650-1200 (dean's office);
603-650-5000 (medical center); 603-650-1202 (dean's fax)
Web site: http://dms.dartmouth.edu/

Dartmouth Medical School, founded as the medical department of Dartmouth College, opened with its first lecture on November 22, 1797. The medical school is a component of the Dartmouth-Hitchcock Medical Center and has facilities on the campus of Dartmouth College and at the medical center in Lebanon, New Hampshire.

Type: private
2008-2009 total enrollment: 316
Clinical facilities: Mary Hitchcock Memorial Hospital, Veterans Affairs Hospital (White River Junction, Vermont), Veterans Affairs Hospital (Manchester, New Hampshire), Hitchcock Clinic, Hartford (Connecticut) Hospital, Mary Imogene Bassett Hospital (Cooperstown, New York), New Hampshire State Hospital (Concord, New Hampshire), Concord Hospital (Concord, New Hampshire), West Central Services (Lebanon; Claremont; Newport, NH), Maine Medical Center (Portland, ME), Cheshire Hospital (Keene, NH), Brown University/Memorial Hospital of Rhode Island (Pawtucket, RI), Indian Health Service Hospital (Tuba City, AZ), South Shore Hospital (Miami, FL), Yukon-Kushokwim Delta Regional Hospital (Bethel, AK), Maine-Dartmouth Family Practice Residency (Augusta, ME), Napier Hospital (Napier, New Zealand), Community-based clinics in southern New Hampshire, northern Vermont, and Maine.

Dartmouth College Officials

President. . . . . James Wright, Ph.D.
Provost . . . . Barry Scherr, Ph.D.

Medical School Administrative Staff

Dean. . . . . William R. Green, Ph.D.
Senior Associate Dean for Academic Affairs . . . . Leslie P. Henderson, Ph.D.
Senior Associate Dean for Medical Education . . . . John F. Modlin, M.D.
Associate Dean and Chief Operating Officer. . . . . Charles R. Mannix, J.D.
Associate Dean of Student and Multicultural Affairs . . . . Lori Arviso Alvord, M.D.
Associate Dean for Health Policy and Clinical Practice . . . . . . Gerald T. O'Connor, Ph.D., D.Sc.
Associate Dean, VA Hospital Affairs . . . . TBA
Assistant Dean of Clinical Affairs . . . . .Jocelyn D. Chertoff, M.D.
Assistant Dean of Continuing Medical Education . . . . Richard I. Rothstein, M.D.
Assistant Dean for Graduate Medical Education . . . . H. Worth Parker, M.D.
Assistant Dean for Medical Education (Clerkships) . . . . Eric A. Shirley, M.D.
Assistant Dean for Medical Education (OCER) . . . . Catherine F. Pipas, M.D.
Assistant Dean for Medical Education (ORIME) . . . . Greg Ogrinc, M.D.
Assistant Dean for Medical Education (Residency Affairs) . . . . Susan N. Harper, M.D.
Assistant Dean of Student Affairs . . . . Sue Ann Hennessy
Senior Advising Dean and Director of Community Programs. . . . . . . .Joseph F. O'Donnell, M.D.
Chief Financial Officer. . . . . Michael F. Wagner
Vice President for Development, DHMC. . . . . Brian T. Lally
Medical Student Registrar . . . . .Joan Monahan
Director of Admissions. . . . . Andrew G. Welch
Director, Animal Care and Use Program. . . . . Brian L. Ermeling, D.V.M.
Director, Biomedical Libraries . . . . William F. Garrity
Director of Communications . . . . Hali Wickner
Director of Computing and Information Technologies . . . . Stephen B. McAllister
Director of Financial Aid . . . . G. Dino Koff

Department and Division or Section Chairs

Basic Sciences

Anatomy . . . . Rand Swenson, M.D.
Biochemistry . . . . Charles K. Barlowe, Ph.D.

Genetics . . . . Jay C. Dunlap, Ph.D.
Microbiology . . . . Randolph J. Noelle, Ph.D. (Acting)
Pharmacology and Toxicology . . . . Joyce A. DeLeo, Ph.D.
Physiology . . . . Hermes H. Yeh, Ph.D.

Clinical Sciences

Anesthesiology . . . . Thomas A. Dodds, M.D. (Acting)
Community and Family Medicine . . . . Michael Zubkoff, Ph.D.
Medicine . . . . Murray Korc, M.D.
   Allergy . . . . Donald Woodmansee, M.D.
   Cardiology . . . . Michael Simons, M.D.
   Clinical Research . . . . Gerald T. O'Connor, Ph.D.
   Clinical Pharmacology . . . . David W. Nierenberg, M.D.
   Dermatology . . . . James G. H. Dinulos, M.D.
   Emergency Medicine . . . . Norman N. Yanofsky, M.D.
   Endocrinology . . . . Richard Comi, M.D.
   Gastroenterology . . . . Richard Rothstein, M.D.
   General Internal Medicine . . . . W. Blair Brooks, M.D.
   Infectious Diseases . . . . Bryan Marsh, M.D. (Acting)
   Nephrology and Hypertension . . . . Brian Remillard, M.D.
   Neurology . . . . Gregory Holmes, M.D.
   Occupational Health . . . . Robert McLellan, M.D.
   Pulmonary and Critical Care . . . . Richard Enelow, M.D.
   Radiation Oncology . . . . Alan Hartford, M.D. (Acting)
   Rheumatology and Connective Tissue Disease . . . . Daniel Albert, M.D.
   VA Medicine . . . . James Geiling, M.D.
Pathology . . . . Wendy A. Wells, M.B.B.S. (Acting)
Pediatrics . . . . John Modlin, M.D.
   Allergy/Immunology . . . . Donald Woodmansee, M.D.
   Cardiology . . . . Michael F. Flanagan, M.D.
   Critical Care . . . . James Filiano, M.D.
   Endocrinology . . . . Samuel Casella, M.D.
   Genetics and Child Development . . . . Lawrence Kaplan, M.D.
   General Academic Pediatrics . . . . Henry Bernstein, M.D.
   Hematology and Oncology . . . . Jack van Hoff, M.D.
   Neonatology . . . . William H. Edwards, M.D.
   Neurology . . . . Richard P. Morse, M.D.
   Pulmonary . . . . TBA
Obstetrics and Gynecology . . . . Richard H. Reindollar, M.D.
Orthopaedics . . . . James N. Weinstein, D.O.
Psychiatry . . . . Alan I. Green, M.D.
Radiology . . . . Peter K. Spiegel, M.D.
Surgery . . . . Richard W. Dow, M.D.
   Cardiothoracic . . . . William C. Nugent, M.D.
   General Surgery . . . . Richard Barth, M.D.
   Neurosurgery . . . . David W. Roberts, M.D.
   Ophthalmology . . . . Christopher Chapman, M.D.
   Oral Surgery . . . . Rocco Addante, M.D.
   Otolaryngology and Audiology . . . . Daniel Morrison, M.D.
   Plastic, Reconstructive . . . . Carolyn L. Kerrigan, M.D.
   Transplantation . . . . David Axelrod, M.D.
   Urology . . . . William Bihrle, M.D.
   Vascular Surgery . . . . Richard J. Powell, M.D.

Centers

Center for Aging . . . . John H. Wasson, M.D.
Center for Health Policy and Clinical Practice . . . . James N. Weinstein, D.O.
Hood Center for Family Support . . . . Madeline Dalton, Ph.D.
New Hampshire Dartmouth Psychiatric Research Center . . . . Robert Drake, M.D.
Norris Cotton Cancer Center . . . . Mark Israel, M.D.

UMDNJ—New Jersey Medical School

185 South Orange Avenue
Newark, New Jersey 07103-2714
973-972-4300; 972-4538/4539 (dean's office); 972-7104 (fax)
Web site: http://njms.umdnj.edu

The UMDNJ-New Jersey Medical School was incorporated on August 6, 1954, as the Seton Hall College of Medicine and Dentistry, and in November 1954, was granted a charter by the New Jersey Department of Education. In 1965, Seton Hall College of Medicine and Dentistry became the New Jersey College of Medicine and Dentistry, a state-supported institution. The New Jersey Medical School is one of eight schools that comprise the statewide UMDNJ (University of Medicine and Dentistry of New Jersey), established in July 1970 under a single board of trustees.

Type: public
2008-2009 total enrollment: 680
Clinical facilities: UMDNJ-University Hospital, Hackensack University Medical Center, Kessler Institute for Rehabilitation, Veterans Affairs Medical Center (East Orange).

University Officials

President. . . . . William F. Owen, Jr., M.D.

Medical School Administrative Staff

Dean. . . . . Robert L. Johnson, M.D. (Interim)
Vice Dean . . . . Maria L. Soto-Greene, M.D.
Associate Dean and Chief Financial Officer . . . . David L. Roe
Executive Director for Administration. . . . . Walter L. Douglas
Senior Associate Dean, Research . . . . William C. Gause, Ph.D.
Senior Associate Dean, Clinical Affairs . . . . Kendall R. Sprott, M.D.
Senior Associate Dean, Academic Affairs. . . . . Lawrence A. Feldman, Ph.D.
Associate Dean, Graduate Medical Education . . . . Stephen R. Baker, M.D.
Associate Dean, Curriculum and Faculty Development . . . . Vacant
Associate Dean, Student Affairs . . . . Ian Thomas Cohen, M.D.
Associate Dean, Admissions and Special Programs. . . . . George F. Heinrich, M.D.
Executive Assistant to the Dean . . . . Michael J. Petti

Department and Division or Section Chairs

Basic Sciences

Biochemistry and Molecular Biology. . . . . Michael B. Mathews, Ph.D.
Cell Biology and Molecular Medicine. . . . . Stephen Vatner, M.D.
Microbiology and Molecular Genetics. . . . . Carol S. Newlon, Ph.D.
Pathology and Laboratory Medicine. . . . . Stanley Cohen, M.D.
Pharmacology and Physiology. . . . . Andrew P. Thomas, Ph.D.

Clinical Sciences

Anesthesiology. . . . . Ellise Delphin, M.D.
Emergency Medicine . . . . Vacant
Family Medicine . . . . Mark S. Johnson, M.D.
Medicine . . . . Bunyad Haider, M.D. (Interim)
  Academic Medicine, Geriatrics, and Community Programs. . . . . Mary Ann Haggerty, M.D.
  Allergy, Immunology, and Rheumatology . . . . Leonard Bielory, M.D.
  Cardiology. . . . . Marc Klapholz, M.D.
  Dermatology . . . . Robert A. Schwartz, M.D.
  Endocrinology and Metabolism. . . . . David Bleich, M.D.
  Gastroenterology . . . . Arun Samanta, M.D. (Interim)
  Hematology and Oncology. . . . . Lillian Pliner, M.D. (Interim)
  Infectious Diseases . . . . David Alland, M.D.
  Nephrology . . . . Leonard Meggs, M.D.
  Pulmonary Diseases and Critical Care . . . . Kevin Fennelly, M.D. (Interim)
Neurological Surgery. . . . . Peter W. Carmel, M.D.
Neurology and Neurosciences . . . . Stephen Kamin, M.D. (Acting)
  Cerebrovascular . . . . Jawad Kirmani, M.D. (Acting)
  Pediatric Neurology . . . . Caroline Hayes-Rosen, M.D.

Obstetrics, Gynecology, and Women's Health . . . . Gerson Weiss, M.D.
   General Obstetrics and Gynecology. . . . . A. Brian Little, M.D.
   Gynecologic Oncology . . . . Bernadette Cracchiolo, M.D.
   Maternal and Fetal Medicine . . . . Joseph Apuzzio, M.D.
   Reproductive Endocrinology and Infertility . . . . Peter McGovern, M.D.
Ophthalmology and Visual Science. . . . . Marco A. Zarbin, M.D., Ph.D.
   Comprehensive Ophthalmology . . . . Suqin Guo, M.D.
   Cornea, External Diseases, and Refractive Surgery . . . . Peter S. Hersh, M.D.
   Glaucoma . . . . Robert Fechtner, M.D.
   Neuro-Ophthalmology . . . . Larry Frohman, M.D.
   Oculopathology . . . . Tatyana Milman, M.D.
   Oculoplastics and Orbital Reconstructive Surgery . . . . Paul Langer, M.D.
   Pediatric Ophthalmology and Strabismus . . . . Rudolph Wagner, M.D.
   Retina and Vitreous Surgery . . . . Neelakshi Bhagat, M.D.
   Uvietis and Infectious Disease . . . . Ronald Rescigno, M.D.
Orthopaedics. . . . . Joseph Benevenia, M.D. (Interim)
   Foot and Ankle . . . . Wayne Berberian, M.D.
   Hand Injuries and Disorders. . . . . John Capo, M.D.
   Musculoskeletal Oncology. . . . . Francis Patterson, M.D.
   Orthopaedic Trauma . . . . Michael Sirkin, M.D.
   Pediatric Orthopaedics. . . . . Sanjeev Sabharwal, M.D.
   Spine Disorders and Surgery . . . . Michael J. Vives, M.D.
   Sports Medicine and Arthroscopic Surgery . . . . Robin Gehrmann, M.D.
   Total Joint Replacement. . . . . Calin Moucha, M.D.
Pediatrics . . . . Kendell Sprott, M.D., J.D. (Acting)
   Adolescent Medicine and Young Adult . . . . Robert L. Johnson, M.D.
   Cardiology. . . . . Joel Hardin, M.D.
   Child Development . . . . Barbie Bier, M.D.
   Emergency Medicine . . . . Robert Barricella, D.O.
   Gastroenterology . . . . Iona Monteiro, M.D.
   General Pediatrics and Pediatric Education . . . . Susan Mautone, M.D.
   Genetics. . . . . Franklin Desposito, M.D.
   Hematology and Oncology . . . . Franklin Desposito, M.D. (Acting)
   Center for Human Development and Aging . . . . Abraham Aviv, M.D.
   Infectious Diseases, Allergy, and Immunology . . . . James Oleske, M.D.
   Nephrology . . . . Constancia Uy, M.D.
   Primary Care . . . . Deborah Johnson, M.D.
   Pulmonology . . . . Helen Aguila, M.D.
Physical Medicine and Rehabilitation . . . . Joel A. DeLisa, M.D.
   Noninvasive Ventilation and Pulmonary Rehabilitation . . . . John R. Bach, M.D.
   Occupational/Musculoskeletal Medicine . . . . Todd P. Stitik, M.D.
   Spinal Cord Injury . . . . Susan V. Garstang, M.D.
Preventive Medicine and Community Health . . . . William E. Halperin, M.D., Dr.PH.
   Biostatistics and Epidemiology . . . . Michael Brimacombe, Ph.D.
   General Preventive Medicine and International Health . . . . Reza Najem, M.D.
   Nutrition and Aging. . . . . John Bogden, Ph.D.
Psychiatry . . . . Giovanni Caracci, M.D. (Interim)
   Child and Adolescent Psychiatry . . . . Charles Cartwright, M.D., and Tolga Taneli, M.D.
Radiation Oncology. . . . . Maria Soto-Greene, M.D. (Interim)
Radiology . . . . Stephen R. Baker, M.D.
   Diagnostic Radiology . . . . Stephen R. Baker, M.D.
   Radiation Research. . . . . Roger Howell, Ph.D.
Surgery . . . . Edwin A. Deitch, M.D.
   Cardiothoracic . . . . Justin Sambol, M.D.
   Critical Care. . . . . Anne Mosenthal, M.D.
   Emergency Services . . . . Hossein Shahidi, M.D.
   General . . . . Edwin A. Deitch, M.D.
   Laparoscopy. . . . . Asha Bale, M.D.
   Oncology. . . . . Lawrence Harrison, M.D.
   Otolaryngology. . . . . Soly Baredes, M.D.
   Pediatric . . . . I. Thomas Cohen, M.D.
   Plastic . . . . Mark Granick, M.D.
   Transplantation . . . . Baburao Koneru, M.D.
   Trauma . . . . David H. Livingston, M.D.
   Urology . . . . Mark Jordan, M.D.
   Vascular. . . . . Justin T. Sambol, M.D. (Interim)

University of Medicine and Dentistry of New Jersey
Robert Wood Johnson Medical School
125 Paterson Street, Suite 1400
New Brunswick, New Jersey 08901
732-235-5600; 235-6300 (dean's office); 235-6315 (fax)
Web site: http://rwjms.umdnj.edu

UMDNJ-Robert Wood Johnson Medical School has campuses in Piscataway, New Brunswick, and Camden, New Jersey. Established as Rutgers Medical School, its name changed to Robert Wood Johnson Medical School in 1986.

Type: public
2008-2009 total enrollment: 670
Clinical facilities: Principal hospitals are Robert Wood Johnson University Hospital and Cooper Hospital/University Medical Center. University hospitals are Jersey Shore University Medical Center and the University Medical Center at Princeton. Major clinical affiliates are Somerset Medical Center and Raritan Bay Medical Center. In addition, there are 27 clinical affiliates.

University Officials

President. . . . . William F. Owen, Jr., M.D.
Executive Vice President, Academic and Clinical Affairs . . . . Denise V. Rodgers, M.D.

Medical School Administrative Staff

Interim Dean and Chief Executive Officer,
   Robert Wood Johnson University Medical
   Group . . . . Peter S. Amenta, M.D., Ph.D.
Senior Associate Dean for Community Health. . . . . Eric G. Jahn, M.D. (Acting)
Senior Associate Dean for Education . . . . Stephen F. Lowry, M.D.
Senior Associate Dean for Research . . . . Arnold Rabson, M.D. (Acting)
Senior Associate Dean for Clinical Affairs. . . . . Anthony T. Scardella, M.D. (Acting)
Associate Dean for Clinical Research . . . . Vacant
Associate Dean for Research. . . . . Celine Gelinas, Ph.D.
Associate Dean for Oncology Programs. . . . . Vacant
Associate Dean for Admissions . . . . Carol A. Terregino, M.D.
Associate Dean for Graduate School of Biological Sciences . . . . Terri Goss-Kinzy, Ph.D.
Associate Dean for Postgraduate Education. . . . . Vacant
Associate Dean for Academic and Student Affairs at Camden . . . . . . Carol A. Terregino (Acting)
Associate Dean for Global Health. . . . . Javier Escobar, M.D.
Associate Dean for Research at Camden . . . . Peter Melera, Ph.D.
Associate Dean for Veterans Affairs . . . . Vacant
Associate Dean for Women's Health. . . . . Gloria A. Bachmann, M.D.
Associate Dean for Graduate Medical Education . . . . Marie C. Trontell, M.D.
Associate Dean for Education. . . . . David Swee, M.D.
Associate Dean for Student Affairs . . . . David Seiden, Ph.D.
Assistant Dean for Student Affairs for the Clinical Years . . . . Susan R. Rosenthal, M.D.
Assistant Dean for Student Affairs. . . . . Sonia Garcia-Laumbach, M.D.
Assistant Dean for Educational Programs . . . . Norma Saks, Ph.D.
Assistant Dean for Student and Multicultural Affairs . . . . Cheryl Dickson, M.D.
Assistant Dean for Curriculum . . . . William Zehring, Ph.D.
Assistant Dean for Education . . . . Archana Pradhan, M.D., M.P.H.
Assistant Dean for Student Affairs at Camden . . . . Robert J. Risimini, M.D.
Assistant Dean for Multicultural and Community Affairs . . . . Jocelyn Mitchell-Williams, M.D.
Chief Operating and Financial Officer . . . . Alice Lustig

Department Chairs

Basic Sciences

Biochemistry . . . . Michael Hampsey, Ph.D. (Acting)
Molecular Genetics, Microbiology, and Immunology . . . . Sidney Pestka, M.D.
Neuroscience and Cell Biology . . . . Cheryl Dreyfus, Ph.D. (Acting)
Pathology and Laboratory Medicine . . . . Peter S. Amenta, M.D., Ph.D.
Pharmacology . . . . Leroy F. Liu, Ph.D.
Physiology and Biophysics . . . . Nicola C. Partridge, Ph.D.

Clinical Sciences

Anesthesia . . . . Christine Hunter, M.D.
Dermatology . . . . Babar Rao, M.D. (Acting)
Environmental and Occupational Medicine . . . . Howard Kiper, M.D. (Acting)
Emergency Medicine . . . . Michael E. Chansky, M.D.
Family Medicine . . . . Alfred F. Tallia, M.D.
Medicine . . . . John B. Kostis, M.D.
Neurology . . . . Suhayl Dhib-Jalbut, M.D.
Obstetrics, Gynecology, and Reproductive Sciences . . . . Gloria A. Bachmann, M.D. (Acting)
Ophthalmology . . . . Stuart N. Green, M.D.
Orthopaedic Surgery . . . . Charles J. Gatt, M.D.
Pediatrics . . . . Patricia N. Whitley-Williams, M.D. (Acting)
Physical Medicine and Rehabilitation . . . . Thomas E. Strax, M.D.
Psychiatry . . . . Matthew Menza, M.D. (Acting)
Radiation Oncology . . . . Bruce G. Haffty, M.D.
Radiology . . . . John Nosher, M.D.
Surgery . . . . Stephen F. Lowry, M.D.

UMDNJ-Robert Wood Johnson Medical School, Camden Campus

856-757-7905 (Associate Dean, Academic and Student Affairs)

Department Heads

Anesthesiology . . . . Michael Goldberg, M.D.
Emergency Medicine . . . . Michael E. Chansky, M.D.
Family Medicine . . . . Dyanne P. Westerberg, D.O.
Medicine . . . . Joseph E. Parrillo, M.D.
Obstetrics and Gynecology . . . . Robin L. Perry, M.D.
Orthopaedic Surgery . . . . Lawrence Miller, M.D.
Pathology . . . . Roland Schwarting, M.D.
Pediatrics . . . . William Sharrar, M.D.
Physical Medicine and Rehabilitation Therapy . . . . Elliot Bodofsky, M.D.
Psychiatry . . . . Thomas Newmark, M.D.
Radiation Oncology and Nuclear Medicine . . . . Vacant
Radiology . . . . Raymond Baraldi, M.D.
Surgery . . . . Steven Ross, M.D. (Acting)

University of New Mexico School of Medicine
MSC 08 4720
Albuquerque, New Mexico 87131
505-272-2321 (dean's office); 272-6581 (fax)
Web site: http://hsc.unm.edu/som

The establishment of the school of medicine at the University of New Mexico was authorized by the board of regents in 1961. The first entering class enrolled in fall 1964. The school of medicine is situated on the university campus and is a part of the University of New Mexico Health Sciences Center.

Type: public
2008-2009 total enrollment: 280
Clinical facilities: University of New Mexico Hospitals, Veterans Administration Medical Center, Bernalillo County Mental Health/Mental Retardation Center, University of New Mexico Children's Psychiatric Hospital, University of New Mexico Cancer Center, Ambulatory Care Center, Center for Non-invasive Diagnosis, Carrie Tingley Hospital.

University Officials

President. . . . . David Schmidly, Ph.D.
Provost and Executive Vice President for Academic Affairs . . . . Viola Florez, Ph.D. (Interim)
Executive Vice President for Administration and
    Vice President for Business and Finance . . . . David W. Harris
Executive Vice President, Health Sciences Center . . . . Paul B. Roth, M.D.
Vice President for Student Affairs. . . . . Eliseo Torres, Ph.D.
Vice President for Advancement. . . . . Michael Kingan
Vice Provost for Research. . . . . Vacant

Medical School Administrative Staff

Dean. . . . . Paul B. Roth, M.D.
Executive Dean . . . . Jeffrey K. Griffith, Ph.D.
Associate Dean for Student Affairs . . . . Eve Espey, M.D.
Assistant Dean for Admissions . . . . David Bear, Ph.D.
Associate Dean, Office of Cultural and Ethnic Programs . . . . Valerie Romero-Leggott, M.D.
Associate Dean for Undergraduate Medical Education . . . . Craig Timm, M.D.
Associate Dean for Graduate Medical Education. . . . . David Sklar, M.D.
Senior Associate Dean for Medical Education . . . . Ellen M. Cosgrove, M.D.
Senior Associate Dean for Academic Affairs . . . . Susan M. Scott, M.D.
Associate Dean for Clinical Affairs . . . . Robert Katz, M.D.
Senior Associate Dean for Research . . . . Richard Larson, M.D.
Associate Vice President, Health Sciences Center
    Library and Informatics Center . . . . Holly Buchanan, Ed.D.

Department and Division or Section Chairs

Basic Sciences

Biochemistry and Molecular Biology. . . . . William Anderson, Ph.D.
Cell Biology and Physiology . . . . Paul McGuire, M.D.
Molecular Genetics and Microbiology. . . . . Vojo Deretic, Ph.D.
Neurosciences . . . . David D. Savage II, Ph.D.
Pathology . . . . Brian Hjelle, Ph.D. (Interim)

Clinical Sciences

Anesthesiology. . . . . John Wills, M.D.
Dermatology . . . . R. Steven Padilla, M.D.
Emergency Medicine . . . . Michael Richards, M.D.
    Pediatric Emergency Care. . . . . Robert Sapien, M.D.
Family and Community Medicine. . . . . Arthur Kaufman, M.D.
    Family Practice. . . . . Vacant
    Geriatrics. . . . . Robert L. Rhyne, Jr., M.D.

Medicine . . . . Pope Moseley, M.D.
   Cardiology . . . . Warren Laskey, M.D.
   Endocrinology . . . . David Schade, M.D.
   Epidemiology and Preventive Medicine . . . . Marianne Berwick
   Gastroenterology . . . . Thomas Ma, M.D.
   General Medicine . . . . Carolyn M. Voss, M.D.
   Gerontology . . . . Carla Herman, M.D.
   Hematology and Oncology . . . . Robert Hromas, M.D.
   Infectious Diseases . . . . Gregory Mertz, M.D.
   Nephrology and Renal . . . . Philip G. Zager, M.D.
   Pulmonary . . . . Richard Crowell, M.D.
   Rheumatology . . . . Arthur D. Bankhurst, M.D.
Neurology . . . . Gary A. Rosenberg, M.D.
   Pediatric Neurology . . . . Leslie Morrison, M.D.
Neurosurgery . . . . Howard Yonas, M.D.
Obstetrics and Gynecology . . . . William F. Rayburn, M.D.
   Breast Disease Program . . . . Kathleen Kennedy, M.D.
   Certified Nurse Midwifery Service . . . . Vacant
   Gynecologic Oncology . . . . Harriett Smith, M.D.
   Gynecology . . . . Maxine H. Dorin, M.D.
   Maternal and Fetal Medicine . . . . Kimberly Leslie, M.D.
   Reproductive Endocrinology and Infertility . . . . Francis W. Byrn, M.D.
Orthopaedics . . . . Robert Schenk, M.D.
   Adult Reconstruction . . . . Dennis P. Rivero, M.D.
   Foot and Ankle Reconstruction . . . . Richard A. Miller, M.D.
   General Orthopaedic Surgery . . . . Paul Echols, M.D.
   Hand Surgery . . . . Moheb S. Moncim, M.D.
   Occupational Therapy . . . . Terry K. Crowe, Ph.D.
   Pediatrics . . . . Frederick Sherman, M.D.
   Physical Therapy . . . . Susan Queen, PT, Ph.D.
   Spine . . . . Jose Reyna, M.D.
   Sports Medicine . . . . Daniel C. Wascher, M.D.
   Trauma . . . . Thomas A. DeCoster, M.D.
Pediatrics . . . . Loretta Cordova de Ortega, M.D. (Interim)
   Adolescent Medicine . . . . Victor S. Strasberger, M.D.
   Ambulatory . . . . Andrew Hsi, M.D.
   Cardiology . . . . M. Beth Goens, M.D.
   Critical Care . . . . Mark Crowley, M.D.
   Pulmonary . . . . Elizabeth Perkett, M.D.
   Developmental Disabilities . . . . Catherine McClain, M.D.
   Dysmorphology . . . . Carol L. Clericuzio, M.D.
   Endocrinology . . . . Nancy Gregor, M.D.
   Hematology and Oncology . . . . Richard Heiderman, M.D.
   Infectious Disease . . . . Gary D. Overturf, M.D.
   Neonatology . . . . Kristi Watterberg
   Pediatrics Rehabilitation Medicine . . . . Denise Taylor, M.D.
Psychiatry . . . . Samuel J. Keith, M.D.
   Child and Adolescent Psychiatry . . . . Robert A. Bailey, M.D.
Radiation Oncology . . . . Vacant
Radiology . . . . Michael R. Williamson, M.D.
   Biomedical Physics . . . . Phillip Heintz, Ph.D.
Surgery . . . . John Russell, M.D.
   Cardiothoracic Surgery . . . . Jorge A. Wernly, M.D.
   General Surgery . . . . Thomas Howdieshell, M.D.
   Ophthalmology . . . . Arup Das, M.D.
   Pediatric Surgery . . . . David Lemon, M.D.
   Plastic Surgery, Head, Neck, and Reconstructive Surgery . . . . Bret Baack, M.D.
   Urology . . . . Anthony Smith, M.D.
   Vascular Surgery . . . . Mark Langsfeld, M.D.

Albany Medical College
47 New Scotland Avenue
Albany, New York 12208
518-262-6008 (dean's office); 262-6515 (fax)
Web site: www.amc.edu

The Albany Medical College, chartered by the legislature of New York, opened on January 2, 1839. The medical college is part of the Albany Medical Center.

Type: private
2008-2009 total enrollment: 513
Clinical facilities: Albany Medical Center Hospital, Samuel Stratton DVA Medical Center, St. Peter's Hospital (Albany), Ellis Hospital (Schenectady), Capital District Psychiatric Center (Albany), Mary Imogene Bassett Hospital, AMC South Clinical Campus, Center for Disabled.

Albany Medical Center Officials

President and Chief Executive Officer .... James J. Barba
Executive Vice President for Health Affairs...................... Vincent P. Verdile, M.D.
Executive Vice President and Chief Operating Officer..................... Gary J. Kochem
Executive Vice President for Integrated Delivery
   Systems and Hospital Systems General
   Director .... Steven M. Frisch, M.D.
Senior Vice President for External Relations........................... Terri Cerveny
Senior Vice President and General Counsel .... Lee R. Hessberg
Senior Vice President for Government Relations and Strategic Planning .... Kim Fine
Senior Vice President and Chief Financial Officer.................. William C. Hasselbarth

Medical School Administrative Staff

Dean... Vincent P. Verdile, M.D.
Vice Dean for Academic Administration.......................... Henry S. Pohl, M.D.
Senior Associate Dean for Clinical Research .... Paul J. Davis, M.D.
Senior Associate Dean for Student Affairs....................... Elizabeth Higgins, M.D.
Associate Dean for Academic Affairs........................... Elizabeth Higgins, M.D.
Associate Dean for Graduate Medical Education..................... Joel Bartfield, M.D.
Associate Dean for Graduate Studies Program................... Thomas Anderson, Ph.D.
Associate Dean for Medical Education .... Jonathan M. Rosen, M.D.
Assistant Dean for Biomedical Informatics and Information Science .... Enid Geyer
Assistant Dean for Student and Minority Affairs .... Open
Executive Associate Dean.. John DePaola
Director, Admissions and Records .... Joanne Nanos
Director, Alumni Office.. Karyn Connolly
Director of Continuing Medical Education .... Jennifer Price
Director of Public Relations..................................... Gregory J. McGarry
Librarian and Director, Schaffer Library of Health Sciences .... Enid Geyer

Department and Division or Section Chairs

Interdisciplinary Research Centers

Cardiovascular Science.. Harold A. Singer, Ph.D.
Cell Biology and Cancer Research .. Paula J. McKeown-Longo, Ph.D., and Paul J. Higgins, Ph.D.
Immunology and Microbial Disease .... Dennis W. Metzger, Ph.D.
Neuropharmacology and Neuroscience..................... Stanley D. Glick, M.D., Ph.D.

Clinical Sciences

Anesthesiology... Kevin W. Roberts, M.D.
Emergency Medicine.. Mara McErlean, M.D.
Family Practice .... Neil Mitnick, D.O.
Medicine.. Ferdinand J. Venditti, Jr., M.D.
   Cardiology... Edward Philbin, M.D.
   Clinical Pharmacology .... Open
   Endocrinology .... Matthew C. Leinung, M.D.
   Gastroenterology .... Cathy Bartholomew, M.D.
   General Internal Medicine .... Alwin F. Steinmann, M.D.
   Geriatric Medicine... Open
   Hematology and Medical Oncology... Open
   HIV Medicine .... Douglas G. Fish, M.D.
   Nutrition .... Lyn J. Howard, M.B.Ch.B.
   Pulmonary Diseases .... Thomas Smith, M.D.
   Renal Diseases .... George Eisele, M.D.
   Rheumatology .... Open
Neurology.. Michael Gruenthal, M.D., Ph.D.
Neurosciences Institute .... A. John Popp, M.D.
Obstetrics, Gynecology, and Reproductive Sciences................... Kevin C. Kiley, M.D.
   General Gynecology and Obstetrics..................... Norman F. Angell, M.D., Ph.D.
   Gynecologic Endocrinology and Infertility... Open
   Gynecologic Oncology .... Patrick Timmins, M.D.
   Maternal and Fetal Medicine .... Camille Kanaar, M.D.
   Urogynecology and Reproductive Pelvic Surgery .... Open
Ophthalmology... John Simon, M.D.
Pathology and Laboratory Medicine.................................... Jeffrey S. Ross, M.D.
Pediatrics .... David A. Clark, M.D.
Physical Medicine and Rehabilitation .... George P. Forrest, M.D.
Psychiatry .... Victoria I. Balkoski, M.D.
   Child Psychiatry .... Victoria I. Balkoski, M.D.
Radiology .... Gary Siskin, M.D.
   Vascular and Interventional Radiology.................................... Gary Siskin, M.D.
Surgery... Steven Stain, M.D.
   Cardiothoracic Surgery.. Lewis Britton, M.D.
   General Surgery... David J. Conti, M.D.
   Neurosurgery... A. John Popp, M.D.
   Orthopaedic Surgery .... Richard Uhl, M.D.
   Otolaryngology.. Steven M. Parnes, M.D.
   Pediatric Surgery .... Open
   Plastic Surgery .... Jerome Chao, M.D.
   Urological Surgery .... Barry A. Kogan, M.D.
   Vascular Surgery.. R. Clement Darling, M.D.
Vascular Institute... Dhiraj M. Shah, M.D.

Albert Einstein College of Medicine of Yeshiva University

1300 Morris Park Avenue
Bronx, New York 10461
718-430-2000; 430-2801 (dean's office); 430-8822 (fax)
Web site: www:aecom.yu.edu

The Albert Einstein College of Medicine admitted its first class in fall 1955. The college of medicine is approximately seven miles from the main campus of the university.

Type: private
2008-2009 total enrollment: 759
Clinical facilities: Beth Abraham Hospital, Beth Israel Medical Center, Bronx-Lebanon Hospital Center, Bronx Psychiatric Center and Bronx Psychiatric Children's Hospital, Four Winds Hospital, Jack D. Weiler Hospital of Albert Einstein College of Medicine (division of Montefiore Medical Center), North Shore-Long Island Jewish Health System, Montefiore Medical Center, North Bronx Care Network (Jacobi Medical Center and North Central Bronx Hospital), Parker Jewish Geriatric Institute.

University Officials

President. . . . . Richard M. Joel, J.D.
Chancellor . . . . Norman Lamm, Ph.D.
Vice President for Medical Affairs. . . . . Allen M. Spiegel, M.D.

Medical School Administrative Staff

Dean. . . . . Allen M. Spiegel, M.D.
Executive Dean . . . . Edward R. Burns, M.D.
Senior Associate Dean for Students . . . . Stephen G. Baum, M.D.
Associate Dean, Public Affairs and Communication. Gordon W. Earle
Associate Dean, Office of Diversity Enhancement . . . . Milton A. Gumbs, M.D.
Associate Dean, Continuing Medical Education. . . . . Victor B. Hatcher, Ph.D.
Associate Dean, Students . . . . Nadine T. Katz, M.D.
Associate Dean, Educational Affairs . . . . Albert S. Kuperman, Ph.D.
Associate Dean, Clinical Research Education. . . . . Paul R. Marantz, M.D.
Associate Dean, Institutional Advancement. . . . . Glenn Miller
Associate Dean, Clinical Affairs and Graduate
 Medical Education . . . . Michael J. Reichgott, M.D., Ph.D.
Associate Dean, Clinical and Translational Research . . . . Harry Shamoon, M.D.
Associate Dean, Finance and Administration. . . . . Jed M. Shivers
Assistant Dean, Montefiore Medical Center. . . . . Brian Currie, M.D.
Assistant Dean, Jacobi Medical Center . . . . Wayne R. Cohen, M.D.
Assistant Dean, Beth Israel Medical Center . . . . Adrienne Fleckman, M.D.
Assistant Dean, Bronx-Lebanon Hospital Center . . . . Joshua M. Rubenstein, M.D.
Assistant Dean, Long Island Jewish Medical Center . . . . Miriam A. Smith, M.D.
Assistant Dean, Educational Informatics . . . . Christopher Cimino, M.D.
Assistant Dean, Clinical Research at Montefiore Medical Center . . . . Brian Currie, M.D.
Assistant Dean, Graduate Studies . . . . Todd R. Evans, Ph.D.
Assistant Dean, Scientific Resources . . . . Harris Goldstein, M.D.
Assistant Dean, Educational Resources . . . . Penny Steiner-Grossman, Ed.D.
Assistant Dean, Faculty Development . . . . Christina M. Coyle, M.D.
Assistant Dean, Scientific Operations . . . . John L. Harb
Assistant Dean, Admissions. . . . . Noreen Kerrigan
Assistant Dean . . . . Stephen H. Lazar, Ed.D.
Assistant Dean, Academic Affairs . . . . Barbara A. Levy
Assistant Dean, Information Technology. Robert C. Lummis, Ph.D.
Assistant Dean, Academic Administration . . . . Shelly Motzkin
Assistant Dean, Office of Diversity Enhancement. . . . . Nilda Soto
Assistant Dean, Biomedical Science Education . . . . Howard M. Steinman, Ph.D.
Director, Medical Scientist Training Program . . . . Myles Akabas, M.D., Ph.D.
Director, Belfer Institute for Advanced Biomedical Studies . . . . Jonathan M. Backer, M.D.
Director, Graduate Programs . . . . Victoria H. Freedman, Ph.D.
Director, Office of Grant Support. . . . . Charles B. Hathaway, Ph.D.
Director, D. Samuel Gottesman Library . . . . Judie Malamud

Albert Einstein College of Medicine of Yeshiva University: NEW YORK

Department and Division or Section Chairs

Basic Sciences

Anatomy and Structural Biology . . . . John S. Condeelis, Ph.D., and Robert H. Singer, Ph.D.
Biochemistry . . . . Vern L. Schramm, Ph.D.
Biological Sciences Division . . . . Arthur I. Skoultchi, Ph.D.
   Cell Biology . . . . Arthur I. Skoultchi, Ph.D.
   Developmental and Molecular Biology . . . . E. Richard Stanley, Ph.D.
   Molecular Genetics . . . . Jack Lenz, Ph.D. (Interim)
   Molecular Pharmacology . . . . Charles S. Rubin, Ph.D., and Susan B. Horwitz, Ph.D.
Microbiology and Immunology . . . . Arturo Casadevall, M.D., Ph.D.
Neuroscience . . . . Donald S. Faber, Ph.D.
Pathology . . . . Michael B. Prystowsky, M.D.
Physiology and Biophysics . . . . Denis L. Rousseau, Ph.D.
Systems and Computational Biology . . . . Aviv Bergman, Ph.D.

Clinical Sciences

Anesthesiology . . . . Albert J. Saubermann, M.D.
Cardiothoracic Surgery . . . . Robert E. Michler, M.D.
Dentistry . . . . Richard A. Kraut, D.D.S.
Emergency Medicine . . . . E. John Gallagher, M.D.
Epidemiology and Population Health . . . . Thomas E. Rohan, M.D., Ph.D.
Family and Social Medicine . . . . Peter A. Selwyn, M.D.
Medicine . . . . Victor L. Schuster, M.D.
Neurological Surgery . . . . Eugene S. Flamm, M.D.
Neurology . . . . Mark F. Mehler, M.D.
Nuclear Medicine . . . . M. Donald Blaufox, M.D., Ph.D.
Obstetrics and Gynecology and Women's Health . . . . Irwin R. Merkatz, M.D.
Ophthalmology and Visual Sciences . . . . Vacant
Otolaryngology . . . . Marvin P. Fried, M.D.
Pediatrics . . . . Phillip Ozuah, M.D.
Physical Medicine Rehabilitation . . . . Avital Fast, M.D.
Psychiatry and Behavioral Sciences . . . . T. Byram Karasu, M.D.
Radiation Oncology . . . . Shalom Kalnicki, M.D.
Radiology . . . . E. Stephen Amis, Jr., M.D.
Surgery . . . . Robert E. Michler, M.D.
   Orthopedic Surgery . . . . Neil J. Cobelli, M.D.
   Plastic and Reconstructive Surgery . . . . David A. Staffenberg, M.D.
Urology . . . . Arnold Melman, M.D.

Columbia University College of Physicians and Surgeons

630 West 168th Street
New York, New York 10032
212-305-3592 (dean's office); 305-3545 (fax)
Web site: www.columbia.edu

Columbia University began as King's College, which was founded in 1754 by royal grant of George II, King of England. In 1814, the medical faculty of Columbia College was merged with the college of physicians and surgeons. In 1860, the college of physicians and surgeons became the medical department of Columbia College. In 1891, the college was incorporated as an integral part of the university. The medical school is part of the Columbia-Presbyterian Medical Center.

Type: private
2008-2009 total enrollment: 659
Clinical facilities: Presbyterian Hospital (Sloane Hospital for Women, Babies and Children's Hospital, Vanderbilt Clinic, Neurological Institute, Eye Institute, New York Orthopedic Hospital, Squier Urological Clinic); New York State Psychiatric Institute; Mary Imogene Bassett Hospital (Cooperstown); Harlem Hospital Center; Helen Hayes Hospital (Haverstraw); Overlook Hospital (Summit, New Jersey); St. Luke's-Roosevelt Hospital Center; Valley Hospital (Ridgewood, New Jersey); Horton Memorial Hospital (Middletown); Lawrence Hospital (Bronxville); White Plains Hospital Center; New Milford Hospital (Connecticut); Stamford Hospital (Connecticut); Nyack Hospital (New York); St. Luke's (Newburgh, New York); St. Mary's Hospital for Children (New York); St. Vincent's Hospital (Connecticut); Cornwall Hospital (New York); Holy Name Hospital (Teaneck, New Jersey).

University Officials

President. . . . . Lee C. Bollinger, J.D.
Provost and Dean of Faculties . . . . Alan Brinkley, Ph.D.
Executive Vice President for Health and Biomedical Sciences . . . . Lee Goldman, M.D.
Executive Vice President for Research . . . . David Hirsh, Ph.D.
Chief Operating Officer. . . . . Lisa Hogarty, M.S.
Chief Financial Officer. . . . . Joanne Quan, M.A.
Chief Human Resources Officer. . . . . Louis Lemieux, M.B.A.
Chief Information Officer . . . . Robert V. Sideli, M.D.
Associate General Counsel. Patricia Sachs Catapano, J.D., M.P.H.
Vice President for Development. . . . . Susan S. Stalcup
Deputy Vice President for Government and Community Affairs. . . . . Ross A. Frommer, J.D.
Controller. . . . . Francine Caracappa, M.B.A., C.P.A.
Associate Vice President for Health Sciences Facilities Management. . . . . Robert Lemieux
Deputy Vice President for Information
   Technology for Health Sciences . . . . George M. Hripcsak, M.D.
Associate Dean for Diversity and Minority Affairs . . . . Hilda Y. Hutcherson, M.D.
Assistant Vice President for Professional Resource Services . . . . Daniel W. Morrissey
Assistant Vice President for Public Safety . . . . James F. McShane
Associate Vice President and Associate Dean for Scholarly Resources. . . . . . . Pat Molholt, Ph.D.
Associate Vice President for Biomedical Communications . . . . Jeffrey Szmulewicz
Associate Vice President, Facilities Management . . . . Amador Centeno, M.S.
Associate Vice President and Chief Communications Officer. . . . . Rosemary Keane
Associate Vice President and Chief Compliance Officer. . . . . Diane Lloyd Yaeger, J.D.
Associate Vice President, Environmental Health and Safety. . . . . Kathleen Crowley, M.P.H.
Assosciate Vice President for HIPAA Compliance/Privacy Officer . . . . Karen Pagliaro-Meyer
Assistant Vice President, Campus Operations . . . . Herman Matte, M.A.
Associate Vice President for Information Technology . . . . Robert V. Sideli, M.D.
Assistant Vice President for Government and Community Affairs. . . . . Sandra Harris
Assistant Vice President for External Relations . . . . Bonita Enochs
Assistant Vice President for Communications
   and Director of Publications . . . . Bonita Eaton Enochs, M.A.
Deputy Vice President for External Relations . . . . Marilyn Castaldi

Medical School Administrative Staff

Dean of the Faculties of Health Sciences and Medicine. . . . . Lee Goldman, M.D.
Senior Vice Dean of the Faculty of Medicine . . . . Steven Shea, M.D.
Vice Dean for Research . . . . Robert Kass, Ph.D.

Columbia University College of Physicians and Surgeons: NEW YORK

Vice Dean for Administration. . . . . Martha Hooven
Vice Dean for Academic Affairs . . . . Anne Taylor, M.D.
Vice Dean for Education . . . . Ronald E. Drusin, M.D.
Senior Associate Dean, Continuing Medical Education . . . . Donald S. Kornfeld, M.D.
Senior Associate Dean for Faculty Affairs and Health and Safety . . . . Robert Lewy, M.D.
Senior Associate Dean for Student Affairs. . . . . Lisa A. Mellman, M.D.
Senior Associate Dean for Harlem Hospital Center. . . . . Alfred Ashford, M.D., M.B.A.
Associate Dean and Chief Operating Officer, Harlem Hospital Center. . . . . Ernest Hart, J.D.
Associate Dean for St. Luke's-Roosevelt Hospital Center . . . . William Rosner, M.D.
Associate Dean for Bassett Healthcare . . . . Walter A. Franck, M.D.
Associate Dean at Stamford Health System . . . . Noel I. Robin, M.D.
Associate Dean at St. Vincent's Hospital in Bridgeport . . . . Michael I. Herman, M.D.
Associate Dean for Admissions . . . . Andrew Frantz, M.D.
Associate Dean for Alumni Relations and Development. . . . . Anke Nolting, Ph.D.
Associate Dean for Gender Equity and Career
  Development . . . . Jeanine D'Armiento, M.D., Ph.D.
Associate Dean for Graduate Affairs . . . . Richard B. Robinson, Ph.D.
Associate Dean for Development and Executive
  Director of Alumni Relations . . . . Anke Lunsman Nolting, Ph.D.
Associate Dean for Diversity and Minority Affairs . . . . Hilda Hutcherson, M.D.
Associate Dean for Scholarly Resources. . . . . Pat Molholt, Ph.D.
Assistant Dean for Graduate Affairs . . . . Fred Loweff, M.P.A.
Director of the Office of Faculty Affairs . . . . Carolyn M. Merten
Director of the Office of Clinical Trials . . . . Eileen Leach
Director of Science and Technology Ventures. . . . . Ofra Weinberger, Ph.D.
Director of Student Activities . . . . Rosemarie Scilipoti
Director of Institutional Review Board . . . . George Gasparis
President, Faculty Practice Organization . . . . Richard U. Levine, M.D.
Executive Director, Faculty Practice Organization . . . . Michael Duncan
Chief Operating Officer, Faculty Practice Organization. . . . . Roe Long, M.B.A., R.N.
Executive Director of Finance . . . . Aren Laljie, M.B.A., C.P.A.

Department and Division or Section Chairs

Basic Sciences

Anatomy and Cell Biology . . . . Michael Shelanski, M.D., Ph.D. (Interim)
Biochemistry and Molecular Biophysics. . . . . Arthur C. Palmer III, Ph.D. (Interim)
Genetics and Development. . . . . Gerard Karsenty, M.D., Ph.D.
Microbiology. . . . . Aaron Mitchell, Ph.D. (Interim)
Pathology and Cell Biology . . . . Michael L. Shelanski, M.D., Ph.D.
Pharmacology . . . . Robert S. Kass, Ph.D.
Physiology and Cellular Biophysics . . . . Andrew Marks, M.D.

Clinical Sciences

Anesthesiology. . . . . Margaret Wood, M.D.
Biomedical Informatics . . . . George M. Hripcsak, M.D.
Dermatology . . . . David R. Bickers, M.D.
Medicine. . . . . Donald W. Landry, M.D., Ph.D.
Neurological Surgery . . . . Robert A. Solomon, M.D.
Neurology . . . . Timothy A. Pedley, M.D.
Neuroscience. . . . . John Koester, Ph.D. (Interim)
Obstetrics and Gynecology. . . . . Mary E. D'Alton, M.D.
Ophthalmology . . . . Stanley Chang, M.D.
Orthopedic Surgery. . . . . Louis U. Bigliani, M.D.
Otolaryngology-Head and Neck Surgery . . . . Lanny Garth Close, M.D.
Pediatrics . . . . Lawrence R. Stanberry, M.D., Ph.D.
Psychiatry . . . . Jeffrey Lieberman, M.D.
Radiation Oncology. . . . . K. S. Clifford Chao, M.D.
Radiology . . . . Ronald L. Van Heertum, M.D. (Interim)
Rehabilitation Medicine. . . . . Joel Stein, M.D.
Surgery . . . . Craig R. Smith, M.D. (Interim)
Urology. . . . . Mitchell Benson, M.D.

Weill Cornell Medical College of Cornell University

New York, New York 10021
212-746-5454; 746-6005 (dean's office); 746-8424 (fax)
E-mail: dean@med.cornell.edu
Web site: www.med.cornell.edu

Cornell University Medical College was established in New York City in 1898, and its graduate school of medical sciences in 1952 by the trustees of Cornell University in order to take advantage of New York City's extensive opportunities for clinical instruction. The medical college moved to its present location in 1932 as the research and educational component of the New York Hospital-Cornell Medical Center. In 1998, the medical college and graduate school were renamed the Joan and Sanford I. Weill Medical College and Graduate School of Medical Sciences of Cornell University, and the college is now known as the Weill Cornell Medical College of Cornell University.

Type: private
2008-2009 total enrollment: 398
Clinical facilities: Amsterdam Nursing Home, Brooklyn Hospital Center, Burke Rehabilitation Hospital, Cayuga Medical Center at Ithaca, Community Health Network, New York Community Hospital, Hospital for Special Surgery, Lincoln Medical and Mental Health Center, Memorial Sloan-Kettering Cancer Center, New York Presbyterian Hospital, New York Downtown Hospital, New York Hospital Medical Center of Queens, New York Methodist Hospital, the Rogosin Institute, Southampton Hospital, The Methodist Hospital (Houston, Texas), Westchester Square Medical Center, University Group Medical Associates, Wyckoff Heights Medical Center.

University Officials

President. . . . . David J. Skorton, M.D.
Provost for Medical Affairs . . . . Antonio M. Gotto, Jr., M.D., D.Phil.

Medical School Administrative Staff

Dean. . . . . Antonio M. Gotto, Jr., M.D., D.Phil.
Dean, Graduate School of Medical Sciences,
   Executive Vice Provost and Senior Executive
   Vice Dean . . . . David P. Hajjar, Ph.D.
Dean, Weill Cornell Medical College (Qatar) . . . . Daniel R. Alonso, M.D.
Senior Associate Dean (Clinical Affairs) . . . . E. Darracott Vaughan, M.D.
Associate Provost and Executive Vice Dean for
   Administration and Finance . . . . Stephen M. Cohen
Associate Provost for International Initiatives and Executive Vice Dean . . . . Steven P. Rosalie
Vice Provost (Development). . . . . Larry Schafer
Vice Provost (Public Affairs). . . . . Myrna Manners
Senior Associate Dean (Education). . . . . Carol Storey-Johnson, M.D.
Associate Dean (Academic Affairs) . . . . Debra Gillers
Associate Dean, Pre-Medical Education (Qatar) . . . . David Robertshaw, Ph.D., D.V.M.
Associate Dean (Admissions) . . . . Charles L. Bardes, M.D.
Associate Dean (Affiliations) . . . . Oliver T. Fein, M.D.
Associate Dean (Billing Compliance) . . . . Stephen J. Thomas, M.D.
Associate Dean (Burke Medical Research Institute). . . . . Mary Beth Walsh, M.D.
Associate Dean (Continuing Medical Education). . . . . Scott J. Goldsmith, M.D.
Associate Dean (Curricular Affairs), Curriculum
   and Educational Development . . . . Peter M. Marzuk, M.D.
Associate Dean (Graduate School of Medical Sciences). . . . . Randi Silver, Ph.D.
Associate Dean (Healthcare System). . . . . Eliot Lazar, M.D.
Associate Dean (MSKCC). . . . . Thomas J. Fahey, Jr., M.D.
Associate Dean (Research Administration) . . . . Harry M. Lander, Ph.D.
Associate Dean (Student Affairs and Equal Opportunity Programs) . . . . Carlyle Miller, M.D.
Librarian. . . . . Carolyn Reid
Assistant Dean (Admissions). . . . . Liliana Montano
Assistant Dean (Departmental Associates). . . . . Marcus M. Reidenberg, M.D.
Assistant Dean (Graduate School) . . . . Francoise Freyre
Assistant Dean (Research Compliance). . . . . Barbara Pifel, R.N., J.D.
Assistant Dean (Intercampus Affairs) . . . . Caren A. Heller, M.D.
Assistant Dean (Research Integrity) . . . . Mary Simmerl
Assistant Dean (Research Planning and Strategic Development) . . . . Eelco A. Slagter
Assistant Dean (Student Affairs). . . . . Elizabeth Wilson Anstey
Deputy University Counsel and Sec. of the Medical College. . . . . James R. Kahn, J.D.
Chief Medical Officer, Physician Organization . . . . Daniel M. Knowles, M.D.
Chief Administrative Officer, Physician Organization. . . . . Nancy L. Farrell
Senior Director, Facilities Management. . . . . Andrew Ryan
Senior Director, Financial Operations. . . . . Edward Walsh
Senior Director, Human Resources. . . . . Lisa Abbott
Senior Director, Office of Technology Development . . . . Brian J. Kelly
Senior Director for Budgets and Financial Planning . . . . Scott Puccino
Director, Office of Faculty Affairs. . . . . Mark A. Albano, Ph.D.
Director, Office of Grants and Contracts. . . . . Barbara Pifel, R.N.
Director, Risk Management . . . . Thomas Lawrence

Weill Cornell Medical College of Cornell University: NEW YORK

Director, Research Animal Resource Center . . . . Neil Lipman, V.M.D.
Chief Information Officer . . . . Virginia McFerran

Department and Division or Section Chairs
Basic Sciences

Biochemistry . . . . Frederick R. Maxfield, Ph.D.
Cell and Developmental Biology . . . . Katherine A. Hajjar, M.D.
Genetic Medicine . . . . Ronald G. Crystal, M.D.
Microbiology and Immunology . . . . Carl F. Nathan, M.D.
Pathology and Laboratory Medicine . . . . Daniel M. Knowles, M.D.
Pharmacology . . . . Lorraine J. Gudas, Ph.D.
Physiology and Biophysics . . . . Harel Weinstein, D.Sc.

Clinical Sciences

Anesthesiology . . . . John J. Savarese, M.D.
Cardiothoracic Surgery . . . . O. Wayne Isom, M.D.
Dermatology . . . . Richard D. Granstein, M.D.
Medicine . . . . Andrew I. Schafer, M.D.
   Cardiology . . . . Bruce B. Lerman, M.D.
   Clinical Pharmacology . . . . Marcus M. Reidenberg, M.D.
   Emergency Medicine . . . . Neal E. Flomenbaum, M.D.
   Endocrinology, Diabetes and Metabolism . . . . Julianne L. Imperato-McGinley, M.D.
   Gastroenterology and Hepatology . . . . Ira M. Jacobson, M.D.
   General Internal Medicine . . . . Mary E. Charlson, M.D.
   Geriatrics and Gerontology . . . . Ronald D. Adelman, M.D., and Mark S. Lachs, M.D.
   Hematology and Medical Oncology . . . . Barbara L. Hempstead, M.D., Ph.D.,
      and David M. Nanus, M.D.
   Immunology . . . . Kendall A. Smith, M.D.
   International Medicine and Infectious Diseases . . . . Warren D. Johnson, Jr., M.D.
   Medical Ethics . . . . Joseph J. Fins, M.D.
   Nephrology and Hypertention . . . . Manikkam Suthanthiran, M.D.
   Pulmonary and Critical Care Medicine . . . . Ronald G. Crystal, M.D.
   Rheumatology . . . . Stephen A. Paget, M.D.
Neurology and Neuroscience . . . . M. Flint Beal, M.D.
Neurological Surgery . . . . Philip E. Stieg, M.D., Ph.D.
Obstetrics and Gynecology . . . . Frank A. Chervenak, M.D., Ph.D.
Ophthalmology . . . . Donald D'Amico, M.D.
Orthopaedic Surgery . . . . Thomas P. Sculco, M.D.
Otorhinolaryngology . . . . Michael G. Stewart, M.D.
Pediatrics . . . . Gerald M. Loughlin, M.D.
Psychiatry . . . . Jack D. Barchas, M.D.
Public Health . . . . Alvin I. Mushlin, M.D.
Radiology . . . . Robert Min, M.D.
Rehabilitation Medicine (Free Standing Division) . . . . Nancy Strauss, M.D. (Acting)
Surgery . . . . Fabrizio Michelassi, M.D.
   Bariatric and Minimally Invasive . . . . Alfons Pomp, M.D.
   Breast . . . . Alex Swistel, M.D.
   Burn Center . . . . Roger W. Yurt, M.D.
   Colon and Rectal . . . . Jeffrey Milsom, M.D.
   Oral and Maxillofacial . . . . David A. Behrman, D.M.D.
   Pediatric . . . . Nitsana Spigland, M.D.
   Plastic . . . . Robert Grant, M.D.
   Transplantation . . . . Sandip Kapur, M.D.
   Trauma and Critical Care . . . . Philip S. Barie, M.D.
   Vascular . . . . K. Craig Kent, M.D.
Urology . . . . Peter Schlegel, M.D.

Centers and Institutes

Ansary Center for Stem Cell Therapeutics . . . . Shahin Rafii, M.D.
Center for Aging Research and Clinical Care . . . . Ronald D. Adelman, M.D.,
      and Mark S. Lachs, M.D.
Center for Complementary and Integrative Medicine . . . . Mary E. Charlson, M.D.
Center for the Study of Hepatitis C . . . . Ira M. Jacobson, M.D. **
Center for Vascular Biology . . . . David P. Hajjar, Ph.D.
Institute for Computational Biomedicine . . . . Harel Weinstein, M.D.
Institute for Reproductive Medicine
   Women's Service Center . . . . Zev Rosenwaks, M.D.
   Men's Service Center . . . . Marc Goldstein, M.D.
Sackler Institute for Developmental Psychobiology . . . . B.J. Casey, Ph.D.
Iris Cantor Women's Health Center . . . . Orli R. Etingin, M.D.
The Arthur and Rochelle Belfer Institute of
   Hematology and Medical Oncology . Barbara Hempstead, M.D., Ph.D., and David Nanus, M.D.
Lehman Brothers Lung Cancer Research Center . . . . Nasser Altorki, M.D.

**Medical Director

Mount Sinai School of Medicine of New York University

One Gustave L. Levy Place
New York, New York 10029-6574
212-241-6500; 241-8884 (dean's office); 824-2302 (fax)
Web site: www.mssm.edu

The school of medicine was granted a provisional charter by the board of regents of the State University of New York in 1963 and an absolute charter on May 24, 1968, to establish a medical school on the campus of the Mount Sinai Hospital. The school matriculated its first students in September 1968. In July 1999, Mount Sinai School of Medicine formally affiliated with New York University.

Type: private
2008-2009 total enrollment: 512
Clinical facilities: The Mount Sinai Hospital, Bronx Veterans Affairs Medical Center, Cabrini Medical Center, Elmhurst Hospital Center, Englewood Hospital and Medical Center, Jamaica Hospital, Jersey City Medical Center, Jewish Home and Hospital, North General Hospital, Phelps Memorial Hospital Center, Pilgrim Psychiatric Center, Queens Hospital Center, Saint Barnabas Health Care System, St. Joseph's Regional Medical Center.

University Officials

President, New York University...................................... John Sexton, Ph.D.
President, Mount Sinai Medical Center.......................... Kenneth L. Davis, M.D.

Medical School Administrative Staff

Dean, Mount Sinai School of Medicine and
  Executive Vice President for Academic Affairs,
  The Mount Sinai Medical Center .... Dennis S. Charney, M.D.
Dean for Basic Science and the Graduate School
  of Biological Sciences .... John Morrison, Ph.D.
Dean for Translational Biomedical Research....................... Hugh Sampson, M.D.
Dean for Medical Education..................................... David Muller, M.D.
Dean for Clinical Affairs....................................... Louis Russo, M.D.
Dean for Graduate Medical Education .... Barry D. Stimmel, M.D.
Dean for Operations .... Jeffrey Silberstein
Dean for QHC/Elmhurst Programs .... Jasmin Moshirpur, M.D.
Senior Vice President for Finance............................ Stephen T. Harvey
Senior Vice President for Development .... Mark Kostegan
Associate Dean and Vice President for Operations .... Maureen Milici
Associate Dean for Education and Translational Research Operations .... Phyllis Schnepf
Associate Dean for Research................................. Jeffrey Silverstein, M.D.
Associate Dean for Research Resources........................ Reginald Miller, D.V.M.
Associate Dean for Diversity Programs and Policy .... Gary C. Butts, M.D.
Associate Dean for Faculty Affairs and Administration.............. Leslie Schneier
Associate Dean for Planning and Resource Management................. Rama Iyengar
Associate Dean for Research................................. Glenn Martin, M.D.
Associate Dean for Sponsored Programs........................ Jessica Moise
Associate Dean for the Graduate School of Biological Sciences .... Miki Rifkin, Ph.D.
Associate Dean for Clinical Research .... Mary Sano, Ph.D.
Associate Dean for Graduate Education in Translational Research........... Lisa Satlin, M.D.
Associate Dean for Academic, Student Affairs,
  and Continuing Medical Education .... Suzanne Rose, M.D.
Associate Dean for Medical Student Research..................... Karen Zier, Ph.D.
Associate Dean for Undergraduate Medical Education .... Erica Friedman, M.D.
Associate Dean for Graduate Medical Education.................... Kevin M. Troy, M.D.
Associate Dean for Admissions................................ Scott Barnett, M.D.
Associate Dean for Information Resources and Systems................ Lynn Kasner Morgan
Associate Dean for Academic Development and Mentoring............. Lakshmi Devi, Ph.D.
Associate Dean for Alliance Development........................ Robert Southwick
Associate Dean for Bronx Veterans Administration Affairs.......... Eric Langhoff, M.D., Ph.D.
Associate Dean QHC/Elmhurst Programs........................ Kenneth Feifer
Associate Dean for North General Hospital...................... Samuel Daniel, M.D.

Associate Dean for Jersey Medical Center . . . . Robert Lahita, M.D.
Associate Dean for Atlantic Health Systems. . . . . Susan Kaye, M.D.

Department Chairs

Basic Sciences

Center for Comparative Medicine and Surgery . . . . Reginald W. Miller, D.V.M.
Gene and Cell Medicine . . . . Savio L. C. Woo, Ph.D.
Genetics and Genomic Sciences . . . . Robert J. Desnick, Ph.D., M.D.
Microbiology . . . . Peter Palese, Ph.D.
Developmental and Regenerative Biology . . . . Marek Mlodzik, Ph.D.
Neuroscience. . . . . Eric J. Nestler, M.D., Ph.D.
Oncological Sciences . . . . Stuart Aaronson, M.D.
Pharmacology and Systems Therapeutics . . . . Ravi Iyengar, Ph.D.
Structural and Chemical Biology . . . . Ming-Ming Zhou, Ph.D.

Clinical Sciences

Anesthesiology. . . . . David Reich, M.D.
Cardiothoracic Surgery . . . . David Adams, M.D.
Cardiovascular Institute . . . . Valentin Fuster, M.D.
Community Medicine. . . . . Philip J. Landrigan, M.D.
Dentistry . . . . John Pfail, D.D.S.
Dermatology . . . . Mark G. Lebwohl, M.D.
Emergency Medicine . . . . Sheldon Jacobson, M.D.
Geriatrics and Adult Development . . . . Albert Siu, M.D.
Health Policy. . . . . Eric A. Rose, M.D.
Medical Education. . . . . David Muller, M.D.
Medicine . . . . Paul Klotman, M.D.
   Cardiology . . . . Valentin Fuster, M.D., Ph.D.
   Clinical Immunology . . . . Lloyd Mayer, M.D.
   Endocrinology . . . . Derek LeRoith, M.D., Ph.D.
   Gastroenterology . . . . Lloyd Mayer, M.D.
   General Medicine. . . . . Thomas McGinn, M.D.
   Hematology and Medical Oncology. . . . . George Atweh, M.D.
   Infectious Diseases . . . . Mary E. Klotman, M.D.
   Liver Diseases. . . . . Scott Friedman, M.D.
   Nephrology . . . . Barbara Murphy, M.D.
   Pulmonary and Critical Care. . . . . Michael Iannuzzi, M.D.
   Rheumatology . . . . Peter D. Gorevic, M.D.
Neurology. . . . . C. Warren Olanow, M.D.
Neurosurgery. . . . . Joshua Bederson, M.D.
Obstetrics, Gynecology, and Reproductive Science . . . . Michael Brodman, M.D.
Ophthalmology . . . . Douglas Jabs, M.D.
Orthopaedics. . . . . Evan Flatow, M.D.
Otolaryngology . . . . Eric Genden, M.D.
Pathology . . . . Alan L. Schiller, M.D.
Pediatrics . . . . Frederick J. Suchy, M.D.
Psychiatry . . . . Eric Hollander, M.D.
Radiation Oncology. . . . . Richard Stock, M.D.
Radiology . . . . Burton P. Drayer, M.D.
Rehabilitation Medicine. . . . . Kristjan T. Ragnarsson, M.D.
Surgery . . . . Michael Marin, M.D.
Transplant Institute . . . . Jonathan Bromberg, M.D., Ph.D.
Urology. . . . . Simon Hall, M.D.

New York Medical College
Administration Building
Valhalla, New York 10595
914-594-4900 (provost and dean's office); 594-4145 (fax)
Web site: www.nymc.edu

New York Medical College was founded by William Cullen Bryant and received its charter from the legislature of New York state in April 1860. New York Medical College is a health sciences university in the Catholic tradition that includes two graduate schools: the graduate school of basic medical sciences and the school of public health. For over 100 years, the college was located in New York City. During the late 1970s, the college moved to its present location in Westchester County.

Type: private
2008-2009 total enrollment: 669
Clinical facilities: Academic Medical Centers - Saint Vincent Catholic Medical Centers, Westchester Medical Center. **University hospitals** - Danbury Hospital, Metropolitan Hospital Center, Our Lady of Mercy Medical Center. **Major affiliated hospital** - Sound Shore Medical Center of Westchester.

University Officials

President and Chief Executive Officer	Karl P. Adler, M.D.
Provost and Dean, School of Medicine	Ralph A. O'Connell, M.D.
Senior Vice President, Chief Financial Officer, and Vice Provost	Stephen J. Piccolo, Jr.
Vice Provost and Senior Associate Dean for Academic Administration	William A. Steadman II
Vice President and General Counsel	Waldemar A. Comas
Vice President for University Development and University Planning	Julie A. Kubaska
Dean, Graduate School of Basic Medical Sciences	Francis L. Belloni, Ph.D.
Dean, School of Public Health	Robert W. Amler, M.D.
Chief Information Officer	John C. Hammond

Medical College Administration

Vice Dean for Graduate Medical Education and Affiliations	Richard G. McCarrick, M.D.
Vice Dean for Westchester Medical Center	Renee Garrick, M.D.
Vice Dean for Medical Education	Martha S. Grayson, M.D.
Senior Associate Dean for Metropolitan Hospital Center	Richard K. Stone, M.D.
Senior Associate Dean for Our Lady of Mercy Medical Center	C. Gene Cayten, M.D.
Senior Associate Dean for Saint Vincent Catholic Medical Centers/Manhattan	Margaret D. Smith, M.D.
Senior Associate Dean for Westchester Medical Center	Paul K. Woolf, M.D.
Senior Associate Dean for Danbury Hospital	Pierre F. Saldinger, M.D.
Senior Associate Dean for Student Affairs	Gladys M. Ayala, M.D.
Senior Associate Dean	Saverio S. Bentivegna, M.D.
Associate Dean for Admissions	Fern Juster, M.D.
Associate Dean for Continuing Medical Education	Joseph F. Dursi, M.D.
Associate Dean for Student Affairs	Elliott N. Perla, M.D.
Associate Dean for Student Financial Planning	Anthony M. Sozzo
Associate Dean for Saint Vincent Catholic Medical Centers/Brooklyn-Queens Region	John R. Denton, M.D.
Associate Dean for Saint Vincent Catholic Medical Centers/Staten Island Region	Edward L. Arsura, M.D.
Associate Dean for Sound Shore Medical Center	Burton Herz, M.D.
Associate Dean for Medical Education	Jennifer Koestler, M.D.
Associate Dean	Joseph T. English, M.D.
Associate Dean for Research Administration	Catharine Crea
Associate Dean and Director of Medical Sciences Library	Diana J. Cunningham
University Registrar and Associate Provost	Judith A. Ehren
Senior Communications Director	Donna Moriarty
Director of Comparative Medicine	Ellen Levee, D.V.M.
Executive Assistant to the Provost and Dean	Vilma E. Bordonaro

Department and Division or Section Chairs

Basic Sciences

Biochemistry and Molecular Biology.......................... Ernest Y. C. Lee, Ph.D.
Cell Biology and Anatomy .... Joseph D. Etlinger, Ph.D.
Microbiology and Immunology.............................. Ira Schwartz, Ph.D.
Pharmacology .... John C. McGiff, M.D.
Physiology .... Thomas H. Hintze, Ph.D.

Clinical Sciences

Anesthesiology.. Kathryn E. McGoldrick, M.D.
  Vice Chair, Saint Vincent Catholic Medical Centers............. George G. Neuman, M.D.
Dental Medicine .... Joseph F. Morales, D.D.S.
Dermatology .... Bijan Safai, M.D., D.Sc.
Emergency Medicine..................................... Gregory L. Almond, M.D.
Family and Community Medicine.......................... Montgomery Douglas, M.D.
Medicine... William H. Frishman, M.D.
  Administrative Vice Chair............................... Stephen J. Peterson, M.D.
  Vice Chair for Education .... Robert G. Lerner, M.D.
  Vice Chair for Research and Scientific Affairs .... Gary P. Wormser, M.D.
  Vice Chair, Saint Vincent Catholic Medical Centers........... Dennis M. Greenbaum, M.D.
Neurology.. Brij Singh Ahluwalia, M.D.
Neurosurgery... Raj Murali, M.D.
  Vice Chair, Saint Vincent Catholic Medical Centers............. Alan D. Hirschfeld, M.D.
Obstetrics and Gynecology............................... Howard Blanchette, M.D.
  Vice Chair, Our Lady of Mercy Medical Center.................. Kevin D. Reilly, M.D.
  Vice Chair, Richmond University Medical Center................. Michael Moretti, M.D.
Ophthalmology .... Joseph B. Walsh, M.D.
Orthopedic Surgery...................................... David E. Asprinio, M.D.
Otolaryngology .... Steven D. Schaefer, M.D.
Pathology .... Iradge Argani, M.D. (Interim)
Pediatrics .... Leonard J. Newman, M.D.
  Vice Chair, Westchester Medical Center .... Michael H. Gewitz, M.D.
Psychiatry and Behavioral Sciences.......................... Joseph T. English, M.D.
  Vice Chair, Westchester Medical Center .... Neil Zolkind, M.D.
  Vice Chair, Saint Vincent Catholic Medical Centers................. Spencer Eth, M.D.
Radiation Medicine .... Chitti R. Moorthy, M.D.
  Vice Chair, Westchester Medical Center .... Chitti R. Moorthy, M.D.
Radiology .... Chitti R. Moorthy, M.D. (Acting)
Rehabilitation Medicine................................... Maria P. de Araujo, M.D.
Surgery .... John A. Savino, M.D.
Urology.. Muhammad S. Choudhury, M.D.
  Vice Chair, Saint Vincent Catholic Medical Centers/Manhattan .... Michael Grasso, M.D.
  Vice Chair, Saint Vincent Catholic Medical
    Centers/Manhattan .... Christopher B. Mills, M.D.
  Vice Chair, Westchester Medical Center .... Patricia A. Sheiner, M.D.

New York University School of Medicine

550 First Avenue
New York, New York 10016
212-263-7300; 263-3269 (dean's office); 263-1828 (fax)
Web site: www.med.nyu.edu/education

The New York University School of Medicine admitted its first class in 1841. The parent university is a private institution, receiving no tax support and having no geographic restrictions on its student body. The medical school is part of the New York University Medical Center.

Type: private
2008-2009 total enrollment: 716
Clinical facilities: Bellevue Hospital Center, Veterans Affairs Medical Center, New York University Hospitals Center, Tisch Hospital, Howard A. Rusk Institute of Rehabilitation Medicine, Hospital for Joint Diseases Orthopaedic Institute, Gouverneur Hospital, Lenox Hill Hospital, North Shore University Hospital, Jamaica Hospital Medical Center.

Medical School Administrative Staff

President. . . . . John Sexton
Dean and Chief Executive Officer . . . . Robert I. Grossman, M.D.
Vice Dean, Chief of Staff . . . . Andrew W. Litt, M.D.
Vice Dean, Chief of Hospital Operations . . . . Bernard A. Birnbaum, M.D.
Vice Dean for External Affairs . . . . Harold S. Koplewicz, M.D.
Vice Dean, Chief Information Officer. . . . . Paul Conocenti
Vice Dean, Chief Financial Officer . . . . Richard R. Crater
Vice Dean for Clinical Affairs and Strategy . . . . Andrew Brotman, M.D.
Vice Dean for Administration. . . . . Kathleen P. Gallagher
Vice Dean and General Counsel. . . . . Annette B. Johnson, Esq.
Vice Dean for Education, Faculty, and Academic Affairs . . . . Steven B. Abramson, M.D.
Vice Dean for Science . . . . Vivian Lee, M.D., Ph.D.
Vice Dean for Human Resources . . . . Nancy Sanchez
Senior Associate Dean for Medical Education and Student Affairs. . . . . Vacant
Senior Associate Dean for Science Administration. . . . . Heidi Aronin, M.P.A.
Senior Associate Dean for Biomedical Sciences. . . . . Joel D. Oppenheim, Ph.D.
Senior Associate Dean for Community Health Affairs . . . . Mariano J. Rey, M.D.
Associate Dean for Graduate Medical Education. . . . . Carol Bernstein, M.D.
Associate Dean for Student Affairs . . . . Lynn Buckvar-Keltz, M.D.
Associate Dean for Postgraduate Programs . . . . Norman Sussman, M.D.
Vice Dean for Real Estate Development and Facilities. . . . . Vicki Match Suna
Associate Dean for Sponsored Programs Administrations. . . . . Tom Marcussen
Associate Dean for Clinical Research . . . . Steven B. Abramson
Associate Dean for Medical Education . . . . Julianne Chase, Ph.D.
Associate Dean for Admissions and Financial Aid . . . . Nancy B. Genieser, M.D.
Associate Dean for Government Affairs. . . . . Gilda Ecroyd
Director, Office of Registration and Student Records . . . . Maureen A. Doran
Executive Director of Development . . . . Lawrence Siegel
Associate Dean for Education (Lenox Hill Hospital) . . . . Michael S. Bruno, M.D.
Associate Dean for Education (North Shore University Hospital). . . . . Lawrence Smith, M.D.
Assistant Dean (VA Medical Center). . . . . Michael S. Simberkoff, M.D.
Assistant Dean for Advanced Applications. . . . . Jonathan H. Weider
Associate Dean for Research Administration . . . . Vacant
Assistant Dean for Admissions and Financial Aid. . . . . Joanne McGrath
Assistant Dean for Diversity and Community Affairs . . . . Mekbib Gemeda

Department and Division or Section Chairs

Basic Sciences

Biochemistry. . . . . Dafna Bar-Sagi, Ph.D.
Cell Biology. . . . . David D. Sabatini, M.D., Ph.D.
Environmental Medicine . . . . Max Costa, Ph.D.
Forensic Medicine . . . . Charles S. Hirsch, M.D.

Medical and Molecular Parasitology . . . . Karen Day, Ph.D.
Microbiology . . . . Claudio Basilico, M.D.
Pathology . . . . David Roth, M.D., Ph.D.
Pharmacology . . . . Herbert H. Samuels, M.D.
Physiology and Neuroscience . . . . Rodolfo Llinas, M.D., Ph.D.

Clinical Sciences

Anesthesiology . . . . Thomas Blanck, M.D.
Cardiothoracic Surgery . . . . Aubrey Galloway, M.D.
Dermatology . . . . Seth Orlow, M.D. (Acting)
Emergency Medicine . . . . Lewis R. Goldfrank, M.D.
Medicine . . . . Martin Blaser, M.D.
    Cardiology* . . . . Glenn Fishman, M.D.
    Clinical Oncology* . . . . Franco M. Muggia, M.D.
    Clinical Pharmacology . . . . Bruce Cronstein, M.D.
    Endocrinology* . . . . Ann Danoff, M.D.
    Gastroenterology* . . . . Robert Raicht, M.D.
    Genetics* . . . . Rochelle Hirschhorn, M.D.
    Geriatrics* . . . . Scott Sherman, M.D. (Interim)
    Hematology* . . . . Simon Karpatkin, M.D.
    Hypertension/Nephrology* . . . . Edward Skolnik, M.D.
    Infectious Diseases and Immunology* . . . . Joel Ernst, M.D.
    Molecular Endocrinology* . . . . Herbert H. Samuels, M.D.
    Pulmonary and Critical Care Medicine* . . . . William N. Rom, M.D.
    Primary Care* . . . . Marc Gourevitch, M.D.
    Rheumatology* . . . . Steven B. Abramson, M.D.
Neurology . . . . Edwin H. Kolodny, M.D.
Neurosurgery . . . . Jafar Jafar, M.D. (Interim)
Obstetrics and Gynecology . . . . Robert F. Porges, M.D. (Interim)
Ophthalmology . . . . Jack Dodick, M.D.
Orthopedic Surgery . . . . Joseph D. Zuckerman, M.D.
Otolaryngology . . . . Anil Lalwani, M.D.
Pediatrics . . . . Bernard Dryer, M.D. (Acting)
Psychiatry . . . . Dolores Malaspina, M.D.
Radiation Oncology . . . . Silvia Formenti, M.D.
Radiology . . . . Robert Grossman, M.D.
Rehabilitation Medicine . . . . Steven Flanagan, M.D.
Surgery . . . . H. Leon Pachter, M.D.
    Endocrine Surgery . . . . Keith Heller, M.D.
    General* . . . . Kenneth Eng, M.D.
    Pediatric Surgery . . . . Howard Ginsburg, M.D.
    Plastic Surgery* . . . . Joseph G. McCarthy, M.D.
    Surgical Oncology . . . . Daniel Roses, M.D.
    Transplant . . . . Lewis Tepperman, M.D.
    Trauma/Critical Care . . . . Ronald Simon, M.D.
    Vascular . . . . Mark Adelman, M.D.
Urology . . . . Herbert Lepor, M.D.

*Specialty without organizational autonomy.

University of Rochester School of Medicine and Dentistry

601 Elmwood Avenue
Rochester, New York 14642
585-275-0017 (deans' office); 256-1131 (fax)
Web site: www.rochester.edu

The school of medicine and dentistry was founded in 1920 and accepted its first class in 1925. The medical center adjoins the university's River campus with its programs in arts and science and major intellectual disciplines.

Type: private
2008-2009 total enrollment: 410
Clinical facilities: The Strong Memorial Hospital, Highland Hospital, Rochester General Hospital, Monroe Community Hospital, St. Mary's Hospital, Parkridge Hospital, Eastman Dental Center.

University Officials

President and Chief Executive Officer .... Joel Seligman
Provost and Executive Vice President .... Ralph W. Kuncl, M.D., Ph.D.
Senior Vice President for Health Sciences and
   Chief Executive Officer, University of
   Rochester Medical Center .... Bradford C. Berk, M.D., Ph.D.
Senior Vice President for Administration and
   Finance and Chief Financial Officer .... Ronald J. Paprocki
Vice Provost and University Dean for Graduate Studies..................... Bruce Jacobs
Vice President and General Secretary, Senior
   Advisor to the President and University Dean .... Paul Burgett
Senior Vice President for Institutional Resources .... Douglas Phillips
Senior Vice President and General Counsel .... Sue S. Stewart

Medical School Administrative Staff

Senior Vice President for Health Sciences and
   Chief Executive Officer, University of
   Rochester Medical Center .... Bradford C. Berk, M.D., Ph.D.
Dean... David S. Guzick, M.D., Ph.D.
President and Chief Executive Officer, Strong
   Memorial Hospital and Highland Hospital .... Steven I. Goldstein
Medical Center Vice President and Chief Operating Officer .... Peter G. Robinson
Medical Center Vice President and Chief Financial Officer .... Michael C. Goonan
Vice President and Chief Medical Officer..................... Raymond J. Mayewski, M.D.
Vice President for Clinical Services............................ Richard I. Fisher, M.D.
Senior Associate Dean for Graduate and Postdoctoral Education........ Edith M. Lord, Ph.D.
Senior Associate Dean for Academic Affairs .... Richard I. Burton, M.D.
Senior Associate Dean for Clinical Research .... Thomas A. Pearson, M.D., Ph.D.
Senior Associate Dean for Basic Research...................... Stephen Dewhurst, Ph.D.
Senior Associate Dean for Clinical Affairs...................... Richard I. Fisher, M.D.
Senior Associate Dean for Medical Education .... David R. Lambert, M.D.
Senior Associate Dean for Graduate Medical Education .... Diane M. Hartmann, M.D.
Senior Director, Finance and Administration .... William P. Passalacqua
Associate Dean for Admissions.................................John T. Hansen, Ph.D.
Associate Dean for Educational Evaluation and Research .... Ronald M. Epstein, M.D.
Associate Dean for Faculty Development-Education............... Denham Ward, M.D., Ph.D.
Associate Dean for Faculty Development-Women and Diversity .... Vivian Lewis, M.D.
Assistant Dean for Medical Education and Student Affairs.................. Brenda D. Lee
Assistant Dean for Medical Simulation .... Linda L. Spillane, M.D.
Director of Continuing Professional Education........................... Paul Lambiase
Director of Admissions.. Pat Samuelson
Director, Edward G. Miner Library.............................. Julia F. Sollenberger

University of Rochester School of Medicine and Dentistry: NEW YORK

Department, Center, and Division or Section Chairs

Basic Sciences

Biochemistry and Biophysics. . . . . Robert A. Bambara, Ph.D.
Biomedical Engineering. . . . . Richard E. Waugh, Ph.D.
Biomedical Genetics . . . . Hartmut Land, Ph.D.
Biostatistics and Computational Biology . . . . David Oakes, Ph.D. (Interim)
Aab Cardiovascular Research Institute . . . . Mark B. Taubman, M.D.
Center for Neural Development and Disease. . . . . Harris Gelbard, M.D., Ph.D.
Center for Pediatric Biomedical Research. . . . . Vacant
Center for Musculoskeletal Research . . . . Regis J. O'Keefe, M.D., Ph.D.
Center for Neurodegenerative and Vascular
   Brain Disorders . . . . Berislav V. Zlokovic, M.D., Ph.D.
Center for Oral Biology. . . . . Robert G. Quivey, Jr., Ph.D.
Center for Translational Neuromedicine . . . . Steven A. Goldman, M.D., Ph.D.,
   and Maiken Nedergaard, M.D., D.M.Sc.
Center for Vaccine Biology and Immunology . . . . Tim R. Mosmann, Ph.D.
Community and Preventive Medicine . . . . Susan Fisher, Ph.D.
Environmental Medicine . . . . Thomas A. Gasiewicz, Ph.D.
Laboratory Animal Medicine* . . . . Jeffrey D. Wyatt, D.V.M.
Microbiology and Immunology. . . . . Barbara H. Iglewski, Ph.D.
Neurobiology and Anatomy . . . . Gary D. Paige, M.D., Ph.D.
Pharmacology and Physiology. . . . . A. William Tank, Ph.D.

Clinical Sciences

Anesthesiology. . . . . James L. Robotham, M.D.
Cancer Center. . . . . Richard I. Fisher, M.D.
Dentistry . . . . Cyril Meyerowitz, D.D.S.
Dermatology . . . . Alice P. Pentland, M.D.
Emergency Medicine . . . . Gregory P. Conners, M.D., M.P.H., M.B.A.
Family Medicine . . . . Thomas L. Cambell, M.D.
Imaging Sciences. . . . . David L. Waldman, M.D., Ph.D.
Medicine. . . . . Mark B. Taubman, M.D.
Neurology. . . . . TBA
Neurosurgery. . . . . Webster H. Pilcher, M.D., Ph.D.
Obstetrics and Gynecology. . . . . James R. Woods, M.D.
Ophthalmology . . . . Steven E. Feldon, M.D.
Orthopaedics and Rehabilitation . . . . Regis J. O'Keefe, M.D., Ph.D.
Otolaryngology-Head and Neck Surgery . . . . Shawn D. Newlands, M.D., Ph.D., M.B.A.
Pathology and Laboratory Medicine . . . . Daniel H. Ryan, M.D.
Pediatrics . . . . Nina F. Schor, M.D., Ph.D.
Physical Medicine and Rehabilitation . . . . K. Rao Poduri, M.D.
Psychiatry . . . . Eric D. Caine, M.D.
Radiation Oncology. . . . . Paul Okunieff, M.D.
Surgery . . . . Jeffrey H. Peters, M.D.
Urology. . . . . Edward M. Messing, M.D.

State University of New York, Downstate Medical Center
College of Medicine
450 Clarkson Avenue, Box 97
Brooklyn, New York 11203-2098
718-270-1000; 270-3776 (dean's office); 270-4074 (fax)
Web site: www.downstate.edu

The college of medicine was founded in 1860 as the teaching division of the Long Island College Hospital in Brooklyn. In 1930, it was incorporated as the Long Island College of Medicine, and in 1950, it was merged with the State University of New York to become the first unit of the Downstate Medical Center.

Type: public
2008-2009 total enrollment: 775
Clinical facilities: Major affiliates—Brookdale Hospital Medical Center, Kings County Hospital Center, Long Island College Hospital, Maimonides Medical Center, Staten Island University Hospital, University Hospital of Brooklyn, VA New York Harbor Healthcare System, Lenox Hill Hospital. **Limited affiliates**—Brooklyn Hospital Center, Coney Island Hospital, Flushing Hospital, Lutheran Medical Center, Kingsboro Psychiatric Center, Kingsbrook Jewish Medical Center, New York Methodist Hospital, Jamaica Hospital, Miami Children's Hospital, Long Island Jewish Medical Center, Northshore University Hospital, St. Vincent's Hospital and Medical Center of New York, St. Vincent's Medical Center of Richmond, Woodhull Medical and Mental Health Center. **Graduate affiliates**—Interfaith Medical Center, Beth Israel Hospital, Memorial Sloan-Kettering Cancer Center, Our Lady of Mercy Medical Center, St. John's Episcopal Hospital—South Shore, NYS Institute for Basic Research in Developmental Disabilities.

University Official
Chancellor . . . . John R. Ryan

Health Science Center Administrative Staff
President. . . . . John C. LaRosa, M.D.
Executive Vice President and Chief Operating Officer. . . . . Ivan M. Lisnitzer
Senior Vice President for Institutional
   Advancement and Philanthropy and Vice
   President for Academic Affairs . . . . Jo Ann Bradley, Ed.D.
Assistant Vice President for Institutional Advancement . . . . Ellen Watson
Assistant Vice President for Planning . . . . Dorothy R. Fyfe
Senior Vice President and Chief Financial Officer. . . . . Frederick J. Hammond, Jr.
Chief Executive Officer . . . . Debra D. Carey
Vice President, Office of Compliance and Audit Services. . . . . Renee Poncet

College of Medicine
Dean, College of Medicine. . . . . Ian L. Taylor, M.D., Ph.D.
Vice Dean . . . . Roger Q. Cracco, M.D.
Vice Dean for Graduate Medical Education . . . . Frank E. Lucente, M.D.
Vice President for Student Affairs and Dean of Students. . . . . Lorraine Terracina, Ph.D.
Senior Associate Dean for Education . . . . Stanley Friedman, M.D.
Associate Dean for Student Affairs . . . . Sophie R. Christoforou
Associate Dean for Administration . . . . Ross Clinchy, Ph.D.
Associate Dean of Minority Affairs . . . . Constance Hill, M.D.
Associate Dean for Graduate Medical Education . . . . George Frangos, Ph.D.
Assistant Dean for Clinical Education . . . . Sheldon Landesman, M.D.
Assistant Dean for Program and Faculty Development. . . . . Fredric Volkert, Ph.D.
Assistant Dean for Student Affairs. . . . . Jeffrey Putman
Registrar . . . . Elaine Billington, J.D.
Director, Academic Fiscal Affairs . . . . Richard D. Katz
Director of Admissions. . . . . Shushawna DeOliveira, D.H.A.
Director, Continuing Medical Education. . . . . Edeline Mitton, M.Ed.
Director, Graduate Medical Education . . . . Monica Dweck, M.D.
Director, Institutional Research and Educational Evaluation . . . . Barbara Lawrence, Ph.D.
Director, Financial Aid. . . . . James Newell
Director, Alumni Affairs. . . . . Jill Ditchik

Department and Division or Section Chairs
Basic Sciences
Anatomy and Cell Biology . . . . M. A. Q. Siddiqui, Ph.D.
Biochemistry . . . . Alfred Stracher, Ph.D.
Microbiology and Immunology. . . . . Maureen V. McLeod, Ph.D. (Interim)
Pathology . . . . Suzanne S. Mirra, M.D.
Physiology and Pharmacology. . . . . Robert Wong, Ph.D.

Clinical Sciences

Anesthesiology. . . . . James E. Cottrell, M.D.
  Ambulatory Surgery . . . . Rebecca Twersky, M.D.
  Cardiac . . . . Ketan Shevde, M.D.
  Critical Care. . . . . Jean Charchaflieh, M.D.
  Neuroanesthesia. . . . . Audree A. Bendo, M.D.
  Obstetrical . . . . David Wlody, M.D., and Alexandru Apostol, M.D.
  Pain Management . . . . Olga Tyuleneva, M.D.
  Pediatrics. . . . . Khosrow Mojdehi, M.D.
  Transplant . . . . Vacant
Dermatology . . . . Alan R. Shalita, M.D.
Emergency Medicine . . . . Michael Lucchesi, M.D.
Family Practice . . . . Miriam T. Vincent, M.D., Ph.D. (Interim)
Medicine. . . . . Edmund Bourke, M.D.
  Allergy and Immunology . . . . Rauno Joks, M.D. (Interim)
  Cardiology. . . . . Luther T. Clark, M.D.
  Digestive Diseases and Hepatology . . . . Nora Bergasa, M.D. (Interim)
  Endocrinology, Hypertension, and Diabetes . . . . Samy McFarlane, M.D.
  Hematology and Oncology. . . . . Gerald Soff, M.D.
  Infectious Diseases . . . . William M. McCormack, M.D.
  Internal Medicine. . . . . Steven Cohn, M.D.
  Pulmonary Medicine and Critical Care . . . . Spiro Demetis, M.D. (Interim)
  Renal Diseases . . . . Moro O. Salifu, M.D., M.P.H.
  Rheumatology . . . . Ellen Ginzler, M.D.
  Student Health. . . . . Marcia Gerber, M.D.
Neurology . . . . Roger Cracco, M.D.
Neurosurgery. . . . . Stephen T. Onesti, M.D.
Obstetrics and Gynecology. . . . . Ovadia Abulafia, M.D.
  Gynecologic Oncology . . . . Yi-Chun Lee, M.D.
  Gynecology . . . . Vacant
  Maternal Fetal Medicine. . . . . David Sherer, M.D.
  Reproductive Endocrinology . . . . Ozgul Muneyyirici, M.D.
Ophthalmology . . . . Douglas Lazzaro, M.D.
Orthopedic Surgery and Rehabilitation Medicine . . . . William P. Urban, Jr., M.D.
Otolaryngology . . . . Frank E. Lucente, M.D.
Pediatrics . . . . Stanley E. Fisher, M.D.
  Adolescent Medicine . . . . Amy Suss, M.D.
  AIDS Program . . . . Hermann Mendez, M.D.
  Allergy and Immunology . . . . Hamid Moallem, M.D.
  Ambulatory Care . . . . Eugene Dinkevich, M.D.
  Asthma Center. . . . . Madu Rao, M.D.
  Cardiology. . . . . Jayendra Sharma, M.D.
  Child Development . . . . Tzipporah Sklar, M.D.
  Critical Care. . . . . Stephen Wadowski, M.D.
  Endocrinology . . . . Salvador Castells, M.D. (Interim)
  Gastroenterology . . . . William Treem, M.D.
  Genetics. . . . . Vacant
  Hematology and Oncology. . . . . S. P. Rao, M.D.
  Infectious Diseases . . . . Margaret Hammerschlag, M.D.
  Neonatology. . . . . Gloria Valencia, M.D. (Interim)
  Nephrology . . . . Morris Schoeneman, M.D.
  Neurology . . . . Joan Cracco, M.D.
  Pulmonology . . . . Madu Rao, M.D.
Preventive Medicine and Community Health . . . . Pascal J. Imperato, M.D.
Psychiatry . . . . Stephen Goldfinger, M.D.
Radiation Oncology. . . . . Marvin Rotman, M.D.
Radiology . . . . Salvatore J. Sclafani, M.D.
Surgery . . . . Michael E. Zenilman, M.D.
  Cardiothoracic Surgery. . . . . Robert C. Lowery, M.D.
  Dental and Oral Medicine . . . . Susan Pugliese, D.D.S.
  General Surgery and Surgical Oncology . . . . Alexander Schwartzman, M.D.
  Pediatric Surgery . . . . Nicholas Shorter, M.D.
  Plastic Surgery . . . . Felix R. Ortega, M.D. (Interim)
  Transplantation Surgery. . . . . Dale A. Distant, M.D.
  Trauma and Surgical Critical Care . . . . Patricia O'Neill, M.D., and Robert Kurtz, M.D.
  Vascular Surgery. . . . . Thomas L. Raftery, M.D.
Urology. . . . . Richard J. Macchia, M.D.

University at Buffalo, School of Medicine and Biomedical Sciences
State University of New York
3435 Main Street
Buffalo, New York 14214
716-829-3955 (dean's office); 829-2179 (fax)
Web site: www.smbs.buffalo.edu

The University of Buffalo School of Medicine was founded in 1846, and in 1898, the school of medicine absorbed the medical department of Niagara University. In September 1962, the University at Buffalo was merged with and became a unit of the State University of New York.

Type: public
2008-2009 total enrollment: 560
Clinical facilities: Erie County Medical Center, KALEIDA Health Buffalo General Division, KALEIDA Health Women's and Children's Hospital of Buffalo, KALEIDA Health Millard Fillmore Health System, Veterans Administration Medical Center, Roswell Park Cancer Institute, Sisters of Charity Hospital, Mercy Hospital.

University Officials

President. . . . . John B. Simpson, Ph.D.
Provost . . . . Satish Tripathi, Ph.D.
Vice President for Health Sciences . . . . David L. Dunn, M.D., Ph.D.

Medical School Administrative Staff

Dean, School of Medicine and Biomedical Sciences . . . . Michael E. Cain, M.D.
Senior Staff Associate. . . . . Nancy Glieco
Senior Associate Dean for Research . . . . Suzanne Laychock, Ph.D.
Senior Associate Dean for Graduate Medical Education . . . . Roseanne C. Berger, M.D.
Senior Associate Dean for Academic Affairs . . . . Nancy H. Nielsen, M.D., Ph.D.
Senior Associate Dean for Advancement. . . . . Kathleen A. Wiater
Senior Associate Dean for Curriculum . . . . Avery Ellis, M.D.
Senior Associate Dean for Resource Management. Sandra Drabek
Associate Dean for Biomedical Rescarch and Education . . . . Mulchand Patel, M.D.
Associate Dean for Development . . . . Eric C. Alcott
Associate Dean for Support Services. . . . . Ray Dannenhoffer, Ph.D.
Assistant Dean and Director of Continuing Medical Education . . . . Lori McMann
Assistant Dean for Undergraduate Education . . . . Mary Anne Rokitka, Ph.D.
Assistant Dean for Multi-Cultural Affairs. . . . . David Milling, M.D.
Associate Dean for Medical Education and Admissions . . . . Charles Severin, Ph.D., M.D.
Assistant Dean for Evaluation: Research . . . . Frank Schimpfhauser, Ph.D.
Registrar . . . . James Rosso
Editor, Buffalo Physician and Biomedical Scientist . . . . Stephanie Unger

Department and Division or Section Chairs

Basic Sciences

Biochemistry . . . . Kenneth Blumenthal, Ph.D.
Biotechnical and Clinical Sciences . . . . Paul Kostyniak, Ph.D.
Microbiology. . . . . John Hay, Ph.D.
Pathology and Anatomical Sciences . . . . Reid Heffner, M.D.
Pharmacology and Toxicology . . . . Ronald P. Rubin, Ph.D.
Physiology and Biophysical Sciences. . . . . Harold Strauss, M.D.
Structural Biology . . . . George DeTitta, Ph.D.

University at Buffalo, School of Medicine and Biomedical Sciences
State University of New York: NEW YORK

Clinical Sciences

Anesthesiology . . . . Mark Lema, M.D., Ph.D.
Dermatology . . . . Allan Oseroff, M.D.
Emergency Medicine . . . . G. Richard Braen, M.D.
Family Medicine . . . . Thomas Rosenthal, M.D.
Gynecology and Obstetrics . . . . John Yeh, M.D.
Medicine . . . . Alan Saltzman, M.D.
Neurology . . . . Frederick Munschauer, M.D.
Neurosurgery . . . . L. Nelson Hopkins III, M.D.
Nuclear Medicine . . . . Hani Abdel-Nabi, M.D., Ph.D.
Ophthalmology . . . . James Reynolds, M.D.
Orthopaedics . . . . Lawrence Bone, M.D.
Otolaryngology . . . . David Sherris, M.D.
Pediatrics . . . . Frederick C. Morin III, M.D.
Psychiatry . . . . Steven Dubovsky, M.D.
Radiation Oncology . . . . Michael Kuettel, M.D., Ph.D.
Radiology . . . . Angelo M. DelBalso, M.D., D.D.S.
Rehabilitation Medicine . . . . John Naughton, M.D. (Interim)
Surgery . . . . Merril Dayton, M.D.
Urology . . . . Gerald Sufrin, M.D.

Stony Brook University Medical Center

Health Sciences Center
HSC Level 4-170
Stony Brook, New York 11794-8430
631-444-1630 (office); 631-444-1785 (dean's office); 631-444-1340 (fax);
631-444-2113 (admissions)
Web site: www.stonybrookmedicalcenter.org

The medical center at Stony Brook University, a union of the school of medicine and University Hospital, is located on the university campus. The first students were accepted into the medical school for the 1971-72 academic year. Instruction takes place in the academic tower, University Hospital, and affiliated institutions.

Type: public
2008-2009 total enrollment: 448
Clinical facilities: Stony Brook University Hospital and affiliated teaching hospitals including Nassau University Medical Center, Winthrop-University Hospital, Brookhaven National Laboratory, and Veterans Administration Medical Center (Northport) provide both clinical and academic facilities for all students. In addition, special teaching programs for students and house staff are provided for in a number of associated community hospitals.

University Official

President . . . . Shirley Strum Kenny, Ph.D.

Medical Center Administrative Staff

Dean . . . . Richard N. Fine, M.D.
Dean, Nassau University Medical Center . . . . Kenneth Steier, D.O. (Acting)
Vice Dean for Academic and Faculty Affairs . . . . Peter Williams, J.D., Ph.D.
Vice Dean for Clinical Affairs . . . . Thomas M. Biancaniello, M.D.
Vice Dean for Scientific Affairs . . . . Wadie Bahou, M.D.
Chief Executive Officer of Stony Brook University Hospital . . . . Steven Strongwater, M.D.
Associate Dean for Academic and Faculty Affairs . . . . Latha Chandran, M.D.
Associate Dean for Admissions . . . . Jack Fuhrer, M.D.
Associate Dean for Continuing Medical Education . . . . Dorothy S. Lane, M.D.
Associate Dean for Student and Minority Affairs . . . . Aldustus E. Jordan, Ed.D.
Associate Dean for Finance and Personnel . . . . John H. Riley
Associate Dean for Medical Education . . . . Frederick Schiavone, M.D.
Associate Dean for Administration . . . . Michael Porembski
Associate Dean for Scientific Affairs . . . . Sharon Nachman, M.D.
Associate Dean for Clinical Affairs . . . . William Greene, M.D.
Associate Dean for VA Medical Center, Northport . . . . Edward J.C. Mack, M.D.
Associate Dean, Winthrop-University Hospital . . . . John F. Aloia, M.D.
Associate Dean for Educational Development and Evaluation . . . . Elza Mylona, Ph.D.
Assistant Dean for Admissions . . . . Grace Agnetti
Assistant Dean for Faculty Personnel . . . . Karen M. Wilk
Assistant Dean for Medical Education . . . . Marilyn London, Ed.D.
Assistant Dean for Student Affairs . . . . Mary Jean Allen
Associate Laboratory Director for Life Sciences,
    Brookhaven National Laboratory . . . . Peter Bond, Ph.D. (Interim)
Director, Health Sciences Library . . . . Spencer Marsh
Director, Laboratory Animal Resources . . . . Thomas Zimmerman
Director of Budget and Finance . . . . Glenn Schmidt
Director of Operations for Scientific Affairs . . . . Glen Itzkowitz

Department and Division or Section Chairs

Basic Sciences

Anatomical Sciences . . . . William Jungers, Ph.D.
Biochemistry and Cell Biology . . . . Robert Haltiwanger, Ph.D. (Interim)
Biomedical Engineering . . . . Clinton Rubin, Ph.D.
Molecular Genetics and Microbiology . . . . Jorge Benach, Ph.D.
Neurobiology and Behavior . . . . Lorna Role, Ph.D.
Pathology . . . . Kenneth R. Shroyer, M.D., Ph.D.
Pharmacological Sciences . . . . Michael Frohman, Ph.D.
Physiology and Biophysics . . . . Peter R. Brink, Ph.D.

Clinical Sciences

Anesthesiology . . . . Peter Glass, M.D.

Dermatology . . . . Evan Jones, M.D. (Acting)
Emergency Medicine . . . . Mark C. Henry, M.D.
Family Medicine . . . . Jeffery S. Trilling, M.D.
Medicine . . . . Margaret Parker, M.D. (Acting)
   Cardiology . . . . David L. Brown, M.D.
   General Medicine/Geriatrics . . . . Suzanne Fields, M.D.
   Hematology . . . . Theodore Gabig, M.D.
   Infectious Diseases . . . . David Tompkins, M.D.
   Medical Oncology . . . . Theodore Gabig, M.D.
   Gastroenterology . . . . Basil Rigas, M.D.
   Nephrology . . . . Edward Nord, M.D.
   Pulmonary and Critical Care . . . . Gerald Smaldone, M.D.
   Rheumatology . . . . Margaret Parker, M.D. (Acting)
   VA Medical Center (Northport) . . . . Mark Graber, M.D.
   Winthrop-University Hospital . . . . Michael S. Niederman, M.D.
Neurological Surgery . . . . Raphael Davis, M.D.
Neurology . . . . Patricia Coyle, M.D. (Acting)
Obstetrics, Gynecology, and Reproductive Medicine . . . . J. Gerald Quirk, M.D., Ph.D.
   Gynecologic Oncology . . . . Michael Pearl, M.D.
   Gynecology and General Obstetrics . . . . Christine A. Conway, M.D.
   Maternal and Fetal Medicine . . . . Paul L. Ogburn, Jr., M.D.
   Midwifery . . . . Christina Kocis
   Reproductive Endocrinology and Infertility . . . . Richard Bronson, M.D.
Ophthalmology . . . . Patrick A. Sibony, M.D.
Orthopaedics . . . . Lawrence Hurst, M.D.
Pediatrics . . . . Margaret M. McGovern, M.D., Ph.D.
   Adolescent Medicine . . . . Joseph Puccio, M.D.
   Allergy and Immunology . . . . Catherine E. Kier, M.D.
   Cardiology . . . . Thomas M. Biancaniello, M.D.
   Critical Care . . . . Margaret M. Parker, M.D.
   Cystic Fibrosis . . . . Catherine E. Kier, M.D.
   Developmental Psychology . . . . Janet E. Fischel, Ph.D.
   Endocrinology . . . . Thomas A. Wilson, M.D.
   Gastroenterology . . . . Anupama Chawla, M.D.
   General Pediatrics . . . . Latha Chandran, M.D.
   Genetics . . . . Patricia A. Galvin-Parton, M.D., and David Tegay, D.O.
   Hematology and Oncology . . . . Robert I. Parker, M.D.
   Infectious Diseases . . . . Sharon A. Nachman, M.D.
   Neonatology . . . . Janet Larson, M.D.
   Nephrology . . . . Dilys Whyte, M.D.
Preventive Medicine . . . . Iris Granek, M.D. (Acting)
Psychiatry and Behavioral Sciences . . . . Mark J. Sedler, M.D., M.P.H.
   Adult Psychiatry (Director) . . . . Mark J. Sedler, M.D., M.P.H.
   Adult Consultation/Liaison . . . . Steven Cole, M.D.
   Adult Inpatient . . . . Andrew Francis, Ph.D.
   Adult Outpatient . . . . Eric Fink, M.D.
   Behavioral Medicine (Director) . . . . Peter Halperin, M.D.
   Child and Adolescent Psychiatry (Director) . . . . Gabrielle Carlson, M.D.
   Child Consultation/Liaison . . . . Darla Broberg, Ph.D.
   Child Inpatient . . . . David Margulies, M.D.
   Child Outpatient . . . . Deborah Weisbrot, M.D.
Radiation Oncology . . . . Allen G. Meek, M.D.
Radiology . . . . John Ferretti, M.D. (Acting)
   Nuclear Medicine . . . . Cora Cabahug, M.D.
Surgery . . . . John J. Ricotta, M.D.
   Cardiothoracic . . . . Todd Rosengart, M.D.
   Otolaryngology . . . . Arnold Katz, M.D.
   Pediatric Surgery . . . . Thomas Lee, M.D.
   Transplantation Surgery . . . . Wayne C. Waltzer, M.D.
   Trauma . . . . Marc Shapiro, M.D.
   Surgical Oncology . . . . Vacant
   Vascular Surgery . . . . John Ricotta, M.D.
   Plastic . . . . Alexander Dagum, M.D.
   Nassau University Medical Center . . . . Gerald Shaftan, M.D.
   VA Medical Center, Northport . . . . Eugene Mohan, M.D.
   Winthrop-University Hospital . . . . William P. Reed, Jr., M.D.
Urology . . . . Wayne C. Waltzer, M.D.

157

State University of New York
Upstate Medical University
College of Medicine
750 East Adams Street
Syracuse, New York 13210-2399
315-464-9720; 464-9721 (fax)
Web site: www.upstate.edu

The college of medicine traces its history back to 1834, when it was organized as the medical department of Geneva College. The college remained in Geneva until 1872, when it moved to Syracuse as the college of medicine of Syracuse University. It became part of the State University of New York (SUNY) in 1950, and was renamed the Upstate Medical Center. In 1986, it was renamed the SUNY Upstate Medical University. The main campus is located in Syracuse, and a satellite clinical campus is in Binghamton. The main office of the State University of New York is located in Albany.

Type: public
2008-2009 total enrollment: 614
Clinical facilities: University Hospital, Crouse Hospital, Veterans Administration Medical Center, St. Joseph's Hospital Health Center, Community-General Hospital, Hutchings Psychiatric Center, United Health Services, Inc., Our Lady of Lourdes Memorial Hospital, Guthrie Medical Center/Robert Packer Memorial Hospital.

University Officials

Chancellor, State University of New York	John B. Clark, Ed.D. (Interim)
President, SUNY Upstate Medical University	David R. Smith, M.D.
Senior Vice President, SUNY Upstate Medical University	Steven J. Scheinman, M.D.
Senior Vice President for Administration and Finance	Steven C. Brady
Chief Executive Officer, University Hospital, and Senior Vice President for Hospital Affairs	Phillip S. Schaengold, J.D.
Associate Senior Vice President for Operations	Wanda M. Thompson, Ph.D.
Vice President for Research	Steven Goodman, Ph.D.
Vice President for Academic Affairs	TBA
Assistant Vice President for Academic Affairs	Paul L. Grover, Ph.D.

Medical School Administrative Staff

Dean, College of Medicine	Steven J. Scheinman, M.D.
Dean for Student Affairs	Julie White, Ph.D.
Dean for Binghamton Campus	Rajesh J. Davé, M.D.
Senior Associate Dean for Education	Lynn M. Cleary, M.D.
Senior Associate Dean for Resource Management	MaryGrace VanNortwick
Associate Dean for Graduate Medical Education	Sara Jo Grethlein, M.D.
Associate Dean for Clinical Affairs	Leonard B. Weiner, M.D.
Associate Dean, VA Medical Center	William Marx, D.O.
Associate Dean, Crouse Hospital	Open
Associate Dean, St. Joseph's Hospital Health Center	Dennis A. Ehrich, M.D.
Associate Dean, Community General Hospital	Daniel Carlson, M.D.
Assistant Dean for Student Affairs	N. Barry Berg, Ph.D.
Assistant Dean for Curriculum	David Turner, Ph.D.
Associate Dean for Continuing Medical Education	Paul L. Grover, Ph.D.
Assistant Vice President, Governmental and Community Relations	Daniel N. Hurley
Director, Vivarium	Robert H. Quinn, D.V.M.
Assistant Dean for Multicultural Resources	TBA
Director, Health Science Library	Cristina A. Pope

State University of New York
Upstate Medical University College of Medicine: NEW YORK

Department and Division or Section Chairs

Basic Sciences

Cell and Developmental Biology. . . . . Joseph W. Sanger, Ph.D.
Biochemistry and Molecular Biology. . . . . Richard L. Cross, Ph.D.
Microbiology and Immunology. . . . . Rosemary Rochford, Ph.D.
Pharmacology . . . . Richard Wojcikiewicz, Ph.D. (Interim)
Neuroscience and Physiology . . . . Michael W. Miller, Ph.D.

Clinical Sciences

Anesthesiology. . . . . Nancy A. Nussmeier, M.D.
Emergency Medicine . . . . John B. McCabe, M.D.
Family Medicine . . . . Andrea T. Manyon, M.D.
Medicine. . . . . Michael Iannuzzi, M.D.
Neurology. . . . . Jeremy M. Shefner, M.D.
Neurosurgery. . . . . Walter A. Hall, M.D.
Obstetrics and Gynecology. . . . . Shawky Z. A. Badawy, M.D.
Ophthalmology . . . . John A. Hoepner, M.D.
Orthopedic Surgery. . . . . Stephen A. Albanese, M.D.
Otolaryngology and Communication Sciences. . . . . Robert M. Kellman, M.D.
Pathology . . . . Gregory A. Threatte, M.D.
Pediatrics . . . . Thomas R. Welch, M.D.
Physical Medicine and Rehabilitation . . . . Robert J. Weber, M.D.
Psychiatry and Behavioral Science . . . . Mantosh J. Dewan, M.D.
Radiation Oncology. . . . . Jeffrey A. Bogart, M.D.
Radiology . . . . David Feiglin, M.D.
Surgery. . . . . Paul R.G. Cunningham, M.D.
Urology. . . . . Firouz Daneshgari, M.D.

Other

Bioethics and Humanities . . . . Kathy Faber-Langendoen, M.D.
Public Health and Preventive Medicine . . . . Donna Bacchi, M.D., M.P.H.

Duke University School of Medicine

P.O. Box 2927
Durham, North Carolina 27710
919-684-2455 (dean's office); 684-0208 (dean's office fax);
684-2255 (chancellor's office); 681-7020 (chancellor's office fax)
Web site: http://medschool.duke.edu

Duke University School of Medicine, which is a part of the Duke University Medical Center, is located on the campus of Duke in Durham. The hospital opened in 1930, and its first medical students were admitted in October 1930.

Type: private
2008-2009 total enrollment: 471
Clinical facilities: Duke University Hospital, Veterans Administration Hospital (Durham), Durham Regional Hospital, Duke Raleigh Hospital, Lenox Baker Hospital, North Carolina Eye and Ear Hospital, Veterans Administration Hospital (Oteen), Murdoch Center, John Umstead Hospital, Dorothea Dix Hospital, Cabarrus Memorial Hospital.

University Officials

President . . . . Richard Brodhead, Ph.D.
Chancellor for Health Affairs and President and
   Chief Executive Officer . . . . Victor J. Dzau, M.D.
Senior Vice Chancellor for Academic Affairs . . . . R. Sanders Williams, M.D.
Vice Chancellor for Academic Affairs . . . . Nancy C. Andrews, M.D., Ph.D.
Vice Chancellor for Development and Alumni Affairs . . . . Michael Morsberger
Associate Vice President, Community Affairs . . . . Mary Ann Black
Vice Chancellor for Corporate and Venture Development . . . . Robert Y. Taber, M.D.
Vice Chancellor for Clinical Research . . . . Robert Califf, M.D.
Vice Chancellor for Integrated Planning . . . . Molly K. O'Neill

Medical School Administrative Staff

Dean, School of Medicine . . . . Nancy C. Andrews, M.D., Ph.D.
Vice Dean for Education . . . . Edward G. Buckley, M.D. (Interim)
Executive Vice Dean for Administration . . . . Scott Gibson
Vice Dean for Clinical Research . . . . Eugene Z. Oddone, M.D.
Vice Dean, Administration and Finance . . . . Billy Newton, Jr.
Vice Dean, Basic Sciences . . . . Sally Kornbluth, Ph.D.
Vice Dean for Faculty Enrichment . . . . Augustus O. Grant, M.B., CH.B.
Vice Dean, Medical Affairs . . . . Michael Cuffe, M.D.
Associate Vice Dean for Faculty Development . . . . Ann J. Brown, M.D.
Associate Dean for Clinical Affairs . . . . Theodore Pappas, M.D.
Associate Dean and Director for Student Affairs . . . . Caroline P. Haynes, M.D., Ph.D.
Associate Dean and Director, Graduate Medical Education . . . . John L. Weinerth, M.D.
Associate Dean, Admissions . . . . Brenda E. Armstrong, M.D.
Associate Dean, Curriculum Development . . . . Colleen O. Grochowski, Ph.D.
Associate Dean, Continuing Medical Education . . . . Katherine Grichnik, M.D.
Assistant Dean, Undergraduate Primary Care Education . . . . Barbara L. Sheline, M.D.

Department and Division or Section Chairs

Basic Sciences

Biochemistry . . . . Kenneth N. Kreuzer, Ph.D. (Interim)
Biostatistics and Bioinformatics . . . . Elizabeth R. DeLong, Ph.D. (Acting)
Cell Biology . . . . Brigid Hogan, Ph.D.
Molecular Genetics and Microbiology . . . . Thomas Petes, Ph.D.
Immunology . . . . Thomas F. Tedder, Ph.D.
Neurobiology . . . . James McNamara, Sr., M.D.
Pharmacology and Cancer Biology . . . . Anthony R. Means, Ph.D.

Clinical Sciences

Anesthesiology . . . . Mark F. Newman, M.D.
   General, Vascular, Transplant Anesthesia . . . . Kerri Robertson, M.D.
   Ambulatory Anesthesia . . . . Stephen Klein, M.D.
   Critical Care Medicine . . . . Chris Young, M.D.
   Cardiothoracic Anesthesia* . . . . Joseph Matthew, M.D.

General Services* .... Cecil O. Borel, M.D.
Women's Anesthesia* .... Holly Muir, M.D.
Pain Clinic* .... Winston Parris, M.D.
Pediatric Anesthesia* .... Allison K. Ross, M.D.
Community and Family Medicine .... J. Lloyd Michener, M.D.
   Community Health .... Susan Yaggy
   Chronic Disease Epidemiology Research .... Truls Ostbye, M.D., Ph.D.
   Clinical Informatics .... David F. Lobach, M.D., Ph.D.
   Doctor of Physical Therapy Education Program .... Jan K. Richardson, P.T., Ph.D.
   Family Medicine .... Samuel W. Warburton, M.D.
   Occupational and Environmental Medicine .... Dennis J. Darcey, M.D.
   Physician Assistant Education Program .... Justine Strand
Medicine .... Harvey Jay Cohen, M.D.
   Cardiology* .... Howard Rockman, M.D.
   Dermatology* .... Russell P. Hall, M.D.
   Endocrinology, Metabolism, and Nutrition* .... Mark N. Feinglos, M.D.
   Gastroenterology* .... Anna M. Diehl, M.D.
   General Internal Medicine* .... Lori Bastian, M.D.
   Geriatrics* .... Kenneth E. Schmader, M.D.
   Hematology* .... Marilyn J. Telen, M.D.
   Infectious Diseases* .... John D. Hamilton, M.D.
   Medical Oncology and Transplantation Division .... Jeffrey Crawford, M.D.
   Nephrology* .... Thomas M. Coffman, M.D.
   Neurology* .... Warren J. Strittmatter, M.D.
   Pulmonary, Allergy, and Critical Care Medicine* .... Paul W. Noble, M.D.
   Rheumatology and Immunology* .... William St. Clair, M.D.
Obstetrics and Gynecology .... Haywood Brown, M.D.
   Clinical and Epidemiologic Research .... Evan Myers, M.D.
   General Obstetrics and Gynecology .... Joanne Piscitelli, M.D.
   Maternal and Fetal Medicine* .... R. Phillip Heine, M.D.
   Minimally Invasive Surgery .... Craig J. Sobolewski, M.D.
   Gynecological Oncology .... Andrew Berchuck, M.D.
   Reproductive Endocrinology and Fertility* .... David Walmer, M.D.
   Urogynecology .... Anthony Visco, M.D.
Ophthalmology .... David L. Epstein, M.D.
Pathology .... Salvatore V. Pizzo, M.D., Ph.D.
Pediatrics .... Joseph W. St. Geme, M.D.
   Allergy and Immunology .... A. Wesley Burks, M.D.
   Blood and Marrow Transplantation .... Joanne Kurtzberg, M.D.
   Cardiology* .... John F. Rhodes, M.D.
   Child Development and Behavioral Health .... Richard D'Alli, M.D.
   Critical Care Medicine .... Ira Cheifetz, M.D.
   Endocrinology* .... Michael S. Freemark, M.D.
   Gastroenterology, Hepatology, and Nutrition .... Martin H. Ulshen, M.D.
   Hematology and Oncology* .... Daniel S. Wechsler, M.D., Ph.D.
   Hospital and Emergency Medicine .... W. Clay Bordley, M.D. (Interim)
   Infectious Diseases* .... Coleen K. Cunningham, M.D.
   Medical Genetics .... Priya Kishnani, M.D.
   Neonatology* .... Ronald N. Goldberg, M.D.
   Nephrology .... John W. Foreman, M.D.
   Neurology* .... Mohamad A. Mikati, M.D.
   Primary Care Pediatrics .... Dennis A. Clements, M.D., Ph.D.
   Pulmonary .... Judith A. Voynow, M.D.
Psychiatry .... K. Ranga R. Krishnan, M.D.
Radiation Oncology .... Christopher Willett, M.D.
Radiology .... Carl E. Ravin, M.D.
Surgery .... Danny O. Jacobs, M.D.
   Speech Pathology and Audiology .... Frank DeRuyter, M.D., Ph.D.
   Emergency Medicine .... Michael Hocker, M.D.
   Thoracic* .... Peter K. Smith, M.D.
   General Surgery* .... Paul Kuo, M.D.
   Neurosurgery* .... Allan H. Friedman, M.D.
   Orthopaedic* .... James Nunley, M.D.
   Otolaryngology* .... Ramon M. Esclamado, M.D.
   Pediatric General Surgery* .... Henry E. Rice, M.D.
   Plastic, Reconstructive, and Oral Surgery .... L. Scott Levin, M.D.
   Urologic* .... Judd W. Moul, M.D.

*Specialty without organizational autonomy.

The Brody School of Medicine at East Carolina University
600 Moye Boulevard, AD-52
Greenville, North Carolina 27834-4354
252-744-1020 (general information); 744-2201 (dean's office); 744-9003 (fax)
Web site: www.ecu.edu

In 1972, East Carolina University enrolled students in a one-year program in medical education. The present four-year school was established in 1975.

Type: public
2008-2009 total enrollment: 293
Clinical facilities: Pitt County Memorial Hospital, Pitt County Mental Health Center, Walter B. Jones Alcoholic Rehabilitation Center, Child Developmental Evaluation Center.

University Officials
Chancellor . . . . Stephen C. Ballard, Ph.D.

Medical School Administrative Staff
Vice Chancellor and Dean . . . . Phyllis N. Horns, R.N., D.S.N.,F.A.AN (Interim)
Vice Dean . . . . Nicholas H. Benson, M.D.
Senior Associate Dean for Academic Affairs . . . . Virginia D. Hardy, Ph.D.
Associate Dean for Admissions . . . . James G. Peden, Jr., M.D.
Associate Dean for Medical Education . . . . David W. Musick, Ph.D.
Associate Dean for Administration and Finance . . . . Gary Vanderpool (Interim)
Associate Dean for Clinical Affairs . . . . Vacant
Associate Dean for Continuing Medical Education . . . . Stephen E. Willis, M.D.
Associate Dean for Graduate Medical Education . . . . Lorraine Basnight, M.D.
Associate Dean for Academic Support and Enrichment Center . . . . Virginia D. Hardy, Ph.D.
Associate Dean for Research and Graduate Studies . . . . John M. Lehman, Ph.D.
Associate Dean for Academic and Faculty Development . . . . Lars C. Larsen, M.D.

Department and Division or Section Chairs
Basic Sciences
Anatomy and Cell Biology . . . . Cheryl B. Knudson, Ph.D.
Biochemistry and Molecular Biology . . . . Phillip H. Pekala, Ph.D. (Interim)
Comparative Medicine . . . . Dorcas P. O'Rourke, D.V.M.
Medical Humanities . . . . Maria C. Clay, Ph.D. (Interim)
Microbiology and Immunology . . . . C. Jeffrey Smith, Ph.D.
Pharmacology and Toxicology . . . . David A. Taylor, Ph.D.
Physiology . . . . Robert M. Lust, Ph.D.
Public Health . . . . Lloyd F. Novick, M.D. (Interim)

Clinical Sciences
Cardiovascular Sciences . . . . T. Bruce Ferguson, M.D.
  Cardiothoracic Surgery . . . . W. Randolph Chitwood, Jr., M.D.
  Vascular Surgery . . . . C. Steven Powell, M.D.
Emergency Medicine . . . . Theodore R. Delbridge, M.D.
  EastCare Air Medical Services . . . . Jeffrey D. Ferguson, M.D.
  Eastern Carolina Injury Prevention Program . . . . Herbert G. Garrison, M.D.
  Emergency Medical Services . . . . Juan A. March, M.D.
  Research . . . . John E. Gough, M.D.
  EM Residency Program . . . . Leigh A. Patterson, M.D.
  EM/IM Residency Program . . . . Charles K. Brown, M.D.
  Toxicology . . . . William J. Meggs, M.D.
Family Medicine . . . . Kenneth K. Steinweg, M.D. (Interim)
  Clinical Services . . . . Robert J. Newman, M.D.
  Dental Residency . . . . Omar Paredes, D.D.S.
  Educational Development . . . . Lars C. Larsen, M.D.
  Firetower Clinic . . . . Tommy Ellis, M.D.
  Geriatric Education . . . . Irene Hamrick, M.D.
  Research . . . . Doyle M. Cummings, Pharm.D.
  Residency Program . . . . Gary Levine, M.D.
  Predoctoral Education . . . . Janice Daugherty, M.D.
  Sports Medicine . . . . Joseph P. Garry, M.D.
  Women's Health . . . . Dorothy Butler, M.D.
Internal Medicine . . . . Paul Bolin, Jr., M.D. (Interim)
  Cardiology . . . . Wayne E. Cascio, M.D.
  Dermatology . . . . Charles Phillips, M.D.
  Endocrinology . . . . Almond J. Drake III, M.D.
  Gastorenterology . . . . Mahfuzul Haque, M.D.
  General Medicine . . . . Gregg M. Talente, M.D. (Interim)
  Hematology and Oncology . . . . Adam Asch, M.D.
  Infectious Disease . . . . Paul Cook, M.D. (Interim)

Nephrology . . . . Paul Bolin, Jr., M.D.
Pulmonary and Critical Care Medicine . . . . Mani S. Kavuru, M.D.
Rheumatology . . . . Vacant
Residency Program . . . . M. Suzanne Kraemer, M.D.
Obstetrics and Gynecology . . . . Edward R. Newton, M.D.
General Obstetrics and Gynecology . . . . Thomas Kraemer, M.D.
Gynecologic Oncology . . . . Howard D. Homesley, M.D.
Maternal-Fetal Medicine . . . . Edward R. Newton, M.D. (Interim)
Reproductive Endocrinology and Infertility . . . . Clifford C. Hayslip, Jr., M.D.
Reproductive Physiology Lab . . . . Charles A. Hodson, Ph.D.
Residency Program . . . . Clifford C. Hayslip, Jr., M.D.
Pathology and Laboratory Medicine . . . . Peter J. Kragel, M.D.
Autopsy and Forensic Pathology . . . . William Oliver, M.D.
Clinical Chemistry and Medical Informatics . . . . Paul G. Catrou, M.D.
Clinical Immunology . . . . Gregory A. Gagnon, M.D.
Coagulation . . . . Arthur P. Bode, Ph.D.
Cytology-Thin Needle Biopsy . . . . James Finley, M.D.
Electron Microscopy . . . . Paul H. Strausbauch, M.D., Ph.D.
Hematology, Coagulation, and Urinalysis . . . . Gregory A. Gagnon, M.D.
HLA-Tissue Transplantation . . . . Lorita Rebellato-deVente, Ph.D.
Immunochemistry and Allergy . . . . Donald R. Hoffman, Ph.D.
Microbiology and Serology . . . . John D. Christie, M.D., Ph.D.
Molecular Pathology . . . . Larry J. Dobbs, Jr., M.D., Ph.D.
Regional Pathology . . . . Gregory A. Gagnon, M.D.
Renal Pathology . . . . Karlene Hewan-Lowe, M.D.
Research and Education . . . . Donald R. Hoffman, Ph.D.
Surgical Pathology . . . . Karen Hewan-Lowe, M.D.
Transfusion Service . . . . Emmanuel Fadeyi, M.D.
Pediatrics . . . . Ronald M. Perkin, M.D.
Adolescent . . . . Sharon Mangan, M.D.
Behavior and Development . . . . Michael Reichel, M.D.
Cardiology . . . . David W. Hannon, M.D.
Critical Care . . . . James Gutai, M.D.
Endocrinology . . . . Ying Chang, M.D.
Gastroenterology . . . . J. Rainer Poley, M.D.
General and Ambulatory . . . . Dale Newton, M.D.
Genetics and Child Development . . . . Berrin Ozturk, M.D.
Hematology and Oncology . . . . Charles Daeschner, M.D.
Infectious Disease . . . . Debra Tristram, M.D.
Neonatology . . . . James Cummings, M.D.
Nephrology . . . . Nour Baltagi, M.D.
Pulmonary . . . . Gerald Strope, M.D.
Residency Program . . . . Karin Hillenbrand, M.D.
Physical Medicine and Rehabilitation . . . . Daniel Moore, M.D.
Pain Medicine . . . . Thurman B. Whitted, M.D.
Residency Program . . . . Raymundo D. Millan, M.D.
Wound Care and Hyperbaric Medicine . . . . Daniel Moore, M.D.
Psychiatric Medicine . . . . Sy Saeed, M.D.
Adult Psychiatry . . . . Stanley Oakley, M.D.
Adult Residency Program . . . . Diana S. Antonacci, M.D.
Child and Adolescent Psychiatry . . . . John Diamond, M.D.
Child and Adult Residency Program . . . . Kaye McGinty, M.D.
Radiation Oncology . . . . Ron R. Allison, M.D.
Radiation Biology Oncology . . . . Ron R. Allison, M.D.
Surgery . . . . Michael F. Rotondo, M.D.
Bariatric and Advanced Laparoscopic Surgery . . . . William H. H. Chapman III, M.D.
Chowan General Surgery . . . . Alden Davis, M.D.
Clinical Effectiveness . . . . Claudia E. Goettler, M.D.
General, Gastrointestinal Endocrine Surgery . . . . Walter E. Pofahl, M.D.
Lenior General Surgery . . . . William L. Rucker, M.D.
Pediatric Surgery . . . . Michael F. Rotondo, M.D.
Plastic Surgery and Reconstructive Surgery . . . . Richard Zeri, M.D.
Surgical Education/Transplantation-Immunology . . . . Carl E. Haisch, M.D.
Surgical Oncology . . . . Emmanuel E. Zervos, M.D.
Trauma, Emergency Surgery and Surgical Critical Care . . . . Scott G. Sagraves, M.D.

University of North Carolina at Chapel Hill School of Medicine

Bondurant Hall, 301 Columbia Street
Campus Box 7000
Chapel Hill, North Carolina 27599
919-966-4161 (dean's office); 919-966-8623 (fax)
Web site: www.med.unc.edu

The school of medicine of the University of North Carolina was established in 1879. It is located on the campus of the University of North Carolina at Chapel Hill.

Type: public
2008-2009 total enrollment: 653
Clinical facilities: UNC Hospitals, Wake Medical Center, Moses H. Cone Memorial Hospital, Carolinas Medical Center, New Hanover Regional Medical Center, Nash General Hospital, Memorial Mission Hospital.

University Officials

President of University System . . . . Erskine B. Bowles
Chancellor, UNC at Chapel Hill. . . . . H. Holden Thorp, Ph.D.
Executive Vice Chancellor and Provost. Bernadette Gray-Little, Ph.D.

Medical School Administrative Staff

Dean of the School of Medicine, Vice
  Chancellor of Medical Affairs, and CEO of
  UNC Health Care System . . . . William L. Roper, M.D.
Associate Vice Chancellor for Strategic Alliances. . . . . Margaret B. Dardess, Ph.D., J.D.
Vice Dean for Academic Affairs . . . . Etta D. Pisano, M.D.
Vice Dean for Clinical Affairs. . . . . Marschall S. Runge, M.D., Ph.D.
President, UNC Hospitals. . . . . Gary L. Park
  Executive Vice President and Chief Operating Officer. . . . . Todd L. Peterson
Chief Financial Officer, UNC Health Care System. . . . . John P. Lewis
Executive Associate Dean for Finance and Administration. . . . . Kevin M. FitzGerald
  Associate Dean for Resource Analysis, Planning, and Management. . . . . . . Robert W. Marriott
  Assistant Dean for Finance and Business Operations . . . . Patricia G. Oliver
  Assistant Dean for Human Resources . . . . Bruce Wicks (Interim)
Executive Associate Dean for Medical Education. . . . . Vacant
  Assistant Dean for Medical Education Operations . . . . Karen Stone
  Associate Dean for Admissions . . . . Robert A. Bashford, M.D.
  Associate Dean for Student Affairs . . . . Georgette A. Dent, M.D.
  Director, Office of Educational Development . . . . Ellen Roberts, Ph.D. (Interim)
  Associate Director, Office of Continuing Medical Education . . . . Deedra Donley
  Assistant Dean for Admissions. . . . . Larry D. Keith
Executive Associate Dean for Faculty Affairs . . . . Eugene P. Orringer, M.D.
  Associate Dean for Faculty Development . . . . Patricia J. Byrns, M.D.
Executive Associate Dean for Clinical Affairs and Chief of Staff. . . . . . . Brian P. Goldstein, M.D.
Executive Associate Dean for Graduate Medical Education . . . . Philip G. Boysen, M.D.
Executive Associate Dean for Research. . . . . William F. Marzluff, Ph.D.
  Assistant Dean for Graduate Education . . . . Virginia Miller, Ph.D.
Executive Associate Dean and Director, North
  Carolina Area Health Education Centers
  Program . . . . Thomas J. Bacon, Dr.P.H.
Associate Dean for Allied Health Sciences . . . . Lee K. McLean, Ph.D.
Associate Dean for Medical Alumni Affairs. . . . . James R. Harper, M.D.
Associate Dean for Advancement . . . . David B. Anderson
  Assistant Dean for Institutional Advancement . . . . Jane M. McNeer
  Assistant Dean for Institutional Advancement . . . . Deborah C. Dibbert
Director, Office of Public Affairs and Marketing. . . . . Karen McCall
Director, Division of Laboratory Animal Medicine. . . . . John F. Bradfield, D.V.M., Ph.D.
Librarian. . . . . Carol G. Jenkins

Department and Division or Section Chairs
Basic Sciences

Biochemistry and Biophysics. . . . . Leslie Parise, Ph.D.
Biomedical Engineering. . . . . H. Troy Nagle, M.D., Ph.D.
Cell and Developmental Biology. . . . . Vytas Bankaitis, Ph.D.
Cell and Molecular Physiology . . . . James M. Anderson, M.D., Ph.D.
Genetics . . . . Terry Magnuson, Ph.D.
Microbiology and Immunology. . . . . William Goldman, Ph.D.

Nutrition . . . . June Stevens, Ph.D.
Pathology and Laboratory Medicine . . . . J. Charles Jennette, M.D.
Pharmacology . . . . Gary L. Johnson, Ph.D.

Clinical Sciences

Allied Health Sciences . . . . Lee K. McLean, Ph.D.
Anesthesiology . . . . Edward A. Norfleet, M.D.
Dermatology . . . . Luis A. Diaz, M.D.
Emergency Medicine . . . . Charles B. Cairns, M.D.
Family Medicine . . . . Warren F. Newton, M.D.
Medicine . . . . Marschall S. Runge, M.D., Ph.D.
  Cardiology . . . . W. Cam Patterson, M.D.
  Endocrinology and Metabolism . . . . John B. Buse, M.D., Ph.D.
  Gastroenterology and Hepatology . . . . Robert S. Sandler, M.D., M.P.H.
  General Medicine and Clinical Epidemiology . . . . Michael Pignone, M.D., M.P.H.
  Geriatric Medicine . . . . Jan Busby-Whitehead, M.D.
  Hematology and Oncology . . . . Richard M. Goldberg, M.D.
  Infectious Diseases . . . . Myron S. Cohen, M.D.
  Nephrology and Hypertension . . . . Ronald J. Falk, M.D.
  Pulmonary and Critical Care Medicine . . . . James F. Donohue, M.D.
  Rheumatology, Allergy, and Immunology . . . . Joanne Jordan, M.D., M.P.H.
Neurology . . . . William Powers, M.D.
Obstetrics and Gynecology . . . . Daniel L. Clarke-Pearson, M.D.
  Advanced Laparoscopy and Pelvic Pain . . . . John F. Steege, M.D.
  Gynecologic Oncology . . . . Wesley C. Fowler, Jr., M.D.
  Maternal and Fetal Medicine . . . . M. Kathryn Menard, M.D.
  Midwifery . . . . Kathy Higgins, C.N.M.
  Reproductive Endocrinology and Infertility . . . . Marc A. Fritz, M.D.
  Urogynecology and Reconstructive Pelvic Surgery . . . . Ellen C. Wells, M.D.
  Women's Primary Health Care . . . . John M. Thorp, M.D.
Ophthalmology . . . . Travis A. Meredith, M.D.
Orthopaedics . . . . Douglas R. Dirschl, M.D.
Otolaryngology-Head and Neck Surgery . . . . Harold C. Pillsbury III, M.D.
Pediatrics . . . . Alan D. Stiles, M.D.
  Developmental Disorders . . . . James Bobfish, M.D.
  General Pediatrics and Adolescent Medicine . . . . Jacob Lohr, M.D. (Interim)
  Neonatal-Perinatal Medicine . . . . Carl L. Bose, M.D.
  Pediatric Cardiology . . . . G. William Henry, M.D.
  Pediatric Critical Care Medicine . . . . G. William Henry, M.D.
  Pediatric Endocrinology and Diabetes . . . . Ali Calikoglu, M.D.
  Pediatric Gastroenterology . . . . Steven N. Lichtman, M.D.
  Pediatric Genetics and Metabolism . . . . Cynthia M. Powell, M.D.
  Pediatric Hematology and Oncology . . . . Stuart Gold, M.D.
  Pediatric Immunology and Infectious Diseases . . . . David B. Peden, M.D.
  Pediatric Nephrology and Hypertension . . . . Debbie S. Gipson, M.D., M.S.
  Pediatric Pulmonary Medicine . . . . Terry L. Noah, M.D.
Physical Medicine and Rehabilitation . . . . Michael Y. Lee, M.D.
Psychiatry . . . . David R. Rubinow, M.D.
  Adult Psychiatry . . . . B. Tony Lindsey, M.D.
  Child Psychiatry . . . . A. Jack Naftel, M.D.
  TEACCH . . . . Gary B. Mesibov, Ph.D.
Radiation Oncology . . . . Lawrence Marks, M.D.
Radiology . . . . Matthew A. Mauro, M.D.
Social Medicine . . . . Alan Cross, M.D.
Surgery . . . . Anthony A. Meyer, M.D., Ph.D.
  Abdominal Transplant . . . . David A. Gerber, M.D.
  Burn Center . . . . Bruce A. Cairns, M.D.
  Cardiothoracic Surgery . . . . Michael R. Mill, M.D.
  G. I. Surgery . . . . Mark J. Koruda, M.D.
  Neurosurgery . . . . Matthew G. Ewend, M.D.
  Pediatric Surgery . . . . Daniel Von Allmen, M.D.
  Plastic Surgery . . . . C. Scott Hultman, M.D.
  Surgical Oncology . . . . Benjamin F. Calvo, M.D.
  Trauma and Critical Care . . . . Preston B. Rich, M.D.
Urology . . . . Culley C. Carson III, M.D.
Vascular Surgery . . . . Blair A. Keagy, M.D.

Wake Forest University Health Sciences School of Medicine

Medical Center Boulevard
Winston-Salem, North Carolina 27157
336-716-2011; 716-5026 (dean's office); 716-5139 (fax)
Web site: www1.wfubmc.edu/school

The school of medicine, established at Wake Forest, North Carolina, in 1902, operated as a two-year medical school until 1941, when it was moved to Winston-Salem and expanded to a four-year medical college. At that time, it was renamed the Bowman Gray School of Medicine of Wake Forest College. The name of the parent institution was officially changed to Wake Forest University in 1967. The medical school and the North Carolina Baptist Hospitals, Inc., were formally organized as the Medical Center of Bowman Gray School of Medicine and North Carolina Baptist Hospital in 1974. The medical center organization became a corporation in 1976. The name of the school was changed to the Wake Forest University School of Medicine in 1997.

Type: private
2008-2009 total enrollment: 452
Clinical facilities: Forsyth Memorial Hospital, North Carolina Baptist Hospitals, Inc., Reynolds Family Health Center, Veterans Administration Medical Center—Salisbury.

University Officials

President, Wake Forest University. . . . . Nathan O. Hatch, Ph.D.
President, Wake Forest University Physicians. . . . . Raymond C. Ray, M.D., Ph.D. (Interim)

Medical School Administrative Staff

Dean. . . . . William B. Applegate, M.D.
Executive Vice President and Chief Operations Officer. . . . . Douglas L. Edgeton
Senior Associate Dean . . . . Steven M. Block, M.B.B.Ch.
Senior Associate Dean for Research . . . . Sally A. Shumaker, Ph.D.
Associate Dean for Academic Computing and
  Information Services . . . . Johannes M. Boehme II
Associate Dean for Medical Student Admissions . . . . Lewis H. Nelson III, M.D.
Associate Dean for Graduate Medical Education. . . . . Patricia H. Petrozza, M.D.
Associate Dean for Education. . . . . K. Patrick Ober, M.D.
Associate Dean for Student Services . . . . Burton Reifler, M.D. (Interim)
Assistant Dean for Education . . . . M. Ann Lambros, Ph.D.
Assistant Dean for Research . . . . Paula Means
Assistant Dean for Resource Management. . . . . Laurie Molloy
Assistant Dean for Student Services and Director
  of Diversity and Development Initiatives . . . . Brenda A. Latham-Sadler, M.D.
Vice President for Development and Alumni Affairs . . . . Norman D. Potter, Jr.
Vice President for Facilities Planning and Construction. . . . . TBN
Vice President for Information Services . . . . Paul M. LoRusso
Vice President for Financial Planning and Chief Financial Officer. . . . . Terry L. Hales, Jr.
Vice President for Human Resources . . . . Ron L. Hoth
Vice President for Government Relations . . . . Joanne C. Ruhland
Dean, Graduate School . . . . Lorna C. Moore, Ph.D.
Director, AHEC. . . . . Michael P. Lischke, Ed.D.
Director, Emeritus Affairs. . . . . M. Robert Cooper, M.D.
Director, Libraries . . . . E. Parks Welch

Department and Division or Section Chairs
Basic Sciences

Biochemistry . . . . Douglas Lyles, Ph.D.
Cancer Biology . . . . Steven A. Akman, M.D. (Acting)
Microbiology and Immunology. . . . . Griffith Parks, Ph.D.
Neurobiology and Anatomy . . . . Barry E. Stein, Ph.D.
Pathology . . . . A. Julian Garvin, M.D., Ph.D.
  Comparative Medicine . . . . Jay R. Kaplan, Ph.D.
  Lipid Sciences . . . . Lawrence L. Rudel, Ph.D.
  Tumor Biology. . . . . Mark C. Willingham, M.D.
Physiology and Pharmacology. . . . . Linda Porrino, Ph.D.
Public Health Sciences. . . . . Gregory L. Burke, M.D.
  Biostatistical Sciences . . . . Mark A. Espeland, Ph.D.
    Biostatistics. . . . . Gregory W. Evans
    Statistical Genetics and Bioinformatics. . . . . Carl D. Langefeld, Ph.D.
  Epidemiology . . . . David C. Goff, Jr., M.D., Ph.D.
  Social Sciences and Health Policy . . . . Doug Easterling, Ph.D.

Health Care Systems and Policy . . . . Ann M. Geiger, Ph.D.
Social and Behavioral Sciences . . . . Michelle J. Naughton, Ph.D.
Society and Health . . . . Mark Wolfson, Ph.D.
Regenerative Medicine (Tissue Engineering) . . . . Anthony Atala, M.D.

Clinical Sciences

Anesthesiology. . . . . Joseph R. Tobin, M.D.
  Section on Ambulatory and Outpatient. . . . . TBN
  Cardiothoracic Anesthesia. . . . . Thomas Slaughter, M.D.
  Section on Chronic Pain
  Critical Care. . . . . David L. Bowton, M.D.
  Section on Inpatient Anesthesia . . . . John E. Reynolds, M.D.
  Neuroanesthesia. . . . . John E. Reynolds, M.D.
  Obstetric Anesthesia. . . . . Robert D'Angelo, M.D.
  Pediatric Anesthesia and Pediatric Critical Care. . . . . Joseph R. Tobin, M.D.
  Section on Regional Anes and Acute Pain. . . . . J.C. Gerancher, M.D.
Dentistry . . . . Raymond S. Garrison, D.D.S.
Dermatology . . . . Alan B. Fleischer, Jr., M.D.
Family and Community Medicine. . . . . Michael L. Coates, M.D.
Internal Medicine . . . . Thomas D. DuBose, Jr., M.D.
  Cardiology. . . . . William C. Little, M.D.
  Endocrinology and Metabolism. . . . . K. Patrick Ober, M.D.
  Gastroenterology . . . . Kenneth L. Koch, M.D.
  General Internal Medicine . . . . Catherine M. Jones, M.D.
  Gerontology and Geriatric Medicine. . . . . Jeff D. Williamson, M.D.
  Hematology and Oncology. . . . . Bayard Powell, M.D.
  Infectious Diseases . . . . Kevin High, M.D.
  Molecular Medicine . . . . Richard F. Loeser, Jr., M.D.
  Nephrology . . . . Barry I. Freeman, M.D.
  Pulmonary and Critical Care Medicine . . . . Eugene Bleecker, M.D.
  Rheumatology . . . . TBN
Neurology. . . . . Allison Brashear, M.D.
  Neuromuscular Diseases. . . . . Open
  Neuropsychology . . . . TBN
  Pediatric Neurology . . . . Cesar C. Santos, M.D.
Obstetrics and Gynecology. . . . . David C. Merrill, M.D., Ph.D.
  General Obstetrics and Gynecology. . . . . Andrea Fernandez, M.D.
  General Gynecology . . . . Robert C. Henderson, M.D.
  Gynecologic Oncology . . . . Brigitte E. Miller, M.D.
  Maternal and Fetal Medicine . . . . David C. Merrill, M.D., Ph.D.
Pediatrics . . . . Jon S. Abramson, M.D.
  Medical Genetics . . . . Deborah A. Meyers, Ph.D.
Physician Assistant Studies . . . . James A. Van Rhee
Psychiatry and Behavioral Medicine . . . . W. Vaughn McCall, M.D.
  Child and Adolescent Psychiatry . . . . Guy K. Palmes, M.D.
  Geriatric Psychiatry. . . . . W. Vaughn McCall, M.D.
Radiation Oncology. . . . . A. William Blackstock, M.D.
  Clinical Radiation. . . . . Allan deGuzman, Ph.D.
  Radiation Physics . . . . J. Daniel Bourland, Ph.D.
  Radiation Biology. . . . . Michael E.C. Robbins, Ph.D.
Radiologic Sciences . . . . Allen D. Elster, M.D.
  Medical Engineering . . . . Peter Santago II, Ph.D.
  Radiology, Diagnostic. . . . . Allen D. Elster, M.D.
Surgical Sciences . . . . J. Wayne Meredith, M.D.
  Cardiothoracic. . . . . Neal D. Kon, M.D.
  Emergency Medical Services . . . . James W. Hoekstra, M.D.
  General . . . . J. Wayne Meredith, M.D.
  Neurosurgery. . . . . Charles L. Branch, M.D.
    Section on Brain Tumor Biology . . . . Waldemar Debinski, M.D., Ph.D.
  Ophthalmology . . . . Craig Greven, M.D.
  Orthopedic . . . . L. Andrew Koman, M.D.
  Otolaryngology. . . . . J. Dale Browne, M.D.
  Plastic and Reconstructive. . . . . Malcolm Marks, M.D.
  Urology . . . . Anthony Atala, M.D.

University of North Dakota School of Medicine and Health Sciences

501 North Columbia Road, Stop 9037
Grand Forks, North Dakota 58202-9037
701-777-2515 (general information); 701-777-2514 (dean's office); 777-3527 (fax)
Web site: www.med.und.nodak.edu

The University of North Dakota School of Medicine was founded in 1905 as a two-year school of basic science. Its expansion to an M.D. degree-granting program was approved in 1973, and its first class graduated in 1976. The first two years of medical education are provided in Grand Forks, while the third and fourth years are provided in Bismarck, Fargo, Grand Forks, Minot, and other communities across the state. The school's name was changed in 1996 to the University of North Dakota School of Medicine and Health Sciences to reflect the diversity of educational and research activities that occur at the school.

Type: public
2008-2009 total enrollment: 242
Clinical facilities: Veterans Administration Center Hospital, Altru Health System, MeritCare Health System, Innovis Health, St. Alexius Hospital, Medcenter One, Trinity Medical Center, Minot Air Force Base Hospital, and community hospitals throughout North Dakota.

University Officials

President	Robert O. Kelley, Ph.D.
Vice President for Academic Affairs and Provost	Greg Weisenstein, Ph.D.
Vice President for Student Affairs and Outreach Services	Robert Boyd, Ph.D.
Vice President for Operations and Finance	Robert Gallager
Vice President for Health Affairs	H. David Wilson, M.D.
Vice President for Research	Gary E. Johnson, Ph.D. (Interim)
Vice President for General Administration	Philip Harmeson

Medical School Administrative Staff

Dean	H. David Wilson, M.D.
Vice Dean	Joshua Wynne, M.D.
Associate Dean, Student Affairs and Admissions	Judy L. DeMers
Associate Dean, Southeast Campus	Julie A. Blehm, M.D.
Associate Dean, Southwest Campus	Nicholas H. Neumann, M.D.
Associate Dean, Administration and Finance	Randy S. Eken
Associate Dean, Research and Program Development	Edward R. Sauter, M.D.
Associate Dean, Academic Affairs	Joshua Wynne, M.D.
Associate Dean, Rural Health	Mary K. Wakefield, Ph.D.
Associate Dean, Clinical Education	Charles E. Christianson, M.D.
Assistant Dean, Graduate Medical Education	David J. Theige, M.D.
Assistant Dean, Veterans Affairs	William P. Newman, M.D.
Assistant Dean, Northeast Campus	Jon W. Allen, M.D.
Assistant Dean, Northwest Campus	Martin L. Rothberg, M.D.
Assistant Dean for Students, Southwest Campus	Steffen P. Christensen, M.D.
Director, Graduate Medical Education	Bruce G. Pitts, M.D.
Director, Medical Education	Thomas M. Hill, M.D.
Director, Center for Rural Health	Mary K. Wakefield, Ph.D.
Director, Communications	Juan Pedraza
Director, Continuing Medical Education and Outreach	Open
Director, Development	Blanche E. Abdallah
Director, Harley French Library of the Health Sciences	Lila Pedersen
Director, Public Affairs	Pamela D. Knudson
Director, Indians Into Medicine (INMED)	Eugene L. Delorme, J.D.
Chief Information Officer	Nasser Hammami

University of North Dakota School of Medicine and Health Sciences:
NORTH DAKOTA
Department and Division or Section Chairs

Basic Sciences

Anatomy and Cell Biology .... Edward C. Carlson, Ph.D.
Biochemistry and Molecular Biology........................ Gene A. Homandberg, Ph.D.
Microbiology and Immunology......................... Kevin D. Young, Ph.D. (Interim)
Occupational Therapy.. Janet Jedlicka, Ph.D.
Pathology .... Mary Ann Sens, M.D., Ph.D.
    Clinical Laboratory Science Program............................... Ruth Pauer
    Cytotechnology Program................................. Katherine Hoffman
Pharmacology, Physiology, and Therapeutics................... Jonathan D. Geiger, Ph.D.
Physical Therapy .... Thomas M. Mohr, Ph.D.

Clinical Sciences

Family and Community Medicine........................... Robert W. Beattie, M.D.
    Athletic Training Program .... Steven Westereng
    Physician Assistant Program .... Mary Ann Laxen
Internal Medicine .... William P. Newman, M.D.
    Ambulatory .... Julie A. Blehm, M.D.
    Cardiology... Jonathan Dickson, M.D.
    Critical Care Medicine .... Mark Tieszen, M.D.
    Endocrinology Metabolism .... William P. Newman, M.D.
    Epidemiology.. Abe E. Sahmoun, M.D.
    Gastroenterology .... Vacant
    General Medicine....................................... Julie A. Blehm, M.D.
    Geriatrics... Darin W. Lang, M.D.
    Hematology and Oncology................................. Ralph Levitt, M.D.
    Hospitalist .... Mohammed Sanaullah, M.D.
    Nephrology .... Byron D. Danielson, M.D.
    Nutrition .... Leslie M. Klevay, M.D.
    Infectious Disease...................................... Tze-Shien Lo, M.D.
    Pulmonary .... Ajay Aggarwall, M.D.
    Rheumatology .... Umbreen Hasan, M.D.
Clinical Neuroscience .... James E. Mitchell, M.D.
    Neurology .... Vacant
    Neuroradiology .... Roger L. Gilbertson, M.D.
    Psychiatry... James E. Mitchell, M.D.
Obstetrics and Gynecology................................. Dennis J. Lutz, M.D.
Pediatrics .... Stephen J. Tinguely, M.D.
Surgery... Robert P. Sticca, M.D.
    Orthopedic Surgery .... J. Donald Opgrande, M.D.

Case Western Reserve University School of Medicine

10900 Euclid Avenue
Cleveland, Ohio 44106-4915
216-368-2000; 368-2825 (dean's office); 368-2820 (dean's office fax)
Web site: http://mediswww.cwru.edu

The school was organized in 1843 as the Cleveland Medical College in cooperation with Western Reserve College, then located at Hudson, Ohio. The school of medicine is now legal successor to all of the regular medical schools that have existed from time to time in Cleveland and is located on the Case Western Reserve University campus. In 2004, the Cleveland Clinic Lerner College of Medicine of Case Western Reserve University, a distinct five-year M.D. program within the Case School of Medicine and based at the nearby Cleveland Clinic Foundation, accepted its first annual class of 32 students. The Cleveland Clinic Lerner College of Medicine offers a unique program designed to prepare its graduates for careers as physician investigators.

Type: private
2008-2009 total enrollment: 712
Clinical facilities: University Hospitals of Cleveland, Cleveland Clinic Foundation, Louis Stokes Cleveland Veterans Affairs Medical Center, MetroHealth Medical Center, St. Vincent Charity Hospital/Saint Luke's Medical Center.

University Officials

President. . . . . Barbara R. Snyder
Provost . . . . Jerold S. Goldberg, D.D.S. (Interim)
Vice President for Medical Affairs. . . . . Pamela B. Davis, M.D., Ph.D.

Medical School Administrative Staff

Dean, School of Medicine . . . . Pamela B. Davis, M.D., Ph.D.
Vice Dean for Clinical Affairs, Case Medical Center . . . . Achilles Demetriou, M.D.
Vice Dean for Education and Academic Affairs. Daniel Ornt, M.D.
Vice Dean for Research . . . . Robert Miller, Ph.D.
Executive Dean, CCLCM . . . . Andrew J. Fishleder, M.D.
Senior Associate Dean for Students . . . . C. Kent Smith, M.D.
Associate Dean and Director of Graduate Medical Education . . . . Jerry M. Shuck, M.D.
Associate Dean for Admissions . . . . Lina Mehta, M.D.
Associate Dean for Admissions and Student Affairs, CCLCM . . . . Kathleen Franco, M.D.
Associate Dean for Curricular Affairs . . . . Terry W. Wolpaw, M.D.
Associate Dean for Curricular Affairs, CCLCM . . . . Alan L. Hull, M.D., Ph.D.
Associate Dean for Faculty Affairs and Human Resources . . . . Daniel E. Anker, Ph.D., J.D.
Associate Dean for Faculty Affairs, CCLCM. . . . . Andrew C. Novick, M.D.
Associate Dean for Finance . . . . Christopher D. Masotti
Associate Dean for Geriatric Medicine . . . . Vacant
Associate Dean for Louis Stokes Veterans Affairs Medical Center. . . . . Murray D. Altose, M.D.
Associate Dean of Medical Student Research. . . . . Vacant
Associate Dean for MetroHealth System . . . . Ben H. Brouhard, M.D.
Associate Dean for Research Administration . . . . Richard Sohn, Ph.D.
Associate Dean for Student Affairs . . . . Robert Haynie, M.D., Ph.D.
Assistant Dean for Space and Facilities Planning. . . . . Jill Stanley
Registrar . . . . Joseph Corrao

Department and Division or Section Chairs

Basic Sciences

Anatomy. . . . . Daniel Ornt, M.D. (Interim)
Biochemistry. . . . . Michael A. Weiss, M.D., Ph.D.
Bioethics . . . . Stuart Youngner, M.D.
Biomedical Engineering. . . . . Jeffrey Duerk, Ph.D.
Environmental Health Sciences . . . . Dorr Dearborn, M.D., Ph.D.
Epidemiology and Biostatistics . . . . Robert Elston, Ph.D. (Interim)
General Medical Sciences. . . . . Pamela B. Davis, M.D., Ph.D.
  Cancer Center . . . . Stanton Gerson, M.D.

Center for the Advancement of Medical Learning . . . . Vacant
Center of the Study of Kidney Biology and Disease . . . . John Sedor, M.D.
Center for Clinical Investigation . . . . Pamela B. Davis, M.D., Ph.D.
Center for Global Health and Diseases . . . . James W. Kazura, M.D.
Center for Mass Spectrometry and Proteomics. . . . . Mark R. Chance, Ph.D.
Center for Psychoanalytic Child Development . . . . Thomas F. Barrett, M.D.
Center for Science, Health and Society . . . . Nathan A. Berger, M.D.
RNA Center. . . . . Timothy W. Nilsen, Ph.D.
Genetics . . . . Joseph H. Nadeau, Ph.D.
Molecular Biology and Microbiology. . . . . Jonathan Karn, Ph.D.
Molecular Medicine, Cleveland Clinic Lerner
    College of Medicine . . . . Paul E. DiCorleto, Ph.D.
Neurosciences . . . . Lynn Landmesser, Ph.D.
Nutrition. . . . . Henri Brunengraber, M.D., Ph.D.
Pathology . . . . Clifford V. Harding, M.D., Ph.D. (Interim)
Pharmacology . . . . Krzysztof Palczewski, Ph.D.
Physiology and Biophysics . . . . Walter Boron, M.D., Ph.D.

Clinical Sciences

Anesthesiology-University Hospitals of Cleveland. . . . . Howard S. Nearman, M.D.
Anesthesiology-Cleveland Clinic Lerner College of Medicine . . . . Michael Roizen, M.D.
Anesthesiology-MetroHealth Medical Center. . . . . Tejbir S. Sidhu, M.D.
Dermatology-University Hospitals of Cleveland . . . . Kevin D. Cooper, M.D.
Dermatology-MetroHealth Medical Center . . . . Marlene Willen, M.D.
Emergency Medicine-University Hospitals of Cleveland . . . . Edward Michelson, M.D.
Emergency Medicine-MetroHealth Medical Center . . . . Charles L. Emerman, M.D.
Family Medicine-University Hospitals of Cleveland . . . . George E. Kikano, M.D.
Family Medicine-MetroHealth Medical Center . . . . James W. Campbell, M.D.
Medicine-University Hospitals of Cleveland. . . . . Richard A. Walsh, M.D.
Medicine-Cleveland Clinic Lerner College of Medicine . . . . James Young, M.D.
Medicine-MetroHealth Medical Center. . . . . Alfred F. Connors, Jr., M.D.
Neurological Surgery-University Hospitals of Cleveland . . . . Warren R. Selman, M.D.
Neurology-University Hospitals of Cleveland . . . . Anthony J. Furlan, M.D.
Neurology-MetroHealth Medical Center . . . . Joseph P. Hanna, M.D.
Ophthalmology and Visual Sciences-University
    Hospitals of Cleveland . . . . Jonathan H. Lass, M.D.
Ophthalmology-Cleveland Clinic Lerner College of Medicine . . . . Hilel Lewis, M.D.
Orthopaedics-University Hospitals of Cleveland. . . . . Randall Marcus, M.D.
Orthopaedics-MetroHealth Medical Center. . . . . Brendan M. Patterson, M.D.
Otolaryngology-Head and Neck Surgery-
    University Hospitals of Cleveland . . . . James E. Arnold, M.D.
Otolaryngology-Head and Neck Surgery-MetroHealth Medical Center . . . . . . Joseph Carter, M.D.
Pathology-University Hospitals of Cleveland . . . . Clifford V. Harding, M.D., Ph.D. (Interim)
Pathology-Cleveland Clinic Lerner College of Medicine. . . . . William Hart, M.D.
Pathology-MetroHealth Medical Center . . . . Joseph Tomashefski, M.D.
Pediatrics-University Hospitals of Cleveland. . . . . Avroy Fanaroff, M.D.
Pediatrics-Cleveland Clinic Lerner College of Medicine. . . . . Robert Wyllie, M.D.
Pediatrics-MetroHealth Medical Center. . . . . Robert C. Cohn, M.D.
Physical Medicine and Rehabilitation-MetroHealth Medical Center . . . . Gary S. Clark, M.D.
Plastic Surgery-University Hospitals of Cleveland . . . . Bahman Guyuron, M.D.
Psychiatry-University Hospitals of Cleveland . . . . Robert Ronis, M.D.
Psychiatry-MetroHealth Medical Center . . . . R. Taylor Segraves, M.D., Ph.D.
Radiation Oncology-University Hospitals of Cleveland . . . . Nathan Levitan, M.D. (Interim)
Radiology-University Hospitals of Cleveland . . . . Charles F. Lanzieri, M.D. (Acting)
Radiology-Cleveland Clinic Lerner College of Medicine. . . . . Michael T. Modic, M.D.
Radiology-MetroHealth Medical Center . . . . Stephen Tamarkin, M.D.
Reproductive Biology-University Hospitals of Cleveland. . . . . James Liu, M.D.
Reproductive Biology-MetroHealth Medical Center . . . . Patrick Catalano, M.D.
Surgery-University Hospitals of Cleveland . . . . Jeffrey Ponsky, M.D.
Surgery-Cleveland Clinic Lerner College of Medicine . . . . Kenneth Ouriel, M.D.
Surgery-MetroHealth Medical Center . . . . Mark A. Malangoni, M.D.
Urology-University Hospitals of Cleveland. . . . . Donald R. Bodner, M.D. (Acting)

Northeastern Ohio Universities College of Medicine

4209 State Route 44
P.O. Box 95
Rootstown, Ohio 44272-0095
330-325-2511; 325-6255 (dean's office); 325-5919 (dean's office fax)
Web site: www.neoucom.edu

The Northeastern Ohio Universities Colleges of Medicine and Pharmacy (NEOUCOM) is a community-based, state medical school established in November 1973. NEOUCOM awards the M.D. degree and, through consortial relationships with the University of Akron, Kent State University, and Youngstown State University, offers a combined B.S./M.D. degree program. The administration, basic sciences, and community health sciences are located on the Rootstown campus, and the clinical sciences are community-based in hospitals in Akron, Canton, Youngstown, and the 19-county area of northeast Ohio. The charter class graduated in May 1981. NEOUCOM also offers the Pharm.D. degree and is a cosponsor of the Consortium of Eastern Ohio Master of Public Health Program.

Type: public
2008-2009 total enrollment: 503
Clinical facilities: Teaching Hospitals (Associated): Akron General Health System, Akron Children's Hospital, Alliance Community Hospital, Summa Health System (Akron); Barberton Citizens Hospital; Aultman Hospital, Mercy Medical Center (Canton); St. Elizabeth Health Center; Forum Health Tod Children's Hospital, Northside Medical Center (Youngstown). **Affiliated Hospitals:** Cleveland Clinic Health System; Edwin Shaw Hospital for Rehabilitation (Akron); Fairview Hospital (Cleveland); Heartland Behavioral Healthcare (Massillon); Kaiser Permanente Health System, Louis Stokes Cleveland Department of Veteran's Affairs, Lutheran Hospital, Marymount Hospital (Cleveland); MedCentral System (Mansfield); Medina General Hospital; Robinson Memorial Hospital (Ravenna); Salem Community Hospital; Wadsworth-Rittman Hospital (Wadsworth); Forum Health Hillside Rehabilitation Hospital, Forum Health Trumbull Memorial Hospital (Warren). **Associated Health Departments:** The Akron Health Department; Stark County Health Department.

College Officials

President	Lois Margaret Nora, M.D., J.D.
Senior Vice President for Academic Affairs	Mark A. Penn, M.D.
Vice President for Administration and Finance	Debra K. Staats
Vice President for Institutional Advancement	Lindsey H. Loftus
Vice President for Strategic Alliances	Kathleen C. Ruff, M.B.A.
General Counsel	Maria R. Schimer, J.D.

Medical School Administration

Dean of Medicine	Lois Margaret Nora, M.D., J.D.
Executive Associate Dean for Medicine	Mark A. Penn, M.D.
Associate Dean for Clinical Sciences	Jay C. Williamson, M.D.
Dean of Pharmacy	David D. Allen, R.Ph., Ph.D., FASHP
Executive Associate Dean for Pharmacy	Robb McGory, R.Ph., Pharm.D.
Vice President for Research	Walter E. Horton, Ph.D.
Associate Dean for Clinical Education (Akron)	Joseph Zarconi, M.D.
Associate Dean for Clinical Education (Akron)	Michael G. Holder, Jr., M.D.
Associate Dean for Clinical Education (Akron)	James M. Dougherty, M.D.
Associate Dean for Clinical Education (Barberton)	J. Randall Richard, M.D.
Associate Dean for Clinical Education (Canton)	Martha W. Magoon, M.D.
Associate Dean for Clinical Education (Canton)	J. Richard Ziegler, Jr., M.D.
Associate Dean for Clinical Education (Youngstown)	Rebecca S. Bailey, M.D.
Associate Dean for Clinical Education (Youngstown)	Michael S. Kavic, M.D.
Associate Dean for Health Professions Education	Clint W. Snyder, Ph.D.
Assistant Dean for Student Affairs and Admissions	Priscilla J. Moss
Chief of Staff	Kathleen C. Ruff
Director, Admissions	Michelle L. Cassetty
Director, Assessment	Margarita D. Kokinova, Ph.D.
Director, Area Health Education Center	Jonathan T. Jenney
Director, Center for Studies of Clinical Performance	Holly A. Gerzina
Director, Chief Medical Librarian	Thomas C. Atwood
Director, Comparative Medicine	Walter I. Horne, D.V.M.
Director, Continuing Professional Education	Lori Gourley Babbey
Director, Curriculum	Martha A. Silling, Ph.D.
Director, Development	Abbe Turner

Director, Governmental Relations. . . . . Richard W. Lewis
Director, Graduate Programs . . . . Walter E. Horton, Ph.D.
Director, Human Resources . . . . Marsha S. Mills
Director, Public Relations and Marketing . . . . Mark S. Bosko
Registrar . . . . Michelle L. Cassetty
Director, Professional Development . . . . Anita R. Pokorny

Basic Medical and Community Health Sciences

Anatomy and Neurobiology . . . . Jeffrey J. Wenstrup, Ph.D.
Behavioral Sciences . . . . Mark L. Savickas, Ph.D.
Community Health Sciences. . . . . Sharon K. Hull, M.D.
Integrative Medical Sciences. . . . . William M. Chilian, Ph.D.

Clinical Sciences

Emergency Medicine . . . . Open
   Pediatric Emergency Medicine* . . . . Jeffrey A. Kempf, D.O.
Family Medicine . . . . Anthony J. Costa, M.D.
Internal Medicine . . . . George I. Litman, M.D.
   Allergy/Immunology*. . . . . Joseph F. Alexander, Jr., M.D.
   Cardiology* . . . . J. Ronald Mikolich, M.D.
   Dermatology*. . . . . Eliot N. Mostow, M.D., M.P.H.
   Endocrinology* . . . . James K. Salem, M.D.
   Gastroenterology* . . . . Nabil M. Fahmy, M.D.
   General Medicine*. . . . . Dale P. Murphy, M.D.
   Geriatric Medicine* . . . . Benjamin M. Hayek, M.D.
   Hematology/Oncology* . . . . John J. Petrus, M.D.
   Infectious Disease*. . . . . Thomas M. File, Jr., M.D.
   Nephrology* . . . . John F. Jacobs, Jr., M.D.
   Neurology* . . . . Christopher A. Sheppard, M.D.
   Pulmonary and Critical Care*. . . . . Rebecca S. Bailey, M.D.
   Rehabilitation Medicine* . . . . Michael J. Delahanty, D.O.
   Rheumatology* . . . . Andrew C. Raynor, M.D.
Obstetrics and Gynecology. . . . . Michael P. Hopkins, M.D.
Orthopaedic Surgery . . . . Mark C. Leeson, M.D.
Pathology . . . . Robert W. Novak, M.D.
Pediatrics . . . . Norman C. Christopher, M.D.
   Neonatology. . . . . Anand D. Kantak, M.D.
Psychiatry . . . . Mark R. Munetz, M.D.
   Community Psychiatry . . . . Mark R. Munetz, M.D.
   Psychology* . . . . Sharon Irwin, Ph.D.
Radiology . . . . J. Eric Blum, M.D.
   Medical Radiation Biophysics* . . . . Dale E. Starchman, Ph.D.
   Nuclear Medicine*. . . . . John M. Lahorra, M.D.
   Pediatric Radiology*. . . . . Godfrey Gaisie, M.D.
   Radiation Oncology* . . . . Michael J. Seider, M.D., Ph.D.
   Sectional Imaging*. . . . . Laura A. Cawthon, M.D., M.P.H.
Surgery . . . . Daniel P. Guyton, M.D.
   Anesthesiology* . . . . Veeraiah C. Perni, M.D.
   Neurosurgery* . . . . Ghassan F. Khayyat, M.D.
   Ophthalmology*. . . . . James H. Bates, M.D.
   Otolaryngology* . . . . Joseph P. Yut, M.D.
   Plastic Surgery* . . . . James A. Lehman, Jr., M.D.
   Thoracic and Cardiovascular*. . . . . Robert W. Kamienski, M.D.
Urology. . . . . Phillip F. Nasrallah, M.D.

*Specialty without organizational autonomy.

Ohio State University College of Medicine

254 Meiling Hall
370 West Ninth Avenue
Columbus, Ohio 43210
614-292-2220; 292-2600 (dean's office); 292-4254 (fax)
Web site: www.medicine.osu.edu

The college of medicine of Ohio State University was established in 1914 by an act of the Ohio legislature.

Type: public
2008-2009 total enrollment: 835
Clinical facilities: Ohio State University Hospitals; Ohio State University Hospital East; Ohio State University Harding Hospital; Arthur G. James Cancer Hospital and Richard J. Solove Research Institute; Richard M. Ross Heart Hospital; Mount Carmel Medical Center; Grant Medical Center; Riverside Methodist Hospitals; Nationwide Children's Hospital; St. Ann's Hospital; Veterans Affairs Medical Center (Dayton); Bethesda Hospital Center of Zanesville (Ohio); Veterans Hospital (Chillicothe, Ohio); Veterans Outpatient Clinic; Medical Center Hospital (Chillicothe, Ohio).

University Officials

President. . . . . E. Gordon Gee
Senior Vice President and Executive Dean for Health Sciences . . . . Steven G. Gabbe, M.D.

Medical School Administrative Staff

Dean. . . . . Wiley W. 'Chip' Souba, Jr., M.D., Sc.D.
Executive Vice Dean . . . . Daniel Sedmak, M.D.
Vice Dean for Clinical Affairs. . . . . E. Christopher Ellison, M.D.
  Associate Dean for Ancillary Services. . . . . Douglas A. Rund, M.D.
  Associate Dean for Medical Services . . . . Michael Grever, M.D.
  Associate Dean for Primary Care. . . . . Mary Jo Welker, M.D.
  Associate Dean for Surgical Services . . . . E. Christopher Ellison, M.D.
Vice Dean for Education . . . . Catherine Lucey, M.D.
  Associate Dean for Admissions and Records . . . . Donald Batisky, M.D.
  Associate Dean for Graduate Medical Education . . . . Andrew M. Thomas, M.D.
  Associate Dean for Student Life. . . . . Linda Stone, M.D.
  Associate Dean for Medical Education and Outreach. . . . . Daniel Clinchot, M.D.
  Assistant Dean, Clinical Skills and Medical Education . . . . Carol Hasbrouck
  Assistant Dean for Medical Education,
    Nationwide Children's Hospital . . . . Mary McIlroy, M.D.
  Assistant Dean for Medical Education, Mount Carmel Hospital. . . . . Patrick Ecklar, M.D.
  Assistant Dean for Medical Education, Grant Hospital . . . . Bruce T. Vanderhoff, M.D.
  Assistant Dean for Medical Education, Ohio Health, Inc. . . . . Pamela Jelly-Boyers, Ph.D.
  Assistant Dean for Rural Medical Education. . . . . Randall Longenecker, M.D.
Vice Dean for Research . . . . Caroline C. Whitacre, Ph.D.
  Associate Dean for Translational and Applied Research. . . . . Chandan Sen, Ph.D.
  Associate Dean for Basic Research. . . . . Joanna Groden, Ph.D.
  Associate Dean for Clinical Research. . . . . Rebecca Jackson, M.D.
  Associate Dean for Outcomes Research. . . . . Michael F. Para, M.D.
  Associate Dean for Research Education and
    Graduate Studies . . . . Ginny Bumgardner, M.D., Ph.D.
  Assistant Dean for Research . . . . James King, Ph.D.
Senior Associate Dean for Academic Affairs and
  Secretary of the College . . . . Robert A. Bornstein, Ph.D.
Assistant Dean for Diversity and Cultural Affairs . . . . Leon McDougle, M.D.
Associate Dean and Director, School of Allied Medical Professions . . . . . Deborah Larsen, Ph.D.
Director, School of Biomedical Science . . . . Caroline C. Whitacre, Ph.D.
Chief Administrative Officer. . . . . Brad Harris
Director, Center for Continuing Medical Education . . . . Barbara Berry

Ohio State University College of Medicine: OHIO

Department and Division or Section Chairs

Basic Sciences

Biomedical Informatics . . . . Joel H. Saltz, M.D., Ph.D.
Molecular and Cellular Biochemistry . . . . Michael Ostrowski, Ph.D.
Molecular Virology, Immunology, and Medical Genetics . . . . Carlo Croce, M.D.
Neuroscience. . . . . James King, Ph.D. (Interim)
Pharmacology . . . . Wolfgang Sadee, Dr.rer.nat
Physiology and Cell Biology . . . . Muthu Periasamy, Ph.D.

Clinical Sciences

Anesthesiology. . . . . David A. Zvara, M.D.
Emergency Medicine . . . . Douglas A. Rund, M.D.
Family Medicine . . . . Mary Jo Welker, M.D.
Internal Medicine . . . . Michael Grever, M.D.
  Cardiovascular Medicine. . . . . William T. Abraham, M.D.
  Dermatology . . . . Mark Bechtel, M.D.
  Digestive Health. . . . . Nicholas Verne, M.D.
  Endocrinology, Diabetes, and Metabolism . . . . Kwame Osei, M.D.
  General Internal Medicine . . . . Catherine Lucey, M.D. (Interim)
  Hematology and Oncology. . . . . Gregory A. Otterson, M.D., and John Byrd, M.D.
  Hospital Medicine . . . . Adrienne Bennett, M.D.
  Human Genetics . . . . Albert de la Chapelle, M.D. (Interim)
  Immunology, Allergy, and Rheumatology . . . . Ronald L. Whisler, M.D.
  Infectious Diseases . . . . Larry S. Schlesinger, M.D.
  Nephrology . . . . Brad Rovin, M.D.
  Pulmonary, Allergy, Critical Care, and Sleep Medicine. . . . . Clay Marsh, M.D.
Neurological Surgery. . . . . E. Antonio Chiocca, M.D., Ph.D.
Neurology. . . . . Michael Racke, M.D.
Obstetrics and Gynecology. . . . . Larry J. Copeland, M.D.
Ophthalmology. . . . . Thomas Mauger, M.D.
Orthopaedics. . . . . Christopher Kaeding, M.D. (Interim)
Otolaryngology . . . . D. Bradley Welling, M.D., Ph.D.
Pathology . . . . Sanford Barsky, M.D.
Pediatrics . . . . Michael Brady, M.D.
Physical Medicine and Rehabilitation . . . . William S. Pease, M.D.
Psychiatry . . . . Radu Saveanu, M.D.
Radiation Medicine . . . . Nina Mayr, M.D.
Radiology. . . . . Daniel D. Sedmak, M.D. (Interim)
  Abdominal Imaging . . . . William Bennett, M.D.
  Interventional Radiology. . . . . William Yuh, M.D.
  Breast Imaging. . . . . Adele Lipari, D.O.
  Imaging Research. . . . . Michael Knopp, M.D., Ph.D.
  Musculoskeletal Radiology . . . . Joe Yu, M.D.
  Neuroradiology . . . . Donald W. Chakeres, M.D.
  Nuclear Medicine. . . . . Nathan Hall, M.D., Ph.D.
  Radiobiology . . . . Altaf Wani, Ph.D.
  Thoracic Imaging. . . . . Mark King, M.D.
  Ultrasound. . . . . Vacant
Surgery. . . . . E. Christopher Ellison, M.D.
  Thoracic and Cardiovascular Surgery . . . . Benjamin Sun, M.D.
  Critical Care, Trauma, and Burns . . . . Steven M. Steinberg, M.D.
  General Surgery. . . . . W. Scott Melvin, M.D.
  Pediatric Surgery . . . . Donna A. Caniano, M.D.
  Plastic Surgery . . . . Michael Miller, M.D.
  Surgical Oncology . . . . William B. Farrar, M.D.
  Transplantation Surgery. . . . . Mitchell Henry, M.D.
  General Vascular Surgery . . . . Patrick Vaccaro, M.D.
Urology. . . . . Robert R. Bahnson, M.D.

University of Cincinnati College of Medicine

P.O. Box 670555
Cincinnati, Ohio 45267-0555
513-558-7391 (dean's office); 558-1165 (fax)
Web site: www.med.uc.edu

The college of medicine is a descendant of the Medical College of Ohio, which was chartered in 1819. In 1896, this college became the medical department of the University of Cincinnati by incorporation into that institution. The medical college is part of the University of Cincinnati Academic Health Center.

Type: public
2008-2009 total enrollment: 634
Clinical facilities: Cincinnati Children's Hospital Medical Center, Christ Hospital, Drake Center, Inc., Good Samaritan Hospital, Jewish Hospital, Shriners Burns Hospital, Veterans Affairs Medical Center, University Hospital, Health Alliance of Greater Cincinnati, Franciscan Hospital.

University Officials

President. . . . . Nancy L. Zimpher, Ph.D.
Vice President for Health Affairs . . . . David M. Stern, M.D.

Medical School Administrative Staff

Dean. . . . . David M. Stern, M.D.
Executive Associate Dean for Clinical Programs . . . . Thomas Boat, M.D.
Senior Associate Dean for Medical Education . . . . Andrew T. Filak, M.D.
Senior Associate Dean for Operations and Finance . . . . Robert F. Ambach, C.F.O.
Senior Associate Dean for Research and Graduate Education . . . . Robert Highsmith, Ph.D.
Senior Associate Dean for Student Affairs and Admissions. . . . . Laura Wexler, M.D.
Associate Dean for Faculty and Legal Affairs. . . . . M. Kathleen Robbins, J.D.
Associate Dean for Diversity and Community Affairs . . . . Charles Collins, M.D.
Associate Dean for Clinical Research . . . . James Heubi, M.D.
Associate Dean for Clinical Research . . . . Joel Tsevat, M.D.
Associate Dean for Collaborative Research
  Activities with Cincinnati Children's Hospital
  Medical Center . . . . Marsha Wills-Karp, Ph.D.
Associate Dean for Hospital Operations . . . . Lee Ann Liska
Assistant Dean for Admissions . . . . R. Stephen Manual, Ph.D.
Assistant Dean for Continuing Medical Education. . . . . John R. Kues, Ph.D.
Assistant Dean for Diversity and Community Affairs . . . . Kenneth Davis, M.D.
Assistant Dean for Medical Education. . . . . Mary Heider, Ph.D., and Michael Sostok, M.D.
Assistant Dean for Graduate Education. . . . . Laura Hildreth
Assistant Dean for Student Affairs and Registrar . . . . Iva Dean Lair-Adolph
Assistant Dean for Student Affairs. . . . . Denise D. Gibson, Ph.D.
Assistant Dean, Office of Faculty and Administrative Affairs. . . . . Lynda L. Price
Assistant Dean, Medical School Financial Aid . . . . Daniel Burr, Ph.D.
Executive Director and Controller . . . . Jan Hawk

Department and Division or Section Chairs

Basic Sciences

Biomedical Engineering. . . . . William S. Ball, M.D.
Cancer and Cell Biology . . . . Jorge Moscat, Ph.D.
Environmental Health . . . . Shuk-Mei Ho, Ph.D.
  Biostatistics and Epidemiology*. . . . . Kim N. Dietrich, Ph.D.
  Industrial Hygiene, Occupational Safety, and Ergonomics* . . . . Carol Rice, Ph.D.
  Molecular Toxicology* . . . . Howard Shertzer, Ph.D.
  Occupational Environmental Medicine* . . . . Andrew Freeman, M.D. (Acting)
Molecular Cellular Physiology. . . . . Marshall Montrose, Ph.D.
Molecular Genetics, Biochemistry, and Microbiology. . . . . Malak Kotb, Ph.D.
Pathology . . . . David Witte, M.D.

Anatomic Pathology* .... Mohammed Nazek, M.D.
Autopsy* .... Fred Lucas, M.D.
Nephropathology .... Lois Arend, M.D.
Neuro-Pathology* .... Ady Kendler, M.D.
Surgical Pathology* .... Fred Lucas, M.D.
Pharmacology and Cell Biophysics .... Evangelia Kranias, Ph.D.

Clinical Sciences

Anesthesiology .... William E. Hurford, M.D.
Barrett Cancer Center .... David M. Stern, M.D. (Acting)
Dermatology .... Diya F. Mutasim, M.D.
Emergency Medicine .... Brian Gibler, M.D.
Family Medicine .... Jeffrey Susman, M.D.
Internal Medicine .... Bradley Britigan, M.D.
   Cardiology* .... Neal Weintraub, M.D.
   Digestive Diseases* .... Kenneth Sherman, M.D.
   General Medicine* .... Mark Eckman, M.D.
   Hematology and Oncology* .... Al Muhleman, M.D. (Acting)
   Infectious Diseases* .... George Deepe, M.D.
   Medical Immunology, Rheumatic Disease, and Allergy* .... Larry Houk, M.D. (Acting)
   Metabolism and Endocrinology* .... David D'Alessio, M.D.
   Nephrology and Hypertension* .... Manoocher Soleimani, M.D.
   Pulmonary Diseases* .... Francis X. McCormack, M.D.
Neurology .... Joseph P. Broderick, M.D.
Neurosurgery .... Raj K. Narayan, M.D.
Obstetrics and Gynecology .... Arthur T. Evans, M.D.
Ophthalmology .... James J. Augsburger, M.D.
Orthopedic Surgery .... Peter Stern, M.D.
Otolaryngology and Head and Neck Surgery .... Myles Pensak, M.D.
Pediatrics .... Arnold Strauss, M.D.
Physical Medicine and Rehabilitation .... Mark Goddard, M.D.
Psychiatry .... Stephen Strakowski, M.D.
Public Health Sciences .... Ronnie Horner, Ph.D.
Radiation Oncology .... William Barrett, M.D.
Radiology .... Mary Gaskill-Shipley, M.D. (Interim)
   Body Imaging .... Jonathan Moulton, M.D.
   Breast Imaging .... Mary Mahoney, M.D.
   Cardiothoracic Imaging .... Ralph Shipley, M.D.
   Diagnostics .... Mary Gaskill-Shipley, M.D. (Acting)
   Interventional Imaging .... Ross Ristagno, M.D.
   Neuroradiology .... Thomas Tomsick, M.D.
   Nuclear Medicine .... Mariano Fernandez-Ulla, M.D.
   Pediatric Radiology .... Lane Donnelly, M.D.
Surgery .... Michael Edwards, M.D.
   Burn .... Richard Kagan, M.D.
   Cardiac* .... Walter Merrill, M.D.
   Colorectal .... Janice Rafferty, M.D.
   General Surgery* .... David Fischer, M.D.
   Oral Surgery* .... Robert Marciani, M.D.
   Pediatric Surgery* .... Richard G. Azizkhan, M.D.
   Plastic Surgery* .... WmJohn Kitzmiller, M.D.
   Surgical Oncology* .... Jeffrey Sussman, M.D.
   Thoracic* .... Walter Merrill, M.D.
   Transplantation and Surgical Immunology* .... E. Steve Woodle, M.D.
   Trauma and Critical Care* .... Jay Johannigman, M.D.
   Urology* .... James Donovan, M.D.
   Vascular Surgery* .... George Meier, M.D.

*Specialty without organizational autonomy.

The University of Toledo, College of Medicine

3045 Arlington Avenue
Toledo, Ohio 43614
419-383-4000; 383-4243 (dean's office); 383-6100 (fax)
Web site: http://hsc.utoledo.edu/

The University of Toledo College of Medicine came into existence July 1, 2006, as a result of the merger of the former Medical University of Ohio, a free-standing, state-supported academic health center, and the University of Toledo, one of 14 state-supported universities in Ohio. The Medical University of Ohio was formerly the Medical College of Ohio. The University of Toledo College of Medicine falls under the policy-making authority of the Ohio Board of Regents. The first class of medical students was admitted in 1969.

Type: public
2008-2009 total enrollment: 586
Clinical facilities: University Medical Center at The University of Toledo, St. Vincent Mercy Medical Center, the Toledo Hospital, Northwest Psychiatric Hospital.

University of Toledo Administrative Staff

President. . . . . Lloyd A. Jacobs, M.D.
Provost and Executive Vice President for Health
    Affairs and Dean of the College of Medicine . . . . Jeffrey P. Gold, M.D.
Senior Vice President for Finance and Strategy. . . . . Scott Scarborough, Ph.D.
Vice President for Institutional Advancement . . . . Vernon Snyder
Administrator and Chief Information Officer . . . . Godfrey Ovwhigo
Vice President for Research Administration . . . . R. Douglas Wilkerson, Ph.D.
Associate Dean, College of Medicine, Graduate Programs . . . . R. Douglas Wilkerson, Ph.D.
Associate Dean for Student Affairs, College of Medicine . . . . Patricia J. Metting, Ph.D.
Director, Institutional Diversity. . . . . Sam Hancock, Ed.D.
Associate Dean for Admissions . . . . James Kleshinski, M.D.
    Assistant Dean for Admissions. . . . . Robert Crissman, Ph.D.
Associate Dean for Clinical Affairs . . . . Ronald McGinnis, M.D.
Associate Dean for Clinical Undergraduate and
    Graduate Medical Education . . . . Mary R. Smith, M.D.
Director, Alumni Affairs and Development . . . . Daniel Saevig
Associate Dean for Preclinical Medical Education . . . . Carol Bennett-Clarke, Ph.D.
Associate Dean, Continuing Medical Education. . . . . William Davis, D.D.S.
Director, Division of Laboratory Animal Medicine. . . . . Brent Martin, D.V.M.
Director, Mulford Library. . . . . Marlene Porter
Director of Communications . . . . John Adams
Director, Financial Aid. . . . . Patricia J. Metting, Ph.D.
Registrar . . . . Patricia J. Metting, Ph.D.
Associate Dean for Faculty Development and
    Curriculum Evaluation . . . . Constance J. Shriner, Ph.D.

The University of Toledo, College of Medicine: OHIO

Department and Division or Section Chairs

Basic Sciences

Biochemistry and Cancer Biology . . . . William Maltese, Ph.D.
Medical Microbiology and Immunology . . . . Akira Takashima, Ph.D.
Neurosciences . . . . Brian Yamamoto, Ph.D.
Physiology, Pharmacology, Metabolism, and Cardiovascular Science . . . . Amir Askari, Ph.D.

Clinical Science

Anesthesiology. . . . . Alan Marco, M.D.
Family Medicine . . . . Linda French, M.D.
Medicine. . . . . Joseph Shapiro, M.D.
  Cardiology. . . . . Christopher Cooper, M.D.
  Dermatology . . . . Lori Gottwald, M.D.
  Endocrinology and Metabolism. . . . . Gregory Tennyson, M.D.
  Gastroenterology . . . . Isam Daboul, M.D.
  General Internal. . . . . Basil Akpunonu, M.D.
  Hematology and Oncology . . . . Iman Mohamed, M.D.
  Hepatology . . . . Thomas Sodeman, M.D.
  Infectious Disease. . . . . Julia Westerink, M.D.
  Nephrology . . . . Deepak Malhotra, M.D.
  Pulmonary. . . . . Jeffrey Hammersley, M.D.
  Rheumatology . . . . M. Bashar Kahaleh, M.D.
Neurology. . . . . Gretchen Tietjen, M.D.
Obstetrics and Gynecology. . . . . Terrence Horrigan, M.D.
Orthopaedic Surgery . . . . Nabil Ebraheim, M.D.
Pathology . . . . Robert Mrak, M.D.
Pediatrics . . . . David Krol, M.D.
Psychiatry . . . . Marijo Tamburrino, M.D.
Radiation Oncology. . . . . John J. Feldmeier, D.O.
Radiology . . . . Lee Woldenberg, M.D.
Surgery . . . . Gerald Zelenock, M.D.
Urology. . . . . Stephen Selman, M.D. (Interim)

Wright State University Boonshoft School of Medicine

3640 Col. Glenn Highway
Dayton, Ohio 45435-0001
937-775-3010; 775-2933 (dean's office); 775-2211 (fax)
E-mail: SOM_dean@wright.edu
Web site: www.med.wright.edu

Wright State University was first established in 1964 as a campus of the Ohio University System operated conjointly by the Ohio State University and Miami University of Ohio; in 1967, independent status as one of 12 state-assisted universities was conferred. The school of medicine was authorized in 1973 by the state of Ohio. The administration and the basic sciences departments are located on the parent university campus in Fairborn, a suburb of Dayton. The clinical sciences departments are community-based in six affiliated hospitals in the Dayton area. The charter class matriculated in September 1976.

Type: public
2008-2009 total enrollment: 370
Clinical facilities: Children's Medical Center, Good Samaritan Hospital and Health Center, Greene Memorial Hospital, Kettering Medical Center, Miami Valley Hospital, Department of Veterans Affairs Medical Center (Dayton), Wright-Patterson Medical Center.

University Officials

President. . . . . David R. Hopkins, Ph.D.
Director, Biomedical Sciences Ph.D. Program . . . . Gerald M. Alter, Ph.D.
Provost . . . . Steven R. Angle, Ph.D.

Medical School Administrative Staff

Dean. . . . . Howard M. Part, M.D.
Executive Associate Dean . . . . Margaret M. Dunn, M.D.
Associate Dean for Academic Affairs. . . . . Dean X. Parmelee, M.D.
Associate Dean for Air Force Affairs . . . . Colonel Kimberly Slawinski, M.D.
Associate Dean for Research Affairs . . . . Robert E. W. Fyffe, Ph.D.
Associate Dean for Fiscal Affairs. . . . . John L. Bale
Associate Dean for Student Affairs and Admissions . . . . Gary LeRoy, M.D.
Associate Dean for Veterans Affairs . . . . Steven M. Cohen, M.D.
Assistant Dean for Admissions . . . . Stephen E. Peterson, Ph.D.
Assistant Dean for Minority Affairs . . . . Gary LeRoy, M.D.
Assistant to the Dean. . . . . Betty Kangas
Associate Vice President for Advancement . . . . Robert S. Copeland
Fordham Health Sciences Librarian . . . . Sheila Shellabarger
Director, Interdisciplinary Teaching Laboratory . . . . Debra M. Hendershot
Director, Laboratory Animal Resources. . . . . Gregory Boivin, D.V.M.
Director of Marketing and Communications . . . . Cindy Young

Department and Division or Section Chairs

Basic Sciences

Neuroscience, Cell Biology and Physiology . . . . Timothy Cope, Ph.D.
Biochemistry and Molecular Biology. . . . . Steven J. Berberich, Ph.D.
Pharmacology and Toxicology . . . . Mariana Morris, Ph.D.

Clinical Sciences

Community Health . . . . Arthur Pickoff, M.D.
   Aerospace Medicine. . . . . Robin Dodge, M.D.
   Center for Global Health Systems, Management, and Policy. . . . . Richard J. Schuster, M.D.
   Center for Intervention, Treatment, and Addictions Research . . . . Robert Carlson, Ph.D.
   Lifespan Health Research Center . . . . Roger M. Siervogel, Ph.D.
   Medical Humanities . . . . Mary T. White, Ph.D.
   Premier Community Health . . . . Pamela Reichel (Exec. Dir.)
Dermatology . . . . Michael P. Heffernan, M.D.
Emergency Medicine . . . . Glenn C. Hamilton, M.D.
Family Medicine . . . . Mark E. Clasen, M.D., Ph.D.
Geriatric Medicine. . . . . Larry Lawhorne, M.D.
Medicine. . . . . Glen D. Solomon, M.D.
   Cardiology . . . . Ajay Agarwal, M.D.

Endocrinology . . . . Thomas Koroscil, M.D., Ph.D.
Gastroenterology . . . . Gregory Beck, M.D.
General Internal Medicine . . . . W. Scott Richardson, M.D.
Hematology and Oncology . . . . Michael Baumann, M.D.
Infectious Disease . . . . John S. Czachor, M.D.
Nephrology . . . . Mohammed Saklayen, M.D.
Neurology . . . . Bradley Jacobs, M.D.
Nuclear Medicine . . . . Joseph C. Mantil, M.D., Ph.D.
Pulmonary . . . . Jeffrey Y. Schnader, M.D.
Rheumatology . . . . William E. Venanzi, M.D.
Obstetrics and Gynecology . . . . Gary Ventolini, M.D.
Gynecologic Oncology . . . . Thomas Reid, M.D.
Gynecology . . . . Mark C. Bidwell, M.D.
Maternal and Fetal Medicine . . . . Christopher Croom, M.D.
Reproductive Endocrinology . . . . Lawrence Amesse, M.D., Ph.D.
Research . . . . Open
Orthopaedic Surgery, Sports Medicine, and Rehabilitation . . . . Richard T. Laughlin, M.D.
Pathology . . . . L. David Mirkin, M.D.
Pediatrics . . . . Arthur Pickoff, M.D.
Cardiology . . . . Joseph Ross, M.D.
Endocrinology and Metabolism . . . . Maria D. Urban, M.D.
Gastroenterology and Nutritional Support . . . . Adam G. Mezoff, M.D.
General and Community Pediatrics . . . . John Pascoe, M.D.
Hematology and Oncology . . . . Emmett Broxson, M.D.
Infectious Disease . . . . Sherman J. Alter, M.D.
Medical Genetics . . . . Marvin Miller, M.D.
Neurology . . . . Daniel J. Lacey, M.D., Ph.D.
Pulmonary Medicine and Cystic Fibrosis . . . . Robert Fink, M.D.
Psychiatry . . . . Jerald Kay, M.D.
Surgery . . . . Alex G. Little, M.D.
Anesthesiology . . . . Nancy Kwon, M.D.
Cardiovascular and Thoracic . . . . Mark P. Anstadt, M.D.
General Surgery . . . . Linda M. Barney, M.D.
Neurosurgery . . . . Cynthia Africk, M.D.
Ophthalmology . . . . Michael J. Besson, M.D.
Otolaryngology . . . . Robert A. Goldenberg, M.D.
Pediatric Surgery . . . . David Meagher, M.D.
Plastic Surgery . . . . R. Michael Johnson, M.D.
Surgical Oncology . . . . Paula Termuhlen, M.D.
Trauma Surgery . . . . Mary C. McCarthy, M.D.
Urology . . . . Open
Vascular . . . . Eugene Simoni, M.D.

University of Oklahoma College of Medicine

P.O. Box 26901, BMSB 357
Oklahoma City, Oklahoma 73126
405-271-2265 (dean's office); 271-3032 (fax)
Web site: www.medicine.ouhsc.edu

The college of medicine is one of seven health professions colleges that make up the University of Oklahoma Health Sciences Center, located 20 miles from its main campus in Norman. The college of medicine was established in 1900 as a two-year preclinical college and merged in 1910 with the Epworth Medical College in Oklahoma City to become a four-year degree-granting college.

Type: public
2008-2009 total enrollment: 646
Clinical facilities: OU Medical Center, Children's Hospital, Veterans Affairs Medical Center, Integris Baptist Medical Center, Saint Anthony Hospital, Bone and Joint Hospital, Griffin Memorial Hospital (Norman), Bass Memorial Hospital (Enid), St. Mary's Hospital (Enid).

University Officials

President. . . . . David L. Boren
Senior Vice President and Provost . . . . Joseph J. Ferretti, Ph.D.
Vice President for Health Affairs . . . . M. Dewayne Andrews, M.D.
Vice President for Administrative Affairs. . . . . Kenneth D. Rowe
Vice President for Research . . . . Joseph L. Waner, Ph.D.

Medical School Administrative Staff

Executive Dean . . . . M. Dewayne Andrews, M.D.
Senior Associate Dean . . . . Robert H. Roswell, M.D.
Associate Dean for Medical Education . . . . Chris Candler, M.D.
Associate Dean for Student Affairs . . . . Phebe Tucker, M.D.
Associate Dean for Graduate Medical Education . . . . John Zubialde, M.D.
Associate Dean for Faculty Development. . . . . Valerie N. Williams, Ph.D.
Associate Dean for Administration and Finance . . . . Anne Barnes
Associate Dean for Clinical Affairs . . . . C. Douglas Folger, M.D.
Associate Dean for Clinical Practice . . . . Brian L. Maddy
Associate Dean for VA Hospital Affairs . . . . D. Robert McCaffree, M.D.
Assistant Dean for Continuing Medical Education. . . . . Roger Sheldon, M.D.

Department and Division or Section Chairs

Basic Sciences

Biochemistry and Molecular Biology. . . . . Paul H. Weigel, Ph.D.
Cell Biology. . . . . Lawrence I. Rothblum, Ph.D.
Microbiology and Immunology. . . . . John J. Iandolo, Ph.D.
Pathology . . . . Michael Talbert, M.D.
Physiology . . . . Robert D. Foreman, Ph.D.

Clinical Sciences

Anesthesiology. . . . . Jane C. K. Fitch, M.D.
Dermatology . . . . Ray Cornelison, Jr., M.D.
Family Medicine . . . . Steven Crawford, M.D.
Geriatric Medicine. . . . . Marie A. Bernard, M.D.
Medicine. . . . . Michael Bronze, M.D.
  Cardiology. . . . . Dwight Reynolds, M.D.
  Digestive Disease and Nutrition. . . . . Courtney W. Houchen, M.D.
  Endocrinology and Diabetes . . . . Timothy Lyons, M.D.
  General Internal Medicine . . . . Michael Bronze, M.D.
  Hematology-Oncology . . . . Howard Ozer, M.D., Ph.D.
  Rheumatology, Immunology, and Allergy . . . . John B. Harley, M.D., Ph.D.
  Infectious Diseases . . . . Douglas Drevets, M.D.
  Nephrology . . . . Benjamin Cowley, Jr., M.D.
  Pulmonary Disease . . . . Gary T. Kinasewitz, M.D.
Neurology. . . . . David Lee Gordon, M.D.
Neurosurgery. . . . . Timothy Mapstone, M.D.

Obstetrics and Gynecology . . . . Robert S. Mannel, M.D.
   Gynecologic Oncology . . . . D. Scott McMeekin, M.D.
   Maternal and Fetal Medicine . . . . Eric Knudtson, M.D.
   Reproductive Endocrinology and Infertility . . . . Karl Hansen, M.D.
Ophthalmology . . . . David W. Parke II, M.D.
Orthopaedic Surgery and Rehabilitation . . . . David C. Teague, M.D.
Otorhinolaryngology . . . . Jesus Medina, M.D.
Pediatrics . . . . Terrence L. Stull, M.D.
   Adolescent Medicine . . . . Philip W. Rettig, M.D.
   Cardiology . . . . Ed Overholt, M.D.
   Critical Care . . . . Morris R. Gessouroun, M.D.
   Developmental and Behavioral Pediatrics . . . . Mark Wolraich, M.D.
   Diabetes and Endocrinology . . . . Kenneth Copeland, M.D.
   Gastroenterology . . . . John E. Grunow, M.D.
   General and Community Pediatrics . . . . Terrence S. Stull, M.D. (Interim)
   Genetics . . . . John Mulvihill, M.D.
   Hematology and Oncology . . . . William Meyer, M.D.
   Infectious Disease . . . . V. SanJoaquin, M.D.
   Neonatology . . . . Marilyn Escobedo, M.D.
   Nephrology . . . . Martin Turman, M.D.
   Pulmonology and Cystic Fibrosis . . . . James Royall, M.D.
   Rheumatology . . . . James Jarvis, M.D.
Psychiatry and Behavioral Sciences . . . . Betty Pfefferbaum, M.D., J.D.
Radiation Oncology . . . . Terence S. Herman, M.D.
Radiological Sciences . . . . Susan M. Edwards, M.D.
Surgery . . . . Russell Postier, M.D.
   General Surgery . . . . Russell Postier, M.D.
   Pediatric Surgery . . . . David Tuggle, M.D.
   Plastic Surgery . . . . Kamal Sawan, M.D.
   Thoracic Surgery . . . . Marvin Peyton, M.D.
   Transplant . . . . Larry R. Pennington, M.D.
Urology . . . . Daniel J. Culkin, M.D.

University of Oklahoma College of Medicine-Tulsa
Schusterman Center
4502 East 41st Street
Tulsa, Oklahoma 74135-2553
918-660-3000; 660-3095 (dean's office); 660-3090 (fax)

The University of Oklahoma College of Medicine-Tulsa was established by legislative action in 1973. Up to 35 students each year may transfer from Oklahoma City to Tulsa after their sophomore year to complete their clinical education.
Clinical facilities: Hillcrest Medical Center, Saint Francis Hospital, St. John Medical Center, Laureate Psychiatric Clinic and Hospital, and O.U. Clinics.

Administrative Staff

Dean . . . . Gerard P. Clancy, M.D.
Senior Associate Dean for Academic Programs . . . . F. Daniel Duffy, M.D.
Senior Associate Dean for Administration and Finance . . . . Leland N. Alexander
Associate Dean for Academic Services . . . . Meredith Davison, Ph.D.
Associate Dean for Academic Development . . . . Ronald B. Saizow, M.D.
Associate Dean for Community Health and Research Development . . . . Mark Fox, M.D.
Assistant Dean for Finance . . . . Jonathan Joiner

Department Chairs

Family Medicine . . . . R. Michael Morse, M.D.
Medicine . . . . Charles J. Foulks, M.D.
Obstetrics and Gynecology . . . . Michael O. Gardner, M.D.
Pediatrics . . . . Robert W. Block, M.D.
Psychiatry . . . . Ondria Gleason, M.D.
Surgery . . . . Thomas A. Broughan, M.D.

Oregon Health & Science University School of Medicine

3181 S.W. Sam Jackson Park Road
Mailcode L102
Portland, Oregon 97239-3098
503-494-7677; 494-8220 (dean's office); 494-3400 (fax)
Web site: www.ohsu.edu/som

The University of Oregon School of Medicine in Portland, Oregon, was established in 1887. In 1913, it was merged with the medical department of Willamette University in Salem, and all students were transferred to Portland. In 1974, the schools of medicine, dentistry, and nursing were combined into the University of Oregon Health Sciences Center. The center was renamed Oregon Health & Science University in 2001.

Type: public
2008-2009 total enrollment: 512
Clinical facilities: University Hospital, Doernbecher Memorial Hospital for Children, Child Development Rehabilitation Center, Outpatient Clinics, Veterans Administration Medical Center, Emanuel Hospital and Health Center, Good Samaritan Hospital and Medical Center, Kaiser Foundation Hospitals - Northwest Region, Portland Adventist Medical Center, Providence Medical Center, Shriners Hospital for Children, St. Charles Medical Center of Bend, St. Vincent Hospital and Medical Center, Cascades East Family Practice Center at Klamath Falls, Merle West Medical Center at Klamath Falls, Family Health Centers at Gabriel Park, Richmond, Sellwood-Moreland, Beaverton, Scappoose, Hillsboro, Oregon City, University Fertility Consultants.

University Officials

President. . . . . Joseph E. Robertson, M.D.
Executive Vice President . . . . Steve Stadum, J.D.
Vice President for Finance. . . . . Brad King
Vice President for Academic Affairs and Provost. . . . . Lesley M. Hallick, Ph.D.
Vice President and Executive Director, OHSU Healthcare. . . . . Peter F. Rapp
Vice President for Government and Community Affairs. . . . . Lois L. Davis
Registrar and Director of Financial Aid. . . . . A. Cherie Honnell

Medical School Administrative Staff

Dean. . . . . Mark A. Richardson, M.D.
Vice Dean. . . . . Open
Dean-Emeritus. . . . . John A. Benson, M.D.
Dean-Emeritus. . . . . Joseph D. Bloom, M.D.
Dean-Emeritus. . . . . John W. Kendall, M.D.
Associate Dean, Basic Research. . . . . Open
Associate Dean, Clinical Affairs. . . . . Neil A. Swanson, M.D.
Associate Dean, Clinical Research. . . . . Eric Orwoll, M.D.
Associate Dean, Faculty Affairs and Development . . . . Patrician Hurn, Ph.D.
Associate Dean, Finance. . . . . Thomas G. Flora, Ed.D.
Associate Dean, Continuing Medical Education
  and Graduate Medical Education . . . . Donald E. Girard, M.D.
Associate Dean, Graduate Studies. . . . . Allison Fryer, Ph.D.
Associate Dean, Health Systems Affairs . . . . A. Roy Magnusson
Associate Dean, Medical Education. . . . . Open
Associate Dean, Planning, Administration, and Diversity Affairs. . . . . Ella C. Booth, Ph.D.
Associate Dean, Student Affairs . . . . Molly L. Osborne, M.D.
Assistant Dean, Administration and Faculty Affairs . . . . Nicole Lockart
Assistant Dean, Admissions. . . . . Cynthia D. Morris, Ph.D.
Assistant Dean, Medical Education . . . . Vicki Fields
Assistant Dean, Primary Care Education . . . . John W. Saultz, M.D.
Assistant Dean, Veterans Affairs . . . . John Dryden

Department and Division or Section Chairs

Basic Sciences

Behavioral Neuroscience . . . . Robert J. Hitzemann, Ph.D.

Biochemistry and Molecular Biology...................... Peter S. Rotwein, M.D., Ph.D.
Cell and Developmental Biology......................... Bruce E. Magun, Ph.D.
Heart Research Center.................................. Kent L. Thornburg, Ph.D.
Molecular and Medical Genetics........................ Susan Hayflick, M.D. (Interim)
Molecular Microbiology and Immunology.............. Mary Stenzel-Poore, Ph.D. (Interim)
Physiology and Pharmacology.......................... David C. Dawson, Ph.D.
Science and Engineering .... Ed W. Thompson, Ph.D.

Clinical Sciences

Anesthesiology and Perioperative Medicine........................... Jeffrey Kirsch, M.D.
Center for Women's Health.............................. Joanna M. Cain, M.D.
Dermatology .... Neil A. Swanson, M.D.
Diagnostic Radiology................................... Frederick S. Keller, M.D.
    Nuclear Medicine.................................. Jeffrey S. Stevens, M.D.
Dotter Interventional Institute .... Frederick S. Keller, M.D.
Emergency Medicine.................................... O. John Ma, M.D.
Family Medicine .... John W. Saultz, M.D.
Medical Informatics and Clinical Epidemiology.................. William R. Hersh, M.D.
Medicine... D. Lynn Loriaux, M.D., Ph.D.
    Allergy and Clinical Immunology .... Anthony Montanaro, M.D. (Interim)
    Arthritis and Rheumatic Diseases .... James T. Rosenbaum, M.D.
    Cardiovascular Medicine.............................. Sanjiv Kaul, M.D.
    Endocrinology, Diabetes, and Clinical Nutrition .... David D. Cook, M.D. (Interim)
    Gastroenterology .... David A. Lieberman, M.D.
    General Internal Medicine and Geriatrics .... Judith Bowen, M.D.
    Health Promotion and Sports Medicine .... Linn Goldberg, M.D.
    Hematology and Medical Oncology........................... Michael Heinrich, M.D.
    Hospital Medicine .... Alan J. Hunter, M.D.
    Infectious Diseases .... Brian Wong, M.D.
    Nephrology and Hypertension .... David H. Ellison, M.D.
    Pulmonary and Critical Care Medicine .... David B. Jacoby, M.D.
Neurological Surgery................................... Kim J. Burchiel, M.D.
Neurology... Dennis N. Bourdette, M.D.
Obstetrics and Gynecology.............................. Joanna M. Cain, M.D.
OHSU Cancer Institute .... Brian Druker, M.D.
Ophthalmology .... David Wilson, M.D.
Orthopaedics and Rehabilitation .... Jung Yoo, M.D.
Otolaryngology, Head, and Neck Surgery .... Ted Cook, M.D. (Acting)
Pathology .... Douglas Weeks, M.D.
    Anatomic Pathology................................ Ken Gatter, M.D.
    Laboratory Medicine .... James D. MacLowry, M.D.
Pediatrics .... H. Stacy Nicholson, M.D.
    Developmental Pediatrics .... Brian T. Rogers, M.D.
    Pediatric Cardiology.............................. Mark D. Reller, M.D.
    Pediatric Neurology .... Thomas K. Koch, M.D.
Physician Assistant Education Division .... Ted Ruback
Psychiatry .... George A. Keepers, M.D.
    Child and Adolescent Psychiatry .... Robert S. McKelvay, M.D.
    Clinical Psychiatry .... George A. Keepers, M.D.
Public Health and Preventive Medicine .... Thomas M. Becker, M.D.
Radiation Medicine .... Charles R. Thomas, M.D.
Surgery .... John G. Hunter, M.D.
    Cardiothoracic Surgery............................ Ross Ungerleider, M.D.
    General Surgery............................. Robert G. Martindale, M.D. (Interim)
    Liver and Pancreas Transplantation .... John G. Hunter, M.D. (Interim)
    Oral and Maxillofacial Surgery .... Leon Assael, D.M.D.
    Pediatric Surgery .... Mark L. Silen, M.D.
    Plastic and Reconstructive Surgery .... Juliana E. Hansen, M.D.
    Surgical Oncology .... Kevin G. Billingsley, M.D.
    Urology.. John M. Barry, M.D.
    Vascular Surgery................................. Gregory L. Moneta, M.D.

Drexel University College of Medicine (Formerly MCP Hahnemann School of Medicine)

245 North 15th Street, MS400
Philadelphia, Pennsylvania 19102
215-991-8560; 991-8566; 843-0214 (ed. & acad. affrs.); 762-8900 (fax);
762-3500 (dean's office);
Web site: www.drexelmed.edu

Drexel University College of Medicine represents the union of the Women's Medical College of Pennsylvania and Hahnemann Medical College, whose roots go back 157 years. In 2002, the combined medical schools—then MCP-Hahnemann-merged with Drexel University, a 100-year-old institution recognized for its focus on technology across the curriculum. Fostering interdisciplinary research between the college of medicine and its other schools and colleges is a university priority.

Type: private
2008-2009 total enrollment: 1,010
Clinical facilities: Abington Memorial Hospital, Allegheny General Hospital, Atlantic Health System, Capital Health System, Forbes Regional Hospital, Eagleville Hospital, Graduate Hospital, Hahnemann University Hospital, Holy Redeemer Hospital and Medical Center, Lehigh Valley Hospital, Medical College of Pennsylvania Hospital, Warminster Hospital, Wyoming Valley Health Care System, St. Christopher's Hospital for Children, Crozer-Chester Medical Center, Easton Hospital, Friends Hospital, Hamot Medical Center, Mercy Catholic Medical Center, Monmouth Medical Center, Pinnacle Hospitals, Montgomery Hospital,Chestnut Hill Hospital, Reading Hospital and Medical Center, St. Peter's University Hospital, Wilkes-Barre Veterans Affairs Medical Center, York Hospital.

University Officials

President. . . . . Constantine Papadakis, Ph.D.
Provost . . . . Mark L. Greenberg, Ph.D. (Interim)
Senior Vice President for Finance and Treasurer . . . . Thomas Elzey
Dean, College of Medicine. . . . . Richard V. Homan, M.D.
Dean, College of Nursing and Health Professions . . . . Gloria Donnelly, Ph.D.
Dean, School of Public Health . . . . Marla Gold, M.D.

Medical School Administrative Staff

Senior Vice President for Health Affairs . . . . Richard Homan, M.D.
Dean. . . . . Richard Homan, M.D.
Associate Dean, External Relations and Strategic Development . . . . Claire A. Tillman
Director of Deans Services . . . . Dyanne J. Glass
Vice Dean, Educational and Academic Affairs. . . . . Barbara A. Schindler, M.D.
  Associate Dean, Admissions. . . . . Cheryl Hanau, M.D.
  Associate Dean, Assessment and Evaluation . . . . Burton J. Landau, Ph.D.
  Associate Dean, Clincal Skills, Education, and Assessment . . . . Dennis H. Novack, M.D.
  Associate Dean, Community Outreach Programs . . . . Vincent Zarro, M.D.
  Assistant Dean, Continuing Medical Education . . . . Cynthia Johnson
  Associate Dean, Information Technology. . . . . Arnold Smolen, Ph.D.
  Assistant Dean, Interdisciplinary Foundations of Medicine . . . . Donna Russo, Ph.D.
  Associate Dean, Student Affairs and Diversity. . . . . Anthony Rodriguez, M.D.
  Associate Dean, Program for Integrated Learning . . . . Susan Zern, M.D.
  Associate Dean, Student Affairs. . . . . Samuel K. Parrish, Jr., M.D.
  Associate Dean, Planning and Operations . . . . Simon W. Abrahms
  Associate Dean, Faculty Affairs and Professional Development . . . . Mary Moran, M.D.
  Senior Associate Dean, Student Affairs and
    Medical Education (AGH) . . . . James Wilberger, M.D.
  Vice Dean for Research . . . . Kenny J. Simansky, Ph.D.
  Vice Dean for Biomedical Graduate Studies. . . . . Barry Waterhouse, Ph.D.
Director of Graduate Medical Education and
  Designated Institutional Official . . . . Jay Yanoff, Ed.D.
  Associate Dean, Graduate Medical Education . . . . Mark Woodland, M.D.

Drexel University College of Medicine (Formerly MCP Hahnemann School of Medicine): PENNSYLVANIA

Department Chairs

Basic Sciences

Biochemistry . . . . Jane Clifford, Ph.D.
Microbiology and Immunology. . . . . Brian Wigdahl, Ph.D.
Neurobiology and Anatomy . . . . Itzhak Fischer, Ph.D.
Pharmacology and Physiology. . . . . John Harvey, Ph.D.

Clinical Sciences

Anesthesiology. . . . . Mian Ahmad, M.D. (Interim)
Cardiovascular Medicine and Surgery. . . . . Andrew S. Wechsler, M.D.
Dermatology . . . . Herbert Allen, M.D.
Emergency Medicine . . . . Richard Hamilton, M.D.
Family, Community, and Preventive Medicine. . . . . Eugene Hong, M.D.
Medicine. . . . . James C. Reynolds, M.D.
Neurology. . . . . Robert J. Schwartzman, M.D.
Obstetrics and Gynecology. . . . . Owen Montgomery, M.D.
Ophthalmology . . . . Myron Yanoff, M.D.
Orthopedic Surgery. . . . . Norman Johanson, M.D.
Otolaryngology-Head and Neck Surgery . . . . Robert Sataloff, M.D.
Pathology and Laboratory Medicine . . . . J. Steve Hou, M.D.
Pediatrics . . . . Daniel V. Schidlow, M.D.
Psychiatry . . . . Susan McLeer, M.D.
Radiation Oncology. . . . . Lydia Komarnicky, M.D.
Radiologic Sciences . . . . Michael Hallowell, M.D.
Surgery. . . . . William C. Meyers, M.D.

Centers and Institute

Director, Institute for Women's Health. . . . . Lynne Yeakel

Jefferson Medical College of Thomas Jefferson University

1025 Walnut Street
Philadelphia, Pennsylvania 19107-5083
215-955-6000; 955-6980 (dean's office); 503-2654 (fax)
E-mail: dean.jmc@mail.tju.edu
Web site: www.tju.edu

Jefferson Medical College was established in 1824; classes have been graduated annually since 1826. It is privately controlled, nondenominational, and coeducational. On July 1, 1969, Thomas Jefferson University was established with the Jefferson Medical College as one of its colleges.

Type: private
2008-2009 total enrollment: 999
Clinical facilities: Thomas Jefferson University Hospital, Thomas Jefferson University Hospital—Methodist Division. **Affiliated hospitals:** Abington Memorial Hospital, A. I. duPont Hospital for Children, Albert Einstein Medical Center, Bryn Mawr Hospital, Christiana Care Health Services, Excela Health Latrobe Hospital, Frankford Hospital, Lankenau Hospital, Magee Rehabilitation Hospital, Mercy Hospital of Pittsburgh, Reading Hospital and Medical Center, Underwood Memorial Hospital, Virtua West Jersey Hospital, Wilmington Veterans Affairs Medical Center, York Hospital.

University Officials

President. . . . . Robert L. Barchi, M.D., Ph.D.
Dean and Senior Vice President. . . . . Michael J. Vergare, M.D. (Interim)
Dean, Jefferson College of Graduate Studies. . . . . James H. Keen, Ph.D.
Dean, Jefferson College of Health Professions. . . . . James B. Erdmann, Ph.D.

Medical School Administrative Staff

Dean. . . . . Michael J. Vergare, M.D. (Interim)
Chief of Staff and Senior Associate Dean, Organizational Development. . . . . Open
Chief Operating Officer. . . . . John Ogunkeye
Senior Associate Dean, Clinical Affairs . . . . William M. Keane, M.D.
Associate Dean, Cancer-related Services . . . . Richard G. Pestell, M.D., Ph.D.
The Lillian H. Brent Dean of Students and Admissions. . . . . Clara A. Callahan, M.D.
   Associate Dean, Student Affairs and Career Counseling . . . . Charles A. Pohl, M.D.
   Assistant Dean, Student Affairs and Career Counseling. . . . . Kristin L. DeSimone, M.D.
   Assistant Dean, Student Affairs and Career Counseling. . . . . Bernard L. Lopez, M.D.
   Assistant Dean, Student Affairs and Career Counseling. . . . . John M. Spandorfer, M.D.
Senior Associate Dean, Continuing Medical
   Education, and Faculty and Alumni Affairs . . . . Joseph L. Seltzer, M.D.
Associate Dean, Alumni Relations, Executive
   Director of Alumni Association . . . . Phillip J. Marone, M.D.
Associate Dean, Faculty Affairs and Faculty Development. . . . . Karen D. Novielli, M.D.
Senior Associate Dean, Graduate Medical
   Education and Affiliations . . . . David L. Paskin, M.D.
   Assistant Dean, Graduate Medical Education . . . . John Caruso, M.D.
   Assistant Dean, Graduate Medical Education . . . . John Kairys, M.D.
Senior Associate Dean, Academic Affairs/
   Undergraduate Medical Education . . . . Susan L. Rattner, M.D., F.A.C.P.
Associate Dean, Academic Affairs/
   Undergraduate Medical Education . . . . Karen M. Glaser, Ph.D.
Associate Dean, Academic Affairs/
   Undergraduate Medical Education . . . . Steven K. Herrine, M.D.
Associate Dean, Diversity and Minority Affairs. . . . . Edward B. Christian, Ph.D.
   Assistant Dean, Diversity and Minority Affairs . . . . Luz Ortiz
Assistant Dean, Medical Education, Albert Einstein Medical Center . . . . . . Douglas McGee, D.O.
Assistant Dean, Medical Education, Mercy Hospital of Pittsburgh. . . . . Irv Freeman, Ph.D.
Assistant Dean, Medical Education, Christiana Care . . . . Brian W. Little, M.D.
Assistant Dean, Medical Education, Main Line Health. . . . . James F. Burke, M.D.
Chief Executive of the Practice, Nemours
   Children's Clinic-Wilmington/A.I. duPont
   Hospital for Children . . . . Bernard J. Clark, M.D.

Jefferson Medical College of Thomas Jefferson University: PENNSYLVANIA

Director, Center for Research in Medical
Education and Health Care . . . . Joseph S. Gonnella, M.D.

Department and Division or Section Chairs

Basic Sciences

Biochemistry and Molecular Pharmacology. . . . . Jeffrey Benovic, Ph.D.
Cancer Biology . . . . Richard G. Pestell, M.D., Ph.D.
Microbiology and Immunology. . . . . Timothy Manser, Ph.D.
Molecular Physiology and Biophysics . . . . Marion J. Siegman, Ph.D.
Pathology . . . . Fred Gorstein, M.D.
Pharmacology and Experimental Therapeutics . . . . Scott Waldman, M.D., Ph.D.

Clinical Sciences

Anesthesiology. . . . . Zvi Grunwald, M.D.
Dermatology and Cutaneous Biology . . . . Jouni J. Uitto, M.D., Ph.D.
Emergency Medicine . . . . Theodore A. Christopher, M.D.
Family and Community Medicine. . . . . Richard C. Wender, M.D.
Health Policy. . . . . David B. Nash, M.D.
Medical Oncology . . . . Neal Flomenberg, M.D.
Medicine. . . . . Arthur M. Feldman, M.D., Ph.D.
Neurology. . . . . Abdolmohamad Rostami, M.D., Ph.D.
Neurosurgery. . . . . Robert H. Rosenwasser, M.D.
Obstetrics and Gynecology. . . . . Louis Weinstein, M.D.
Ophthalmology. . . . . Julia A. Haller, M.D.
Orthopaedic Surgery. . . . . Todd J. Albert, M.D.
Otolaryngology-Head and Neck Surgery . . . . William M. Keane, M.D.
Pediatrics . . . . Jay S. Greenspan, M.D.
Psychiatry and Human Behavior. . . . . Michael J. Vergare, M.D.
Radiation Oncology. . . . . Adam P. Dicker, M.D. (Interim)
Radiology . . . . Vijay M. Rao, M.D.
Rehabilitation Medicine. . . . . John L. Melvin, M.D.
Surgery. . . . . Charles J. Yeo, M.D.
Urology. . . . . Leonard G. Gomella, M.D., F.A.C.S.

Institute Directors

Farber Institute for Neurosciences . . . . Lorraine Iacovitti, Ph.D. (Interim)
Kimmel Cancer Institute . . . . Richard G. Pestell, M.D., Ph.D.

Pennsylvania State University College of Medicine

500 University Drive
P.O. Box 850
Hershey, Pennsylvania 17033
717-531-8521; 531-8323 (dean's office); 531-5351 (fax)
E-mail: hpaz@psu.edu
Web site: www.hmc.psu.edu

The Milton S. Hershey Medical Center of the Pennsylvania State University was established in August 1963 and admitted its first class of medical students in 1967. Located on a 549-acre campus on the western edge of Hershey, the medical center is 12 miles from the state capital, Harrisburg, and approximately 105 miles from the university's main campus at University Park.

Type: public
2008-2009 total enrollment: 579
Clinical facilities: A 504-bed university hospital is located on the campus as part of a single, continuous structure housing both the hospital and the Medical Sciences Building. Core clinical clerkships and elective clerkships are given at the medical center hospital and at affiliated hospitals.

University Officials

President. . . . . Graham B. Spanier

Medical School Administrative Staff

Senior Vice President for Health Affairs and Dean . . . . Harold L. Paz, M.D.
Associate Vice President for Health Finance and Business and Controller . . . . . Wayne W. Zolko
Vice Dean for Clinical Affairs. . . . . A. Craig Hillemeier, M.D.
Vice Dean for Faculty and Administrative Affairs. . . . . R. Kevin Grigsby, D.S.W.
Vice Dean for Educational Affairs. . . . . Richard J. Simons, M.D.
Vice Dean for Research Affairs. . . . . Alan J. Snyder, Ph.D. (Interim)
Associate Dean for Academic Achievement. . . . . Alphonse E. Leure-duPree, Ph.D.
Associate Dean for Primary Care . . . . James M. Herman, M.D.
Associate Dean for Admissions and Student Affairs . . . . Dwight Davis, M.D.
Associate Dean for Education (Lehigh Valley Hospital). . . . . Vacant
Associate Dean for Graduate Studies . . . . Michael Verderame, Ph.D.
Associate Dean for Graduate Medical Education. . . . . Ronald Domen, M.D.
Associate Dean for Clinical Education . . . . Maryellen E. Gusic, M.D.
Associate Dean for Technology and Development. . . . . Alan J. Snyder, Ph.D.
Associate Dean for Basic Science Research . . . . Sheila L. Vrana, Ph.D.
Associate Dean for Professional Development . . . . Luanne E. Thorndyke, M.D.
Associate Dean for Preclinical Curriculum . . . . Carol Whitfield, Ph.D.
Associate Dean for Medical Education (York Hospital) . . . . Richard Sloan, M.D.
Associate Dean for Clinical Science Research . . . . Thomas Terndrup, M.D.
Associate Vice President for Development. . . . . Kristen B. Rozansky

Department and Division or Section Chairs
Basic Sciences

Biochemistry and Molecular Biology. . . . . Judith S. Bond, Ph.D.
Cellular and Molecular Physiology . . . . Leonard S. Jefferson, Ph.D.
Comparative Medicine . . . . Ronald P. Wilson, V.M.D.
Public Health Sciences. . . . . Vernon M. Chincilli, Ph.D.
Humanities . . . . John Neely, M.D. (Interim)
Microbiology and Immunology. . . . . Richard J. Courtney, Ph.D.
Neural and Behavioral Sciences . . . . Colin J. Barnstable, D.Phil.
Pharmacology . . . . Kent Vrana, Ph.D.

Clinical Sciences

Anesthesiology. . . . . Berend Mets, M.B., Ch.B., Ph.D.
Cardiac Anesthesia . . . . Kane High, M.D.
Critical Care Medicine . . . . John K. Stene, Jr., M.D., Ph.D., and Kane High, M.D.
Pain Medicine . . . . Vitaly Gordin, M.D.
Pediatric Anesthesia . . . . Patrick McQillan, M.D.
Regional Anesthesia . . . . J. Eric Greensmith, M.D.
Simulation Development and Cognitive Science . . . . Elizabeth Sinz, M.D.
Dermatology . . . . James Marks, M.D.
Emergency Medicine . . . . Thomas Terndrup, M.D.
Family and Community Medicine. . . . . James M. Herman, M.D.
Medicine. . . . . Robert C. Aber, M.D.
Cardiology . . . . Gerald V. Naccarelli, M.D.

190

Endocrinology . . . . Andrea Manni, M.D.
Gastroenterology . . . . Thomas J. McGarrity, M.D.
Hematology and Oncology . . . . David Claxton, M.D. (Interim)
Infectious Diseases . . . . Leslie J. Parent, M.D.
Internal Medicine. . . . . Christopher N. Sciamanna, M.D.
Pulmonary. . . . . Kevin Gleeson, M.D. (Interim)
Renal Medicine . . . . William Reeves, M.D.
Rheumatology . . . . Barbara E. Ostrov, M.D.
Neurology. . . . . David C. Good, M.D.
Neurosurgery. . . . . Robert E. Harbaugh, M.D.
Obstetrics, Gynecology, and Women's Health . . . . John T. Repke, M.D.
Gynecologic Oncology . . . . Edward Podczaski, M.D. (Interim)
Maternal and Fetal Medicine . . . . Serdar H. Ural, M.D.
Reproductive Endocrinology. . . . . William C. Dodson, M.D.
Women's Health . . . . Matthew F. Davies, M.D.
Ophthalmology. . . . . David Quillen, M.D.
Orthopaedics and Rehabilitation . . . . Kevin Black, M.D.
Pathology . . . . Dani S. Zander, M.D.
Anatomic Pathology. . . . . Catherine S. Abendroth, M.D.
Clinical Laboratories . . . . Michael B. Bongiovanni, M.D.
Pediatrics . . . . A. Craig Hillemeier, M.D.
Adolescent Medicine . . . . Richard Levine, M.D.
Cardiology. . . . . Stephen E. Cyran, M.D.
Critical Care. . . . . Steven E. Lucking, M.D.
Endocrinology . . . . Steven Wassner, M.D. (Interim)
Gastroenterology and Nutrition . . . . Douglas Field, M.D.
General Pediatrics . . . . Mark Widome, M.D. (Interim)
Genetics. . . . . Roger Ladda, M.D.
Hematology and Oncology. . . . . Barbara Miller, M.D.
Infectious Diseases . . . . John H. Dossett, M.D.
Nephrology . . . . Steven J. Wassner, M.D.
Neurology . . . . William Trescher, M.D.
Newborn Medicine. . . . . Charles Palmer, M.D.
Pulmonology . . . . Gavin Graff, M.D.
Rheumatology . . . . Barbara E. Ostrov, M.D.
Psychiatry . . . . James Hegarty, M.D. (Interim)
Anxiety, Stress, and Trauma . . . . Deborah Beidel, Ph.D.
Behavioral Health Clinic. . . . . Steven Sinderman, M.D.
Behavioral Neuroimaging . . . . Gregory J. Moore, M.D.
Education and Training Programs. . . . . Errol M. Aksu, M.D.
Molecular Neuropharmacology Research. . . . . John Ellis, Ph.D.
Sleep Medicine Research . . . . Edward O. Bixler, Ph.D.
Child and Adolescent Psychiatry . . . . Michael Murray, M.D.
Radiology . . . . Kathleen Dunne Eggli, M.D.
Abdominal Imaging . . . . Thomas Dykes, M.D.
CVI . . . . Peter N. Waybill, M.D.
Diagnostic Radiology . . . . Rickhesvar P.M. Mahraj, M.D.
Musculoskeletal . . . . Timothy J. Mosher, M.D.
Health Physics . . . . Kenneth L. Miller
Neuroradiology . . . . Dan Nguyen, M.D.
Nuclear Medicine. . . . . Douglas F. Eggli, M.D.
Pediatric Radiology. . . . . Danielle K. Boal, M.D.
Radiation Oncology . . . . Henry Wagner, M.D.
Thoracic Imaging. . . . . Rickhesvar R.M. Mahraj, M.D.
Surgery . . . . Peter W. Dillon, M.D.
Cardiothoracic Surgery. . . . . Walter E. Pae, Jr., M.D.
Colon and Rectal Surgery. . . . . Walter Koltun, M.D.
General Surgery . . . . Robert N. Cooney, M.D.
Otolaryngology-Head and Neck Surgery . . . . Fred Fedok, M.D.
Pediatric Surgery . . . . Robert E. Cilley, M.D.
Plastic and Reconstructive Surgery . . . . Donald Mackay, M.D.
Transplantation . . . . Zakiyah Kadry, M.D.
Trauma and Critical Care. . . . . Robert A. Cherry, M.D.
Vascular Surgery. . . . . Robert G. Atnip, M.D.
Urology . . . . Ross M. Decter, M.D.
Surgical Oncology . . . . Gordon L. Kauffman, Jr., M.D.

Temple University School of Medicine

3420 North Broad Street
Philadelphia, Pennsylvania 19140
215-707-7000; 707-8773 (dean's office); 707-8431 (fax)
E-mail: tusmdean@temple.edu
Web site: www.temple.edu/medschool

The school of medicine was opened as a department of Temple University in 1901.

Type: private
2008-2009 total enrollment: 716
Clinical facilities: Major facilities—Abington Memorial Hospital, Crozer-Chester Medical Center, Western Pennsylvania, Conemaugh Valley Memorial Hospital (Johnstown), Fox Chase Cancer Center, Geisinger Health System, Jeanes Hospital, Lancaster General Hospital, Lehigh Valley Medical Center, Mercy Hospital (Scranton), Moses Taylor Hospital (Scranton), Montgomery Hospital (Norristown), Moss Rehabilitation Hospital, Reading Hospital and Medical Center, St. Francis Hospital (Wilmington), St. Luke's Hospital (Bethlehem), Sacred Heart Hospital (Allentown), Shriner's Hospital for Children, Temple University Children's Medical Center, Temple University Hospital.

University Officials

President. . . . . Ann Weaver Hart, Ph.D.
Provost . . . . Lisa Staiano-Coico, Ph.D.
Senior Executive Vice President of Health Sciences. . . . . Edmond F. Notebaert
President and Chief Executive Officer, Temple
    University Health System . . . . Joseph W. Marshall III

Medical School Administrative Staff

Dean. . . . . John M. Daly, M.D.
Executive Associate Dean. . . . . Richard J. Kozera, M.D.
    Assistant Dean and Director of the RAR Program . . . . Raul A. Dela Cadena, M.D.
Senior Associate Dean for Education . . . . Ronald F. Tuma, Ph.D.
    Associate Dean for Admissions . . . . Audrey Uknis, M.D.
    Associate Dean for Student Affairs . . . . Kathleen Reeves, M.D.
    Associate Dean for Medical Education. . . . . Gerald H. Sterling, Ph.D.
    Associate Dean for Graduate Studies. . . . . Barrie Ashby, Ph.D.
    Associate Dean for the M.D./Ph.D. Program . . . . Dianne Soprano, Ph.D.
    Assistant Dean for Academic Affiliations . . . . Stephen R. Permut, M.D., J.D.
        Assistant Dean for Affiliate and Liaison Activities . . . . William F. Schulze
Senior Associate Dean for Research . . . . Richard Coico, Ph.D.
Senior Associate Dean for Faculty Affairs . . . . Joanne M. Orth, Ph.D.
Vice Dean for Finance and Administration and
    Executive Director, Temple University
    Physicians . . . . Thomas Kupp
    Chief Operating Officer, Temple University Physicians . . . . Lisa Fino
Vice Dean for Information Technology, School
    of Medicine, and Chief Information Officer,
    Temple University Physicians . . . . Frank Erdlen
Associate Dean at Abington Memorial Hospital. . . . . David Gary Smith, M.D.
Associate Dean at Crozer Chester Medical Center. . . . . Susan L. Williams, M.D.
Associate Dean at Geisinger Medical Center . . . . Linda Famiglio, M.D.
Associate Dean at St. Luke's Hospital . . . . Joel C. Rosenfeld, M.D.
Associate Dean at Western Pennsylvania Hospital . . . . Elliot Goldberg, M.D.
Assistant Dean, Continuing Medical Education . . : . . . . Melinda M. Somasekhar, Ph.D.
Assistant Dean for Institutional Advancement . . . . Eric Abel
Assistant Dean for Minority Affairs . . . . Donald Parks, M.D.
Vice Dean for Clinical Operations . . . . Vacant
Director, Center for Minority Health . . . . Ala S. Frey, M.D.
Director of Bioresources . . . . Milton April, D.V.M.
Director, Health Sciences Library. . . . . Mark-Allen Taylor

Department Chairs and Section Chiefs

Basic Science Departments and Research Centers

Anatomy and Cell Biology . . . . Steven N. Popoff, Ph.D.
Biochemistry . . . . Donald Gill, Ph.D.
Cardiovascular Research Center . . . . Steven Houser, Ph.D.
Center for Substance Abuse . . . . Martin Adler, Ph.D.
Fels Institute for Cancer Research and Molecular Biology . . . . E. Premkumar Reddy, Ph.D.
Microbiology and Immunology. . . . . Doina Ganea, Ph.D.
Pathology and Laboratory Medicine . . . . Yuri Persidsky, M.D.
Pharmacology . . . . Nae Dun, Ph.D.
Physiology. . . . . Steven Houser, Ph.D.
Thrombosis Research Center . . . . A. Koneti Rao, M.D.

Clinical Science Departments

Anesthesiology. . . . . Rodger Barnette, M.D.
Emergency Medicine . . . . Robert McNamara, M.D.
Family Practice and Community Health . . . . Stephen R. Permut, M.D.
Internal Medicine . . . . Joel Richter, M.D.
   Cardiology. . . . . Jose C. Missri, M.D.
   Endocrinology and Metabolism. . . . . Guenther H. Boden, M.D.
   Gastroenterology . . . . Robert S. Fisher, M.D.
   General Internal Medicine . . . . Lawrence Kaplan, M.D.
   Hematology. . . . . A. Koneti Rao, M.D.
   Infectious Diseases . . . . Thomas Fekete, M.D.
   Nephrology . . . . Patricio Silva, M.D. (Acting)
   Oncology. . . . . Richard II. Creech, M.D.
   Pulmonary Diseases . . . . Gerard J. Criner, M.D.
   Rheumatology . . . . Philip Cohen, M.D.
Neurology. . . . . S. Ausim Azizi, M.D.
Neurosurgery. . . . . Christopher Loftus, M.D.
Obstetrics, Gynecology, and Reproductive Science . . . . Enrique Hernandez, M.D.
Ophthalmology. . . . . Jeffrey Henderer, M.D.
Orthopedic Surgery. . . . . Joseph Thoder, M.D.
Otorhinolaryngology-Head and Neck Surgery . . . . Wasyl Szeremeta, M.D. (Acting)
Pediatrics . . . . Stephen Aronoff, M.D.
   Ambulatory Pediatrics. . . . . Stephen Aronoff, M.D. (Acting)
   Critical Care Pediatrics. . . . . Barry Evans, M.D.
   Hospital-based Pediatrics . . . . Michael Del Vecchio, M.D.
Physical Medicine and Rehabilitation . . . . Ian Maitin, M.D.
Psychiatry and Behavioral Science . . . . David Baron, D.O.
Radiation Oncology. . . . . Curtis Miyamoto, M.D.
Radiology . . . . Charles Jungreis, M.D.
Surgery . . . . Daniel Dempsey, M.D.
   Cardiac and Thoracic. . . . . Satoshi Furukawa, M.D.
   General . . . . Daniel Dempsey, M.D.
   Trauma . . . . Amy Goldberg, M.D.
   Vascular. . . . . John Blebea, M.D.
Urology. . . . . Jack Mydlo, M.D.

University of Pennsylvania School of Medicine

3620 Hamilton Walk
Philadelphia, Pennsylvania 19104-6055
215-898-8034 (academic programs); 898-6796 (dean's office); 573-2030 (fax)
Web site: www.med.upenn.edu

Founded in 1765, the school of medicine of the University of Pennsylvania has the distinction of being the oldest medical school in the United States. It is located on the campus of the university in west Philadelphia.

Type: private
2008-2009 total enrollment: 720
Clinical facilities: Hospital of the University of Pennsylvania, Children's Hospital of Philadelphia, Veterans Administration Medical Center, Penn Presbyterian Medical Center (including Scheie Eye Institute), Children's Seashore House, Philadelphia Child Guidance Clinic, Chestnut Hill Hospital, Englewood Hospital, York Hospital, Pennsylvania Hospital, Chester County Hospital, St. Luke's Hospital-Bethlehem, Virtua-Burlington Hospital, Underwood Memorial Hospital

University Officials

President. . . . . Amy Gutmann, Ph.D.
Provost . . . . Ronald J. Daniels, LL.M.
Executive Vice President for the Health System
   and Dean, School of Medicine . . . . Arthur H. Rubenstein, M.B.B.Ch.
Chief Executive Officer, Health System. . . . . Ralph W. Muller

Medical School Administrative Staff

Executive Vice President and Dean. Arthur H. Rubenstein, M.B.B.Ch.
   Senior Vice President for Public Affairs and
   Chief of Staff to Executive Vice President/
   Dean . . . . Susan E. Phillips
Special Assistant to the Dean . . . . Thomas R. Hecker, Ph.D.
Senior Associate Dean, Program Development. . . . . Alfred P. Fishman, M.D.
Associate Dean, Health Promotion and Disease Prevention . . . . . . Shiriki K. Kumanyika, Ph.D.
Senior Medical Officer, HUP, and Senior
   Associate Dean for Diversity and
   Community Outreach . . . . Bernett L. Johnson, Jr., M.D.
Vice Dean, Education . . . . Gail Morrison, M.D.
Associate Dean for Curriculum . . . . Stanley Goldfarb, M.D.
Associate Dean, Graduate Medical Education . . . . Lisa M. Bellini, M.D.
Associate Dean for Clinical Research . . . . Susan S. Ellenberg, Ph.D.
Assistant Dean, Office of Diversity. . . . . Karen E. Hamilton, Ph.D.
Associate Dean, Student Affairs. . . . . Jon B. Morris, M.D.
Associate Dean, Continuing Medical Education. . . . . Zalman S. Agus, M.D.
Associate Dean, Medical Education Research
   and Director, Evaluation and Assessment . . . . Judy A. Shea, Ph.D.
Assistant Dean, IT for Academic Programs . . . . Michael D. Feldman, M.D., Ph.D.
Associate Dean, Professionalism and Humanism . . . . Paul N. Lanken, M.D.
Chief Administrative Officer and Director, Curriculum Office . . . . Anna T. Delaney
Director of Admissions and Financial Aid . . . . Gaye W. Sheffler
Director, Continuing Medical Education. . . . . Mila Kostic
Director, Office of the Registrar . . . . Helene Weinberg
Director, Standardized Patient Program . . . . Denise LaMarra
Director, Office of Student Affairs. . . . . Barbara R. Wagner
Director, Nutrition Education. . . . . Lisa A. Hark, Ph.D.
Vice Dean, Faculty Affairs. . . . . Alan G. Wasserstein, M.D.
Executive Vice Dean and Chief Scientific Officer . . . . Glen N. Gaulton, Ph.D.
Associate Dean, Combined Degree and Physician Scholars. . . . . Lawrence F. Brass, M.D., Ph.D.
Associate Dean for Research Program Development . . . . Jonas H. Ellenberg, Ph.D.
Associate Dean for Clinical Research. . . . . Susan S. Ellenberg, Ph.D.
Associate Dean for Graduate Education and
   Director, Biomedical Graduate Studies . . . . Susan R. Ross, Ph.D.
Associate Dean, Postdoctoral Research Training . . . . Yvonne Paterson, Ph.D.
Associate Dean, Global Health Programs. Neal Nathanson, M.D.
Executive Director, Office of Human Research . . . . Gregg J. Fromell, M.D.
Director, Office of Corporate Alliances. . . . . Terry J. Fadem
Senior Executive Director, Research and Research Training. . . . . Susan R. Passante

Vice Dean, Professional Services and Senior Vice President. . . . . . Peter D. Quinn, D.M.D., M.D.
   Executive Director, Clinical Practices of the
     University of Pennsylvania . . . . Elizabeth B. Johnston
Vice Dean, Administration and Finance . . . . Christopher P. Kops
   Executive Director, School of Medicine Administration . . . . Robert J. Dugan
   Executive Director of Finance, School of Medicine . . . . Kathleen F. Bramwell
   Executive Director, Office of Research Compliance and Integrity. . . . . Debbi Gilad, J.D.
   Executive Director, Information Services. Mary Alice Annecharico
   Executive Director, Space Planning and Operations. . . . . Eric M. Weckel
   Executive Director, Research Support Services. . . . . Marianne Achenbach
   Executive Director, Faculty Affairs and Professional Development . . . . Victoria A. Mulhern
   Director, Decision Support and Analysis . . . . Lynn K. Meaney
   Director, Resource Planning and Analysis . . . . Daniel J. McCollum
   Director, Health Sciences Library . . . . Anne Seymour (Interim)
Assistant Vice Dean and Chief Advancement Officer. . . . . Armando Chardiet
   Senior Director, Alumni Development and Alumni Relations. . . . . Vanessa Marinari
Senior Vice President for Public Affairs for the Health System. . . . . Susan E. Phillips

Department and Division or Section Chairs

Basic Sciences

Biochemistry and Biophysics. . . . . P. Leslie Dutton, Ph.D.
Biostatistics and Epidemiology . . . . Brian L. Strom, M.D.
Cancer Biology . . . . Lewis A. Chodosh, M.D., Ph.D. (Interim)
Cell and Developmental Biology. . . . . Jonathan A. Epstein, M.D.
Genetics . . . . Thomas R. Kadesch, Ph.D. (Interim)
Medical Ethics. . . . . Arthur L. Caplan, Ph.D.
Microbiology . . . . Robert W. Doms, M.D., Ph.D.
Neuroscience. . . . . Irwin B. Levitan, Ph.D.
Pharmacology . . . . Garret A. FitzGerald, M.D.
Physiology . . . . H. Lee Sweeney, Ph.D.

Clinical Sciences

Anesthesiology and Critical Care . . . . Lee A. Fleisher, M.D.
Dermatology . . . . John R. Stanley, M.D.
Emergency Medicine . . . . William G. Baxt, M.D.
Family Medicine and Community Health . . . . Marjorie A. Bowman, M.D.
Medicine. . . . . Richard P. Shannon, M.D.
   Cardiology. . . . . Michael S. Parmacek, M.D.
   Endocrinology, Diabetes, and Metabolism . . . . Mitchell A. Lazar, M.D., Ph.D.
   Experimental Therapeutics. . . . . Garret A. FitzGerald, M.D.
   Gastroenterology . . . . Anil K. Rustgi, M.D.
   General Medicine. . . . . Sankey V. Williams, M.D.
   Geriatrics. . . . . Jerry C. Johnson, M.D.
   Hematology and Oncology. Lynn M. Schuchter, M.D. (Interim)
   Medical Genetics . . . . Reed E. Pyeritz, M.D., Ph.D.
   Infectious Diseases . . . . Harvey M. Friedman, M.D.
   Pulmonary and Critical Care. . . . . John H. Hansen-Flaschen, M.D.
   Renal Electrolyte . . . . Jeffrey S. Berns, M.D. (Interim)
   Rheumatology . . . . Sharon L. Kolasinski, M.D. (Interim)
   Sleep Medicine. . . . . Allan I. Pack, M.D., Ph.D.
Neurology. . . . . Francisco Gonzalez-Scarano, M.D.
Neurosurgery. . . . . M. Sean Grady, M.D.
Obstetrics and Gynecology. . . . . Deborah A. Driscoll, M.D.
Ophthalmology . . . . Stuart L. Fine, M.D.
Orthopaedic Surgery . . . . Richard D. Lackman, M.D.
Otorhinolaryngology-Head and Neck Surgery . . . . Bert W. O'Malley, M.D.
Pathology and Laboratory Medicine . . . . Mark L. Tykocinski, M.D.
Pediatrics . . . . Alan R. Cohen, M.D.
Physical Medicine and Rehabilitation . . . . Richard Salcido, M.D.
Psychiatry . . . . Dwight L. Evans, M.D.
Radiation Oncology. . . . . Stephen Hahn, M.D.
Radiology . . . . R. Nick Bryan, M.D., Ph.D.
Surgery . . . . James L. Mullen, M.D.

University of Pittsburgh School of Medicine
Alan Magee Scaife Hall of the Health Professions
3550 Terrace Street
Pittsburgh, Pennsylvania 15261
412-648-9891 (admissions); 648-9040 (student affairs); 648-8975 (dean's office);
648-1236 (fax)
Web site: www.medschool.pitt.edu

The school of medicine was originally chartered in 1886 as the Western Pennsylvania Medical College and, in 1892, became affiliated with the Western University of Pennsylvania. In 1908, its name was changed to the school of medicine of the University of Pittsburgh. The University of Pittsburgh became a state-related institution in 1966. The medical school is located on the university campus.

Type: private
2008-2009 total enrollment: 582
Clinical facilities: University of Pittsburgh Medical Center (UPMC) includes: Presbyterian, Montefiore, Shadyside, Southside, Western Psychiatric Institute and Clinic, Children's Hospital of Pittsburgh, Magee Women's Hospital, Veterans Affairs Medical Center, University of Pittsburgh Cancer Institute, Thomas E. Starzl Transplantation Institute, Eye and Ear Institute, and 12 community hospitals.

University Officials

Chancellor . . . . Mark A. Nordenberg
Provost and Senior Vice Chancellor . . . . James V. Maher, Ph.D.
Senior Vice Chancellor for Health Sciences . . . . Arthur S. Levine, M.D.
Associate Senior Vice Chancellor for Health Sciences . . . . Loren H. Roth, M.D.
Associate Senior Vice Chancellor for Health Sciences Administration . . . . Jeffrey L. Masnick
Associate Vice Chancellor for Cancer Research . . . . Ronald B. Herberman, M.D.
Associate Vice Chancellor for Basic Biomedical Research . . . . Michelle S. Broido, Ph.D.
Associate Vice Chancellor for Clinical Research . . . . Steven E. Reis, M.D.
Associate Vice Chancellor for Academic Affairs. . . . . Margaret C. McDonald, Ph.D.
Associate Vice Chancellor for Academic Career Development . . . . Joan M. Lakoski, Ph.D.
Associate Vice Chancellor for Industry Relations
  and Continuing Education . . . . Barbara E. Barnes, M.D.
Assistant Vice Chancellor for Diversity . . . . Paula K. Davis

Medical School Administrative Staff

Dean. . . . . Arthur S. Levine, M.D.
Vice Dean . . . . Steven L. Kanter, M.D.
Senior Associate Dean . . . . Charles F. Reynolds III, M.D.
Associate Dean for Admissions and Financial Aid . . . . Beth M. Piraino, M.D.
Associate Dean for Faculty Affairs. . . . . Ann E. Thompson, M.D.
Associate Dean for Graduate Medical Education. . . . . Rita M. Patel, M.D.
Associate Dean for Graduate Studies . . . . John P. Horn, Ph.D.
Associate Dean for Medical Education . . . . John F. Mahoney, M.D.
Associate Dean for the Medical Scientist Training Program . . . . Clayton A. Wiley, M.D., Ph.D.
Associate Dean for Medical Student Research . . . . Michael L. Boninger, M.D.
Associate Dean for Student Affairs . . . . Joan Harvey, M.D.
Assistant Dean for Graduate Medical Education . . . . Frank J. Kroboth, M.D.
Assistant Dean for Student Affairs and Director,
  Diversity Programs . . . . Chentis Pettigrew, Ph.D.
Assistant Dean for Veterans Administrative Affairs. Rajiv Jain, M.D.

Department and Division or Section Chairs

Centers and Institutes

Thomas E. Starzl Transplantation Institute . . . . Fadi G. Lakkis, M.D. (Sci. Dir.)
University of Pittsburgh Cancer Institute. . . . . Ronald B. Herberman, M.D. (Director)
McGowan Institute for Regenerative Medicine . . . . Alan Russell, Ph.D. (Director)
Cardiovascular Institute. . . . . Barry London, M.D., Ph.D. (Director)
Drug Discovery Institute. . . . . John S. Lazo, Ph.D. (Director)
Systems Neuroscience Institute. . . . . Peter L. Strick, Ph.D. (Director)

Basic Sciences

Biomedical Informatics . . . . Michael J. Becich, M.D., Ph.D.

University of Pittsburgh School of Medicine: PENNSYLVANIA

Cell Biology and Physiology . . . . Raymond A. Frizzell, Ph.D.
Computational Biology. . . . . Ivet Bahar, Ph.D.
Developmental Biology . . . . Open
Immunology . . . . Olivera J. Finn, Ph.D.
Microbiology and Molecular Genetics. . . . . Joseph C. Glorioso III, Ph.D.
Neurobiology. . . . . Susan G. Amara, Ph.D.
Pharmacology and Chemical Biology . . . . Bruce A. Freeman, Ph.D.
Structural Biology . . . . Angela M. Gronenborn, Ph.D.

Clinical Sciences

Anesthesiology. . . . . John P. Williams, M.D.
Critical Care Medicine. . . . . Derek Angus, M.D.
Dermatology . . . . Louis D. Falo, M.D., Ph.D.
Emergency Medicine . . . . Paul M. Paris, M.D.
Family Medicine . . . . Jeannette E. South-Paul, M.D.
Medicine. . . . . Steven D. Shapiro, M.D.
   Clinical Pharmacology . . . . Robert A. Branch, M.D.
   Endocrinology and Metabolism. Andrew F. Stewart, M.D.
   Gastroenterology . . . . David C. Whitcomb, M.D., Ph.D.
   General Internal Medicine . . . . Wishwa N. Kapoor, M.D.
   Geriatric Medicine . . . . Neil M. Resnick, M.D.
   Hematology and Oncology . . . . Ronald B. Herberman, M.D.
   Infectious Diseases . . . . John W. Mellors, M.D.
   Pulmonary and Critical Care. . . . . Mark T. Gladwin, M.D.
   Renal-Electrolyte . . . . Thomas R. Kleyman, M.D.
   Rheumatology . . . . Larry Moreland, M.D.
Neurological Surgery. . . . . Amin Kassam, M.D.
Neurology. . . . . Lawrence R. Wechsler, M.D. (Interim)
Obstetrics, Gynecology, and Reproductive Sciences. . . . . W. Allen Hogge, M.D.
Ophthalmology . . . . Joel S. Schuman, M.D.
Orthopedic Surgery. . . . . Freddie H. Fu, M.D.
Otolaryngology . . . . Jonas T. Johnson, M.D.
Pathology . . . . George K. Michalopoulos, M.D., Ph.D.
Pediatrics . . . . David H. Perlmutter, M.D.
   Adolescent Medicine . . . . Pamela J. Murray, M.D.
   Cardiology . . . . Steven Webber, M.B.Ch.B., M.R.C.P.
   Child Neurology. . . . . Ira Bergman, M.D.
   Endocrinology and Metabolism. . . . . Dorothy J. Becker, M.D. (Acting)
   Gastroenterology . . . . Mark E. Lowe, M.D., Ph.D.
   General Academic Pediatrics. Alejandro Hoberman, M.D.
   Genetics. . . . . Gerard Vockley, M.D., Ph.D.
   Hematology and Oncology . . . . A. Kim Ritchey, M.D.
   Infectious Disease. . . . . Toni Darville, M.D.
   Neonatology and Developmental Biology. . . . . Gary Silverman, M.D., Ph.D.
   Nephrology . . . . Demetrius Ellis, M.D.
   Obesity and Metabolism . . . . Silva Arstanian, M.D.
   Pulmonology, Allergy, and Immunology . . . . Jay K. Kolls, M.D.
   Rheumatology . . . . Raphael Hirsch, M.D.
Physical Medicine and Rehabilitation . . . . Michael L. Boninger, M.D. (Interim)
Psychiatry . . . . David J. Kupfer, M.D.
   Adult Psychiatry . . . . Roger Haskett, M.D.
   Child and Adolescent Psychiatry, Autism, and
      Developmental Disorders . . . . Martin J. Lubetsky, M.D.
   Geriatrics . . . . Jules R. Rosen, M.D.
   Services for Research and Recovery in Serious Mental Illness . . . . . K. N. Roy Chengappa, M.D.
Radiation Oncology. . . . . Joel S. Greenberger, M.D.
Radiology . . . . Scott A. Mirowitz, M.D.
Surgery. . . . . Timothy R. Billiar, M.D.
   Cardiothoracic Surgery. . . . . Ronald Pellegrini, M.D.
   General Surgery. . . . . Andrew Peitzman, M.D.
   Pediatric Surgery . . . . George K. Gittes, M.D.
   Plastic Surgery . . . . W. P. Andrew Lee, M.D.
   Surgical Oncology . . . . David Bartlett, M.D.
   Thoracic and Foregut Surgery. . . . . James Luketich, M.D.
   Transplant Surgery. . . . . Wallis Marsh, M.D. (Interim)
   Vascular Surgery. . . . . Michel Makaroun, M.D.
Urology. . . . . Joel B. Nelson, M.D.

Ponce School of Medicine

P.O. Box 7004
Ponce, Puerto Rico 00732
787-840-2575 (general information); 844-3710 (dean's office); 840-9756 (fax)
E-mail: malbors@psm.edu (admin. assist.)
Web site: www.psm.edu

The Ponce School of Medicine was established in 1977 by the Catholic University of Puerto Rico, but since 1980 has been operated independently under the auspices of the private not-for-profit foundation, the Ponce Medical School Foundation Inc. The administration and basic sciences are located in a series of modern facilities inaugurated on January 1995 in the southern part of the city of Ponce, Puerto Rico. The clinical sciences are community based in eight affiliated hospitals in the southern area of Puerto Rico. Its charter class graduated in May 1981.

Type: private
2008-2009 total enrollment: 574
Clinical facilities: Damas Hospital, Dr. Pila Hospital, Dr. Tito Mattei Metropolitan Hospital, La Concepción Hospital, San Lucas Hospital, Hospital Oncológico Andrés Grillasca, First Hospital Panamericano, San Cristobal Hospital, La Playa Diagnostic and Treatment Center, San Antonio Hospital, Dr. Ramón E Betances University Hospital; VA Medical Center (San Juan), PSM Outpatient Clinics, CSCO Aguadilla General Hospital, CSCO Mayaguez Hospital, Cristo Redentor Hospital, Castañer Clinic, Castañer Hospital, VA Clinic-Ponce, La Casa del Veterano, Centro de Medicina de Familia.

Medical School Administrative Staff

President and Dean . . . . Raúl A. Armstrong, M.D.
Associate Dean for Academic Affairs . . . . Olga Rodriguez, M.D.
Associate Dean for Faculty and Clinical Affairs . . . . Agustín Fernández-Cabrero, M.D.
Medical Director, Ambulatory Clinics . . . . Ricardo Barnes, M.D.
Associate Dean for Graduate Studies and Research . . . . José Torres, Ph.D.
Executive Dean for Administration and Finance . . . . Reinaldo Díaz
Assistant Dean for Student Affairs . . . . Arvin Báez
Director of Admissions . . . . Wanda Vélez, M.D.
Assistant Dean for Education . . . . Gladys Pereles, Ed.D.
Director, Office of Continued Medical Education . . . . José R. Ubieta
Director, Office of Graduate Medical Education (Ponce) . . . . Olga Rodriguez, M.D.
Director, Office of Graduate Medical Education
   (Mayaguez) . . . . Elba Morales de Román, M.D.
Finance Director . . . . Héctor Pérez
Registrar . . . . Segundina Caraballo
Librarian . . . . Carmen G. Malavet
Director of Student Financial Aid . . . . Pedro Barnés
Director of Personnel . . . . Evelyn Lugo
Budget Director and Legal Counselor . . . . Waleska Murphy, Esq.

Department and Division or Section Chairs

Basic Sciences

Anatomy . . . . Juan B. Fernández, Ph.D.
    Cell Biology . . . . Maritza La Paix, M.D.
Biochemistry . . . . José Torres, Ph.D.
Microbiology . . . . Nilda Zapata, M.D.
    Infectious Diseases . . . . Nilda Zapata, M.D.
Physiology, Pharmacology, and Toxicology . . . . León Ferder, M.D.

Clinical Sciences

Family and Community Medicine . . . . Marta Febo, M.D.
    Preventive Medicine . . . . Iván Iriarte, M.D.
Medicine . . . . Miguel Magraner, M.D.
Obstetrics and Gynecology . . . . Joaquin Laboy, M.D.
Pathology . . . . Adalberto Mendoza, M.D.
Pediatrics . . . . Ivonne Galarza, M.D.
Psychiatry . . . . Pedro Castaing, M.D.
Surgery . . . . Aníbal Torres, M.D. (Acting)

Ph.D. Program in Biomedical Sciences

Director . . . . José Torres, Ph.D.

Public Health Program

Director . . . . Juan C. Orengo-Valverde, M.D.

Psy.D. Program

Director . . . . José Pons, Ph.D.

Special Programs

Clinical Research Center . . . . Elizabeth Barranco, M.D.

*Includes all programs: M.D., Ph.D., Psy.D., and M.P.H.

Universidad Central del Caribe School of Medicine

P.O. Box 60-327
Bayamón, Puerto Rico 00960-6032
787-798-3001; 269-4510 (dean's office); 269-1352 (fax)
E-mail: jose.ginel@uccaribe.edu
Web site: www.uccaribe.edu

The school of medicine of Universidad Central del Caribe started operations in September 1976. All basic science and clinical facilities are located on the grounds of the Dr. Ramón Ruiz Arnau University Hospital at Bayamón, Puerto Rico. The new Basic Sciences Building started operation in August 1990.

Type: private
2008-2009 total enrollment: 243
Clinical facilities: Dr. Ramón Ruiz Arnau University Hospital, San Juan City Hospital, San Pablo Hospital, First Hospital Panamericano, Family Practice Centers Northeast Health Region, San Jorge Children's Hospital, Veteran's Administration Hospital, Hospital Interamericano de Medicina Avanzada.

University Officials

President of the University . . . . José Ginel Rodríguez, M.D. (Acting)
President of the Board of Trustees . . . . Jorge Colón-Nevares
Dean of Academic Affairs . . . . Arístides Cruz, Ph.D.
Dean for Admissions and Student Affairs . . . . Nereida Diaz, Ph.D.

Medical School Administrative Staff

Dean . . . . José Ginel Rodríguez, M.D.
Associate Dean of Medicine . . . . Zilka Ríos
Dean of Administration . . . . Emilia Soto
Associate Dean for Research and Graduate Studies . . . . Luis Cubano, Ph.D.
Director of CME . . . . Frances García, M.D.
Director of GME . . . . Frances García, M.D.
Admissions Officer . . . . Irma Cordero
Counselor . . . . Yari M. Marrero
Financial Aid Officer . . . . Ana Galán
Registrar . . . . Irma I. Irizarry
Librarian . . . . Mildred Rivera
Office of Evaluation and Educational Research . . . . Michael Vélez
Office of Curriculum and Faculty Development . . . . Elsa Gilbes
Director of Learning Resources Center . . . . Alfredo Calderón

Universidad Central del Caribe School of Medicine: PUERTO RICO

Department and Division or Section Chairs

Basic Sciences

Anatomy . . . . Sofía Jiménez, Ph.D.
Biochemistry, Cellular Biology, and Nutrition . . . . Richard M. Hann, M.D.
Microbiology and Immunology. . . . . Eddy O. Ríos-Olivares, Ph.D.
Pharmacology . . . . Hector Maldonado, Ph.D.
Physiology . . . . Priscila Sanabria, Ph.D.

Clinical Sciences

Family Medicine and Community Health . . . . Ramón Suárez, M.D.
   Community Health* . . . . Eric González, M.D.
   Family Medicine* . . . . Ramón Suárez, M.D.
Internal Medicine . . . . Melba Colón, M.D.
   Cardiovascular* . . . . José Rivera del Río, M.D.
   Critical Care* . . . . Juan Ruiz, M.D.
   Dermatology* . . . . Limarie Aguila, M.D.
   Endocrinology* . . . . Luis M. Reyes, M.D.
   Gastroenterology* . . . . Ivelisse Ramirez, M.D.
   Hematology and Oncology* . . . . Robert Hunter, M.D.
   Infectious Disease* . . . . Melba Colón, M.D.
   Nephrology* . . . . Luis Quesada, M.D.
   Neurology* . . . . Damaris Torres, M.D.
   Pneumology* . . . . Miriam Melendez-Rosa, M.D.
   Rheumatology* . . . . Salvador Vila, M.D.
Obstetrics and Gynecology . . . . Stanley Asensio, M.D.
Pathology and Laboratory Medicine . . . . Angelissa Franceschini, M.D. (Acting)
Pediatrics . . . . Fermín Sánchez, M.D.
   Allergy* . . . . Carmen Acantilado, M.D.
   Cardiology* . . . . Julio Bauzá, M.D.
   Critical Care* . . . . Juan del Rio, M.D.
   Developmental Pediatrics* . . . . Jorge Arzola-Rivera, M.D.
   Endocrinology* . . . . Fermín Sánchez, M.D.
   Gastroenterology* . . . . Jaime Rosado, M.D.
   Hematology and Oncology* . . . . Carmen L. Bartolomei, M.D.
   Infectology* . . . . Haydeé Garcia, M.D.
   Neonatology* . . . . Juan del Rio, M.D.
   Nephrology* . . . . Open
   Neurology* . . . . Carlos R. Lao, M.D.
   Pneumology* . . . . William de la Paz, M.D.
Psychiatry . . . . José A. Franceschini, M.D.
Radiology . . . . Mercedes de Choudens, M.D.
Surgery . . . . Julio Soto, M.D.
   Anesthesiology* . . . . Open

*Specialty without organizational autonomy.

University of Puerto Rico School of Medicine

Medical Sciences Campus
P.O. Box 365067
San Juan, Puerto Rico 00936-5067
787-758-2525; 765-2363 (dean's office); 756-8475 (dean's fax)
E-mail: wfrontera@rcm.upr.edu
Web site: www.md.rcm.upr.edu/

The University of Puerto Rico School of Medicine accepted its first class in August 1950. The school of medicine developed originally from the school of tropical medicine of the university (which had been established under joint auspices with Columbia University in 1924). Since 1972, the school of medicine has been located on the medical sciences campus on the grounds of the Puerto Rico Medical Center, two miles from the main university campus at Rio Piedras.

Type: public
2008-2009 total enrollment: 432
Clinical facilities: University Hospital, University Pediatric Hospital, Veterans Administration Medical Center, U.P.R. University Hospital, Pavia Hospital, Auxillo Mutuo Hospital, Perea Hospital, De La Concepción Hospital, San Pablo Hospital, First PanAmerican Hospital, San Antonio Hospital, San Juan Oncological Hospital, Cardiovascular Center, San Juan City Hospital and Puerto Rico Medical Center. Nineteen primary care settings located throughout the island are also in use.

University Officials

President, Board of Trustees . . . . Carlos Del Rios, Eng.
President, University of Puerto Rico . . . . Antonio García-Padilla, J.D.

Medical Sciences Campus Officials

Chancellor . . . . José Carlo, M.D.
Dean of Academic Affairs . . . . Delia Camacho, Ph.D.
Dean of Students . . . . Ilka Rios, D.M.D.
Dean of Administration . . . . Irving Jiménez
Librarian . . . . Victoria Delgado
Registrar . . . . Maria Otero

Medical School Administrative Staff

Dean . . . . Walter R. Frontera, M.D., Ph.D.
Associate Dean for Clinical Affairs . . . . Yolanda Gómez, M.D.
Associate Dean for Academic Affairs . . . . Guido E. Santacana, Ph.D.
Associate Dean for Biomedical Sciences and Director Graduate School . . . . . . Walter Silva, Ph.D.
Director, Curriculum Office . . . . Debora Silva, M.D.
Assistant Dean for Student Affairs . . . . Gladys González, M.D.
Chair, Admissions Committee . . . . Gladys González, M.D.
Assistant Dean for Graduate Medical Education . . . . Yolanda Gómez, M.D.
Director, Office of Continuing Medical Education . . . . Roberto Acevedo, M.H.S.A. (Acting)
Director, Evaluation and Research in
    Medical Education Office . . . . Irma Rivera
Chair, Planning and Development Committee . . . . Walter R. Frontera, M.D., Ph.D.
Associate Dean for Administrative Affairs . . . . Roberto Acevedo, M.H.S.A

Department and Division or Section Chairs

Basic Sciences

Anatomy and Neurobiology . . . . Maria Sosa, Ph.D.
Biochemistry and Nutrition . . . . José Rodríguez, Ph.D.
Microbiology and Medical Zoology . . . . Guillermo Vázquez, M.D.
Pathology . . . . Maria Marcos, M.D. (Acting)
Pharmacology and Toxicology . . . . Walmor C. De Mello, M.D., Ph.D.
Physiology and Biophysics . . . . Nelson Escobales, Ph.D.

Clinical Sciences

Anesthesiology . . . . Miguel Marrero, M.D.
Dermatology . . . . Néstor Sanchez, M.D.
Family Medicine . . . . Richard de Andino, M.D.
Medicine . . . . Esther Torres, M.D.
   Cardiology* . . . . Mario R. García-Palmieri, M.D.
   Endocrinology* . . . . Miriam Allende, M.D.
   Gastroenterology* . . . . Pablo Costas, M.D.
   General Internal Medicine* . . . . Carlos González, M.D.
   Geriatrics . . . . Juan Rosado, M.D.
   Hematology* . . . . Eileen Pacheco, M.D. (Acting)
   Infectious Diseases* . . . . Carlos Sánchez, M.D.
   Nephrology* . . . . Rafael Burgos-Calderón, M.D.
   Neurology . . . . Maritza Arroyo, M.D. (Acting)
   Pulmonary Diseases* . . . . Angel F. Laureano, M.D. (Acting)
   Rheumatology* . . . . Luis M. Vilá, M.D.
Obstetrics and Gynecology . . . . Juana Rivera, M.D.
Ophthalmology . . . . Luis Serrano, M.D.
Pediatrics . . . . Clemente Diaz, M.D.
   Cardiology . . . . Angel F. Espinosa, M.D.
   Emergency Care* . . . . Milagros Pumarejo, M.D.
   Endocrinology* . . . . Lilliam González-Pijem, M.D.
   Gastroenterology . . . . David Fernández, M.D.
   General Pediatrics* . . . . Rosario González, M.D.
   Hematology and Oncology . . . . Pedro J. Santiago Borrero, M.D.
   Infectious Diseases . . . . Haydeé Garcia, M.D.
   Intensive Care . . . . Alicia Fernandez-Seins, M.D.
   Medical Genetics* . . . . Maria del Carmen González, M.D.
   Neonatology* . . . . Marta Valcárcel, M.D.
   Nephrology* . . . . Juan O. Peréz, M.D.
   Neurology . . . . Marisel Vázquez, M.D.
   Pneumology* . . . . Maria Alvarez, M.D.
Physical Medicine, Rehabilitation, and Sports Medicine . . . . William Micheo, M.D.
Psychiatry . . . . Lelis Nazario, M.D.
   Child Psychiatry* . . . . Lelis Nazario, M.D.
   General Psychiatry* . . . . Luz N. Colón, M.D.
Radiological Sciences . . . . Frieda Silva, M.D.
   Diagnostic Radiology . . . . Edgar Colón, M.D.
   Nuclear Medicine . . . . Frieda Silva, M.D.
   Radiotherapy . . . . José Santana, M.D.
Surgery . . . . Juan J. Lojo, M.D.
   Neurosurgery . . . . Ricardo Brau, M.D.
   Orthopedics . . . . Manuel Garcia, M.D.
   Otolaryngology . . . . Juan Trinidad, M.D.
   Urology . . . . Antonio Puras, M.D.
Emergency Medicine . . . . Juan González, M.D.

Special Programs

Animal Resources Unit . . . . Malween Martinez, D.V.M.
Biomedical Sciences Core Laboratories . . . . Walter Silva, Ph.D.
Caribbean Primate Research Center . . . . Edmundo Kraiselburd, M.D.
Clinical Research Center . . . . Julio Benabe, M.D.
Clinical Skills Laboratory . . . . Nerian Ortiz, M.D.
Comprehensive Cancer Center . . . . Reynold López, M.D.
Center for Informatic and Technology . . . . José L. Quiñones
Neurobiology Laboratory . . . . Mark Miller, Ph.D. (Acting)
Raffucci Surgical Research Laboratory . . . . Reynold López, M.D.
Trauma Center . . . . Pablo Rodriguez, M.D.

*Specialty without organizational autonomy.

San Juan Bautista School of Medicine

P.O. Box 4968
Caguas, Puerto Rico 00726-4968
787-743-3038; 746-3093 (fax)
Web site: www.sanjuanbautista.edu

San Juan Bautista School of Medicine was founded in 1978 in San Juan, Puerto Rico, as a nonprofit corporation under the laws of the Commonwealth of Puerto Rico. On June 20, 1979, it was authorized by the Council of Higher Education of Puerto Rico to offer studies pertinent to the M.D. degree.

Type: private
2008-2009 total enrollment: 200
Clinical facilities: San Juan Bautista Medical Center

University Officials

President and Dean . . . . Yocasta Brugal-Mena, M.D.
President, Board of Trustees . . . . Raul Morales Borges, M.D.
Medical Director . . . . Iris Pérez, M.D.
Administrator . . . . Amaury Lluveras, R.N., M.H.A.
Chief Financial Officer. . . . . José A. Colón
Dean of Administration and Human Resources. . . . . Carlos Fco. Abreu, B.B.A.
Associate Dean for Research. . . . . Irvin M. Maldonado-Rivera, Ph.D.
Dean of Students. . . . . Vacant
Library Director. . . . . Carlos A. Altamirano
Office of Financial Aid. . . . . Beatriz De Leon Rivera
Office of Registrar. . . . . Lissette Torres
Admissions Officer. . . . . Jaymi Sánchez
Technology Services and Purchasing. . . . . Juan Fco. Flores

Medical Faculty

Associate Dean of Biomedical Sciences. . . . . Gualberto Borrero
Associate Dean of Clinical Sciences . . . . Miriam Ramos, M.D.

Department Chairs

Basic Sciences

Anatomy. . . . . Ramonita Correa, Ph.D.
Biochemistry and Pharmacology. . . . . Olga I. Claudio Cortes, Ph.D.
Clinical Skills. . . . . Mirella Rodriguez Rodriguez, M.D.
Microbiology. . . . . Shirley D. Valentin, Ph.D.
Physiology and Pathology. . . . . Cariluz Santiago Ortiz, Ph.D.

Clinical Sciences

Anesthesiology. . . . . Luis R. Novoa, M.D.
Emergency Medicine . . . . Guillermo Campos, M.D.
Family Medicine . . . . Luis Izquierdo Mora, M.D.
Internal Medicine . . . . Edgardo Cartagena, M.D.
Obstetrics and Gynecology. . . . . Frances T. Serra, M.D.
Pathology . . . . Yocasta Brugal Mena, M.D.
Pediatrics . . . . Norma J. Arciniegas-Medina, M.D., F.A.A.P.
Neonatology and Pediatric Intensive Care Unit. . . . . Edgar Diaz, M.D.
Pediatric Clerkship Coordinator. . . . . Carmen Otero, M.D., F.A.A.P.
Psychiatry and Behavioral Sciences. . . . . Victor Santiago Noa, M.D.
Clinical Administrator . . . . Amaury Lluveras, R.N., M.H.A.
Academic Coordinator. . . . . Myrta N. Sifonte, M.D.
Radiology . . . . Francisco Gomez Goytia, M.D.
Surgery . . . . Jorge L. Cordero Soto, M.D.

Training Programs

Director, Graduate Medical Education . . . . Luis A. Medina, M.D.
Director, Pediatrics . . . . Myrna L. Borges, M.D.
Director, Transitional Year . . . . Lawrence C. Olsen, M.D.
Director, Internal Medicine . . . . José Martinez, M.D.
Director, Psychiatry . . . . José Torres
Director, Primary Medicine and Management. . . . . Luis Izquierdo, M.D.

The Warren Alpert Medical School of Brown University

97 Waterman Street
Providence, Rhode Island 02912
401-863-3991; 863-3330 (dean's office); 863-3431 (fax)
Web site: http://bms.brown.edu

Brown University was founded in 1764. Its first M.D. program, initiated in 1811, was temporarily suspended in 1827. The master of medical science program was begun in 1963, and the M.D.-conferring program started in 1973. Its first class of physicians was graduated in June 1975. The medical school operates in conjunction with seven hospitals in the Providence metropolitan area.

Type: private
2008-2009 total enrollment: 306
Clinical facilities: Butler Hospital, Memorial Hospital of Rhode Island, Miriam Hospital, Women and Infants Hospital, Rhode Island Hospital, Veterans Administration Medical Center, Bradley Hospital.

University Officials

President. . . . . Ruth J. Simmons, Ph.D.
Provost . . . . David I. Kertzer, Ph.D.
Dean of the Faculty . . . . Rajiv Vohra, Ph.D.

Medical School Administrative Staff

Dean of Medicine and Biological Sciences . . . . Edward J. Wing, M.D.
Executive Dean for Administration. . . . . John M. Deeley
Executive Dean for Advancement. . . . . Larry L. Zeiber
Associate Dean for Biology. . . . . Edward Hawrot, Ph.D.
Associate Dean of Medicine (Public Health and Public Policy) . . . . Terrie Wetle, Ph.D.
Associate Dean for Medical Education . . . . Philip A. Gruppuso, M.D.
Associate Dean for Faculty Affairs. . . . . Jane L. Eisen, M.D.
Associate Dean for Graduate and Postdoctoral Studies . . . . Nancy L. Thompson, Ph.D.
Associate Dean of Medicine (Minority Affairs) . . . . Vacant
Associate Dean of Medicine (Clinical Faculty). . . . . Arthur Frazzano, M.D.
Associate Dean of Medicine (Women in
    Medicine and Graduate Medical Education) . . . . Michele G. Cyr, M.D.
Associate Dean of Medicine (Minority
    Recruitment and Retention) . . . . Mercedes Domenech, M.D., Ph.D.
Associate Dean of Medicine (Program in Liberal Medical Education) . . . . . . Julianne Y. Ip, M.D.
Associate Dean of Medicine (Continuing
    Medical Education) . . . . Patrick J. Sweeney, M.D., Ph.D.
Associate Dean of Medicine (Primary Care) . . . . Vacant
Associate Dean of Medicine (Humanities and Social Sciences Curriculum) . . . . Vacant
Assistant Dean of Medicine (Advising) . . . . Anne Cushing-Brescia, M.D.
Assistant Dean of Medicine (Advising) . . . . Timothy M. Empkie, M.D.
Assistant Dean for Veterans Affairs . . . . Vacant
Director, Animal Care Facilities . . . . James S. Harper III, V.M.D.
Director, Financial Services . . . . Thomas Michael, C.P.A.
Director, Medical Student Affairs . . . . Alexandra Morang-Jackson
Director, Admissions and Financial Aid . . . . Kathleen A. Baer
Associate Dean of Biological Sciences. . . . . Marjorie Thompson, Ph.D.
Assistant Dean of Medicine (Admissions) . . . . Arnold-Peter C. Weiss, M.D.
Executive Director of Biomed Development . . . . Susan B. Mouradian
Director of Biomed Advancement Communications . . . . Sarah Baldwin-Beneich

The Warren Alpert Medical School of Brown University: RHODE ISLAND

Department and Division or Section Chairs

Basic Sciences

Ecology and Evolutionary Biology. . . . . Mark D. Bertness, Ph.D.
Molecular Biology, Cell Biology, and Biochemistry . . . . John M. Sedivy, Ph.D.
Molecular Microbiology and Immunology. . . . . Christine A. Biron, Ph.D.
Molecular Pharmacology, Physiology, and Biotechnology. . . . . Wayne Bowen, Ph.D.
Neuroscience. . . . . Barry W. Connors, Ph.D.

Clinical Sciences

Clinical Neurosciences. . . . . J. Donald Easton, M.D.
Community Health . . . . Vincent Mor, Ph.D.
Dermatology . . . . Charles J. McDonald, M.D.
Diagnostic Imaging . . . . John J. Cronan, M.D.
Emergency Medicine. . . . . Brian J. Zink, M.D.
Family Medicine . . . . Jeffrey M. Borkan, M.D., Ph.D.
Medicine. . . . . Lance Dworkin, M.D. (Interim)
    The Memorial Hospital of Rhode Island . . . . Lance Dworkin, M.D. (Interim)
    The Miriam Hospital . . . . Lance Dworkin, M.D. (Interim)
    Rhode Island Hospital . . . . Lance Dworkin, M.D. (Interim)
    Veterans Administration Medical Center. . . . . Lance Dworkin, M.D. (Interim)
    Women and Infants Hospital . . . . Lance Dworkin, M.D. (Interim)
Obstetrics and Gynecology. . . . . Donald R. Coustan, M.D.
Orthopaedics. . . . . Michael Ehrlich, M.D.
    The Miriam Hospital . . . . Michael Ehrlich, M.D.
    Rhode Island Hospital . . . . Michael Ehrlich, M.D.
    Veterans Administration Medical Center. . . . . Richard M. Terek, M.D.
Pathology and Laboratory Medicine . . . . Agnes B. Kane, M.D., Ph.D.
    The Memorial Hospital of Rhode Island . . . . Noubar Kessimian, M.D.
    The Miriam Hospital . . . . Ronald A. DeLellis, M.D.
    Rhode Island Hospital . . . . Ronald A. DeLellis, M.D.
    Women and Infants Hospital . . . . W. Dwayne Lawrence, M.D.
Pediatrics . . . . Robert B. Klein, M.D. (Interim)
Psychiatry and Human Behavior. . . . . Martin B. Keller, M.D.
    Bradley Hospital. . . . . Gregory K. Fritz, M.D.
    Butler Hospital. . . . . Martin B. Keller, M.D.
    The Miriam Hospital . . . . Bess H. Marcus, M.D.
    Rhode Island Hospital . . . . Richard J. Goldberg, M.D.
    Veterans Administration Medical Center. . . . . Robert G. M. Johnston, M.D.
Radiation Medicine . . . . David E. Wazer, M.D.
Surgery. . . . . William G. Cioffi, M.D.
    The Miriam Hospital . . . . Harry C. Sax, M.D.
    Rhode Island Hospital . . . . William G. Cioffi, M.D.
    Veterans Administration Medical Center. . . . . Michael P. Vezeridis, M.D.

Medical University of South Carolina College of Medicine

171 Ashley Avenue
Charleston, South Carolina 29425
843-792-2300; 792-2081 (dean's office); 792-2967 (fax)
Web site: www2.musc.edu

Founded in 1824, the Medical College of South Carolina graduated its first class in 1825. In 1969, its name was changed to the Medical University of South Carolina.

Type: public
2008-2009 total enrollment: 570
Clinical facilities: Charleston Memorial Hospital, Greenville Hospital System, McLeod Regional Medical Center, Medical University Hospital, Naval Regional Medical Center, Richland Memorial Hospital, Roper Hospital, St. Francis Xavier Hospital, Veterans Administration Medical Center (Charleston), Anderson Area Medical Center, Self Memorial Hospital, Spartanburg Regional Medical Center, Allendale County Hospital, Hampton General Hospital.

University Officials

President. . . . . Raymond S. Greenberg, M.D., Ph.D.
Vice President for Academic Affairs and Provost. . . . . John Richard Raymond, M.D.
Vice President for Medical Affairs. . . . . J. G. Reves, M.D.
Vice President for Finance and Administration. . . . . Lisa P. Montgomery
Vice President for Clinical Operations and
 Executive Director of the Medical Center . . . . W. Stuart Smith
Vice President for Development. . . . . Jim Fisher
Director of Libraries and Learning Resource Center. . . . . Thomas G. Basler, Ph.D.
Director of Office of Diversity . . . . Willette Burnham
Executive Director, Enrollment Services . . . . Open
University Counsel. . . . . Joseph C. Good, Jr.

Medical School Administrative Staff

Dean. . . . . J. G. Reves, M.D.
Senior Associate Dean for Medical Education . . . . Jeffrey G. Wong, M.D.
Senior Associate Dean, Diversity. . . . . Deborah Deas, M.D.
Senior Associate Dean, Clinical Affairs . . . . Bruce M. Elliott, M.D.
Associate Dean, Diversity . . . . Thaddeus J. Bell, M.D.
Associate Dean, Admissions . . . . Paul B. Underwood, M.D.
Associate Dean for Minority Recruitment . . . . Aljoeson Walker, M.D.
Associate Dean, Curriculum and Evaluation . . . . Lynn Manfred, M.D., Ed.D.
Associate Dean, Students . . . . Christopher G. Pelic, M.D.
Associate Dean, Finance and Administration. . . . . C. Maurice Snook
Associate Dean for Planning, Implementation, and Evaluation. . . . . Edward F. Cousineau
Associate Dean for Finance . . . . Fred A. Crawford, Jr., M.D.
Associate Dean, Faculty Development. Marc I. Chimowitz, M.B.Ch.B.
Associate Dean, Graduate Medical Education . . . . Harry S. Clarke, M.D., Ph.D.
Associate Dean for Continuing Medical Education . . . . Robert J. Malcolm, M.D.
Associate Dean, Veteran Affairs . . . . Florence N. Hutchison, M.D.
Associate Dean, Area Health Education Consortium . . . . David R. Garr, M.D.
Associate Dean, International Activities. . . . . Peter B. Cotton, M.D.
Associate Dean, Greenville. . . . . Jerry R. Youkey, M.D.
Associate Dean, Columbia . . . . James I. Raymond, M.D.
Associate Dean, Spartanburg . . . . Otis L. Baughman III, M.D.
Associate Dean, Greenwood. . . . . Gary R. Goforth, M.D.
Associate Dean, Florence . . . . William H. Hester, M.D.
Associate Dean, Anderson . . . . Stoney A. Abercrombie, M.D.
Chief Executive Officer, University Practice Plan. . . . . Bruce A. Quinlan
Associate Dean, Development. . . . . Terry Stanley
Associate Dean, Community and Alumni Advocacy . . . . Melissa Henshaw, M.D.
Associate Dean for Interdisciplinary Research . . . . Andrew Kraft, M.D.
Associate Dean for Interdisciplinary Clinical Programs . . . . Michael Gold, M.D., Ph.D.
Associate Dean, Statewide Clinical Effectiveness Education . . . . John Schaefer, M.D.

Associate Dean for Clinical Research .... Kathleen T. Brady, M.D., Ph.D.
Associate Dean, Communication Development .... Linda S. Austin, M.D.

Department and Division or Section Chairs

Basic Sciences

Biochemistry and Molecular Biology........................... Yusuf A. Hannun, M.D.
Biostatistics, Bioinformatics, and Epidemiology................... Barbara C. Tilley, Ph.D.
Cell and Molecular Pharmacology and
    Experimental Therapeutics .... Kenneth D. Tew, Ph.D., D.Sc.
Cell Biology and Anatomy .... Roger R. Markwald, Ph.D.
Comparative Medicine.................................. M. Michael Swindle, D.V.M.
Microbiology and Immunology............................... James S. Norris, Ph.D.
Neurosciences (Research) .... Peter W. Kalivas, Ph.D.
Pathology and Laboratory Medicine............................ Janice M. Lage, M.D.

Clinical Sciences

Anesthesia and Perioperative Medicine........................... Scott T. Reeves, M.D.
Dermatology .... Bruce H. Thiers, M.D.
Family Medicine .... William J. Hueston, M.D.
Medicine.. John R. Feussner, M.D.
    Cardiovascular .... Michael R. Gold, M.D., Ph.D.
    Emergency Medicine .... Laurence H. Raney, M.D.
    Endocrinology, Metabolism, and Nutrition .... Louis M. Luttrell, M.D., Ph.D.
    Gastroenterology .... Mark Payne, M.D.
    General Internal Medicine and Gerontology .... William Moran, M.D.
    Hematology and Oncology........................... Harry Drabkin, M.D.
    Infectious Diseases .... Michael Kilby, M.D.
    Nephrology .... David W. Ploth, M.D.
    Pulmonary and Critical Care.......................... Steven Sahn, M.D.
    Rheumatology and Immunology........................ Richard M. Silver, M.D.
Neurosciences (Clinical) .... Sunil J. Patel, M.D.
Obstetrics and Gynecology........................... J. Peter VanDorsten, M.D.
Ophthalmology .... M. Edward Wilson, M.D.
Orthopaedic Surgery .... Langdon Hartsock, M.D.
Otolaryngology and Communicative Sciences .... Paul R. Lambert, M.D.
Pediatrics .... L. Lyndon Key, M.D.
Psychiatry and Behavioral Sciences...................... Thomas W. Uhde, M.D.
Radiation Oncology................................ Joseph M. Jenrette III, M.D.
Radiology .... Philip Costello, M.D.
Surgery... David J. Cole, M.D.
    Cardiothoracic................................. Fred A. Crawford, Jr., M.D.
    Pediatric Surgery .... Andre Hebra, M.D.
    Plastic and Maxillofacial............................ John Robinson, M.D. (Interim)
Urology... Thomas E. Keane, M.B.B.Ch.

University of South Carolina School of Medicine

Columbia, South Carolina 29208
803-733-3188 (dean's office); 253-5873 (fax)
Web site: www.med.sc.edu

The University of South Carolina School of Medicine was authorized by the South Carolina legislature in June 1973 and is established under the Veterans Administration Medical School Assistance and Health Manpower Training Act of 1972. The new school of medicine campus, located approximately four-and-a-half miles from the main campus of the University of South Carolina, was completed in 1983 and houses basic science departments, administrative offices, and the medical library. Most clinical departments are located at affiliated hospitals in the Columbia area. The school's first class matriculated in September 1977.

Type: public
2008-2009 total enrollment: 315
Clinical facilities: Dorn Veterans Administration Medical Center, Palmetto Health, South Carolina Department of Mental Health, Moncrief Army Hospital, Greenville Hospital System.

University Officials

President. . . . . Andrew Sorensen, Ph.D.
Provost . . . . Mark P. Becker, Ph.D.

Medical School Administrative Staff

Dean. . . . . Donald J. DiPette, M.D.
Associate Dean for Basic Science . . . . Prakash Nagarkatti, Ph.D.
Associate Dean for Clinical Affairs . . . . O. Marion Burton, M.D.
Associate Dean for Clinical Research and Special Projects . . . . Stanley D. Fowler, Ph.D.
Associate Dean for Medical Education and Academic Affairs . . . . . . Richard A. Hoppmann, M.D.
Assistant Dean for Continuing Medical Education. . . . . Morris J. Blachman, Ph.D.
Assistant Dean for Preclinical Curriculum. Lynn K. Thomas, Dr. P.H.
Assistant Dean for Clinical Assessment . . . . Nancy A. Richeson, M.D.
Assistant Dean for Clinical Curriculum. Joshua T. Thornhill IV, M.D.
Associate Dean (Dorn VA Medical Center) . . . . Alfred B. Boykin, Jr., M.D.
Associate Dean (Greenville Hospital System). Jerry R. Youkey, M.D.
Associate Dean (Palmetto Health Alliance) . . . . James I. Raymond, M.D.
Assistant Dean for Medical Education
    (Greenville Hospital System) . . . . Paul V. Catalana, M.D.
Assistant Dean for Minority Affairs . . . . Carol L. McMahon, M.D.
Assistant Dean for Medical Humanities. . . . . Charles S. Bryan, M.D.
Administrator, Office of Admissions and Registrar . . . . Jeanette H. Ford, Ed.D.
Chief Business Officer and Senior Director of
    Budget, Finance, Facilities, and Research
    Administration . . . . Jeffrey L. Perkins
Chief Operating Officer. . . . . Alfred A. Dunn
Director of Information Technology. . . . . D. Lindsie Cone, M.D.
Director of Legal Affairs. . . . . Linda T. Moore, J.D.
Director of Medical Library . . . . Ruth A. Riley
Director of Student Services. . . . . Donald J. Kenney, Ph.D.

University of South Carolina School of Medicine: SOUTH CAROLINA

Department and Division or Section Chairs

Basic Sciences

Biochemistry . . . . James M. Sodetz, Ph.D.
Cell and Developmental Biology and Anatomy . . . . Joseph S. Janicki, Ph.D.
Pathology, Microbiology, and Immunology . . . . Mitzi Nagarkatti, Ph.D.
Pharmacology, Physiology, and Neuroscience . . . . Marlene A. Wilson, Ph.D.

Clinical Sciences

Family and Preventive Medicine . . . . Elizabeth G. Baxley, M.D.
Internal Medicine . . . . Shawn A. Chillag, M.D.
  Allergy and Immunology . . . . David J. Amrol, M.D.
  Cardiology . . . . Donald E. Saunders, Jr., M.D.
  Dermatology . . . . Annette W. Lynn, M.D.
  Endocrinology . . . . Tu Lin, M.D.
  General Internal Medicine . . . . Allan S. Brett, M.D.
  Geriatrics . . . . G. Paul Eleazer, M.D.
  Infectious Diseases . . . . Helmut Albrecht, M.D.
  Nephrology . . . . Steven J. Rosansky, M.D.
  Pulmonary and Critical Care Medicine . . . . James A. Barker, M.D.
  Rheumatology . . . . James W. Fant, Jr., M.D.
Neuropsychiatry and Behavioral Science . . . . Richard K. Harding, M.D.
  Child and Adolescent Psychiatry . . . . Steven P. Cuffe, M.D.
  Forensic Psychiatry . . . . Richard L. Frierson, M.D.
  Neurology . . . . Richard K. Harding, M.D.
  Psychoanalysis . . . . Clyde H. Flanagan, Jr., M.D.
  Rehabilitation Counseling . . . . Linda C. Leech, Ph.D.
Obstetrics and Gynecology . . . . Janice L. Bacon, M.D.
  Ambulatory Obstetrics and Gynecology . . . . Janice L. Bacon, M.D.
  Clinical Genetics . . . . Robert G. Best, Ph.D.
  Gynecology . . . . Janice L. Bacon, M.D.
  Maternal Fetal Medicine . . . . Anthony R. Gregg, M.D.
  Ultrasonography . . . . Anthony R. Gregg, M.D.
Ophthalmology . . . . Richard M. Davis, M.D.
Orthopaedic Surgery . . . . John J. Walsh IV, M.D. (Interim)
Pediatrics . . . . R. Caughman Taylor, M.D.
Radiology . . . . Francis H. Neuffer, M.D.
Surgery . . . . Richard M. Bell, M.D.
  Anesthesiology . . . . Open
  Cardiothoracic Surgery . . . . Reid W. Tribble, M.D.
  General Surgery . . . . Richard M. Bell, M.D.
  Neurosurgery . . . . Lenwood P. Smith, Jr., M.D.
  Otolaryngology . . . . James R. Wells, M.D.
  Pediatric Surgery . . . . P. Prithvi Reddy, M.D.
  Plastic Surgery . . . . Harold I. Friedman, M.D., Ph.D.
  Trauma . . . . Raymond P. Bynoe, M.D.
  Vascular Surgery . . . . Robert R. M. Gifford, M.D.

Sanford School of Medicine of The University of South Dakota

1400 West 22nd Street
Sioux Falls, South Dakota 57105-1570
605-357-1300 (dean's office); 357-1311 (fax)
Web site: www.usd.edu/med

Medical course work began at the University of South Dakota in 1907 with the organization of the college of medicine offering the first two years of the standard four-year medical degree program. The program was expanded in 1974 to degree-granting status and graduated its first class in 1977. The school has a community-based philosophy, and clinical training (Years 3 and 4) is conducted in the community facilities affiliated with the program throughout South Dakota.

Type: public
2008-2009 total enrollment: 209
Clinical facilities: Avera Sacred Heart Hospital, South Dakota Human Services Center, Avera McKennan Hospital and University Health Center, Sanford USD Medical Center, Sioux Falls Veterans Administration Hospital, Children's Care Hospital, Rapid City Regional Hospital, Fort Meade Veterans Administration Hospital.

University Officials

President. . . . . James Abbott
Vice President of Health Affairs . . . . Rodney R. Parry, M.D.

Medical School Administrative Staff

Dean. . . . . Rodney R. Parry, M.D.
Executive Dean . . . . Ron Lindahl, Ph.D.
Dean, Student Affairs. . . . . Paul C. Bunger, Ph.D.
Dean of Clinical Faculty. . . . . Tim Ridgway, M.D.
Dean, Graduate Medical Education . . . . G. Michael Tibbitts, M.D.
Assistant Dean, Graduate Medical Education. Amy Jacobson, Ed.D.
Dean, Health Sciences . . . . Brian Kaatz, Pharm.D.
Dean, Medical Student Education . . . . Janet C. Lindemann, M.D.
Dean, West River Campus . . . . Norman Neu, M.D.
Dean, Yankton Campus . . . . Lori Hansen, M.D.
Dean, Sioux Falls Campus . . . . Tim Ridgway, M.D.
Dean, Vermillion Campus . . . . Ron Lindahl, Ph.D.
Medical Director, Continuing Medical Education . . . . William Held, M.D.
Director of Finance . . . . Julie Kriech
Director of Evaluation and Assessment . . . . Edward G. Simanton, Ph.D.
Associate Director of Education Services. . . . . Brian R. Dzwonek, Ed.D.
Director, Wegner Center Library . . . . Carolyn Warmann, M.A.

Sanford School of Medicine of The University of South Dakota: SOUTH DAKOTA

Department and Division or Section Chairs

Basic Biomedical Sciences

Dean . . . . Ron Lindahl, Ph.D.
Associate Dean . . . . Steve Waller, Ph.D.
Laboratory Medicine . . . . Michael Koch, M.D.

Clinical Sciences

Family Medicine . . . . H. Bruce Vogt, M.D.
   Center for Rural Health Improvement . . . . Open
   Nutrition . . . . Roger Shewmake, Ph.D.
Internal Medicine . . . . LuAnn Eidsness, M.D.
   Allergy and Immunology . . . . R. Maclean Smith, M.D.
   Cardiology . . . . Scott Pham, M.D.
   Critical Care . . . . Ashraf Elshami, M.D.
   Dermatology . . . . Brian Knutson, M.D.
   Endocrinology . . . . J. Michael McMillin, M.D.
   Ethics and Palliative Care . . . . Joann Bennett, D.O.
   Gastroenterology . . . . Larry Schafer, M.D.
   Geriatrics . . . . David Sandvik, M.D.
   Hematology and Oncology . . . . Michael McHale, M.D., and David Elson, M.D.
   Hospitalist Medicine . . . . Aman Khurana, M.D.
   Infectious Diseases . . . . Veronica Soler, M.D.
   Nephrology . . . . Richard Jensen, M.D.
   Pulmonology . . . . Brian Hurley, M.D.
   Research . . . . Karen Munger, Ph.D.
   Rheumatology . . . . Joseph Fanciullo, M.D.
Neurosciences . . . . Jerome Freeman, M.D.
Obstetrics and Gynecology . . . . Keith Hansen, M.D.
Pediatrics . . . . H. Eugene Hoyme, M.D.
   Cardiology . . . . Theresa Stamato, M.D.
   Child Advocacy . . . . Jerome Blake, M.D.
   Clinical Services . . . . James Wallace, M.D.
   Critical Care . . . . Joseph Segeleon, M.D.
   Developmental Pediatrics . . . . Jerome Blake, M.D.
   Education . . . . Lawrence Wellman, M.D.
   Endocrinology, Genetics, and Metabolic Disease . . . . Laura Keppen, M.D.
   Gastroenterology . . . . Gary Neidich, M.D.
   Hematology and Oncology . . . . Linda Stout, M.D.
   Neonatology . . . . David Munson, M.D.
   Neurology . . . . Bonnie Bunch, M.D., Ph.D.
   Palliative Care . . . . Lawrence Fenton, M.D.
   Physical Medicine and Rehabilitation . . . . Julie Johnson, M.D.
   Pulmonology . . . . James Wallace, M.D.
   Research . . . . Amy Elliott, Ph.D.
   Surgery . . . . Adela Casas-Melley, M.D.
Psychiatry . . . . Timothy Soundy, M.D.
Surgery . . . . John Ryan, M.D.
   Anesthesiology . . . . Open
   Neurosurgery . . . . Quentin J. Durward, M.D.
   Ophthalmology . . . . Gregory D. Osmundson, M.D.
   Orthopedic Surgery . . . . Robert Van Demark, Jr., M.D.
   Otolaryngology . . . . Craig Hedges, M.D.
   Urology . . . . Matthew Witte, M.D.

East Tennessee State University
James H. Quillen College of Medicine
P.O. Box 70694
Johnson City, Tennessee 37614
423-439-1000; 439-6315 (dean's office); 439-2033 (admissions); 439-8090 (fax)
E-mail: medcom@com.etsu.edu
Web site: http://com.etsu.edu

The James H. Quillen College of Medicine of East Tennessee State University was authorized by the Tennessee legislature in March 1974 and is established under the Veterans Administration Medical School Assistance and Health Manpower Training Act of 1972. Consistent with its mission, the Quillen College of Medicine is noted for its emphasis on primary care and rural medicine training, placing 75 to 85 percent of its graduates in medically underserved and/or rural communities.

Type: public
2008-2009 total enrollment: 240
Clinical facilities: ETSU Physicians and Associates, Family Practice Centers (Kingsport, Bristol, Johnson City); Johnson City Medical Center; Indian Path Medical Center; Bristol Regional Medical Center; Holston Valley Medical Center (Kingsport); Frontier Health; Woodridge Hospital; James H. Quillen Veterans Affairs Medical Center (Mountain Home); Ambulatory Clinics (Mountain City, Rogersville).

University Officials

President. . . . . Paul E. Stanton, Jr., M.D.
Vice President for Health Affairs . . . . Wilsie S. Bishop, D.P.A.

Medical School Administrative Staff

Dean. . . . . Philip C. Bagnell, M.D.
Executive Associate Dean for Academic and Faculty Affairs . . . . Kenneth E. Olive, M.D.
Executive Associate Dean for Clinical Affairs. . . . . I. William Browder, M.D.
Associate Dean for Student Affairs . . . . Thomas E. Kwasigroch, Ph.D.
Associate Dean for Finance and Administration . . . . Gregory L. Wilgocki
Associate Dean for Graduate Studies . . . . Mitchell E. Robinson, Ph.D.
Associate Dean for Learning Resources. . . . . Biddanda (Suresh) Ponnappa
Assistant Dean and Director of Operations . . . . M. David Linville, M.D.
Assistant Dean for Academic Affairs . . . . Penny Little Smith, Ed.D.
Assistant Dean for Admissions and Records. . . . . Edwin D. Taylor
Assistant Dean for Continuing Medical Education. . . . . Barbara Sucher
Assistant Dean and Director of Medical Education-VAMC . . . . Felix A. Sarubbi, M.D.
Assistant Dean for Women in Medicine . . . . Theresa F. Lura, M.D.
Assistant Dean for Graduate Medical Education . . . . Debra A. Shaw
Assistant Dean for Finance and Administration. . . . . Sue Taylor
Director for Government Relations. . . . . Robert V. Acuff, Ph.D.
Office Manager for Dean's Office. . . . . Donna D. Gage
Media Relations Coordinator . . . . Joseph E. Smith

Department and Division or Section Chairs

Basic Sciences

Anatomy and Cell Biology . . . . Richard G. Skalko, Ph.D.
    Cell and Tissue Biology . . . . Fred E. Hossler, Ph.D.
    Gross Anatomy. . . . . Thomas E. Kwasigroch, Ph.D.
    Neurobiology. . . . . Ronald H. Baisden, Ph.D.
Biochemistry and Molecular Biology. . . . . W. Scott Champney, Ph.D.
Microbiology. . . . . Priscilla B. Wyrick, Ph.D.
Pharmacology . . . . Gregory A. Ordway, Ph.D.
Physiology. . . . . William L. Joyner, Ph.D.

Clinical Sciences

Family Medicine .... John P. Franko, M.D.
    Division of Education .... Forrest Lang, M.D.
    Division of Primary Care Research .... Fraser (Fred) G. Tudiver, M.D.
    Division of Rural Programs .... Joseph A. Florence IV, M.D.
    Family Medicine Residency-Kingsport .... Reid Blackwelder, M.D.
    Family Medicine Residency-Bristol. .... TBA
    Family Medicine Residency-Johnson City .... Max Bayard, M.D.
Internal Medicine .... Gene D. LeSage, M.D.
    Allergy .... Guha Krishnaswamy, M.D.
    Basic Sciences .... David Chi, Ph.D.
    Cardiology .... Philip D. Henry, M.D.
    Dermatology .... Stuart S. Leicht, M.D.
    Endocrinology .... Charles Stuart, M.D., and Alan Peiris, M.D., Ph.D.
    Gastroenterology .... Mark Young, M.D.
    General Internal Medicine .... Roger Smalligan, M.D.
    Hematology and Oncology .... Koyamangalath Krishnan, M.D.
    Immunology. .... Guha Krishnaswamy, M.D.
    Infectious Disease. .... Jonathan P. Moorman, M.D.
    Preventive Medicine and Epidemiology .... Jay B. Mehta, M.D.
    Pulmonary .... Thomas M. Roy, M.D.
    Rheumatology .... William Wason, M.D.
Obstetrics and Gynecology. .... Martin E. Olsen, M.D.
    Gynecologic Oncology .... Janet Drake, M.D.
    Maternal Fetal Medicine. .... Uchenna Nwosu, M.D., and Jessica DeMay, M.D.
Pathology .... John B. Schweitzer, M.D.
Pediatrics .... David K. Kalwinsky, M.D.
    Adolescent Medicine .... David Chastain, M.D.
    Developmental and Behavioral .... H. Patrick Stern, M.D.
    Research .... William L. Stone, Ph.D.
    Cardiology .... Rajani Anand, M.D.
    Gastroenterology .... Ayman Abdel-Wahab, M.D.
    General Pediatrics .... Debra Quarles Mills, M.D.
    Genetics. .... Jack Rary, Ph.D.
    Hematology and Oncology .... David K. Kalwinsky, M.D., and Kathryn Klopfenstein, M.D.
    Neonatology. .... W. Michael DeVoe, M.D.
    Nephrology .... Ahmad Wattad, M.D.
    Pulmonary and Intensive Care .... Ricky T. Mohon, M.D.
Psychiatry .... Merry N. Miller, M.D.
    VA Psychiatry Services. .... George R. Brown, M.D.
    Child and Adolescent Psychiatry .... TBA
Surgery .... I. William Browder, M.D.
    Cardiovascular and Thoracic Surgery .... William Messerschmidt, M.D.
    Critical Care. .... Tiffany Lasky, M.D.
    Ophthalmology .... Barbara O. Kimbrough, M.D.
    General Surgery. .... Carlos Floresguerra, M.D.
    Plastic Surgery .... Daniel F. Haynes, M.D.
    Research .... David Williams, Ph.D.
    Surgical Oncology .... Mary A. Hooks, M.D.
    Trauma Surgery-Johnson City .... Julie Dunn, M.D.
    Trauma Surgery-Kingsport .... Corydon Siffring, M.D.
    Vascular Surgery. .... Dan Rush, M.D.

Meharry Medical College School of Medicine
1005 Dr. D. B. Todd Jr. Boulevard
Nashville, Tennessee 37208
615-327-6204 (dean's office); 327-6568 (fax); 327-6111 (general information)
Web site: www.mmc.edu/medschool

Meharry Medical College was organized in 1876 as the medical department of Central Tennessee College. In 1900, Central Tennessee College was reorganized as Walden University, and the medical department became known as Meharry Medical College of Walden University. Later, a separate corporate existence was sought, and in 1915, a new charter was granted by the state of Tennessee. Through contributions from various sources, property was acquired in northwest Nashville, and the present school and hospital were erected in 1930-31. The school of medicine is the oldest and largest of the college's three schools.

Type: private
2008-2009 total enrollment: 368
Clinical facilities: Alvin C. York Veterans Administration Medical Center (Murfreesboro), Meharry Ambulatory Care Center, Matthew Walker Comprehensive Health Center, Middle Tennessee Mental Health Institute, Nashville General Hospital at Meharry, Blanchard Army Community Hospital (Fort Campbell, Kentucky), Columbia Centennial Medical Center and Baptist Hospital.

Medical College Officials

President . . . . Wayne J. Riley, M.D., F.A.C.P.
Senior Vice President for Health Affairs and
  Dean, School of Medicine . . . . Valerie Montgomery Rice, M.D.
Vice President for Finance . . . . LaMel Bandy-Neal
General Counsel and Corporate Secretary . . . . Benjamin Rawlins, J.D.
Executive Vice President . . . . Angela Walker Franklin, Ph.D.
Dean, School of Graduate Studies and Research . . . . Maria F. Lima, Ph.D.
Dean, School of Dentistry . . . . William B. Butler, D.D.S.

Medical School Administrative Staff

Executive Vice Dean . . . . Pamela C. Williams, M.D.
Assistant Dean for Student and Academic Affairs . . . . Brenda Merritt
Associate Dean, Graduate Medical Education . . . . Billy R. Ballard, M.D., D.D.S.
Associate Dean for Administration and Chief of Staff . . . . Cassandra S. Ward, Ed.D.
Associate Dean, Faculty Affairs and Development . . . . Patricia Matthews-Juarez, Ph.D.
Associate Dean, Curriculum Evaluation. . . . . Etheleen McGinnis-Hill, Ph.D.
Associate Dean, Academic Services . . . . Vacant
Student Counselor . . . . Sharda D. Mishra, Ph.D.
Assistant Dean, Special Programs . . . . Sharon Turner-Friley
Associate Dean, Finance . . . . Dennis Saucerman
Associate Dean, Academic Computing . . . . Vicky Mosley
Associate Dean, Clinical Affairs . . . . Chike M. Nzerue, M.D.
Associate Dean, Clinical Affiliations . . . . Susanne Tropez-Sims, M.D.
Associate Dean, Biomedical Sciences . . . . James G. Townsel, Ph.D.
Associate Vice President, Student Support
  Services, and Director, Center for Education
  Development and Support . . . . Jacqueline 'Dee' Gardner
Associate Dean, Continuing Medical Education. . . . . Renee Bowen, J.D.

Meharry Medical College School of Medicine: TENNESSEE

Department Chairs

Biomedical Sciences

Cancer Biology . . . . Samuel E. Adunyah, Ph.D.
Cardiovascular Biology . . . . ZhongMao Guo, M.D., Ph.D. (Interim)
Microbial Pathogenesis and Immune Response . . . . Fernando Villalta, Ph.D.
Neurobiology and Neurotoxicology . . . . Clivel Charlton, Ph.D.

Clinical Sciences

Family and Community Medicine . . . . Roger Zoorob, M.D.
Internal Medicine . . . . Steven Wolff, M.D.
Neurology . . . . Patrick Griffith, M.D.
Obstetrics and Gynecology . . . . Gloria Richard-Davis, M.D.
Pathology . . . . Billy R. Ballard, M.D., D.D.S.
Pediatrics . . . . Xylina Bean, M.D.
Radiology . . . . Anthony Disher, M.D.
Surgery . . . . Derrick Beech, M.D.
Professional and Medical Education . . . . George Breaux, M.D.
Psychiatry and Behavioral Sciences . . . . Rahn K. Bailey, M.D.

Center Directors

Center for Health Disparities Research . . . . James Hildreth, M.D., Ph.D.
Center for Women's Health Research . . . . Valerie Montgomery Rice, M.D.

*Specialty without organizational autonomy.

University of Tennessee Health Science Center, College of Medicine

62 South Dunlap, Room 400
Memphis, Tennessee 38163
901-448-5529 (dean's office); 448-7683 (fax)
Web site: www.utmem.edu

The University of Tennessee College of Medicine was established in 1851 as the medical department of the University of Nashville. Later, by mergers and agreements, it became part of the University of Tennessee and was moved to Memphis in 1911. It is one of six colleges comprising the University of Tennessee Health Science Center, and has programs in Chattanooga, Jackson, Knoxville, and Nashville as well as in Memphis.

Type: public
2008-2009 total enrollment: 671
Clinical facilities: Regional Medical Center at Memphis, Baptist Memorial Hospital, Le Bonheur Children's Medical Center, Memphis Mental Health Institute, Department of Veterans' Affairs Medical Center, St. Jude Children's Research Hospital, Methodist University Hospital, the University of Tennessee Medical Center (James K. Dobbs Research Institute, Doctors Office Building), Saint Francis Hospital (Memphis), Baroness Erlanger and T. C. Thompson Hospitals (Chattanooga), University of Tennessee Medical Center (Knoxville), Jackson-Madison County General Hospital (Jackson), Baptist Hospital (Nashville).

University Officials

President . . . . John Petersen, Ph.D.
Chancellor, Health Science Center, and Vice
    President for Health Affairs . . . . Hershel P. Wall, M.D. (Interim)
Executive Dean, College of Medicine . . . . Steve J. Schwab, M.D.
Dean, College of Medicine - Chattanooga. . . . . David C. Seaberg, M.D.
Dean, College of Medicine - Knoxville . . . . James J. Neutens, Ph.D., FASHA
Dean, College of Medicine - Memphis . . . . Steve J. Schwab, M.D.

Medical School Administrative Staff

Executive Dean . . . . Steve J. Schwab, M.D.
Executive Associate Dean for Finance and Administration . . . . J. Timothy Mashburn, M.B.A.
Executive Associate Dean for Graduate Medical
    Education and Continuing Medical Education. . . . . Eugene Mangiante, M.D.
Associate Dean for Clinical Affairs . . . . James Lacey Smith, M.D.
Associate Dean, Medical Education. . . . . Robert G. Shreve, Ed.D.
Associate Dean, Faculty Affairs . . . . Mary Ann Watson, Ph.D.
Associate Dean, Student Affairs . . . . Owen Phillips, M.D.
Associate Dean, Academic Programs at Methodist University Hospital . . . . Steve Miller, M.D.
Assistant Dean, Academic Programs at St. Jude
    Children's Research Hospital . . . . P. Joan Chesney, M.D.
Assistant Dean, Admissions and Enrollment Services . . . . E. Nelson Strother, Jr.
Assistant Dean, Baptist Hospital - Nashville . . . . Vacant
Assistant Dean, Continuing Medical Education
    and Graduate Medical Education . . . . Mary Ann Watson, Ph.D.

University of Tennessee Health Science Center, College of Medicine: TENNESSEE

Department Chairs

Basic Sciences - Memphis Campus

Anatomy and Neurobiology . . . . Matthew Ennis, Ph.D.
Biomedical Engineering and Imaging . . . . Steve Bares, Ph.D., M.B.A. (Interim)
Molecular Sciences . . . . Gerald Byrne, Ph.D.
Pharmacology . . . . Burt M. Sharp, M.D.
Physiology . . . . Gabor J. Tigyi, Ph.D.

Clinical Sciences - Memphis Campus

Anesthesiology . . . . John Zanella, M.D., Ph.D.
Comparative Medicine . . . . Timothy D. Mandrell, D.V.M.
Family Medicine . . . . David L. Maness, D.O., M.S.S., FAAFP
Human Values and Ethics . . . . Terrence Ackerman, Ph.D.
Medicine . . . . Guy L. Reed, M.D.
Neurology . . . . William A. Pulsinelli, M.D., Ph.D.
Neurosurgery . . . . Jon H. Robertson, M.D.
Obstetrics and Gynecology . . . . Veronica T. Mallett, M.D.
Ophthalmology . . . . Barrett G. Haik, M.D.
Orthopaedic Surgery . . . . S. Terry Canale, M.D.
Otolaryngology-Head and Neck Surgery . . . . Jerome W. Thompson, M.D.
Pathology . . . . Charles Handorf, M.D., Ph.D.
Pediatrics . . . . Russell W. Chesney, M.D.
Preventive Medicine . . . . Grant W. Somes, Ph.D.
Psychiatry . . . . James A. Greene, M.D., and Kenneth A. Sakauye, M.D.
Radiology . . . . Barry Gerald, M.D. (Acting)
Surgery . . . . Timothy C. Fabian, M.D.
Urology . . . . Robert Wake, M.D.

Chattanooga Campus

Family Medicine . . . . J. Mack Worthington, M.D.
Medicine . . . . Mukta Panda, M.D. (Acting)
Obstetrics and Gynecology . . . . J. Michael Breen, M.D.
Orthopaedic Surgery . . . . Thomas W. Currey, M.D.
Pediatrics . . . . Marvin Hall, M.D. (Acting)
Plastic Surgery . . . . Larry A. Sargent, M.D.
Radiology . . . . R. Kent Hutson, M.D.
Surgery . . . . R. Phillip Burns, M.D.
Emergency Medicine . . . . R. Phillip Burns, M.D.

Knoxville Campus

Anesthesiology . . . . Jerry L. Epps, M.D.
Family Medicine . . . . Gregory H. Blake, M.D.
Medicine . . . . Timothy J. Panella, M.D.
Obstetrics and Gynecology . . . . Robert F. Elder, M.D.
Pathology . . . . Stuart Van Meter, M.D.
Pediatrics . . . . Eddie S. Moore, M.D.
Radiology . . . . J. Mark McKinney, M.D.
Surgery . . . . Mitchell H. Goldman, M.D.

Vanderbilt University School of Medicine

21st Avenue South at Garland Avenue
Nashville, Tennessee 37232
615-322-5000 (general information); 322-5191 (dean's office); 343-7286 (fax)
E-mail: jeff.balser@vanderbilt.edu
Web site: www.mc.vanderbilt.edu/medschool

Vanderbilt University issued its first M.D. degrees in 1875. During a reorganization in 1925, the medical school was moved to the main campus of Vanderbilt University. The medical school is part of the Vanderbilt University Medical Center.

Type: private
2008-2009 total enrollment: 430
Clinical facilities: Vanderbilt University Hospital, Vanderbilt Stallworth Rehabilitation Hospital, Veterans Administration Medical Center, Middle Tennessee Mental Health Institute, St. Thomas Hospital, Baptist Hospital, Vanderbilt Psychiatric Hospital, Nashville Metropolitan General Hospital, Monroe Carell Jr. Children's Hospital at Vanderbilt.

University Official

Chancellor . . . . Nicholas S. Zeppos

Medical Center Officials

Vice Chancellor for Health Affairs . . . . Harry R. Jacobson, M.D.
Associate Vice Chancellor for Research. . . . . Jeffrey R. Balser, M.D., Ph.D.
Associate Vice Chancellor for Health Affairs and
    Director, Informatics Center . . . . William W. Stead, M.D.
Executive Associate Vice Chancellor, Medical Center Development . . . . Randy L. Farmer
Executive Director for Medical Alumni Affairs . . . . Ann H. Price, M.D.
Associate Vice Chancellor for Clinical Affairs
    and Chief Medical Officer . . . . C. Wright Pinson, M.D.
Chief Financial Officer . . . . J. Richard Wagers, Jr.
Associate Vice Chancellor for Hospital Affairs. . . . . Martin P. Sandler, Ch.B.
Chief Executive Officer, Vanderbilt University Hospital. . . . . Larry M. Goldberg
Associate Vice Chancellor, Medical Center Communications . . . . Joel G. Lee
Corporate Compliance Officer . . . . Robert H. Ossoff, M.D.
Executive Director and Chief Executive Officer,
    Vanderbilt Children's Hospital . . . . Kevin B. Churchwell, M.D.

Medical School Administrative Staff

Dean. . . . . Jeffrey R. Balser, M.D., Ph.D. (Interim)
Senior Associate Dean for Biomedical Research,
    Education, and Training . . . . G. Roger Chalkley, D.Phil.
Associate Dean for Diversity in Graduate Medical
    Education and Faculty Affairs . . . . André L. Churchwell, M.D.
Associate Dean for Diversity in Medical Education . . . . George C. Hill, Ph.D.
Associate Dean for Graduate Medical Education . . . . Donald W. Brady, M.D.
Associate Dean for Undergraduate Medical Education . . . . Bonnie M. Miller, M.D.
Associate Dean for Clinical and Translational
    Scientist Development . . . . Nancy J. Brown, M.D.
Associate Dean for Medical Students . . . . Scott M. Rodgers, M.D.
Associate Dean for Faculty Affairs. . . . . David S. Raiford, M.D.
Associate Dean of Admissions. . . . . John A. Zic, M.D.
Associate Dean for Clinical Affairs . . . . Gerald B. Hickson, M.D.
Chief of Staff for Veterans Administration . . . . George Arana, M.D.
Director of Continuing Medical Education . . . . Donald E. Moore, Jr., Ph.D.
Director of Office for Teaching and Learning in Medicine . . . . John H. Shatzer, Ph.D.
Director of Finance . . . . Craig R. Carmichel
Director of Medical School Financial Services. . . . . Vicky L. Cagle
Chief of Staff. . . . . Lynn E. Webb, Ph.D.

Department and Division or Section Chairs

Basic Sciences

Biochemistry . . . . Michael R. Waterman, Ph.D.

Biomedical Informatics .... Daniel R. Masys, M.D.
Biostatistics .... Frank E. Harrell, Jr., Ph.D.
Cancer Biology .... Harold L. Moses, M.D. (Interim)
Cell and Development Biology............................... Susan R. Wente, Ph.D.
Microbiology and Immunology............................ Jacek J. Hawiger, M.D., Ph.D.
Molecular Physiology and Biophysics .... Roger D. Cone, Ph.D.
Pathology .... Samuel A. Santoro, M.D., Ph.D.
Pharmacology .... Heidi E. Hamm, Ph.D.

Clinical Sciences

Anesthesiology.................................... Michael S. Higgins, M.D.
Cardiac Surgery (Surgical Sciences) .... John G. Byrne, M.D.
Emergency Medicine....................................... Corey M. Slovis, M.D.
General Surgery (Surgical Sciences) .... Naji N. Abumrad, M.D.
Hearing and Speech Sciences................................ Fred H. Bess, Ph.D.
Medicine.. Eric G. Neilson, M.D.
   Allergy, Pulmonary, and Critical Care .... Gordon R. Bernard, M.D.
   Cardiovascular Medicine........................ Douglas B. Sawyer, M.D., Ph.D.
   Clinical Pharmacology .... Jason D. Morrow, M.D.
   Dermatology .... George P. Stricklin, M.D., Ph.D.
   Endocrinology and Diabetes........................ Stephen N. Davis, M.D.
   Gastroenterology .... Richard M. Peek, Jr., M.D.
   General Internal Medicine .... Robert S. Dittus, M.D.
   Genetic Medicine........................... Alfred L. George, Jr., M.D.
   Hematology and Oncology .... David H. Johnson, M.D.
   Infectious Disease........................... Richard T. D'Aquila, M.D.
   Nephrology .... Raymond C. Harris, Jr., M.D.
   Rheumatology and Clinical Immunology.............. James Ward Thomas II, M.D.
Neurology...................................... Robert L. Macdonald, M.D., Ph.D.
Neurosurgery (Surgical Sciences) .... George S. Allen, M.D., Ph.D.
Obstetrics and Gynecology...................... Howard W. Jones III, M.D. (Interim)
Ophthalmology and Visual Sciences .... Paul Sternberg, Jr., M.D.
Oral Surgery and Dentistry (Surgical Sciences) .... Samuel J. McKenna, D.D.S., M.D., FACS
Orthopaedics and Rehabilitation .... Dan M. Spengler, M.D.
Otolaryngology .... Robert H. Ossoff, M.D.
Pediatrics .... Jonathan D. Gitlin, M.D.
   Adolescent Medicine .... Lynn Walker, Ph.D.
   Cardiology................................... H. Scott Baldwin, M.D.
   College Health and Young Adult Medicine .... John W. Greene, M.D.
   Critical Care..................................... Rick Barr, M.D.
   Developmental Pediatrics and Cognition..................... Tyler Reimschisel, M.D.
   Endocrinology .... William E. Russell, M.D.
   Gastroenterology and Nutrition .... D. Brent Polk, M.D.
   General Pediatrics .... Shari L. Barkin, M.D.
   Genetics.................................... John A. Phillips III, M.D.
   Hematology and Oncology .... James A. Whitlock, M.D.
   Infectious Disease............................. Terence S. Dermody, M.D.
   Neonatology.................................. Judy L. Aschner, M.D.
   Nephrology .... Kathy Jabs, M.D.
   Pulmonary................................ Jayant K. Deshpande, M.D. (Interim)
   Rheumatology and Immunology.................. Alexander R. Lawton III, M.D.
Pediatric Surgery (Surgical Sciences) .... Wallace W. Neblett III, M.D.
Plastic Surgery (Surgical Sciences) .... Bruce Shack, M.D.
Preventive Medicine................................. William Schaffner, M.D.
   Pharmacoepidemiology............................. Wayne A. Ray, Ph.D.
Psychiatry .... Stephan H. W. Heckers, M.D.
   Addiction Psychiatry.............................. Peter R. Martin, M.D.
   Adult Psychiatry .... Richard C. Shelton, M.D.
   Child and Adolescent Psychiatry...................... George C. Bolian, M.D.
   Clinical Psychopharmacology .... Herbert Y. Meltzer, M.D.
   Forensic Psychiatry.............................. William Bernet, M.D.
   Geriatric Psychiatry............................ Harry E. Gwirtsman, M.D.
Radiation Oncology.................................. Dennis E. Hallahan, M.D.
Radiology and Radiological Sciences............................ Jeremy J. Kaye, M.D.
Section of Surgical Sciences.......................... R. Daniel Beauchamp, M.D.
Thoracic Surgery (Surgical Sciences) .... Joe B. Putnam, Jr., M.D.
Urologic Surgery (Surgical Sciences) .... Joseph A. Smith, Jr., M.D.

Baylor College of Medicine

One Baylor Plaza
Houston, Texas 77030
713-798-4951 (general information); 798-4800 (president's office); 798-6353 (fax)
Web site: www.bcm.edu

Baylor College of Medicine, founded in Dallas in 1900, is the only private medical school in the greater Southwest. The college moved to Houston in 1943 to become the educational cornerstone of the new Texas Medical Center. In 1903, the medical school began an affiliation with Baylor University that lasted until 1969, when Baylor College of Medicine became an independent institution.

Type: private
2008-2009 total enrollment: 666
Clinical facilities: DeBakey Veterans Affairs Medical Center, Harris County Hospital District and Community Health Program (Ben Taub General Hospital and Quentin Mease Community Hospital), Menninger Clinic, St. Luke's Episcopal Hospital, Texas Children's Hospital, The Institute for Research and Rehabilitation and The Methodist Hospital. **Other affiliated clinical institutions:** Cullen Bayou Place, DePelchin Children's Center, Houston Child Guidance Center, Jewish Family Service Cancer Center, Kelsey-Seybold Clinic, Park Plaza Hospital, Seven Acres Jewish Geriatric Center, Shriners Hospital for Children, The University of Texas M.D. Anderson Cancer Center and The Woman's Hospital of Texas.

Medical College Officials

President, Chief Executive Officer, and Executive Dean . . . . Peter G. Traber, M.D.
Chancellor . . . . Bobby R. Alford, M.D.
Chancellor Emeritus . . . . William T. Butler, M.D.
Executive Vice President and Chief Executive
    Officer, Baylor Clinic and Hospital . . . . Donna K. Sollenberger
Senior Vice President and General Counsel . . . . Cyndi M. Baily, J.D., M.P.H.
Senior Vice President for Graduate Sciences and
    Dean, Graduate School of Biomedical
    Sciences . . . . William R. Brinkley, Ph.D.
Senior Vice President and Dean, Medical Education . . . . Stephen B. Greenberg, M.D.
Senior Vice President and Dean, School of
    Allied Health Sciences . . . . J. David Holcomb, Ed.D.
Senior Vice President for Institutional
    Advancement and Executive Administration
    and Chief Development Officer . . . . Lisa Kennedy
Senior Vice President of Finance, Baylor Clinic and Hospital. . . . . David C. Salsberry
Vice President for Public Affairs and Federal Government Relations . . . . Claire M. Bassett
Vice President of Human Resources . . . . Rachel H. Caillouet, Ph.D.
Vice President for Finance and Planning and
    Chief Financial Officer . . . . Kim David, C.P.A., M.B.A. (Acting)
Vice President for Clinic and Hospital
    Operations, Baylor Clinic and Hospital . . . . Lynn Fischer, R.N., M.B.A.,
                    Tracy Giacoma, R.N., M.B.A., M.S.N., and Tom Riley, M.B.A.
Vice President for Medical Affairs, Baylor Clinic and Hospital . . . . William Lunn, M.D.
Vice President for Information Technology and Chief Information Officer . . . . . . Jenifer Jarriel
Vice President for Human Resources, Baylor Clinic and Hospital . . . . Anne Speed, B.B.A.
Vice President of Marketing. . . . . Jenny Dudley
Vice President of Development. . . . . Angela Hodson
Vice President for Operations and Finance. . . . . Bernice Joseph
Vice President of Strategic Capital Projects. . . . . Robert G. McCleskey
Vice President for Business Operations. . . . . Carlos Rodriguez, M.B.A.

Medical College Academic Administration

Vice President and Chief Investment Officer. . . . . William D. Walker, J.D., M.B.A.
President, Chief Executive Officer, and Executive Dean . . . . Peter G. Traber, M.D.
Dean of the Graduate School of Biomedical Sciences . . . . William R. Brinkley, Ph.D.
Senior Vice President and Dean, Medical Education . . . . Stephen B. Greenberg, M.D.
Senior Associate Dean, Graduate Medical Education . . . . Linda B. Andrews, M.D.

Dean of the School of Allied Health Sciences . . . . J. David Holcomb, Ed.D.
Senior Associate Dean, Student Affairs . . . . Donald T. Donovan, M.D.
Senior Associate Dean, Continuing Medical Education . . . . C. Michael Fordis, Jr., M.D.
Senior Associate Dean for Academics and
  Admissions, Graduate School of Biomedical
  Sciences . . . . Hiram F. Gilbert, Ph.D.
Senior Associate Dean, Admissions . . . . Lloyd H. Michael, Ph.D.
Senior Associate Dean, Undergraduate Medical Education . . . . Elizabeth A. Nelson, M.D.
Senior Associate Dean . . . . James L. Phillips, M.D.
Associate Dean, Extramural Affairs . . . . Scott F. Basinger, Ph.D.
Associate Dean for Research Assurances . . . . Stacey L. Berg, M.D.
Associate Dean for Clinical Affairs . . . . John W. Burruss, M.D.
Associate Dean, Student Affairs . . . . Florence F. Eddins-Folensbee, M.D.
Associate Dean, Undergraduate Medical Education . . . . J. Clay Goodman, M.D.
Associate Dean for Clinical Research . . . . Placido B. Grino, M.D.
Associate Dean, Admissions . . . . Graciela B. Villarreal, M.D.
Assistant Dean, Graduate Medical Education . . . . Jacqueline E. Levesque, A.Ed.
Assistant Dean for Clinical Affairs . . . . William W. Lunn, M.D.
Assistant Dean, Graduate Education . . . . Gayle R. Slaughter, Ph.D.
Assistant Dean, Continuing Medical Education . . . . William A. Thomson, Ph.D.
Director, Human Genome Sequencing Center . . . . Richard A. Gibbs, Ph.D.
Director, Smith Breast Center . . . . C. Kent Osborne, M.D.
Director, Huffington Center on Aging . . . . Gretchen Darlington, Ph.D. (Acting)
Director, Center for Medical Ethics and Health Policy . . . . Baruch A. Brody, Ph.D.
Director, Dan L. Duncan Cancer Center . . . . C. Kent Osborne, M.D.
Director, Center for Cell and Gene Therapy . . . . Malcolm K. Brenner, M.D., Ph.D.

Department and Division or Section Chairs

Basic Sciences

Biochemistry and Molecular Biology . . . . Adam Kuspa, Ph.D.
Immunology . . . . Richard G. Cook, Ph.D. (Interim)
Molecular and Cellular Biology . . . . Bert W. O'Malley, M.D.
Molecular and Human Genetics . . . . Arthur L. Beaudet, M.D.
Molecular Physiology and Biophysics . . . . Susan L. Hamilton, Ph.D.
Molecular Virology and Microbiology . . . . Janet S. Butel, Ph.D.
Neuroscience . . . . Michael J. Friedlander, Ph.D.
Pathology . . . . Thomas M. Wheeler, M.D.
Pharmacology . . . . Timothy G. Palzkill, Ph.D.

Clinical Sciences

Anesthesiology . . . . Maya S. Suresh, M.D.
Dermatology . . . . John E. Wolf, Jr., M.D.
Family and Community Medicine . . . . Stephen J. Spann, M.D.
Medicine . . . . David J. Tweardy, M.D. (Interim)
Neurology . . . . Eli M. Mizrahi, M.D.
Neurosurgery . . . . Raymond A. Sawaya, M.D.
Obstetrics and Gynecology . . . . Dale Brown, Jr., M.D. (Interim)
Ophthalmology . . . . Dan B. Jones, M.D.
Orthopedic Surgery . . . . Michael H. Heggeness, M.D.
Otolaryngology-Head and Neck Surgery . . . . Bobby R. Alford, M.D.
Pediatrics . . . . Morey Haymond, M.D. (Acting)
Physical Medicine and Rehabilitation . . . . Martin Grabois, M.D.
Psychiatry and Behavioral Sciences . . . . Stuart C. Yudofsky, M.D.
  Child and Adolescent Psychiatry . . . . Florence Eddins, M.D.
  Psychology . . . . Melinda Stanley, Ph.D.
Radiology . . . . Michel E. Mawad, M.D.
Surgery . . . . F. Charles Brunicardi, M.D.
Urology . . . . Michael Coburn, M.D. (Acting)

Texas A&M Health Science Center College of Medicine

147 Joe H. Reynolds Medical Building
College Station, Texas 77843-1114
979-845-3431 (dean's office); 847-8663 (fax)
Web site: http://medicine.tamhsc.edu

The Texas A&M University College of Medicine was authorized by the Texas legislature in 1971. Its first class was graduated in June 1981. In January 1991, the board of regents of the Texas A&M University System created the Texas A&M University System Health Science Center, of which the college is an integral part. The college is located on the main campus of the parent university with clinical facilities in affiliated institutions.

Type: public
2008-2009 total enrollment: 353
Clinical facilities: Scott and White Memorial Hospital and Clinic (Temple); Central Texas Veterans' Health Care System; (Temple, Waco, Marlin, Austin); Brazos Family Medicine Residency; Lone Star Circle of Care; Memorial Family Medicine Residency Program, Seton Medical Center Williamson; St. David's Round Rock Medical Center; Carl R. Darnall Army Medical Center (Fort Hood); Driscoll Children's Hospital (Corpus Christi); Christus Spohn Memorial Hospital (Corpus Christi); St. Joseph's Health System (Bryan-College Station); College Station Medical Center (College Station).

Health Science Center Officials

President and Vice Chancellor for Health Affairs . . . . Nancy W. Dickey, M.D.
Vice President for Academic Affairs . . . . Roderick E. McCallum, Ph.D.
Vice President for Finance and Administration . . . . Barry C. Nelson, Ph.D.
Vice President for External Affairs and Development . . . . Russ Gibbs
Vice President for Governmental Affairs . . . . Jenny E. Young
Vice President for Research and Graduate Studies . . . . David S. Carlson, Ph.D.
Vice President for Communication and Program Development . . . . Alicia M. Dorsey, Ph.D.
Vice President for Information Technology and CIO . . . . David A. Cantrell

Medical School Administrative Staff

Dean . . . . Christopher C. Colenda, M.D.
Vice Dean, Houston Campus . . . . David Huston, M.D.
Vice Dean, Temple Campus . . . . Donald E. Wesson, M.D.
Vice Dean for Academic Affairs . . . . Robert Hash, M.D.
Vice Dean for Program Development-Temple Campus . . . . Jules B. Puschett, M.D.
Executive Associate Dean for Finance and Administration . . . . Douglas P. Venuti
Associate Dean for Faculty Development . . . . R. Kelly Hester, Ph.D.
Associate Dean for Student Affairs and Admissions . . . . Kathleen Fallon, M.D.
Associate Dean for Veterans Affairs . . . . Ed J. Sherwood, M.D.
Associate Dean for Coastal Bend Affairs . . . . Juan F. Castro, M.D.
Associate Dean for Research and Graduate Studies . . . . Van Wilson, Ph.D.
Associate Dean, Bryan/College Station Campus . . . . Jonathan Friedman, M.D.
Associate Dean, Round Rock Campus . . . . Kathryn Kotrla, M.D.
Assistant Dean for Academic Affairs . . . . José F. Pliego, M.D.
Assistant Dean for Student Affairs . . . . Gary McCord, M.D.
Assistant Dean for Admissions . . . . Filomeno Maldonado
Assistant Dean for Faculty Development . . . . Ed W. Childs, M.D.
Assistant Dean for Planning, Evaluation, and
    External Affairs . . . . Annette R. Tommerdahl, Ph.D.
Director of Institutional Advancement . . . . Brian Hervey

Department and Division or Section Chairs

Basic Sciences

Humanities in Medicine . . . . Charles W. Sanders, M.D.
Microbial and Molecular Pathogenesis . . . . John M. Quarles, Ph.D.
Molecular and Cellular Medicine . . . . J. Martin Scholtz, Ph.D.
Neuroscience and Experimental Therapeutics . . . . William H. Griffith, Ph.D.
Systems Biology and Translational Medicine . . . . Harris J. Granger, Ph.D.

Clinical Sciences

Anesthesiology . . . . Timothy M. Bittenbinder, M.D.

Emergency Medicine . . . . C. Keith Stone, M.D.
Family and Community Medicine . . . . Glen R. Couchman, M.D.
Internal Medicine . . . . Alejandro Arroliga, M.D. (Interim)
  Allergy and Immunology . . . . John Dvoracek, M.D.
  Cardiology . . . . Greg Dehmer, M.D.
  Molecular Cardiology . . . . Kenneth Baker, M.D.
  Dermatology . . . . David F. Butler, M.D.
  Endocrinology . . . . Veronica K. Piziak, M.D., Ph.D.
  Internal Medicine (College Station) . . . . Mark Richards, M.D.
  General Gastroenterology . . . . Richard Erickson, M.D.
  Geriatrics . . . . Vacant
  Hematology and Oncology . . . . Arthur E. Frankel, M.D.
  Infectious Diseases . . . . John Carpenter, M.D.
  Inpatient Medicine . . . . Luis Camarillo, M.D., and Steven Sibbitt, M.D.
  Nephrology and Hypertension . . . . Charles J. Foulks, M.D.
  Occupational and Environmental Medicine . . . . Don Mackey, M.D.
  Physical Medicine and Rehabilitation . . . . Thomas K. Joseph, M.D.
  Pulmonary and Critical Care . . . . Alejandro Arroliga, M.D.
  Rheumatology . . . . Marilyn Clark, M.D.
  Neurology . . . . Richard P. Lenehan, M.D.
Obstetrics and Gynecology . . . . Robert Shull, M.D. (Interim)
  Obstetrics . . . . Steve Allen, M.D.
  Oncology . . . . Charles Capen, M.D.
Pathology . . . . John Greene, M.D.
Pediatrics . . . . David Easley, M.D. (Interim)
  Emergency and Critical Care . . . . David R. Hardy, M.D., and Madhava Beeram, M.D.
  General Pediatrics . . . . M. C. Smith, M.D.
  Pediatric Subspecialists . . . . David Easley, M.D.
  Regional Pediatrics . . . . M. C. Smith, M.D.
  Endocrinology . . . . William Bryant, M.D.
  Gastroenterology . . . . David Easley, M.D.
  Hematology and Oncology . . . . Dick Suh, M.D.
  Hospital Based . . . . James Brien, D.O.
  Infectious Diseases . . . . James Brien, D.O.
  Intensive Care Pediatrics . . . . David R. Hardy, M.D.
  Neonatology . . . . Madhava Beeram, M.D.
  Nephrology . . . . Ronald Hogg, M.D.
  Pediatric Allergy . . . . George W. Brasher, M.D.
  Pediatric Neurology . . . . Darrell E. Crisp, M.D.
  Pulmonary . . . . John Saito, M.D.
Psychiatry and Behavioral Science . . . . Kathryn Kotrla, M.D.
  Adult Psychiatry . . . . James Flack, M.D.
  Child and Adolescent Psychiatry/Psychology . . . . James Flack, M.D.
Radiology . . . . L. Gill Naul, M.D.
  Diagnostic Radiology . . . . Michael Nipper, M.D.
  Interventional Radiology . . . . Mark L. Montgomery, M.D.
  Neuroradiology . . . . Walter S. Lesley, M.D.
  Nuclear Radiology and Advanced Molecular Imaging . . . . Michael L. Middleton, M.D.
  Physics . . . . Arthur Boyer, Ph.D.
  Radiation Oncology . . . . A.Y. C. Cheung, M.D.
Surgery . . . . W. Roy Smythe, M.D.
  Cardiothoracic Surgery . . . . Charles Reiter, M.D.
  Dentistry . . . . Lance Reed, D.D.S.
  Surgery (College Station) . . . . Dirk Boysen, M.D.
  General Surgery . . . . Sam Snyder, M.D.
  Neurosurgery . . . . Frank S. Harris, M.D.
  Ophthalmology . . . . Glen O. Brindley, M.D.
  Orthopedic Surgery . . . . Robert Probe, M.D.
  Otolaryngology . . . . Reginald Baugh, M.D.
  Pediatric Surgery . . . . Donald R. Cooney, M.D.
  Plastic Surgery . . . . Charles N. Verheyden, M.D.
  Surgical Oncology . . . . Terry C. Lairmore, M.D.
  Transplant Surgery . . . . Greg Jaffers, M.D.
  Urology . . . . Phil Reily, Jr., M.D.
  Vascular Surgery . . . . C. J. Buckley, M.D.
  Podiatry . . . . Matt Lynch, D.P.M. (Interim)
  Trauma/Critical . . . . Ed Childs, M.D.

Texas Tech University Health Sciences Center
School of Medicine
3601 4th Street, MS 6207
Lubbock, Texas 79430
806-743-3000 (dean's office); 743-3021 (fax)
E-mail: som@ttuhsc.edu
Web site: www.ttuhsc.edu

In May 1969, the Texas legislature and governor authorized the establishment of an M.D. degree-granting school of medicine on the campus of Texas Tech University in Lubbock. The school is governed by the board of regents of Texas Tech University and the Texas Tech University Health Sciences Center, which meets in separate sessions for each institution. Each is subject to the supervision and regulations of the coordinating board, Texas College and University System. The medical school, with regional academic health centers in Amarillo, El Paso, and Odessa, is part of the Texas Tech University Health Sciences Center.

Type: public
2008-2009 total enrollment: 568
Clinical facilities: Texas Tech University Health Sciences Center Ambulatory Clinics, University Medical Center, Covenant Medical Center, Texas Tech Southwest, Highland Medical Center, Lubbock City/County Maternity Clinic, Veterans Administration Outpatient Clinics (in Lubbock and El Paso), Northwest Texas Hospital and Psychiatric Pavilion, Baptist St. Anthony's Hospital, Harrington Cancer Center, Veterans Administration Hospital (in Amarillo and Big Spring), R.E. Thomason General Hospital, William Beaumont Army Medical Center, El Paso State Center, St. Joseph's Hospital, Family Services of El Paso, Medical Center Hospital, Texas Department of Criminal Justice (Clements Unit and Montford Unit).

University Officials

President. . . . . John C. Baldwin, M.D.
Executive Vice President . . . . Elmo Cavin
Vice President for Medical Affairs. . . . . Steven L. Berk, M.D.
Vice President for Diversity and Multicultural Affairs. German Núñez
Vice President for Rural and Community Health . . . . Vacant
Vice President and Chief Information Officer. . . . . Michael T. Phillips
Director of Libraries . . . . Richard Wood
Director of Student Services and Registrar . . . . Mike Smith

Medical School Administrative Staff (Lubbock)

Dean, School of Medicine . . . . Steven L. Berk, M.D.
Associate Dean for Research. . . . . C. Patrick Reynolds, M.D., Ph.D.
Associate Dean for Oncology Programs. . . . . Everardo Cobos, M.D.
Associate Dean for Health Services Management. . . . . Cynthia Jumper, M.D.
Associate Dean for Educational Programs. . . . . Terry McMahon, M.D.
Associate Dean for Clinical Affairs . . . . Dale M. Dunn, M.D.
Associate Dean for Faculty Affairs and Development . . . . Thomas Tenner, Ph.D.
Associate Dean for Curriculum. . . . . William Simon, Ph.D.
Associate Dean for Admissions . . . . Bernell K. Dalley, Ph.D.
Assistant Dean for Administration. . . . . Bryce McGregor
Associate Dean for Medical Practice Income Plan (MPIP) . . . . Brent Magers
Assistant Dean for Graduate Medical Education . . . . Jim Watters

Department and Division or Section Chairs
Basic Sciences

Cell Biology and Biochemistry . . . . Harry M. Weitlauf, M.D.
Microbiology and Immunology. . . . . Ronald Kennedy, Ph.D.
Pharmacology . . . . Reid Norman, Ph.D.
Cell Physiology and Molecular Biophysics . . . . Luis Reuss, Ph.D.

Clinical Sciences

Anesthesiology. . . . . Mark Boswell, M.D.
Dermatology . . . . Cloyce Stetson, M.D.
Family and Community Medicine . . . . Michael Ragain, M.D.
Internal Medicine . . . . Cynthia Jumper, M.D. (Interim)
Neurology . . . . Cynthia Jumper, M.D.
Obstetrics and Gynecology. . . . . Edward Yeomans, M.D.
Ophthalmology and Visual Sciences . . . . David McCartney, M.D.
Orthopaedic Surgery . . . . Robert Schutt, M.D.
Pathology . . . . Dale M. Dunn, M.D.
Pediatrics . . . . Richard M. Lampe, M.D.
Psychiatry . . . . Terry McMahon, M.D. (Interim)
Surgery. . . . . John A. Griswold, M.D.
Urology. . . . . Werner deRiese, M.D.

Texas Tech University Health Sciences Center at Amarillo
1400 South Coulter
Amarillo, Texas 79106
806-354-5401

Regional Dean. . . . . Richard Jordan, M.D.
Assistant Academic Dean . . . . Marita A. Sheehan, M.D.
Associate Regional Dean of Faculty Development . . . . Fredrick A. McCurdy, M.D.
Assistant Regional Dean for Finance and Administration. . . . . Deborah Cain
Assistant Regional Dean for Research . . . . Thomas Hale, Ph.D.
Assistant Dean for Quality Improvement. . . . . Charles Wright, M.D.
Family Medicine . . . . Rodney Young, M.D.
Internal Medicine . . . . J. Rush Pierce, M.D.
Obstetrics and Gynecology. . . . . Robert Cummings, M.D.
Pediatrics . . . . Bonna Benjamin, M.D. (Interim)
Psychiatry . . . . Michael Jenkins, M.D.
Surgery. . . . . Dennis B. Dove, M.D.

Texas Tech University Health Sciences Center at El Paso
4800 Alberta Avenue
El Paso, Texas 79905
915-545-6510

Regional Dean. . . . . Robert Suskind, M.D.
Assistant Regional Dean for Finance and Administration. . . . . Larry Elkins
Assistant Dean for Research . . . . Vacant
Assistant Dean for Medical Education. . . . . Manual Schydlower, M.D.
Assistant Dean for Faculty Development . . . . Hoi Ho, M.D.
Anesthesiology. . . . . Swapna Chaudhuri, M.D., Ph.D. (Interim)
Emergency Medicine . . . . Vacant
Family Medicine . . . . Mary Spalding, M.D.
Internal Medicine . . . . Manuel Rivera, M.D.
Neuropsychiatry and Behavioral Sciences . . . . James Wilcox, M.D. (Interim)
Obstetrics and Gynecology. . . . . Bahij Nuwayhid, M.D.
Orthopaedic Surgery. . . . . Miguel Pirela-Cruz, M.D.
Pathology . . . . Darius Boman, M.D. (Interim)
Pediatrics . . . . Gilbert Handal, M.D.
Radiology . . . . Arvin Robinson, M.D. (Interim)
Surgery. . . . . Alan H. Tyroch, M.D.

Texas Tech University Health Sciences Center at the Permian Basin
800 West 4th Street
Odessa, Texas 79763
432-335-5113

Regional Dean. . . . . John Jennings, M.D.
Executive Associate Regional Dean for Hospital
  and Community Affairs and Vice President for
  Fiscal Affairs . . . . William D. Finical
Family Medicine . . . . Peter Valenzuela, M.D.
Internal Medicine . . . . William R. Davis, M.D.
Obstetrics and Gynecology. . . . . R. Moss Hampton, M.D.
Pediatrics . . . . Denise Fitzsimon, M.D.
Psychiatry . . . . Judi Stonedale, D.O.
Surgery. . . . . Shelton Viney, M.D.

University of Texas Health Science Center at San Antonio
School of Medicine
7703 Floyd Curl Drive
San Antonio, Texas 78229
210-567-4420 (dean's office); 567-3435 (fax)
Web site: www.uthscsa.edu

The University of Texas Medical School at San Antonio was established in 1959 by the Texas legislature as a separate component unit of the University of Texas System. The medical school opened at its present site in September 1968. In October 1972, the Board of Regents of the University of Texas System directed the establishment of the University of Texas Health Science Center at San Antonio. The School of Medicine is an integral part of the center, which also consists of the dental school, graduate school of biomedical sciences, school of nursing, and school of allied health sciences.

Type: public
2008-2009 total enrollment: 800
Clinical facilities: University Health System (University Hospital and University Health Center Downtown), Audie L. Murphy Memorial Veterans Hospital, Santa Rosa Medical Center, Cancer Therapy and Research Center, St. Luke's Hospital, Wilford Hall USAF Medical Center, Brooke Army Medical Center, USAF School of Aerospace Medicine, Community Guidance Center, San Antonio Children's Center, Baptist Memorial Hospital System.

University Officials

Chancellor (Austin) . . . . Mark G. Yudof
Executive Vice Chancellor for Health Affairs (Austin) . . . . Kenneth I. Shine, M.D. (Interim)

Health Science Center Administrative Staff

President . . . . Francisco Cigarroa, M.D.
Senior Executive Vice President and Chief Operating Officer . . . . Michael E. Black, M.D.
Chief of Staff and Chief Communications Officer . . . . Mary Etlinger DeLay
Executive Vice President for Facility Planning and Administration . . . . James D. Kazen
Executive Vice President for Business Affairs and Chief Financial Officer. . . . . . . H. Steve Lynch
Vice President and Chief Information Officer . . . . A. Jerome York
Vice President for Development . . . . Deborah Morrill
Vice President for Governmental Relations . . . . Armando Diaz
Vice President for Research . . . . Brian Herman, Ph.D.
Dean of School of Medicine and Vice President
   for Medical Affairs . . . . William L. Henrich, M.D.
Dean of School of Allied Health Sciences . . . . Marilyn S. Harrington, Ph.D.
Dean of Graduate School of Biomedical Sciences . . . . Merle S. Olson, Ph.D.
Dean of Dental School . . . . Kenneth L. Kalkwarf, D.D.S.
Dean of School of Nursing . . . . Eileen Breslin, Ph.D., R.N.
Vice President for Academic Administration . . . . Theresa Chiang, Ed.D.
President and Chief Executive Officer of University Health System . . . . George Hernandez
Director of the VA Hospital . . . . Richard Baltz
Chief of Staff of the VA Hospital . . . . Richard L. Bauer, M.D.

School of Medicine Administrative Staff

Dean of Medical School and Vice President for Medical Affairs . . . . William L. Henrich, M.D.
Vice Dean for Clinical Affairs . . . . Lewis Greenberg, M.D.
Senior Associate Dean for Academic Affairs . . . . C. Nanette Clare, M.D.
Regional Academic Health Center Dean . . . . Leonel Vela, M.D., Ph.D.
Regional Assistant Dean for Medical Education . . . . Adela Valdez, M.D.
Associate Dean for Administration . . . . Jan Wilson, Ed.D.
Associate Dean for Admissions . . . . David J. Jones, Ph.D.
Associate Dean for Student Affairs . . . . Lee D. Jones, M.D.
Assistant Dean for Student Affairs . . . . Thomas L. Matthews, M.D.
Associate Dean for VA Hospital Affairs . . . . Richard L. Bauer, M.D.
Associate Dean for Finance . . . . William R. Allen
Associate Dean for Graduate Medical Education . . . . Lois L. Bready, M.D.
Associate Dean for Continuing Medical Education . . . . Martha Medrano, M.D.
Associate Dean for Research . . . . Robin Brey, M.D.
Assistant Dean for M.D./M.P.H. Program . . . . Claudia Miller, M.D.
Associate Dean for Professionalism and Faculty Development . . . . Pedro L. Delgado, M.D.
Assistant Dean for Ambulatory Services . . . . Carlayne Jackson, M.D.
Assistant Dean for Oncology . . . . Tyler Curiel, M.D.

University of Texas Health Science Center at San Antonio
School of Medicine: TEXAS

Department and Division or Section Chairs
Clinical Sciences

Anesthesiology. . . . . J. Jeffrey Andrews, M.D.
Epidemiology and Biostatistics . . . . Bradley Pollock, Ph.D.
Family and Community Health. . . . . Carlos R. Jaén, M.D., Ph.D.
Medicine. . . . . L. David Hillis, M.D.
   Cardiology. . . . . Steven Bailey, M.D. (Interim)
   Clinical Epidemiology. . . . . Vacant
   Clinical Immunology and Rheumatology. . . . . Michael D. Fischbach, M.D.
   Clinical Pharmacology . . . . Alexander M. Shepherd, M.D., Ph.D.
   Dermatology . . . . Eric W. Kraus, M.D. (Interim)
   Diabetes. . . . . Ralph De Fronzo, M.D.
   Gastroenterology and Human Nutrition . . . . Glenn W. Gross, M.D.
   General Medicine. . . . . Andrew K. Diehl, M.D.
   Geriatrics and Gerontology. . . . . Michael J. Lichtenstein, M.D.
   Hematology and Oncology. . . . . Francis Giles, M.D.
   Infectious Diseases . . . . Thomas F. Patterson, M.D.
   Nephrology . . . . Hanna Abboud, M.D.
   Pulmonary Diseases . . . . Jay I. Peters, M.D. (Interim)
Neurology. . . . . C. Akos Szabo, M.D. (Interim)
Neurosurgery. . . . . David F. Jimenez, M.D.
Obstetrics and Gynecology. . . . . Robert S. Schenken, M.D.
   Gynecology . . . . Kevin Hall, M.D.
   Maternal and Fetal Medicine . . . . Elly M. J. Xenakis, M.D.
   Reproductive Endocrinology and Infertility. . . . . Robert Brzyski, M.D.
Ophthalmology . . . . Carlos Rosende, M.D.
Orthopaedics. . . . . Daniel W. Carlisle, M.D. (Interim)
   Podiatry . . . . Thomas Zgonis, D.P.M. (Interim)
Otolaryngology-Head and Neck Surgery . . . . Randall Otto, M.D.
Pediatrics . . . . Thomas C. Mayes, M.D.
   Cardiology . . . . James H. Rogers, Jr., M.D.
   Child Abuse Pediatrics . . . . Nancy Kellogg, M.D.
   Community Pediatrics. . . . . Victor F. German, M.D.
   Critical Care. . . . . Richard P. Taylor, M.D.
   Endocrinology . . . . Daniel Hale, M.D.
   Gastroenterology . . . . Vacant
   Genetics and Metabolism Disorders. . . . . Jannine D. Cody, Ph.D. (Interim)
   Hematology-Oncology . . . . Gail Tomlinson, M.D., Ph.D.
   Infectious Diseases . . . . Anthony J. Infante, M.D., Ph.D.
   Neonatology. . . . . Steven Seidner, M.D.
   Nephrology . . . . Mazen Arar, M.D.
   Pulmonology . . . . Victor German, M.D. (Interim)
Rehabilitation Medicine. . . . . Nicolas E. Walsh, M.D.
Psychiatry . . . . Pedro L. Delgado, M.D.
   Alcohol and Drug Addiction. . . . . John D. Roache, Ph.D. (Interim)
   Child and Adolescent Psychiatry. . . . . Stephen R. Pliszka, M.D.
   Education . . . . Kenneth L. Matthews, M.D.
   Mood and Anxiety Disorders. . . . . Charles L. Bowden, M.D. (Interim)
   Schizophrenia and Related Disorders . . . . Alexander L. Miller, M.D.
Radiology . . . . Michael J. McCarthy, M.D. (Interim)
   Diagnostic Radiology . . . . Ralph Blumhardt, M.D.
   Imaging Research Center . . . . Peter T. Fox, M.D.
   Radiological Sciences . . . . Gary D. Fullerton, Ph.D.
Radiation Oncology. . . . . Chul S. Ha, M.D.
Surgery . . . . Stephen M. Cohn, M.D.
   Thoracic Surgery . . . . John H. Calhoon, M.D.
   Emergency Medicine . . . . David A. Hnatow, M.D.
   General Surgery VA (GSVA). . . . . Peter Lopez, M.D.
   General Surgery B (GSB) . . . . Wayne H. Schwesinger, M.D.
   General Surgery A (GSA) . . . . Kenneth R. Sirinek, M.D.
   Organ Transplant. . . . . Glenn A. Halff, M.D.
   Plastic and Reconstructive Surgery . . . . Howard Wang, M.D. (Interim)
   South Texas Poison Center. Miguel Fernandez, M.D.
   Trauma Surgery. . . . . Ronald M. Stewart, M.D.
   Vascular Surgery. . . . . Boulos Toursarkissian, M.D.
Urology. . . . . Ian M. Thompson, M.D.

University of Texas Southwestern Medical Center at Dallas
Southwestern Medical School

5323 Harry Hines Boulevard
Dallas, Texas 75390
214-648-3111; 648-2509 (dean's office); 648-8955 (dean's office fax)
Web site: www.utsouthwestern.edu

The University of Texas Southwestern Medical Center at Dallas was founded as Southwestern Medical College in 1943, affiliated with the University of Texas System in 1949, and was given health center form in 1972. The three components of the Southwestern Medical Center are Southwestern Medical School, the graduate school of biomedical sciences, and the allied health sciences school.

Type: public
2008-2009 total enrollment: 922
Clinical facilities: UT Southwestern University Hospitals and Clinics, Parkland Memorial Hospital, Children's Medical Center, Dallas VA Medical Center, Baylor University Medical Center, Callier Center for Communication Disorders, John Peter Smith Hospital, Presbyterian Hospital of Dallas, Richardson Regional Medical Center, Southwestern Institute of Forensic Sciences, Texas Scottish Rite Hospital for Crippled Children, Terrell State Hospital, Methodist Hospitals of Dallas, Methodist Charlton Medical Center, University of Texas Health Center at Tyler, McLennan County Family Practice Center (Waco), Wichita General Hospital (Wichita Falls).

University Officials

Chancellor (Austin) . . . . Mark G. Yudof
Executive Vice Chancellor for Health Affairs (Austin) . . . . Kenneth I. Shine, M.D.

Medical Center Administrative Staff

President. . . . . Daniel K. Podolsky, M.D.
Executive Vice President for Health System Affairs . . . . John D. McConnell, M.D.
Executive Vice President for Academic Affairs and Provost . . . . . . Alfred G. Gilman, M.D., Ph.D.
Executive Vice President for Business Affairs. . . . . John A. Roan
Executive Vice President for Clinical Affairs . . . . Willis C. Maddrey, M.D.
Dean, Medical School . . . . Alfred G. Gilman, M.D., Ph.D.
Dean, Graduate School of Biomedical Sciences. Melanie Cobb, Ph.D.
Dean, Allied Health Sciences School . . . . Raul Caetano, M.D., Ph.D.
Vice President for Clinical Operations . . . . John D. Rutherford, M.D.
Vice President for Corporate and Community Relations . . . . Ruben E. Esquivel
Vice President for Human Resources . . . . William Behrendt, Ph.D.
Vice President for Legal Affairs . . . . Leah A. Hurley, J.D.
Vice President for Medical Affairs. . . . . Bruce Meyer, M.D.
Vice President for Technology Development. . . . . Dennis K. Stone, M.D.
Vice President for External Relations . . . . Cynthia B. Bassel
Vice President for Facilities Management . . . . Kirby Vahle
Vice President for Information Resources. . . . . Kirk A. Kirksey
Vice President for Student and Alumni Affairs . . . . J. Wesley Norred
Assistant Vice President for Public Affairs . . . . John Walls

Medical School Administrative Staff

Dean. . . . . Alfred G. Gilman, M.D., Ph.D.
Senior Associate Dean for Academic Administration . . . . Charles Ginsburg, M.D.
Associate Dean for Undergraduate Medical Education . . . . Lynne M. Kirk, M.D.
Associate Dean for Graduate Medical Education. . . . . Lynne M. Kirk, M.D.
Associate Dean for Student Affairs . . . . James M. Wagner, M.D.
Associate Dean for Student Affairs . . . . Angela P. Mihalic, M.D.
Associate Dean for Minority Student Affairs . . . . Byron L. Cryer, M.D.
Associate Dean for Medical Education . . . . Susan Cox, M.D.
Associate Dean for Oncology Programs. . . . . James K.V. Willson, M.D.
Associate Dean for Academic Planning. . . . . James E. Griffin, M.D.
Associate Dean for Research. . . . . Perrie M. Adams, Ph.D.
Associate Dean for M.D.-Ph.D. Training Program . . . . Andrew R. Zinn, M.D., Ph.D.

Department and Division or Section Chairs

Basic Sciences

Biochemistry . . . . Steven L. McKnight, Ph.D.
Cell Biology. . . . . Richard G. W. Anderson, Ph.D.
Developmental Biology . . . . Luis F. Parada, Ph.D.
Immunology . . . . Edward K. Wakeland, Ph.D.
Microbiology. . . . . Michael V. Norgard, M.D.
Molecular Biology . . . . Eric N. Olson, Ph.D.
Molecular Genetics . . . . Joseph L. Goldstein, M.D.
Neuroscience. . . . . Jane E. Johnson, Ph.D. (Acting)
Pharmacology . . . . David J. Mangelsdorf, Ph.D.
Physiology . . . . James T. Stull, Ph.D.

Clinical Sciences

Anesthesiology. . . . . Charles W. Whitten, M.D. (Acting)
Cardiovascular and Thoracic Surgery . . . . W. Steves Ring, M.D.
Clinical Sciences . . . . Milton Packer, M.D.
Dermatology . . . . Kim B. Yancey, M.D.
Family and Community Medicine. . . . . Alison Dobbie, M.D.
Internal Medicine . . . . J. Gregory Fitz, M.D.
  Allergy. . . . . Rebecca Gruchalla, M.D., Ph.D.
  Cardiology. . . . . Joseph Hill, M.D., Ph.D.
  Clinical Genetics . . . . Helen H. Hobbs, M.D.
  Digestive and Liver Diseases . . . . Don Rockey, M.D.
  Endocrinology and Metabolism. . . . . Keith Parker, M.D., Ph.D.
  Epidemiology. . . . . Robert W. Haley, M.D.
  General Internal Medicine . . . . Lynne M. Kirk, M.D. (Acting)
  Hematology-Oncology . . . . Joan Schiller, M.D.
  Nutrition and Metabolic Diseases . . . . Abhimanyu Garg, M.D.
  Hypertension. . . . . Ronald G. Victor, M.D.
  Infectious Disease. . . . . Beth Levine, M.D.
  Mineral Metabolism . . . . Khashayar Sakhaee, M.D.
  Nephrology . . . . Peter Igarashi, M.D.
  Pulmonary Disease . . . . Lance S. Terada, M.D.
  Rheumatology . . . . David Karp, M.D., Ph.D.
  Transplant Immunology . . . . Peter Stastny, M.D.
Neurological Surgery. . . . . Duke S. Samson, M.D.
Neurology . . . . Stephen C. Cannon, M.D., Ph.D.
Obstetrics-Gynecology . . . . Steven L. Bloom, M.D.
Ophthalmology . . . . James P. McCulley, M.D.
Orthopaedic Surgery . . . . Joseph Borrelli, Jr., M.D.
Otolaryngology-Head and Neck Surgery . . . . Peter S. Roland, M.D.
Pathology . . . . Errol C. Friedberg, M.D.
Pediatrics . . . . George Lister, M.D.
Physical Medicine and Rehabilitation . . . . Karen J. Kowalske, M.D.
Plastic Surgery. . . . . Rodney J. Rohrich, M.D.
Psychiatry . . . . Carol A. Tamminga, M.D. (Acting)
  Psychology. . . . . C. Munro Cullum, Ph.D.
Radiation Oncology. . . . . Hak Choy, M.D.
Radiology . . . . Robert W. Parkey, M.D.
Surgery . . . . Robert Rege, M.D.
  Burn/Trauma/Critical Care . . . . Robert Rege, M.D. (Acting)
  Emergency Medicine . . . . Paul Pepe, M.D.
  GI/Endocrine . . . . Edward Livingston, M.D.
  Oral Surgery . . . . John Zuniga, D.D.S., Ph.D.
  Pediatric Surgery . . . . Robert Foglia, M.D.
  Surgical Oncology . . . . Roderich Schwarz, M.D., Ph.D.
  Transplant Surgery. . . . . Juan Arenas, M.D.
  Vascular Surgery. . . . . G. Patrick Clagett, M.D.
Urology. . . . . Claus Roehrborn, M.D.

University of Texas Medical Branch
University of Texas Medical School at Galveston

301 University Boulevard
Galveston, Texas 77555-0133
409-772-1011; 772-2671 (dean's office); 772-9598 (fax)
E-mail: ganderso@utmb.edu
Web site: www.utmb.edu

The University of Texas Medical Branch at Galveston was established in 1881 as a branch of the University of Texas and accepted its first class in 1891. In addition to the medical school, the campus includes the graduate school of biomedical sciences, school of allied health sciences, school of nursing, Marine Biomedical Institute, Institute for the Medical Humanities, and the Institute for Human Infections and Immunity.

Type: public
2008-2009 total enrollment: 837
Clinical facilities: John Sealy Hospital, Children's Hospital, Rebecca Sealy Hospital, Primary Care Pavillion, Texas Department of Criminal Justice Hospital. **Other facility:** Shriners Burns Institute.

University Officials

Chancellor (Austin) . . . . Kenneth I. Shine, M.D. (ad interim)
Executive Vice Chancellor for Health Affairs (Austin) . . . . Kenneth I. Shine, M.D.

Medical Branch Administrative Staff

President . . . . David L. Callender, M.D., F.A.C.S.
Executive Vice President and Provost . . . . Garland D. Anderson, M.D.
Executive Vice President and Chief Executive
    Officer for the UTMB Health System . . . . Karen Sexton, Ph.D. (ad interim)
Senior Vice President for Health Care Policy and Legislative Affairs . . . . . . Ben G. Raimer, M.D.
Vice President for Education . . . . Pamela G. Watson, Sc.D.
Director, Moody Medical Library . . . . Brett A. Kirkpatrick

Medical School Administrative Staff

Dean of Medicine . . . . Garland D. Andersen, M.D.
Vice Dean for Academic Affairs . . . . Steven A. Lieberman, M.D.
Chief Physician Executive, Faculty Group Practice . . . . Donald S. Prough, M.D.
Chief Financial and Administrative Officer,
    Academic Enterprise . . . . Cameron Slocum, M.B.A.
Chief Communications Officer . . . . Jacqueline M. Genovese
Dean, Austin Programs . . . . T. Samuel Shomaker, M.D., J.D.
Senior Associate Dean for Faculty Affairs . . . . Linda G. Phillips, M.D.
Associate Dean for Graduate Medical Education . . . . Thomas A. Blackwell, M.D.
Associate Dean for Regional Medical Education . . . . Michael A. Ainsworth, M.D.
Associate Dean for Research Services Administration . . . . William New
Associate Dean for Research . . . . David G. Gorenstein, Ph.D.
Associate Dean for Student Affairs and Admissions . . . . Lauree Thomas, M.D.
Assistant Dean for Student Affairs and Admissions . . . . Jeffrey P. Rabek, Ph.D.
Associate Dean for Continuing Medical Education . . . . David K. Rassin, Ph.D.
Assistant Dean for Educational Affairs . . . . Gregory K. Asimakis, Ph.D.
Assistant Dean for Educational Affairs . . . . Judith L. Rowen, M.D.
Assistant Dean for Educational Development . . . . Ann W. Frye, Ph.D.

Department and Division or Section Chairs

Basic Sciences

Biochemistry and Molecular Biology........................ J. Regino Perez-Polo, Ph.D.
Microbiology and Immunology............................... David W. Niesel, Ph.D.
Neuroscience and Cell Biology............................. Henry F. Epstein, M.D.
Pathology .... David H. Walker, M.D.
Pharmacology and Toxicology .... Kathryn A. Cunningham, Ph.D. (ad interim)
Preventive Medicine and Community Health .... Billy U. Philips, Jr., Ph.D.

Clinical Sciences

Anesthesiology... Donald S. Prough, M.D.
Dermatology .... Sharon S. Ramier, M.D.
Family Medicine .... Barbara L. Thompson, M.D.
Internal Medicine .... Randall J. Urban, M.D.
  Allergy, Pulmonary, Immunology, Critical Care, and Sleep......... Victor J. Cardenas, M.D.
  Cardiology... Charles Y. Lui, M.D. (ad interim)
  Endocrinology .... Nicola Abate, M.D.
  Gastroenterology .... Don W. Powell, M.D. (ad interim)
  General Medicine....................................... Thomas Blackwell, M.D.
  Geriatrics... Neil Nussbaum, M.D., J.D.
  Hematology and Oncology................................ Avi Markowitz, M.D.
  Infectious Diseases.................................... A. Clinton White, M.D.
  Nephrology and Hypertension .... Robert E. Beach, M.D.
  Rheumatology .... Emilio B. Gonzalez, M.D.
Neurology.. Tetsuo Ashizawa, M.D.
Obstetrics and Gynecology................................ Gary Hankins, M.D., D.V.
Ophthalmology and Visual Sciences .... Bernard F. Godley, M.D., Ph.D.
Orthopaedics and Rehabilitation .... Ronald W. Lindsey, M.D.
Otolaryngology .... Sharon S. Raimer, M.D. (ad interim)
Pediatrics .... C. Joan Richardson, M.D. (ad interim)
Psychiatry and Behavioral Sciences....................... Robert M. A. Hirschfeld, M.D.
Radiation Oncology....................................... Martin Colman, M.D.
Radiology .... Gregory L. Katzman, M.D.
Surgery .... Courtney M. Townsend, Jr., M.D.
  Cardiovascular and Thoracic............................ Vincent R. Conti, M.D.
  Emergency Medicine .... Brian S. Zachariah, M.D.
  General Surgery.. Courtney M. Townsend, Jr., M.D.
  Neurosurgery... Haring J. W. Nauta, M.D., Ph.D.
  Oral Surgery .... Elgene G. Mainous, D.D.S.
  Plastic Surgery .... Linda G. Phillips, M.D.
  Urology .... Eduardo Orihuela, M.D.

University of Texas Medical School at Houston

6431 Fannin
Houston, Texas 77030
713-500-5160 (student affairs); 500-5010 (dean's office); 500-0602 (fax)
Web site: www.med.uth.tmc.edu

The University of Texas Medical School at Houston was authorized by the Texas legislature in May 1969 as a component of the University of Texas System. With cooperation of the other three University of Texas medical schools, the first class enrolled in September 1970 and was graduated in 1973. The medical school is a part of the University of Texas Health Science Center at Houston with schools of dentistry, public health, nursing, health information sciences, and the graduate school of biomedical sciences.

Type: public
2008-2009 total enrollment: 875
Clinical facilities: Memorial Hermann Hospital, The University of Texas M. D. Anderson Cancer Center, Lyndon B. Johnson General Hospital/Harris County Hospital District, Memorial Hermann Hospital System, Shriners Hospital for Crippled Children, St. Joseph Hospital, Harris County Psychiatric Center, St. Luke's Episcopal Hospital-Texas Heart Institute.

University Officials

Chancellor (Austin) . . . . Kenneth I. Shine, M.D. (Interim)
Executive Vice Chancellor for Health Affairs (Austin) . . . . Kenneth I. Shine, M.D.

Health Science Center Administrative Staff

President. . . . . Larry R. Kaiser, M.D.
Executive Vice President, Chief Operating and Financial Officer. . . . . Kevin Dillon
Executive Vice President for Academic Affairs. . . . . L. Maximilian Buja, M.D.
Executive Vice President for Clinical Affairs . . . . Richard J. Andrassy, M.D.
Executive Vice President for Research . . . . Peter J. Davies, M.D., Ph.D.

Medical School Administrative Staff

Dean. . . . . Giuseppe N. Colasurdo, M.D.
Executive Vice Dean for Clinical Affairs . . . . Brent R. King, M.D.
Associate Dean for Admissions and Student Affairs . . . . Margaret C. McNeese, M.D.
Associate Dean for Educational Programs. . . . . Patricia M. Butler, M.D.
Associate Dean for Faculty Affairs. . . . . Henry W. Strobel, Ph.D.
Associate Dean for Harris County Programs . . . . Steven D. Brown, M.D.
Associate Dean for Information Technology . . . . William A. Weems, Ph.D.
Associate Dean for Institutional Advancement. . . . . Stanley G. Schultz, M.D.
Assistant Dean for Clinical Research. . . . . Jon E. Tyson, M.D.
Assistant Dean for Admissions . . . . Wallace A. Gleason, M.D.
Assistant Dean for Admissions . . . . Judianne Kellaway, M.D.
Assistant Dean for Student Affairs. . . . . Sheela L. Lahoti, M.D.
Assistant Dean for Educational Programs . . . . R. Andrew Harper, M.D.
Assistant Dean for Educational Programs . . . . Gary C. Rosenfeld, Ph.D.
Assistant Dean for Educational Programs . . . . Margaret O. Uthman, M.D.
Assistant Dean for Graduate Medical Education . . . . John R. Potts, M.D.
Assistant Dean for Faculty Affairs . . . . Katherine A. Loveland, Ph.D.
Assistant Dean for Research Affairs. . . . . John H. Byrne, Ph.D.
Director, Graduate Medical Education . . . . David E. Kusnerik
Director, Biomedical Information Technology . . . . Stephen J. Fath, Ph.D.
Director, Center for Laboratory Animal
 Medicine and Care . . . . Bradford S. Goodwin, Jr., D.V.M.
Executive Director of Administration . . . . Nancy O. McNiel, Ph.D.
Executive Director of Finance . . . . Angela M. Hintzel
Director, Management Services . . . . Claire Brunson
Executive Director, Development and Alumni Relations . . . . Jacquelyn Callies
Director, Student Affairs . . . . Patricia E. Caver
Coordinator, Faculty Affairs . . . . Faye W. Viola
Coordinator, Postdoctoral Affairs . . . . Leslie Shields

Department Chairs and Division Directors

Basic Sciences

Biochemistry and Molecular Biology . . . . Rodney E. Kellems, Ph.D.
Integrative Biology and Pharmacology . . . . John F. Hancock, Ph.D.
Microbiology and Molecular Genetics . . . . Samuel Kaplan, Ph.D.
Neurobiology and Anatomy . . . . John H. Byrne, Ph.D.

Clinical Sciences

Anesthesiology . . . . Carin A. Hagberg, M.D.
Cardiothoracic and Vascular Surgery . . . . Hazim J. Safi, M.D.
Dermatology . . . . Ronald P. Rapini, M.D.
Diagnostic and Interventional Imaging . . . . Susan D. John, M.D.
Emergency Medicine . . . . Brent R. King, M.D.
Family and Community Medicine . . . . Carlos A. Moreno, M.D.
Internal Medicine . . . . Philip R. Orlander, M.D. (Interim)
   Cardiology . . . . David D. McPherson, M.D.
   Endocrinology, Diabetes, and Metabolism . . . . Philip R. Orlander, M.D.
   Gastroenterology, Hepatology, and Nutrition . . . . Gene S. LeSage, M.D.
   General Medicine . . . . Philip C. Johnson, M.D.
   Geriatric Medicine . . . . Carmel B. Dyer, M.D.
   Hematology . . . . Harinder S. Juneja, M.D.
   Infectious Diseases . . . . Barbara E. Murray, M.D.
   Medical Genetics . . . . Dianna M. Milewicz, M.D., Ph.D.
   Oncology . . . . Joan M. C. Bull, M.D.
   Pulmonary, Critical Care Medicine, and Sleep Medicine . . . . Richard J. Castriotta, M.D., Ph.D.
   Renal Diseases and Hypertension . . . . Kevin W. Finkel, M.D.
   Rheumatology and Clinical Immunogenetics . . . . John D. Reveille, M.D.
Neurology . . . . James C. Grotta, M.D.
Neurosurgery . . . . Dong H. Kim, M.D.
Obstetrics, Gynecology, and Reproductive Sciences . . . . Susan M. Ramin, M.D.
Ophthalmology and Visual Science . . . . Robert M. Feldman, M.D. (Interim)
Orthopaedic Surgery . . . . Kyle Dickson, M.D.
Otolaryngology-Head and Neck Surgery . . . . Martin J. Citardi, M.D.
Pathology and Laboratory Medicine . . . . Robert L. Hunter, Jr., M.D., Ph.D.
Pediatric Surgery . . . . Kevin P. Lally, M.D.
Pediatrics . . . . Giuseppe N. Colasurdo, M.D.
   Adolescent Medicine . . . . William L. Risser, M.D.
   Cardiology . . . . Syamasundar Rao, M.D.
   Children's Learning Institute . . . . Susan H. Landry, Ph.D.
   Clinical Neurosciences . . . . Andrew C. Papanicolaou, Ph.D.
   Community and General . . . . Robert J. Yetman, M.D.
   Dermatology . . . . Adelaide A. Hebert, M.D.
   Endocrinology . . . . Michael Yafi, M.D.
   Gastroenterology . . . . J. Marc Rhoads, M.D.
   Genetics . . . . Hope Northrup, M.D.
   Hematology . . . . Keith Hoots, M.D.
   Infectious Diseases . . . . Gloria P. Heresi, M.D.
   Neonatology . . . . Kathleen A. Kennedy, M.D., M.P.H.
   Nephrology . . . . Michael C. Braun, M.D. (Interim)
   Neurology . . . . Ian J. Butler, M.D.
   Pulmonology and Critical Care . . . . Giuseppe N. Colasurdo, M.D.
Physical Medicine and Rehabilitation . . . . Gerard E. Francisco, M.D. (Interim)
Psychiatry and Behavioral Sciences . . . . Pedro Ruiz, M.D.
Surgery . . . . Richard J. Andrassy, M.D.
   General . . . . David W. Mercer, M.D.
   Immunology and Organ Transplantation . . . . Charles T. VanBuren, M.D.
   Oral and Maxillofacial . . . . James W. Wilson, D.D.S.
   Plastic and Reconstructive . . . . Donald H. Parks, M.D.
   Urology . . . . O. Lenaine Westney, M.D.

University of Utah School of Medicine
30 North 1900 East
Salt Lake City, Utah 84132-2101
801-581-7201; 581-6436 (dean's office); 585-3300 (fax)
Web site: http://medicine.utah.edu

Founded as a two-year school in 1905, the college of medicine was expanded to a four-year program in 1943. In 1965, it became completely integrated into the university with the completion of the University of Utah Medical Center on the upper campus. In 1981, the name was changed formally to the University of Utah School of Medicine.

Type: public
2008-2009 total enrollment: 412
Clinical facilities: University Hospital and Clinics, LDS Hospital, Salt Lake Regional Medical Center, Cottonwood Hospital, St. Mark's Hospital, Shriners Hospitals for Crippled Children, Primary Children's Medical Center, McKay-Dee Hospital Center, Veterans Affairs Medical Center (Salt Lake City), University of Utah Neuropsychiatric Institute.

University Officials

President . . . . Michael K. Young, J.D.
Senior Vice President, Academic Affairs . . . . David W. Pershing, Ph.D.
Senior Vice President for Health Sciences. A. Lorris Betz, M.D., Ph.D.
Chief Executive Officer, University Hospital . . . . David Entwistle

Medical School Administrative Staff

Executive Dean . . . . A. Lorris Betz, M.D., Ph.D.
Dean. . . . . David J. Bjorkman, M.D.
Associate Dean for Finance . . . . Cathy Anderson
Associate Dean for Student Affairs . . . . Barbara Cahill, M.D.
Associate Dean for Veteran's Affairs . . . . Ronald Gebhart, M.D.
Associate Dean for Admissions . . . . Wayne M. Samuelson, M.D.
Associate Dean for Curriculum and Graduate Medical Education . . . . Larry Reimer, M.D.
Assistant Dean for Continuing Medical
   Education; Medical Graphics/Photography;
   Idaho; International Medical Education . . . . DeVon C. Hale, M.D.
Assistant Dean for Dental Education. . . . . G. Lynn Powell, D.D.S.
Assistant Dean for Diversity and Community Outreach . . . . Edward Junkins, M.D.
Director of Administration . . . . Karen Anastasopoulos
Director of Admissions. . . . . Kathy Z. Doulis
Director of Diversity and Community Outreach . . . . Candi Ramos
Director of Faculty Administration . . . . Jennifer Allie
Director of Financial Aid and Medical Education . . . . Rita Litsas
Director of Student Affairs. . . . . Julia Clayton
Director of Learning Resources . . . . Steven Baumann, Ed.D.

Department and Division or Section Chairs

Basic Sciences

Biochemistry . . . . Dana Carroll, Ph.D.
Human Genetics, Co-Chairs . . . . Mark F. Leppert, Ph.D., and Mario R. Capecchi, Ph.D.
Human and Molecular Biology and Genetics . . . . Guy Zimmerman, M.D.
Biomedical Informatics . . . . Joyce Mitchell, Ph.D.
Neurobiology and Anatomy . . . . Monica Vetter, Ph.D. (Interim)
Oncological Sciences . . . . Barbara J. Graves, Ph.D.
Pathology . . . . Peter Jensen, M.D.
Physiology . . . . Ed Dudek, Ph.D.

Clinical Sciences

Anesthesiology. . . . . Michael K. Cahalan, M.D.
Dermatology . . . . John J. Zone, M.D.
Family and Preventive Medicine . . . . Michael K. Magill, M.D.
   Family Medicine Division . . . . Michael K. Magill, M.D.
   Physician Assistant Program . . . . Donald M. Pedersen, Ph.D.
   Public Health. . . . . Stephen C. Alder, Ph.D.

Rocky Mountain Center for Occupational and
   Environmental Health .... Kurt Hegmann, M.D.
Internal Medicine .... John R. Hoidal, M.D.
   Cardiology.. Ivor J. Benjamin, M.D.
   Endocrinology .... E. Dale Abel, M.B.B.S.
   Gastroenterology .... Curt Hagedorn, M.D.
   General Internal Medicine .... Barry M. Stults, M.D.
   Geriatrics.. Mark A. Supiano, M.D.
   Hematology.. James P. Kushner, M.D.
   Infectious Disease................................... John B. Hibbs, Jr., M.D.
   Nephrology .... Donald Kohan, M.D., Ph.D.
   Oncology... John H. Ward, M.D.
   Pulmonary.. Robert Paine, M.D.
   Rheumatology .... Daniel O. Clegg, M.D.
Neurology.. Stefan M. Pulst, M.D.
Neurosurgery.. William T. Couldwell, M.D.
Obstetrics and Gynecology............................... C. Matthew Peterson, M.D.
   General Obstetrics and Gynecology....................... Howard T. Sharp, M.D.
   Gynecologic Oncology .... Andrew Soison, M.D.
   Maternal-Fetal Medicine................................ Robert M. Silver, M.D.
   Reproductive Endocrinology and Infertility................... Mark Gibson, M.D.
   Urogynecology and Pelvic Reconstructive Surgery .... Peggy A. Norton, M.D.
Ophthalmology and Visual Sciences .... Randall J. Olson, M.D.
Orthopedics .... Charles Saltzman, M.D.
Pediatrics .... Edward B. Clark, M.D.
   Critical Care.. J. Michael Dean, M.D.
   Emergency Medicine .... Jeffrey E. Schunk, M.D.
   Endocrinology and Metabolism........................... Mary Murray, M.D.
   General Clinical Pediatrics .... Chuck Norlin, M.D.
   Genetics.. Nicola Longo, M.D., Ph.D.
   Inpatient Medicine................................. Chris Maloney, M.D., Ph.D.
   Neonatology.. J. Ross Milley, M.D.
   Pediatric Behavioral Health .... D. Richard Martini, M.D.
   Pediatric Cardiology .... Lloyd Y. Tani, M.D.
   Pediatric Clinical Immunology and Rheumatology................. John Bohnsack, M.D.
   Pediatric Gastroenterology .... Linda S. Book, M.D.
   Pediatric Hematology and Oncology.................... Richard S. Lemons, M.D., Ph.D.
   Pediatric Infectious Diseases .... Andrew T. Pavia, M.D.
   Pediatric Nephrology .... Raoul D. Nelson, M.D.
   Pediatric Neurology .... Francis M. Filloux, M.D.
   Pediatric Pulmonology .... John Bohnsack, M.D. (Interim)
   Pediatric Surgery .... Rebecka Meyers, M.D.
   Safe and Healthy Families............................... David Corwin, M.D.
Physical Medicine and Rehabilitation .... Joe Webster, M.D. (Interim)
Psychiatry .... William M. McMahon, M.D.
Radiation Oncology.................................... Dennis C. Shrieve, M.D., Ph.D.
   Medical Physics .... Bill J. Salter, Ph.D.
   Radiation Therapy .... David K. Gaffney, M.D., Ph.D.
Radiology .... Edwin A. Stevens, M.D.
   Chest Radiology....................................... Howard Mann, M.D.
   General Radiology, Body Imaging...................... David E. Avrin, M.D., Ph.D.
   Interventional Radiology................................. James Carlisle, M.D.
   Medical Imaging Research Laboratory...................... Dennis Parker, Ph.D.
   Musculoskeletal Radiology .... Julia R. Crim, M.D.
   Neuroradiology .... Karen Salzman, M.D. (Acting)
   Nuclear Medicine...................................... John Hoffman, M.D.
   Women's Radiology .... Anne Kennedy, M.D.
Surgery.. Sean J. Mulvihill, M.D.
   Cardiothoracic Surgery.................................. John Hawkins, M.D.
   Emergency Medicine .... Erik Barton, M.D.
   General Surgery...................................... Edward W. Nelson, M.D.
   Otolaryngology-Head and Neck Surgery .... Clough Shelton, M.D.
   Pediatric Surgery .... Rebecka Meyers, M.D.
   Plastic and Reconstructive Surgery .... W. Bradford Rockwell, M.D.
   Urology.. Patrick C. Cartwright, M.D.
   Vascular Surgery...................................... Larry Kraiss, M.D.

University of Vermont College of Medicine
E126 Given Building 89, Beaumont Avenue
Burlington, Vermont 05405
802-656-2156 (general information); 656-2156 (dean's office); 656-8577 (fax)
Web site: www.med.uvm.edu

Instruction in what was to become the University of Vermont College of Medicine was initiated in 1803, when Dr. John Pomeroy was appointed to the staff to teach chirurgery (surgery) and anatomy. The first full and regular course of medical lectures, however, was not offered until fall 1822. In 1836, the medical department was forced to close because of lack of students and professors. The school was reorganized and reopened in 1853. In 1899, the medical college became a coordinate department of the university under the control of its board of trustees. In 1911, the college of medicine became an intergal part of the university.

Type: public
2008-2009 total enrollment: 403
Clinical facilities: Fletcher Allen Health Care, Inc., Maine Medical Center (Portland). Cooperating hospitals: Champlain Valley Physicians Hospital, Vermont State Hospital.

University Officials

President. . . . . Daniel M. Fogel, Ph.D.
Provost . . . . John M. Hughes, Ph.D.
Librarian, Health Sciences. . . . . Marianne D. Burke
Director, Sponsored Programs . . . . Ruth A. Farrell
Associate Director, Sponsored Programs. . . . . Beverly A. Blakeney

Medical School Administrative Staff

Dean. . . . . Frederick C. Morin III, M.D.
Executive Assistant to the Dean . . . . Maura L. Randall
Senior Associate Dean for Clinical Affairs. . . . . Paul Taheri, M.D.
Senior Associate Dean for Research and Academic Affairs. . . . . Russell P. Tracy, Ph.D.
Senior Associate Dean for Medical Education . . . . Lewis R. First, M.D.
Associate Dean for Faculty and Staff
    Development and Diversity . . . . Karen Richardson-Nassif, Ph.D.
Associate Dean for Student Affairs . . . . G. Scott Waterman, M.D.
Associate Dean for Continuing Medical Education . . . . Jeffrey Klein, M.D.
Associate Dean for Primary Care . . . . Open
Associate Dean for Patient Oriented Research. . . . . Richard Galbraith, M.D., Ph.D.
Associate Dean for Graduate Medical Education . . . . David Adams, M.D.
Associate Dean for Public Health . . . . Jan K. Carney, M.D.
Associate Dean for Admissions . . . . Janice M. Gallant, M.D.
Associate Dean for Maine Affairs . . . . George L. Higgins III, M.D.
Associate Dean for Finance and Administration . . . . Brian L. Cote
Director Clinical Trials Research . . . . Kimberly Luebbers
Assistant Dean for Communications and Planning . . . . Carole L. Whitaker
Assistant Dean for Development and Alumni Affairs . . . . Richard J. Blount
Executive Secretary of Medical Alumni Association . . . . John P. Tampas, M.D.
Assistant Dean for Facilities Administration and Planning . . . . Susan W. Ligon

Department and Division or Section Chairs

Basic Sciences

Anatomy and Neurobiology . . . . Rodney L. Parsons, Ph.D.
Biochemistry . . . . Paula B. Tracy, Ph.D. (Interim)
Microbiology and Molecular Genetics. . . . . Susan S. Wallace, Ph.D.
Molecular Physiology and Biophysics . . . . David M. Warshaw, Ph.D.
Pathology . . . . Edwin G. Bovill, M.D.
    Clinical Pathology*. . . . . Edwin G. Bovill, M.D.
Pharmacology . . . . Mark T. Nelson, Ph.D.
    Clinical Pharmacology . . . . Richard Galbraith, M.D., Ph.D.

Clinical Sciences

Anesthesiology . . . . Howard M. Schapiro, M.D.
Family Practice . . . . Thomas C. Peterson, M.D. (Interim)
Medicine . . . . Polly E. Parsons, M.D.
   Cardiology* . . . . David J. Schneider, M.D.
   Dermatology* . . . . Paul A. Krusinski, M.D.
   Endocrinology and Metabolism* . . . . John L. Leahy, M.D.
   Gastroenterology* . . . . James Vecchio, M.D.
   General Internal Care* . . . . Benjamin Littenberg, M.D.
   Gerontology* . . . . Naomi Fukagawa, M.D. (Acting)
   Hematology-Oncology* . . . . Marie Wood, M.D. (Interim)
   Human Medical Genetics* . . . . Open
   Immunobiology . . . . Ralph C. Budd, M.D.
   Infectious Diseases* . . . . Christopher J. Grace, M.D.
   Nephrology* . . . . Richard J. Solomon, M.D.
   Pulmonary* . . . . Polly E. Parsons, M.D.
   Rheumatology* . . . . Sheldon Cooper, M.D.
   Vascular Biology . . . . David J. Schneider, M.D.
Neurology . . . . Robert W. Hamill, M.D.
Obstetrics and Gynecology . . . . Mark Phillippe, M.D.
Orthopedics and Rehabilitation . . . . Claude E. Nichols, M.D.
Pediatrics . . . . Lewis R. First, M.D.
   Ambulatory Pediatrics* . . . . Jerry G. Larrabee, M.D.
   Cardiology* . . . . Scott B. Yeager, M.D.
   Critical Care* . . . . Barry W. Heath, M.D.
   Endocrinology . . . . Paul J. Zimakas, M.D.
   Gastrointestinal* . . . . Richard B. Colletti, M.D.
   Genetics* . . . . Leah W. Burke, M.D.
   Hematology-Oncology* . . . . Alan C. Homans, M.D.
   Immunology* . . . . Barry A. Finette, M.D., Ph.D.
   Infectious Disease* . . . . William V. Raszka, M.D.
   Neonatal* . . . . Roger F. Soll, M.D.
   Nephrology* . . . . Ann P. Guillot, M.D.
   Pulmonary* . . . . Thomas Lahiri, M.D.
   Rheumatology . . . . Leslie S. Abramson, M.D.
Psychiatry . . . . Robert A. Pierattini, M.D.
Radiology . . . . Steven P. Braff, M.D.
Surgery . . . . David W. McFadden, M.D.
   Emergency Medicine* . . . . Stephen M. Leffler, M.D.
   General* . . . . Neil H. Hyman, M.D.
   Maxillofacial* . . . . Paul A. Danielson, M.D.
   Neurosurgery* . . . . Bruce I. Tranmer, M.D.
   Ophthalmology* . . . . Terry Wood, M.D.
   Otolaryngology* . . . . William Brundage, M.D.
   Pediatric* . . . . Open
   Plastic* . . . . David W. Leitner, M.D.
   Surgical Oncology* . . . . Seth P. Harlow, M.D.
   Thoracic and Cardiac* . . . . Frank P. Ittleman, M.D.
   Transplantation* . . . . Antonio Di Carlo, M.D.
   Trauma and Surgical Critical Care* . . . . Bruce Crookes, M.D.
   Urology* . . . . Samuel J. Trotter, M.D.
   Vascular* . . . . Andrew Stanley, M.D.

*Specialty without organizational autonomy.

Eastern Virginia Medical School
P.O. Box 1980
Norfolk, Virginia 23501
757-446-5200 (president's office); 446-5600 (general); 446-5800 (dean's office);
446-8444 (fax)
Web site: www.evms.edu

Eastern Virginia Medical School (EVMS) is governed by the Eastern Virginia Medical School Board of Visitors and was established by the General Assembly of the Commonwealth of Virginia in 1964. In September 1976, the medical school graduated 23 physicians in its first class. With the support of the communities of Norfolk, Virginia Beach, Chesapeake, Hampton, Portsmouth, Newport News, Suffolk, and other cities and counties throughout eastern Virginia, the medical school gained recognition as an academic health center. Now, in addition to M.D. and graduate medical education programs, EVMS offers programs in biomedical sciences, clinical psychology, public health, art therapy, physician assistant, clinical embryology, ophthalmic technology, and surgical assistant. Over the years, EVMS has grown into a nationally recognized center for biomedical research, especially in the areas of reproductive medicine, diabetes, geriatrics, pediatrics, and cancer.

Type: public
2008-2009 total enrollment: 800
Clinical facilities: Eastern Virginia Medical School Health Services, Bon Secours DePaul Medical Center, Bon Secours Maryview Medical Center, Chesapeake General Hospital, Children's Hospital of The King's Daughters, Lake Taylor Transitional Care Hospital, Naval Hospital (Portsmouth), Riverside Regional Medical Center, Sentara Bayside Hospital, Sentara Leigh Hospital, Sentara Norfolk General Hospital, Sentara Obici Hospital, Sentara Virginia Beach General Hospital, Veterans Administration Center (Hampton), Williamsburg Community Hospital, Eastern State Hospital.

Eastern Virginia Medical School

President. . . . . Harry T. Lester
Dean and Provost . . . . Gerald J. Pepe, Ph.D.
Vice President for Administration and Finance . . . . Mark R. Babashanian
Vice President of External Affairs . . . . Claudia Keenan Hough

Medical School Administrative Staff

Dean and Provost . . . . Gerald J. Pepe, Ph.D.
Associate Dean, Academic Affairs . . . . Michael J. Solhaug, M.D.
Associate Dean, Graduate Medical Education . . . . Linda R. Archer, Ph.D.
Associate Dean, U.S. Naval Hospital Programs . . . . Rdml. Matthew Nathan
Associate Dean, Business Management . . . . David E. Huband
Assistant Dean, Minority Affairs . . . . Gail C. Williams
Assistant Dean, Women's Affairs . . . . Bonnie J. Dattel, M.D.
Associate Dean, Library and Director, Educational Technology . . . . Judith G. Robinson
Associate Dean, Research . . . . William Wasilenko, Ph.D.
Associate Dean, Human Research Subjects Protection . . . . Robert F. Williams, Ph.D.
Associate Dean, Planning and Health Professions . . . . C. Donald Combs, Ph.D.
Associate Dean, Clinical Affairs. . . . . Alfred Z. Abuhamad, M.D.
Assistant Dean, Faculty Affairs . . . . Alice E. Fretwell
Associate Dean, Education . . . . Thomas R. Pellegrino, M.D.

Department and Division or Section Chairs

Basic Sciences

Microbiology and Molecular Cell Biology . . . . Edward M. Johnson, Ph.D.
Pathology and Anatomy . . . . Nancy F. Fishback, M.D.
Physiological Sciences . . . . Russell L. Prewitt, Ph.D. (Interim)

Clinical Sciences

Dermatology . . . . Antoinette F. Hood, M.D.
Emergency Medicine . . . . Francis L. Counselman, M.D.
Family and Community Medicine . . . . Christine C. Matson, M.D.
Internal Medicine . . . . Jerry L. Nadler, M.D.
Neurology . . . . Thomas R. Pellegrino, M.D.
Obstetrics and Gynecology . . . . Alfred Z. Abuhamad, M.D.
Ophthalmology . . . . Earl R. Crouch, M.D.
Otolaryngology . . . . Barry Strasnick, M.D.
Pediatrics . . . . Donald Lewis, M.D.
Physical Medicine and Rehabilitation . . . . Jean E. Shelton, M.D.
Psychiatry and Behavioral Sciences . . . . Robert P. Archer, Ph.D. (Interim)
Radiation Oncology and Biophysics . . . . Mark S. Sinesi, M.D., Ph.D.
Radiology . . . . Lester S. Johnson, M.D.
Surgery . . . . L.D. Britt, M.D.
Urology . . . . Donald F. Lynch, M.D.

Virginia Commonwealth University
School of Medicine

P.O. Box 980565
Richmond, Virginia 23298
804-828-9000 (general); 828-9788 (dean's office); 828-9629 (admissions);
828-7628 (dean's office fax)
Web site: www.medschool.vcu.edu

The Medical College of Virginia was established in 1838 as a department of Hampden-Sydney and was conducted as such until 1860 when it became a state institution. In 1913, it was consolidated with the University College of Medicine, and in 1914, all students were transferred to the Medical College of Virginia. The 1969 General Assembly of Virginia created, as of July 1, 1968, Virginia Commonwealth University through merging of Richmond Professional Institute-which became the general academic division-and the Medical College of Virginia. The official school name is Virginia Commonwealth University School of Medicine.

Type: public
2008-2009 total enrollment: 750
Clinical facilities: VCU Medical Center, VCU Treatment Center for Children, McGuire Veterans Administration Medical Center. **Affiliated hospitals:** Riverside Hospital, Chippenham Medical Center, INOVA Fairfax Hospital, INOVA Fair Oaks Hospital, Bon Secours St. Mary's Hospital, Children's Hospital, Eastern State Hospital, Piedmont Geriatric Hospital, Reston Hospital Center..

University Officials

President. . . . . Eugene P. Trani, Ph.D.
Vice President for Health Sciences and Chief
   Executive Officer, VCU Health System . . . . Sheldon M. Retchin, M.D.

Medical School Administrative Staff

Executive Vice President for Medical Affairs,
   VCU Health System, and Dean . . . . Jerome F. Strauss III, M.D., Ph.D.
Senior Associate Dean, Faculty Affairs. . . . . PonJola Coney, M.D.
Senior Associate Dean, Medical Education and Student Affairs . . . . Isaac K. Wood, M.D.
Associate Dean, Admissions . . . . Michelle Whitehurst-Cook, M.D.
Associate Dean, Clinical Activities. . . . . Ralph R. Clark, M.D.
Associate Dean, Clinical Affairs. . . . . John D. Ward, M.D.
Associate Dean, Continuing Medical Education. . . . . Paul E. Mazmanian, Ph.D.
Associate Dean, Development. . . . . Thomas E. Holland
Associate Dean, Faculty and Instructional Development. . . . . Carol L. Hampton
Associate Dean, Finance and Administration. . . . . Amy S. Sebring
Associate Dean, Graduate Education. . . . . Jan F. Chlebowski, Ph.D.
Associate Dean, Graduate Medical Education . . . . Mary Alice O'Donnel, Ph.D.
Associate Dean, McGuire Vet Affairs. . . . . Judy L. Brannen, M.D.
Associate Dean, Medical Education-INOVA Campus . . . . Russell P. Seneca, M.D.
Associate Dean, Practice Plan. . . . . James J. Potyraj
Associate Dean, Research. . . . . Gordon L. Archer, M.D.
Associate Dean, School of Public Health. . . . . Tilahun Adera, Ph.D.
Associate Dean, Student Affairs . . . . Christopher M. Woleben, M.D.
Assistant Dean, Medical Education . . . . Allan W. Dow III, M.D.
Assistant Dean, Medical Education-INOVA Campus. . . . . Craig E. Cheifetz, M.D.
Assistant Dean, Medical Education . . . . Linda S. Costanzo, Ph.D.
Assistant Dean, Sponsored Programs . . . . George F. Ford, Ph.D.
Assistant Dean, Student Affairs. . . . . Glenda U. Palmer, Ph.D.
Assistant Dean, Technology Services. . . . . Meenu Tolani
Assistant to the Dean . . . . Joan M. Barrett

Department and Division or Section Chairs

Basic Health Sciences

Anatomy and Neurobiology . . . . John T. Povlishock, Ph.D.
Biochemistry and Molecular Biology . . . . Sarah Spiegel, Ph.D.
Biostatistics . . . . Shumei S. Sun, Ph.D.
Epidemiology and Community Health . . . . Kate Lapane, Ph.D.
Human and Molecular Genetics . . . . Paul Fisher, Ph.D. (Interim)
Microbiology and Immunology . . . . Dennis E. Ohman, Ph.D.
Pharmacology and Toxicology . . . . William Dewey, Ph.D. (Interim)
Physiology . . . . Diomedes E. Logothetis, Ph.D.
Social and Behavioral Health . . . . Laura A. Siminoff, Ph.D.

Clinical Sciences

Anesthesiology . . . . Carlos Arancibia, M.D.
Dermatology . . . . Algin B. Garrett, M.D.
Emergency Medicine . . . . Joseph P. Ornato, M.D.
Family Practice . . . . Anton J. Kuzel, M.D.
Internal Medicine . . . . Richard P. Wenzel, M.D.
Legal Medicine . . . . Marcella F. Fierro, M.D.
Massey Cancer Center . . . . Gordon D. Ginder, M.D.
Neurology . . . . Alan R. Towne, M.D.
Neurosurgery . . . . Harold F. Young, M.D.
Obstetrics and Gynecology . . . . John W. Seeds, M.D.
Ophthalmology . . . . William H. Benson, M.D.
Orthopaedic Surgery . . . . Robert S. Adelaar, M.D.
Otolaryngology . . . . Aristides Sismanis, M.D.
Pathology . . . . David S. Wilkinson, M.D., Ph.D.
Pediatrics . . . . William Moskowitz, M.D. (Interim)
Physical Medicine and Rehabilitation . . . . David X. Cifu, M.D.
Psychiatry . . . . Joel J. Silverman, M.D.
Radiation Oncology . . . . Mitchell S. Anscher, M.D.
Radiology . . . . Ann S. Fulcher, M.D.
Surgery . . . . James P. Neifeld, M.D.

University of Virginia School of Medicine

Health System, P.O. Box 800793
McKim Hall
Charlottesville, Virginia 22908-0793
434-924-5118 (dean's office); 982-0874 (fax)
Web site: www.healthsystem.virginia.edu

According to Thomas Jefferson, medical education was to become part of the curriculum and of general education at the University of Virginia. A school of anatomy and medicine was one of the original eight schools authorized by the General Assembly on January 25, 1819. The school opened on March 7, 1825, and is located on the grounds of the University of Virginia. The medical school is part of the University of Virginia Health System.

Type: public
2008-2009 total enrollment: 555
Clinical facilities: Centra Health, Inc., Martha Jefferson Hospital, Carilion Roanoke Community Hospital, Carilion Roanoke Memorial Hospital, University of Virginia—Health South Rehabilitation Hospital, University of Virginia Kluge Children's Rehabilitation Center, University of Virginia Hospital, Veterans Affairs Medical Center (Salem), Western State Hospital, Winchester Memorial Hospital, Woodrow Wilson Rehabilitation Center, INOVA Fairfax Hospital.

University Officials

President. . . . . John T. Casteen III, Ph.D.
Executive Vice President and Chief Operating Officer. . . . . Leonard W. Sandridge, Jr.
Executive Vice President and Provost . . . . Arthur Garson, Jr., M.D.

Medical Center Administrative Staff

Vice President and Chief Executive Officer,
    University of Virginia Medical Center . . . . R. Edward Howell
Chief Operations Officer . . . . Vacant
Chief Clinical Officer and Chief Nursing Officer. . . . . Pamela F. Cipriano, Ph.D.
Chief Environmental of Care Officer . . . . Thomas A. Harkins
Chief Executive Officer, Health Services Foundation. Marc Dettmann
Chief Financial and Business Development Officer . . . . Larry L. Fitzgerald
Chief Marketing and Strategic Relations Officer . . . . Patricia L. Cluff
Chief Information Officer . . . . Barbara S. Baldwin
Chief Technology and Health Information Officer . . . . Marshall Ruffin, M.D.
President, Clinical Staff . . . . John B. Hanks, M.D.
President, Health Services Foundation . . . . William D. Steers, M.D.
Associate Vice President for Health System Development . . . . Karen Rendleman
Special Advisor to the Vice President and Chief
    Executive Officer of the Medical Center . . . . Sally N. Barber
Compliance Officer . . . . Lori Strauss (Interim)

School of Medicine Administrative Staff

Vice President and Dean . . . . Steven T. DeKosky, M.D.
Senior Associate Dean . . . . Sharon L. Hostler, M.D.
Senior Associate Dean for Clinical Affairs . . . . Jonathon D. Truwit, M.D.
Senior Associate Dean for Continuing Medical
    Education and External Affairs . . . . Karen S. Rheuban, M.D.
Senior Associate Dean for Education . . . . Randolph J. Canterbury, M.D.
Senior Associate Dean for Finance and Administration . . . . Bradley E. Haws
Senior Associate Dean for Research . . . . Erik L. Hewlett, M.D.
Associate Dean for Admissions . . . . Randolph J. Canterbury, M.D.
Associate Dean for Basic Research . . . . Margaret A. Shupnik, Ph.D.
Associate Dean and Director, Claude Moore Health Sciences Library. . . . . . Gretchen M. Arnold
Associate Dean for Clinical Research . . . . Ronald B. Turner, M.D.
Associate Dean for Curriculum. . . . . Donald J. Innes, Jr., M.D.
Associate Dean for Diversity . . . . M. Norman Oliver, M.D.
Associate Dean for Graduate and Medical Scientist Programs . . . . Brian R. Duling, Ph.D.

Associate Dean of Graduate Medical Education. . . . . Susan E. Kirk, M.D.
Associate Dean for International Programs . . . . Leigh Grossman, M.D.
Associate Dean for Medical Alumni Affairs . . . . Barry J. Collins
Associate Dean for Medical Education Support. . . . . Jerry G. Short, Ph.D.
Associate Dean for the Roanoke Program. . . . . Daniel P. Harrington, M.D.
Associate Dean for Administrative Affairs-Salem, Veterans Affairs. . . . . John Patrick
Associate Dean for Student Academic Support
    and Strategic Programs . . . . Moses K. A. Woode, Ph.D.
Associate Dean for Student Affairs . . . . Richard D. Pearson, M.D.
Assistant Dean for Administration. . . . . Polly E. King
Assistant Dean for Admissions . . . . Vacant
Associate Dean for Faculty Development. . . . . Susan M. Pollart, M.D.
Assistant Dean for Clinical Affairs. . . . . Keri K. Hall, M.D.
Assistant Dean for Finance and Human Resources . . . . Anne C. Kromkowski
Assistant Dean for Graduate Research and Training . . . . Joel W. Hockensmith, Ph.D.
Assistant Dean for Medical Education. . . . . Wendi El-Amin, M.D.
Assistant Dean for Medical Education. . . . . Christine M. Peterson, M.D.
Assistant Dean for Research and Scientific
    Director of the Research Advisory Committee . . . . Steven S. Wasserman, Ph.D.
Assistant Dean for Research Support . . . . Jay W. Fox, Ph.D.
Assistant Dean for Student Affairs. . . . . Allison H. Innes, Ph.D.
Director, Faculty and Administrator Development Programs . . . . Vacant
Director, Institutional Analysis and Computing. . . . . Leah Goswell
Director, Research Administration . . . . Stewart P. Craig (Interim)
Director, Space Management . . . . Richard B. Allen

Department and Division or Section Chairs

Basic Sciences

Biochemistry and Molecular Genetics. . . . . Joyce L. Hamlin, Ph.D.
Biomedical Engineering. . . . . Michael B. Lawrence, Ph.D. (Interim)
Cell Biology. . . . . Barry M. Gumbiner, Ph.D.
Microbiology . . . . J. Thomas Parsons, Ph.D.
Molecular Physiology and Biological Physics . . . . Mark Yeager, M.D., Ph.D.
Neuroscience. . . . . Kevin S. Lee, Ph.D.
Pharmacology . . . . Douglas A. Bayliss, Ph.D.

Clinical Sciences

Anesthesiology . . . . George F. Rich, M.D., Ph.D.
Dentistry. . . . . Thomas E. Leinbach, D.D.S.
Dermatology . . . . Thomas G. Cropley, M.D.
Emergency Medicine . . . . Robert E. O'Connor, M.D.
Family Medicine . . . . Sim S. Galazka, M.D.
Internal Medicine . . . . Robert M. Strieter, M.D.
Neurology . . . . Karen C. Johnston, M.D.
Neurosurgery. . . . . Mark E. Shaffrey, M.D.
Obstetrics and Gynecology. . . . . William N. P. Herbert, M.D.
Ophthalmology . . . . Brian P. Conway, M.D.
Orthopaedic Surgery . . . . Mark F. Abel, M.D.
Otolaryngology-Head and Neck Surgery . . . . Paul A. Levine, M.D.
Pathology . . . . Dennis J. Templeton, M.D., Ph.D.
Pediatrics . . . . Robert L. Chevalier, M.D.
Physical Medicine and Rehabilitation . . . . D. Casey Kerrigan, M.D.
Plastic and Maxillofacial Surgery. . . . . Raymond F. Morgan, M.D., F.A.C.S.
Psychiatry and Neurobehavioral Sciences . . . . Bankole A. Johnson, D.Sc., M.D., Ph.D.
Public Health Sciences. . . . . William A. Knaus, M.D.
Radiation Oncology. . . . . James M. Larner, M.D.
Radiology . . . . Alan H. Matsumoto, M.D. (Interim)
Surgery . . . . Irving L. Kron, M.D.
Urology. . . . . William D. Steers, M.D.

University of Washington School of Medicine
Box 356340
Seattle, Washington 98195
206-543-1515 (dean's office); 616-3341 (fax)
E-mail: askuwsom@u.washington.edu
Web site: www.uwmedicine.org

The University of Washington School of Medicine was established in 1945 as a unit of the division of health sciences and an integral part of the total university campus. The school serves the five-state WWAMI (Washington, Wyoming, Alaska, Montana, and Idaho) region.

Type: public
2008-2009 total enrollment: 806
Clinical facilities: Overlake Hospital Medical Center (Bellevue, WA); Evergreen Hospital (Kirkland, WA); Good Samaritan Hospital and Medical Center (Puyallup, WA); Valley Medical Center (Renton, WA); Children's Hospital and Regional Medical Center, Group Health Cooperative Hospitals, Harborview Medical Center, Northwest Hospital, Fred Hutchinson Cancer Research Center, Pacific Medical Center, Swedish Medical Center/First Hill Campus, Swedish Medical Center/Providence Campus, University of Washington Medical Center, VA Puget Sound Health Care System, Virginia Mason Medical Center (Seattle, WA); Deaconess Medical Center, Sacred Heart Medical Center (Spokane, WA); American Lake VA Hospital, Madigan Army Medical Center, Mary Bridge Children's Hospital and Health Center (Tacoma, WA); Alaska Native Medical Center, Providence Alaska Medical Center (Anchorage, AK); Deaconess Medical Center, Saint Vincent Hospital and Health Center (Billings, MT); Saint Patrick Hospital (Missoula, MT); St. Lukes Regional Medical Center, Boise VA Medical Center (Boise, ID); University of Washington Residency Network (WA, WY, AK, MT, ID).

University Officials

President of the University . . . . Mark A. Emmert, Ph.D.
Provost . . . . Phyllis M. Wise, Ph.D.
Executive Vice President for Medical Affairs . . . . Paul G. Ramsey, M.D.

Medical School Administrative Staff

Dean . . . . Paul G. Ramsey, M.D.
Vice Dean, Academic Affairs . . . . Thomas E. Norris, M.D.
Vice Dean, Clinical Affairs . . . . Lawrence R. Robinson, M.D.
Vice Dean, Regional Affairs, Rural Health, and GME . . . . John B. Coombs, M.D.
Vice Dean, Research and Graduate Education . . . . John T. Slattery, Ph.D.
Vice Dean, Administration and Finance . . . . Ruth M. Mahan
Associate Dean, Curriculum . . . . Susan G. Marshall, M.D.
Associate Dean and Chief Administrative Officer, Student Affairs . . . . E. Peter Eveland, Ed.D.
Associate Dean and Director, Multicultural Affairs . . . . David A. Acosta, M.D.
Associate Dean, Graduate Medical Education . . . . Joseph W. York, Ph.D.
Associate Dean, Admissions . . . . Carol C. Teitz, M.D.
Associate Dean for Translational Science . . . . Nora L. Disis, M.D.
Assistant Dean, Faculty Development . . . . Christina M. Surawicz, M.D.
Assistant Dean for Research, CHRMC . . . . James Hendricks, M.D.
Assistant Dean for Research, HMC . . . . Sheila A. Lukehart, Ph.D.
Assistant Dean for Planning and New Initiatives . . . . Richard A. Meisinger, Ph.D.
Associate Vice President for Compliance . . . . Sue Clausen
Associate Vice President for Medical Affairs and
  Director, Health Sciences/UW Medicine News
  & Community Relations . . . . Tina Mankowski
Senior Advisor to the Dean . . . . Harry R. Kimball, M.D.
Director, Medex Program . . . . Ruth Ballweg
Associate Dean and Medical Director, University
  of Washington Medical Center . . . . Thomas O. Staiger, M.D. (Acting)
Associate Dean and Medical Director,
  Harborview Medical Center . . . . J. Richard Goss, M.D. (Interim)
Associate Dean and Medical Director, Children's
  Hospital and Regional Medical Center . . . . David Fisher, M.D.

246

Associate Dean and Chief of Staff, VA Puget
  Sound Health Care System (Seattle and
    American Lake, Tacoma) .... Gordon A. Starkebaum, M.D.
Vice President and Chief Financial Officer .... Bruce Ferguson
Vice President and Chief Operations Officer .... Johnese M. Spisso
Associate Vice President, Development and Alumni Relations .... Lynn K. Hogan, Ph.D.
Director, Medical Policy Affairs .... Jackie L. Der
Assistant to the Executive Vice President and Dean................... Barbara A. Mahoney
Executive Assistant to the Executive Vice President and Dean .... Julie A. Monteith
WWAMI Coordinators and Assistant Deans
  Washington State University (Pullman) and
    University of Idaho (Moscow) .... Andrew Turner, Ph.D.
  Montana State University (Bozeman) .... Linda E. Hyman, Ph.D.
  University of Alaska (Anchorage) .... Dennis P. Valenzeno, Ph.D.
  University of Wyoming (Laramie) .... Sylvia I. Moore, Ph.D., R.D.
  Clinical Medicine Education (Spokane) .... Deborah J. Harper, M.D.
  Family Practice Residency of Idaho.......................... Suzanne Allen, M.D.
  Clinical Phase Coordinator (Whitefish)...................... Jay Erickson, M.D.
  Clinical Phase Coordinator (Montana) .... J. Richard Hillman, M.D., Ph.D.
  Clinical Medical Education (Spokane) .... John McCarthy, M.D.
  Medical Education Program (Washington State-Riverpoint) .... Kenneth Roberts, Ph.D.

Department Chairs

Basic Sciences

Biochemistry....................................... Alan M. Weiner, Ph.D.
Bioengineering .... Paul Yager, Ph.D. (Acting)
Biological Structure................................. John I. Clark, Ph.D.
Comparative Medicine....................... H. Denny Liggitt, D.V.M., Ph.D.
Immunology .... Christopher B. Wilson, M.D.
Medical Education and Biomedical Informatics.................. Fredric M. Wolf, Ph.D.
Medical History and Ethics......................... Wylie G. Burke, M.D., Ph.D.
Microbiology.. James J. Champoux, Ph.D.
Genome Sciences................................ Robert H. Waterston, M.D., Ph.D.
Global Health .... King K. Holmes, M.D., Ph.D.
Pathology .... Nelson Fausto, M.D.
Pharmacology .... William A. Catterall, Ph.D.
Physiology and Biophysics .... Stanley C. Froehner, Ph.D.

Clinical Sciences

Anesthesiology..................................... Debra A. Schwinn, M.D.
Family Medicine .... Alfred O. Berg, M.D.
Laboratory Medicine .... James S. Fine, M.D.
Medicine.. William J. Bremner, M.D., Ph.D.
Neurological Surgery.............................. Richard G. Ellenbogen, M.D.
Neurology.. Bruce R. Ransom, M.D., Ph.D.
Obstetrics and Gynecology........................ David A. Eschenbach, M.D.
Ophthalmology .... Russell N. Van Gelder, M.D., Ph.D.
Orthopaedics and Sports Medicine.................. Frederick A. Matsen III, M.D.
Otolaryngology-Head and Neck Surgery .... Neal D. Futran, M.D.
Pediatrics .... F. Bruder Stapleton, M.D.
Psychiatry and Behavioral Sciences................. Richard C. Veith, M.D.
Radiation Oncology............................. George E. Laramore, M.D., Ph.D.
Radiology .... Norman J. Beauchamp, M.D.
Rehabilitation Medicine........................... Peter C. Esselman, M.D.
Surgery .... Carlos A. Pellegrini, M.D.
Urology.. Hunter Wessells, M.D.

Joan C. Edwards School of Medicine at Marshall University

1600 Medical Center Drive, Suite 3400
Huntington, West Virginia 25701-3655
304-691-1700 (dean's office); 691-1726 (fax)
Web site: http://musom.marshall.edu/

The Joan C. Edwards School of Medicine at Marshall University was developed under the Veterans Administration Medical School Assistance and Health Manpower Training Act (Public Law 92-541), enacted by Congress in 1972. The school of medicine received provisional accreditation from the Liaison Committee on Medical Education, and the first class of 24 students enrolled in January 1978. The school of medicine received full accreditation in 1981, and the charter class was graduated in May of that year. Present enrollment is 65 students per class. Marshall University is located in Huntington, which is situated on the Ohio River. The school of medicine's administrative and clinical facility is adjacent to Cabell Huntington Hospital, and the school has educational facilities at the Veterans Affairs Medical Center. Community hospitals in Huntington provide additional educational and clinical facilities.

Type: public
2008-2009 total enrollment: 195
Clinical facilities: Cabell-Huntington Hospital, St. Mary's Medical Center, Mildred Mitchell-Bateman Hospital, Veterans Affairs Medical Center; University Physicians and Surgeons, Village Medical Center (ambulatory care centers).

University Officials

President. . . . . Stephen J. Kopp, Ph.D.
Vice President for Health Sciences. . . . . Charles H. McKown, Jr., M.D.
Vice President for Academic Affairs . . . . Open
Senior Vice President of Finance and Administration . . . . Anita Lockridge
Vice President for Alumni Development. . . . . Lance West
Vice President of Multicultural Affairs . . . . Shari Clarke, Ph.D.
Dean, Student Affairs. . . . . Stephen W. Hensley

Medical School Administrative Staff

Dean. . . . . Charles H. McKown, Jr., M.D.
Executive Vice Dean . . . . Robert B. Walker, M.D.
Associate Dean for Academic Affairs. . . . . Sarah A. McCarty, M.D.
Associate Dean for Student Affairs . . . . Marie Veitia, Ph.D.
Associate Dean for Admissions and Development . . . . John B. Walden, M.D.
Senior Associate Dean for Clinical Affairs . . . . Gretchen E. Oley, M.D.
Senior Associate Dean for Finance and Administration . . . . James J. Schneider
Senior Associate Dean for Research and Graduate Education . . . . Richard M. Niles, Ph.D.
Senior Associate Dean for Graduate Medical Education . . . . Daniel D. Cowell, M.D.
Associate Dean for External Affairs. . . . . Karen Bledsoe
Senior Associate Dean for Medical Student Education. . . . . Aaron McGuffin, M.D.
Assistant Dean for Professional Development in Medical Education . . . . . . Darshana Shah, Ph.D.
Assistant Dean for Academic Affairs and Rural Programs. . . . . JoAnn Raines
Assistant Dean for Information Technology and Medical Informatics. . . . . Michael McCarthy
Assistant Dean and Director of Continuing Medical Education . . . . David N. Bailey
Assistant Dean and Director of Center for Rural Health . . . . Jennifer T. Plymale
Director of Animal Resources. . . . . Billy Howard, D.V.M.
Director of Health Science Libraries. . . . . Edward M. Dzierzak
Assistant Dean for Admissions . . . . Cynthia A. Warren
Director of Development and Alumni Affairs . . . . Linda Holmes
Director of Forensic Sciences . . . . Terry Fenger, Ph.D.

Department and Division or Section Chairs

Basic Sciences

Biochemistry and Molecular Biology. . . . . Richard M. Niles, Ph.D.
    Microbiology, Immunology, and Molecular Genetics . . . . Donald Primerano, Ph.D.
Pharmacology . . . . Gary O. Rankin, Ph.D.
    Physiology . . . . Open

Joan C. Edwards School of Medicine at Marshall University: WEST VIRGINIA

Clinical Sciences

Cardiovascular Services .... Mark A. Studeny, M.D.
   Cardiovascular Medicine........................... Mark A. Studeny, M.D.
   Interventional Cardiology......................... Mark A. Studeny, M.D.
   Cardio-Thoracic Surgery........................... Edward R. Setser, M.D.
Family and Community Health............................ Robert B. Walker, M.D.
   Community Medicine*........................... Richard Crespo, Ph.D.
   Family Medicine*.................................. Stephen Petrany, M.D.
   Geriatrics*... Open
   International Health.............................. John B. Walden, M.D.
   Occupational Health*........................ Mohammed I. Ranavaya, M.D.
   Sports Medicine*.................................. Ross Patton, M.D.
Medicine... Kevin Yingling, M.D.
   Endocrinology*.......................... Henry K. Driscoll, M.D. (Acting)
   Gastroenterology*................................ Waseem Shora, M.D.
   General Internal Medicine*...................... Kevin Yingling, M.D.
   Geriatrics*..................................... Shirley M. Neitch, M.D.
   Hematology-Oncology*........................... Marie R. Tirona, M.D.
   Infectious Diseases*............................ Thomas Rushton, M.D.
   Nephrology*................................... M. Arif Goreja, M.D.
   Neurology*.................................... Carl F. McComas, M.D.
   Pulmonary Diseases*........................... Imran T. Khawaja, M.D.
   Rheumatology*.................................. Ralph W. Webb, M.D.
Neuroscience.. Bryan R. Payne, M.D.
Obstetrics-Gynecology.................................. Robert C. Nerhood, M.D.
   Endocrine Infertility............................ David C. Jude, M.D.
   Gynecologic Oncology............................ Gerard J. Oakley, M.D.
   Maternal-Fetal Medicine......................... David B. Chafin, M.D.
Orthopedics.. Ali Oliashirazi, M.D.
Pathology.. David Porter, M.D.
   Anatomical Pathology*........................... David Porter, M.D.
   Anatomy, Cell, and Neurobiology............. Laura Richardson, Ph.D.
   Clinical Pathology*............................ David Porter, M.D.
Pediatrics.. Joseph W. Werthammer, M.D.
   Adolescent Medicine*............................ Patricia Kelly, M.D.
   Behavioral Pediatrics.......................... James T. Binder, M.D.
   Cardiology*................................ Mahmood Heydarian, M.D.
   Emergency Medicine*............................ Joseph Evans, M.D.
   Endocrinology*................................ James R. Bailes, M.D.
   Gastroenterology*.............................. Yoram Elitsur, M.D.
   General Pediatrics*............................. Isabel Pino, M.D.
   Hematology-Oncology*...................... Andrew L. Pendleton, M.D.
   Infectious Diseases*........................... Open
   Intensive Care*............................ J. Michael Waldeck, M.D.
   Mental Health*.............................. Charlotte Jones, M.D.
   Neonatology*........................... Joseph W. Werthammer, M.D.
   Nephrology*................................... Open
Psychiatry and Behavioral Medicine.............. Samuel Januszkiewcz, M.D.
Radiology... Peter A. Chirico, M.D.
Surgery... David A. Denning, M.D.
   General Surgery*............................. David A. Denning, M.D.
   Breast Specialists............................. Douglas Henson, M.D.
   Burn Care/Trauma.............................. Sirous Arya, M.D.
   Pediatric Surgery*............................. Bonnie Beaver, M.D.
   Plastic Surgery*........................... William M. Cocke, M.D.
   Vascular Surgery............................... Open
   Oral and Maxillofacial Surgery.......... Raj K. Khanna, D.M.D., M.D.
   Thoracic Surgery.............................. Rebecca Wolfer, M.D.
   Urology....................................... Louis R. Molina, M.D.

*Specialty without organizational autonomy.

West Virginia University School of Medicine
Ste. 1040, Box 9100
Robert C. Byrd Health Sciences Center South
Morgantown, West Virginia 26506-9100
304-293-6607 (dean's office); 293-6627 (dean's office fax); 293-2408 (student affairs)
E-mail: lmiele@hsc.wvu.edu
Web site: www.hsc.wvu.edu

In 1902, West Virginia University (WVU) initiated a two-year medical curriculum, and in 1912, the WVU Board of Regents recognized a separate division of the university to be known as the school of medicine. In 1960, the school was expanded to a four-year program. Currently, the Robert C. Byrd Health Sciences campus is comprised of the 522-bed Ruby Memorial Hospital, Physicians Office Center, WVU Eye Institute, Mary Babb Randolph Cancer Center, WVU Children's Hospital, Betty Puskar Breast Care Center, Chestnut Ridge Psychiatric Hospital, and Mountainview Rehabilitation Center. The Charleston Division was established in October 1972, and is affiliated with Charleston Area Medical Center. The Eastern Division, located in Martinsburg, West Virginia, was established in 2001 as a two-year clinical campus. The Educational and Administrative Building (Erma Byrd Center) was completed in March 2006.

Type: public
2008-2009 total enrollment: 440
Clinical facilities: WVU Hospitals, Monongalia General Hospital, HealthSouth Rehabilitation Hospital, Mary Babb Randolph Cancer Center, and WVU Eye Institute, all in Morgantown; Charleston Area Medical Center, WVU School of Medicine, and Thomas Memorial Hospital in Charleston; United Hospital Center and Louis A. Johnson VA Medical Center in Clarksburg; Martinsburg VA Center, City Hospital in Martinsburg, WV; and Jefferson Memorial Hospital in Ranson, WV.

University Officials
President. . . . . Michael S. Garrison
Vice President for Health Sciences . . . . Fred Butcher, Ph.D. (Interim)

Medical School Administrative Staff
Dean. . . . . James E. Brick, M.D. (Interim)
Chief Administrative Officer. . . . . Leslie Miele
Senior Associate Dean for Medical Education . . . . Norman D. Ferrari III, M.D.
Associate Dean, Student Services and Professional Development . . . . G. Anne Cather, M.D.
Associate Dean, Research and Graduate Studies . . . . Thomas M. Saba, Ph.D.
Associate Dean, Clinical Services. . . . . Jeffrey Neely, M.D.
Associate Dean, Development. . . . . James M. Stevenson, M.D.
Associate Dean, Finance. . . . . Timothy Palencik
Associate Dean, Medical Education. . . . . James M. Shumway, Ph.D.
Associate Dean for Professional Programs. . . . . MaryBeth Mandich, Ph.D.
Assistant Dean, Veterans Administration Affairs. . . . . Maria Kolar, M.D.
Chairperson, Committee on Admissions . . . . Bruce Freeman, M.D.

Institute Directors
Mary Babb Randolph Cancer Center . . . . Scot Remick, M.D.
Center for Health Ethics and Law . . . . Alvin H. Moss, M.D.
Center for Rural Emergency Medicine . . . . Jeffrey H. Coben, M.D.
Institute for Health Policy Research . . . . Sally Richardson
Center of Excellence Women's Health . . . . Barbara Ducatman, M.D.

Department and Division or Section Chairs
Basic Sciences
Biochemistry . . . . James O'Donnell, Ph.D. (Interim)
Microbiology, Immunology, and Cell Biology . . . . John B. Barnett, Ph.D.
Neurobiology and Anatomy . . . . Richard D. Dey, Ph.D.
Physiology amd Pharmacology . . . . Robert L. Goodman, Ph.D.

Clinical Sciences
Anesthesiology. . . . . David Wilks, M.D.
Behavioral Medicine and Psychiatry . . . . James M. Stevenson, M.D.
Community Medicine. . . . . Alan Ducatman, M.D.
Emergency Medicine . . . . Todd J. Crocco, M.D.
Family Medicine . . . . James Arbogast, M.D.
Human Performance and Applied Exercise Science . . . . MaryBeth Mandich, Ph.D.
    Exercise Physiology. . . . . Stephen Always, Ph.D.
    Occupational Therapy . . . . Randy P. McCombie, Ph.D.
    Physical Therapy . . . . MaryBeth Mandich, Ph.D.

Medicine . . . . Kevin Halbritter, M.D. (Interim)
    Cardiology . . . . Robert Beto, M.D.
    Dermatology . . . . Rodney Kovach, M.D.
    Digestive Diseases . . . . Uma Sundaram, M.D.
    General Internal Medicine . . . . Richard D. Layne, M.D.
    Hematology-Oncology . . . . Jame Abraham, M.D.
    Infectious Diseases . . . . Rashida Khakoo, M.D.
    Metabolism-Endocrinology . . . . Tim Jackson, M.D.
    Nephrology . . . . Rebecca Schmidt, D.O.
    Pulmonary and Critical Care . . . . John Parker, M.D.
    Rheumatology . . . . Joann Hornsby, M.D. (Interim)
Neurosurgery . . . . Julian E. Bailes, M.D.
Neurology . . . . John F. Brick, M.D.
Obstetrics and Gynecology . . . . Michael Vernon, Ph.D.
Ophthalmology . . . . Judie Charlton, M.D.
Orthopedic Surgery . . . . Sanford E. Emery, M.D.
Otolaryngology . . . . Stephen J. Wetmore, M.D.
Pathology . . . . Barbara S. Ducatman, M.D.
    Clinical Pathology . . . . Patricia Canfield, M.D.
    Medical Technology Program . . . . Martha Lake, Ed.D.
    Surgical Pathology and Cytopathology . . . . Harold James Williams, M.D.
Pediatrics . . . . Giovanni Piedimonte, M.D.
    Adolescent Medicine . . . . Kathaleen Perkins, M.D.
    Birth Score . . . . Martha Mullet, M.D.
    Cardiology . . . . Larry A. Rhodes, M.D.
    Critical Care . . . . Michael J. Romano, M.D.
    Endocrinology . . . . Evan Jones, M.D., Ph.D.
    Gastroenterology . . . . Wikrom Karnsakul, M.D.
    Genetics and Metabolic . . . . Marybeth Hummel, M.D.
    Hematology and Oncology . . . . Open
    Infectious Diseases . . . . Kathryn Moffett, M.D.
    Neonatal . . . . Janet É. Graeber, M.D.
    Neurology and Child Development . . . . Margaret Jaynes, M.D.
    Section for Allergy, Immunology, and Pulmonary Medicine . . . . Kathryn Moffett, M.D.
Radiology . . . . Mathis Frick, M.D.
    Advanced Imaging and M.R.I. . . . . Jeffrey S. Carpenter, M.D.
    Breast Imaging . . . . Judith S. Schreiman, M.D.
    Diagnostic . . . . Gary D. Marano, M.D.
Surgery . . . . Richard Vaughan, M.D.
    Cardiovascular Thoracic Surgery . . . . Jose Cruzzavala, M.D.
    Urology . . . . Stanley Kandzari, M.D.

Charleston Division
Charleston, WV 25304-1299
304-347-1298; 347-1209 (fax); 347-1206 (dean's office)

Associate Vice President for Health Sciences,
    Dean Clinical Campus . . . . L. Clark Hansbarger, M.D.
Associate Dean for Student Services . . . . James Griffith, M.D.
Behavioral Medicine and Psychiatry . . . . Martin Kommor, M.D.
Family Medicine . . . . Jeffrey V. Ashley, M.D.
Internal Medicine . . . . Gregory Rosencrance, M.D.
Obstetrics and Gynecology . . . . Stephen Bush, M.D.
Pediatrics . . . . John Udall, M.D.
Surgery . . . . James P. Boland, M.D.

Eastern Division
Martinsburg, WV 25402
304-264-9202 (dean's office); 264-9042 (fax)

Associate Vice President for Health Services,
    Dean Clinical Campus . . . . C. H. Mitch Jacques, M.D.
Family Medicine . . . . K. C. Nau, M.D.

Medical College of Wisconsin

8701 Watertown Plank Road
Milwaukee, Wisconsin 53226
414-456-8296; 456-8213 (dean's office); 456-6560 (fax)
Web site: www.mcw.edu

The Medical College of Wisconsin originated in 1913 as the medical department of Marquette University. In 1918, a corporation was chartered by the state of Wisconsin to operate the Marquette University School of Medicine as a component of Marquette University. In 1967, the school of medicine separated from Marquette and was reorganized to become a totally freestanding corporation. In 1970, the name of the college was changed to the Medical College of Wisconsin.

Type: private
2008-2009 total enrollment: 807
Clinical facilities: Major affiliates: Froedtert Memorial Lutheran Hospital, Children's Hospital of Wisconsin, Milwaukee County Mental Health Complex, Curative Rehabilitation Services, Clement J. Zablocki Veterans Affairs Medical Center and the Blood Center of Southeastern Wisconsin. **Community Affiliates:** Columbia Hospital, St. Joseph's Hospital, St. Mary's Hospital (Milwaukee), St. Mary's Hospital (Racine), Aurora Psychiatric Hospital, Sacred Heart Rehabilitation Institute, St. Francis Hospital, St. Luke's Medical Center, Sinai-Samaritan Medical Center, Waukesha Memorial Hospital (Waukesha), West Allis Memorial Hospital, Community Memorial Hospital (Menomonee Falls), St. Luke's Hospital (Racine), Howard Young Medical Center (Woodruff).

Medical School Administrative Staff

President. . . . . T. Michael Bolger, J.D.
Dean and Executive Vice President. . . . . Jonathan I. Ravdin, M.D.
Senior Vice President for Finance and Administration. . . . . Douglas R. Campbell
Chief Financial Officer. . . . . Marjorie M. Spencer
Vice President for Institutional Advancement . . . . James W. Heald
Senior Associate Dean for Academic Affairs . . . . Kenneth B. Simons, M.D.
Associate Dean for Student Affairs . . . . Richard L. Holloway, Ph.D.
Associate Dean for Curriculum. . . . . Philip N. Redlich, M.D., Ph.D.
Assistant Dean, Student Affairs/Diversity. . . . . Dawn S. Bragg, Ph.D.
Senior Associate Dean, Public and Community Health . . . . Cheryl A. Maurana, Ph.D.
Senior Associate Dean for Clinical Affairs - MCP. . . . . Peter J. Plantes, M.D.
Senior Associate Dean for Clinical Affairs - CSG . . . . Joseph E. Kerschner, M.D.
Senior Associate Dean for Graduate Medical Education . . . . Mahendar S. Kochar, M.D.
Associate Dean for the Zablocki Veterans Affairs
   Medical Center . . . . Michael D. Erdmann, M.D.
Senior Associate Dean for Research . . . . David D. Gutterman, M.D.
Associate Dean for Research. . . . . David R. Harder, Ph.D.
Dean, Graduate School . . . . Owen W. Griffith, Ph.D.
Director of Admissions. . . . . Michael Istwan
Executive Director of Alumni Relations . . . . William A. Schultz
Director of Biomedical Resource Center. . . . . Joseph Thulin, D.V.M.
Assistant Vice President, Corporate Compliance . . . . Daniel Wickeham
Director of Continuing Medical Education . . . . Michael D. O'Donnell
Associate Dean for Educational Support and Evaluation . . . . Deborah E. Simpson, Ph.D.
Director of Financial Aid . . . . Linda L. Paschal
Registrar . . . . Lesley A. Mack
Assistant Vice President of Development. . . . . Pamela J. Garvey
Associate Dean for Faculty Affairs. . . . . Alan K. David, M.D.
Director of Libraries . . . . Mary B. Blackwelder
Vice President of Human Resources. . . . . Sherri Ducharme-White
Vice President, Operations. . . . . Tye V. Minckler
Vice President of Planning and Government Affairs . . . . Donna K. Gissen
Assistant Vice President of Public Affairs. . . . . Richard N. Katschke
General Counsel . . . . Sarah D. Cohn

Department Chairs and Division Chiefs

Basic Sciences

Biochemistry . . . . Robert J. Deschenes, Ph.D.
Biophysics . . . . Balaraman Kalyanaraman, Ph.D.
Cell Biology, Neurobiology, and Anatomy. Joseph L. Besharse, Ph.D.
Microbiology and Molecular Genetics. . . . . Paula Traktman, Ph.D.
Pathology . . . . Saul Suster, M.D.
Pharmacology and Toxicology . . . . William B. Campbell, Ph.D.
Physiology. . . . . Allen W. Cowley, Jr., Ph.D.
Population Health . . . . Cheryl A. Maurana, Ph.D. (Interim)

Clinical Sciences

Anesthesiology. . . . . David C. Warltier, M.D., Ph.D.
Dermatology . . . . Thomas J. Russell, M.D. (Interim)
Emergency Medicine . . . . Stephen W. Hargarten, M.D.
Family and Community Medicine. . . . . Alan K. David, M.D.
Medicine. . . . . G. Richard Olds, M.D.
   Cardiovascular Medicine. . . . . Michael P. Cinquegrani, M.D. (Interim)
   Endocrinology, Metabolism, and Clinical Nutrition . . . . Ahmed H. Kissebah, M.D.
   Gastroenterology and Hepatology. . . . . Reza Shaker, M.D.
   General Internal Medicine . . . . Ann B. Nattinger, M.D.
   Geriatrics and Gerontology. . . . . Edmund H. Duthie, Jr., M.D.
   Neoplastic Diseases and Related Disorders. . . . . James C. Wade, M.D.
   Infectious Diseases . . . . Mark A. Bielke, M.D.
   Nephrology . . . . Sundaram Hariharan, M.D.
   Pulmonary and Critical Care. . . . . Elizabeth R. Jacobs, M.D.
   Rheumatology . . . . Lawrence M. Ryan, M.D.
Neurology . . . . Safwan S. Jaradeh, M.D.
Neurosurgery. . . . . Thomas A. Gennarelli, M.D.
Obstetrics and Gynecology. . . . . Dwight P. Cruikshank, M.D.
Ophthalmology . . . . Dale K. Heuer, M.D.
Orthopaedic Surgery . . . . Jeffrey P. Schwab, M.D.
Otolaryngology and Communication Sciences. . . . . Phillip A. Wackym, M.D.
Pediatrics . . . . Robert M. Kliegman, M.D.
Physical Medicine and Rehabilitation . . . . Timothy R. Dillingham, M.D.
Plastic and Reconstructive Surgery . . . . David Larson, M.D.
Psychiatry and Behavioral Medicine . . . . Laura W. Roberts, M.D.
Radiation Oncology. . . . . J. Frank Wilson, M.D.
Radiology . . . . James E. Youker, M.D.
Surgery . . . . Keith T. Oldham, M.D. (Interim)
   Cardiothoracic . . . . James S. Tweddell, M.D.
   Oral and Maxillofacial . . . . Steven R. Sewall, D.D.S.
   Pediatric . . . . Keith T. Oldham, M.D.
   Transplant . . . . Christopher P. Johnson, M.D.
   Trauma/Critical Care. . . . . John Weigelt, M.D.
   Vascular. . . . . Gary R. Seabrook, M.D.
Urology. . . . . William A. See, M.D.

Institutes

Clinical Translational Science Institute . . . . Reza Shaker, M.D.

University of Wisconsin School of Medicine and Public Health
750 Highland Avenue
Madison, Wisconsin 53705-2221
608-263-4900; 263-4910 (dean's office)
Web site: www.med.wisc.edu

The school of medicine and public health is located on the Madison campus of the University of Wisconsin in clinical facilities, occupied since April 1, 1979, adjoining the Madison Veterans Administration Hospital. The school was established in 1907, offering a two-year program. With the construction of Wisconsin General Hospital in 1925, a four-year program was initiated. Its first four-year class graduated in 1927.

Type: public
2008-2009 total enrollment: 600
Clinical facilities: University of Wisconsin Hospital and Clinics, William S. Middleton Veterans Administration Hospital, St. Mary's Hospital Medical Center, Meriter Hospital, Mendota Mental Health Institute, Central Wisconsin Center for the Developmentally Disabled, Sinai Samaritan Medical Center (Milwaukee), Gundersen Clinic-Lutheran Hospital (LaCrosse), Marshfield Clinic and Foundation-St. Joseph's Hospital (Marshfield).

University Officials

President, University of Wisconsin System . . . . Kevin P. Reilly, Ph.D.
Chancellor, University of Wisconsin-Madison . . . . Carolyn A. Martin, Ph.D.

School of Medicine and Public Health Administrative Staff

Vice Chancellor for Medical Affairs and Dean. Robert N. Golden, M.D.
Senior Associate Dean, Academic Affairs. . . . . Susan E. Skochelak, M.D., M.P.H.
Senior Associate Dean, Clinical Affairs . . . . Jeffrey E. Grossman, M.D.
Senior Associate Dean, Translational and Clinical Research. . . . . Marc Drezner, M.D.
Associate Vice Chancellor for Medical Affairs
  and Senior Associate Dean, Administration
  and Finance . . . . Gordon T. Ridley
Associate Dean, Medical Education. . . . . Christine S. Seibert, M.D.
Associate Dean, Hospital Affairs . . . . Carl J. Getto, M.D.
Vice Dean and Associate Dean, Research and
  Graduate Studies . . . . Paul M. DeLuca, Jr., Ph.D.
Associate Dean, Rural and Community Health . . . . Byron J. Crouse, M.D.
Associate Dean, Students . . . . Patrick E. McBride, M.D., M.P.H.
Associate Dean, Marshfield Academic Campus . . . . Erik J. Stratmon, M.D.
Associate Dean, Milwaukee Academic Campus . . . . Jeffrey A. Stearns, M.D.
Assistant Dean, Clinical Affairs, Meriter Hospital. . . . . Geoffrey R. Priest, M.D.
Assistant Dean, Clinical Affairs, VA Hospital . . . . Alan J. Bridges, M.D.
Associate Dean, Clinical Affairs, Western Academic Campus . . . . David H. Chestnut, M.D.
Assistant Dean, Community Programs. . . . . Nancy Sugden
Assistant Dean, Facilities. . . . . Mark C. Wells
Associate Dean, Fiscal Affairs . . . . Kenneth J. Mount
Associate Dean, Administrative Affairs. . . . . Elizabeth T. Bolt
Associate Dean, Continuing Professional Development . . . . George C. Mejicano, M.D., M.S.
Associate Dean, Faculty Development and Affairs . . . . Patricia K. Kokotailo, M.D.
Assistant Dean, Multicultural Affairs . . . . Gloria V. Hawkins, Ph.D.
Assistant Dean, Student Affairs. . . . . Patricia C. DeMarse
Assistant Dean, Technology Transfer . . . . Stephen G. Harsy, Ph.D.
Director, Medical Alumni Association and
  Assistant Dean, Alumni Relations . . . . Karen S. Peterson
Assistant Dean, Health Professions Programs. Beverly Bawden, Ph.D.
Vice President, Health and Life Sciences . . . . Mark Lefebvre
Assistant Dean, Admissions. . . . . Lucy Wall
Director, Health Sciences Library. . . . . Terrance M. Burton

University of Wisconsin School of Medicine and Public Health: WISCONSIN

Department and Division or Section Chairs

Basic Sciences

Anatomy . . . . John K. Harting, Ph.D.
Biomolecular Chemistry . . . . Robert H. Fillingame, Ph.D.
Biostatistics and Medical Informatics . . . . Vacant
Medical Genetics . . . . Michael R. Culbertson, Ph.D.
Medical History and Bioethics . . . . Susan E. Lederer, Ph.D.
Medical Microbiology and Immunology . . . . Rodney A. Welch, Ph.D.
Medical Physics . . . . James A. Zagzebski, Ph.D.
Oncology . . . . F. Michael Hoffmann, Ph.D. (Interim)
Pathology and Laboratory Medicine . . . . Michael N. Hart, M.D.
Pharmacology . . . . Arnold E. Ruoho, Ph.D.
Physiology . . . . Richard L. Moss, Ph.D.
Population Health Sciences . . . . F. Javier Nieto, M.D., Ph.D.

Clinical Sciences

Anesthesiology . . . . Robert A. Pearce, M.D., Ph.D.
Dermatology . . . . Gary S. Wood, M.D.
Family Medicine . . . . Valerie J. Gilchrist, M.D.
Human Oncology . . . . Paul Harari, M.D.
  Biotherapy . . . . Soren Bentzen, Ph.D.
  Radiation Biology . . . . Soren Bentzen, Ph.D.
  Radiation Physics . . . . Bhudatt R. Paliwal, Ph.D.
  Radiation Therapy . . . . Kristin Bradley, M.D.
Medicine . . . . William W. Busse, M.D.
  Allergy, Pulmonary, and Critical Care . . . . Nizar Jarjour, M.D.
  Cardiovascular Medicine . . . . Matthew R. Wolff, M.D.
  Division of Primary Care, Internal Medicine . . . . Elizabeth Trowbridge, M.D.
  Emergency Medicine . . . . Joseph Cline, M.D.
  Endocrinology, Diabetes, and Metabolism . . . . Marc K. Drezner, M.D.
  Gastroenterology and Hepatology . . . . Michael R. Lucey, M.D.
  General Internal Medicine, Scholars Program . . . . Mark Linzer, M.D.
  Geriatrics and Gerontology . . . . Sanjay Asthana, M.D.
  Hematology and Oncology . . . . George Wilding, M.D.
  Infectious Disease . . . . George Mejicano, M.D. (Acting)
  Nephrology . . . . Bryan N. Becker, M.D.
  Rheumatology, Co-Heads . . . . Carolyn L. Bell, M.D., and Kevin McKown, M.D.
Neurological Surgery . . . . Robert J. Dempsey, M.D.
Neurology . . . . Thomas P. Sutula, M.D., Ph.D.
Obstetrics and Gynecology . . . . Laurel W. Rice, M.D.
Ophthalmology and Visual Sciences . . . . Paul L. Kaufman, M.D.
Pediatrics . . . . Ellen R. Wald, M.D.
Psychiatry . . . . Ned H. Kalin, M.D.
Radiology . . . . Thomas M. Grist, M.D.
  Nuclear Medicine . . . . Scott Perlman, M.D.
Orthopedics and Rehabilitation . . . . Thomas A. Zdeblick, M.D.
Surgery . . . . K. Craig Kent, M.D.
  Cardiothoracic . . . . Niloo M. Edwards, M.D.
  General . . . . Dennis P. Lund, M.D.
  Otolaryngology-Head and Neck . . . . Timothy M. McCulloch, M.D.
  Plastic/Reconstructive . . . . Michael L. Bentz, M.D.
  Transplantation . . . . Hans Sollinger, M.D., Ph.D.
Urology . . . . Stephen Y. Nakada, M.D.

Provisional Medical School Members

2008–2009

University of Central Florida College of Medicine

University Tower, Suite 300
12201 Research Parkway
Orlando, Florida 32826-0116
407-823-1841; 823-1856 (fax)
Web site: www.med.ucf.edu

The University of Central Florida College of Medicine was established in 2006 by the Florida Board of Governors, Florida legislature, and governor to increase opportunities for medical education in Florida and address the future need for physicians in the state. The college currently offers undergraduate and graduate programs in biomedical sciences, biotechnology, medical laboratory sciences, and molecular biology and microbiology, and will offer a doctor of medicine (M.D.) degree program beginning fall 2009. The M.D. program will enroll an initial class of 40 students and eventually produce about 120 medical graduates each year. The M.D. program learning experience at the University of Central Florida is a unique and exciting blend of state-of-the-art technology, virtual patients, clinical and laboratory experiences, research, facilitator-directed small-group sessions, and interactive didactic lectures. The M.D. program integrates basic and clinical sciences across all four years. The first two years of the curriculum are structured into modules, with the first year focusing on a fundamental understanding of how the various basic science disciplines relate to the normal human body. The second year takes an organ system-based approach and applies the basic knowledge of the first year to the study of clinical disease, pathological processes, and treatment. The third and fourth years of the curriculum are devoted to clinical experience through clerkships. During each of the clerkships, the fundamental knowledge from the first two years is reinforced through lectures, simulations, journal clubs, and conferences. The four-year medical program capitalizes on the school's existing strengths in biomedical sciences, modeling and simulation, and optics and photonics.

Type: public
2008-2009 total enrollment:
Clinical facilities: Nemours Children's Hospital, Orlando VA Medical Center, Florida Hospital, Orlando Health, Burnham Institute for Medical Research, M.D. Anderson Cancer Research Institute, Orange County Health Department, Lakeside Behavioral Healthcare.

University Officials

President. . . . . John C. Hitt, Ph.D.
Executive Vice President and Provost . . . . Terry L. Hickey, Ph.D.
Vice President and Chief of Staff . . . . Beth Barnes, Ph.D.
Senior Executive Assistant to the President. . . . . Amy Barnickel
Assistant Chief of Staff . . . . Nancy L. Marshall, Ed.D.
Chair, Board of Trustees . . . . Rick Walsh, M.S.
Vice Chair, Board of Trustees. . . . . Tom Yochum

Medical School Administrative Staff

Dean, College of Medicine.................................. Deborah C. German, M.D.
Special Assistant to the Dean .... Karen Smith, M.S.
Director, Burnett School of Biomedical Sciences.............. Pappachan Kolattukudy, Ph.D.
Associate Dean, Faculty and Academic Affairs.................... Richard Peppler, Ph.D.
Associate Dean, Administration and Finance...................... Scott Sumner, M.B.A.
Associate Dean, Planning and Knowledge Management............. Julia Pet-Armacost, Ph.D.
Associate Dean, Special Projects and Chief Legal Counsel........... Jeanette Schreiber, J.D.
Associate Dean, Students .... Randolph Manning, Ed.D.
Assistant Vice President, Development .... Charles Roberts
Special Projects for the Dean .... Robert Armacost, D.Sc.
Assistant Dean, Graduate Medical Education........................ Diane Davey, M.D.
Assistant Dean, Undergraduate Medical Education .... Lynn Crespo, Ph.D.
Registrar .... Teresa Lyons-Oten
Director, Admissions .... Robert Larkin
Director, Accreditation and Assessment .... Basma Selim, Ph.D.
Director, Clinical Skills Center.............................. Laura Cuty-Ruiz, Ph.D.
Director, Finance and Accounting .... Steven Omli, M.B.A., C.M.A.
Director, Harriet F. Ginsburg Health Sciences Library................ Nadine Dexter, M.L.S.
Director, Human Resources................................. Allen Abramson, S.P.H.R.
Director, Information Technologies .... Henry Glaspie, M.S.I.E.
Director, Facilities and Campus Operations .... Barbara O'Hara, M.P.A.
Director, Knowledge Management .... Matthew Gerber, Ph.D.
Director, Student Financial Services .... Ruthanne Madsen, M.B.A.
Associate Director, Burnett School of Biomedical Sciences .... Roseann White, Ph.D.
Assistant Director, Marketing .... Stephen Toth
Coordinator, Event Planning .... Kelley Melendez

Florida International University College of Medicine
11200 S.W. Eighth Street, HLS II 693
Miami, Florida 33199
305-348-0570; 348-0123 (fax)
Web site: http://medicine.fiu.edu/about.php?

Florida International University College of Medicine, south Florida's only public medical school, was created in 2006 amid pressing community health concerns and a projected critical shortage of physicians nationally. The college of medicine is developing a curriculum that reflects an innovative, twenty-first century approach to health care and medical education. The medical school will provide quality, affordable medical education and education physicians who are culturally sensitive to south Florida's diverse demographics. It will help advance south Florida's health care dynamic by facilitating improved access to first-rate medical care among our medically underserved populations and lead an economic impact that will eventually reach more than $1 billion each year. The college will admit its first class in fall 2009. The number of students expected in its inaugural class is 40; the number of students at full capacity will be 480.

Type: public
2008-2009 total enrollment:
Clinical facilities: Jackson Memorial Hospital, Mount Sinai Medical Center, Miami Children's Hospital, Mercy Hospital.

University Officials

President. . . . . Modesto A. 'Mitch' Maidique, Ph.D.
Provost, Executive Vice President, and Chief Operating Officer. . . . . Ronald Berkman, Ph.D.
Chief Financial Officer and Senior Vice President of Administration . . . . Vivian Sanchez
Chief Information Officer and Vice President of Information Technology . . . . . . Min Yao, Ph.D.
Vice President of Academic Affairs. . . . . Douglas Wartzok, Ph.D.
Vice President of Audit and Compliance and General Counsel . . . . Cristina Mendoza
Vice President of Enrollment Services. . . . . Corinne Webb
Vice President of Government Relations. . . . . Steve Sauls
Vice President of Human Resources. . . . . Jaffus Hardrick, Ed.D.
Director of Intercollegiate Athletics . . . . Pete Garcia
Vice President of Research and Dean, University Graduate School. . . . . . . George Walker, Ph.D.
Vice President of Student Affairs and Undergraduate Education . . . . Rosa L. Jones, Ph.D.
Vice President of University and Community Relations . . . . Sandra Gonzalez-Levy

Florida International University College of Medicine: FLORIDA

Medical School Administrative Staff

Founding Dean and Senior Vice President for Medical Affairs. . . . . John A. Rock, M.D.
Founding Director of the College of Medicine Library . . . . David W. Boilard, A.M.L.S.
Executive Associate Dean of Academic Affairs. . . . . Joe Leigh Simpson, M.D.
Executive Associate Dean of Clinical Affairs . . . . J. Patrick O'Leary, M.D.
Executive Associate Dean of Finance and Administration . . . . Larry Bagby, M.B.A.
Executive Associate Dean of Student Affairs . . . . Sanford Markham, M.D.
Associate Dean for Curriculum. . . . . George Dambach, Ph.D.
Assistant Dean of Academic Affairs. . . . . Pedro Jose 'Joe' Greer, Jr., M.D.
Assistant Dean for Community and Clinical Affairs . . . . Fernando J. Valverde, M.D.
Assistant Deans of Student Affairs. . . . . Robert Dollinger, M.D., and Barbra Roller, Ph.D.
Director, Accreditation. . . . . Rodolfo Bonnin, Ph.D.
Director, Admissions and Records . . . . Betty L. Monfort, M.P.H.
Director, Financial Aid. . . . . Pemra Cetin, M.B.A.
Director, Operations . . . . Khaleel Seecharan, M.S.M.I.S.

Department and Division or Section Chairs

Cellular Biology. . . . . Georg Petrolanu, M.D., Ph.D.
Molecular Microbiology and Immunology. . . . . Kalai Mathee, Ph.D. (Interim)
Obstetrics and Gynecology. . . . . Manuel A. Penalver, M.D.
Pathology . . . . Robert J. Poppiti, M.D.

The Commonwealth Medical College

150 North Washington Avenue
Scranton, Pennsylvania 18503
570-504-7000 (campus); 504-7290 (dean's office); 504-7289 (fax)
E-mail: rdalessandri@tcmedc.org
Web site: http://thecommonwealthmedical.com

The Commonwealth Medical College is a new medical school that will serve all of northeastern Pennsylvania and expects to accept 60 medical students and 30 Master of Biomedical Sciences students in 2009. The college has been granted degree-granting authority from the Pennsylvania Department of Education and preliminary accreditation from the Liaison Committee on Medical Education. The college has campuses in Scranton, Wilkes-Barre, and Williamsport, Pennsylvania. The Commonwealth Medical College broke ground on its medical sciences building, featuring state-of-the-art research space, in August 2008. The college will be using temporary facilities during the first two years that feature a new clinical skills and simulation center and a gross anatomy laboratory.

Type: private
2008-2009 total enrollment:
Clinical facilities: Moses Taylor Hospital; Mercy Hospital; Community Medical Center, Scranton; Wyoming Valley Health Care System; Geisinger Wyoming Valley Medical Center; Susquehanna Health System and Guthrie Clinic.

University Official

President, The Commonwealth Medical College . . . . Robert D'Alessandri, M.D.

Medical School Administrative Staff

Dean. . . . . Robert D'Alessandri, M.D.
Vice Dean for Faculty and Clinical Affairs. . . . . Paul Katz, M.D.
Associate Dean for Academic Affairs. . . . . Barry Linger, Ed.D.
Associate Dean for Student Affairs . . . . Louis Binder, M.D.
Associate Dean for Research, Technology
  Transfer, and Economic Development . . . . Daniel Flynn, Ph.D.
Associate Dean for Educational Development . . . . Raymond Smego, M.D.
Associate Dean for Planning and Chief of Staff. . . . . Virginia Hunt, M.U.A.
Associate Dean for Finance and Chief Financial Officer . . . . John Monnier, M.B.A.
Vice President, Social Justice and Diversity . . . . Ida Castro, M.A., J.D.
Associate Dean for Regional Campus Development, Williamsport . . . . . . Keith Shenberger, M.D.
Associate Dean for Regional Campus Development, Wilkes-Barre . . . . Richard English, M.D.
Associate Dean for Regional Campus Development, Scranton . . . . Gerald Tracy, M.D.

The Commonwealth Medical College: PENNSYLVANIA

Department and Division or Section Chairs

Basic Sciences

Chair of the Basic Sciences . . . . Gerald Litwack, Ph.D.

Clinical Sciences Chairs

Family Medicine . . . . Janet Townsend, M.D.
Medicine. . . . . Vacant
Obstetrics and Gynecology. . . . . Vacant
Pediatrics . . . . Vacant
Psychiatry . . . . Vacant
Surgery . . . . Vacant

Texas Tech University Health Sciences Center
Paul L. Foster School of Medicine
4800 Alberta Avenue
El Paso, Texas 79905
915-545-6510
Web site: www.ttuhsc.edu/fostersom

On December 9, 2003, the ground breaking for El Paso Medical Science Building I took place, and two years later, January 31, 2006, a ribbon-cutting ceremony followed. The 93,000-square-foot facility houses research on diabetes, cancer, environmental health and infectious diseases, as well as a repository dedicated to data on Hispanic health and a genomic facility to link hereditary diseases in families. In December 2005, a ground breaking was held for the medical classroom building, which opened in November 2007. The 125,000-square-foot building has four floors and a partial penthouse. Included are classrooms, a library, small group rooms, a clinical skills area for students, faculty and administrative areas, basic sciences labs, a gross anatomy lab, a student services area, and food services.

Type: public
2008-2009 total enrollment:

University Officials

President. . . . . John C. Baldwin, M.D.
Chief of Staff. . . . . Mary Croyle, M.S., C.P.M.
Senior Executive Assistant to the President. . . . . Pureza (Didit) Martinez
Special Assistant to the President . . . . Cindy Gutierrez
Presidential Aide . . . . William Davis
Executive Vice President for Finance and Administration . . . . Elmo M. Cavin
Executive Vice President for Research . . . . Douglas M. Stocco, Ph.D.

Medical School Administrative Staff

Regional and Founding Dean. . . . . Jose Manuel de la Rosa, M.D.
Senior Associate Dean for Medical Education . . . . David J. Steele, Ph.D.
Associate Dean . . . . Hal S. Larsen, Ph.D.
Associate Academic Dean for Admissions and
    Continuing Medical Education . . . . Manuel Schydlower, M.D.
Associate Dean for Accreditation . . . . Darryl M. Williams, M.D., M.P.H.
Associate Dean for Education Outcomes and Technologies. . . . . Robin Satterwhite, Ed.D.
Associate Dean for Medical Education . . . . Brian W. Tobin, Ph.D.
Associate Dean for Faculty Affairs and Development. Hoi Ho, M.D.
Associate Dean for Student Affairs . . . . Kathryn V. Horn, M.D.
Associate Academic Dean for Admissions . . . . Manuel Schydlower, M.D.
Associate Dean for Graduate Medical Education . . . . Jose L. Gonzalez-Sanchez, M.D.
Assistant Dean for Research . . . . Rajinder Koul, Ph.D.
Assistant Dean of Admissions and Student Affairs . . . . Lindsay Roberts
Dean of the School of Allied Health Sciences. . . . . Paul P. Brooke, Jr., Ph.D.
Dean of the School of Medicine. . . . . Steven L. Berk, M.D.
Dean of the School of Nursing. . . . . Alexia Green, R.N., Ph.D., F.A.A.N.
Dean of the School of Pharmacy . . . . Arthur A. Nelson, Jr., R.Ph., Ph.D.
Dean of the Graduate School of Biomedical Sciences . . . . Luis Reuss, M.D.
Vice President for Academic Services . . . . Rial Rolfe, Ph.D., M.B.A.
Vice President for International and Multicultural Affairs . . . . Germń R. Núñez, Ph.D.
Vice President for Information Technology and
    Chief Information Officer . . . . Michael T. Phillips
Vice President for Medical Affairs. . . . . Steven L. Berk, M.D.
Vice President for Rural and Community Health . . . . Steven L. Berk, M.D. (Interim)

Texas Tech University Health Sciences Center
Paul L. Foster School of Medicine: TEXAS

Department Chairs

Clinic Administration and Rehabilitation Counseling . . . . Robin Satterwhite, Ed.D.
Laboratory Science and Primary Care. . . . . Hal S. Larsen, Ph.D.
Rehabilitation Sciences . . . . Steven Sawyer, Ph.D.
Speech, Language, and Hearing Sciences . . . . Rajinder Koul, Ph.D.

Clinical Sciences

Anesthesiology. . . . . Ahmed E. Badr, M.D., F.C.C.M.
Emergency Medicine . . . . Brian K. Wilson, M.D., F.A.C.E.P.
Family Medicine . . . . Mary C. Spalding, M.D.
Community Partnership. . . . . Vacant
Internal Medicine . . . . Harry E. Davis II, M.D. (Interim)
   General Medicine. . . . . Vani Shukla, M.D.
   Gastroenterology . . . . Marc C. Zuckerman, M.D.
   Infectious Diseases . . . . Armando D. Meza, M.D.
   Nephrology . . . . Azikiwe Nwosu, Ph.D.
   Pulmonary and Critical Care. . . . . Manuel Rivera, M.D.
   Rheumatology . . . . Kanchan Pema, M.D.
Neonatology . . . . Carlos Antonio Jesurun, M.D.
Neuropsychiatry. . . . . James A. Wilcox, D.O., Ph.D. (Interim)
Obstetrics and Gynecology. . . . . Bahij S. Nuwayhid, M.D., Ph.D.
Ophthalmology . . . . Vacant
Orthopaedic Surgery and Rehabilitation. Miguel E. Pirela-Cruz, M.D.
Pathology . . . . Darius Boman, M.D.
Pediatrics . . . . Gilberto Aboukalil Handal, M.D.
Radiology . . . . Arvin Robinson, M.D., M.P.H.
Surgery and Neurosurgery . . . . Alan Henry Tyroch, M.D.

Affiliate Medical School Members

2008–2009

University of Alberta Faculty of Medicine and Dentistry

2J2 Walter Mackenzie Health Sciences Centre
8440 112th Street
Edmonton, Alberta Canada T6G 2R7
780-492-6350 (general"M.D. program); 492-6621 (dean's office); 492-7303 (fax)
Web site: www.med.ualberta.ca

The faculty of medicine at the University of Alberta was founded in 1913. The first complete M.D. degrees were granted in 1925. The faculty of dentistry merged with the faculty of medicine on April 1, 1996, to form the new faculty of medicine and dentistry.

Type: public
2008-2009 total enrollment: 523
Clinical facilities: University of Alberta Hospitals, Royal Alexandra Hospitals, Grey Nuns Hospital, Edmonton Misericordia Hospital, Glenrose Rehabilitation Hospital, Alberta Hospital (Edmonton), Alberta Hospital (Ponoka), Cross Cancer Institute, St. Mary's Hospital (Camrose), and Red Deer General Hospital (Red Deer).

University Officials

Chancellor of the University	L. Evans
President and Vice Chancellor	I. V. Samerasekera, Ph.D.
Vice President (Academic)	C. Amrhein, Ph.D.
Vice President (Finance and Administration)	P. Clark
Vice President (Research)	L. Babiuk, Ph.D., D.Sc.
Vice President (External Relations)	S. Conn
Registrar	C. Byrne

Medical School Administrative Staff

Dean	T. J. Marrie, M.D.
Vice Dean	V. Yiu, M.D. (Acting)
Executive Director	V. Wulff, C.A., C.M.C.
Associate Dean, Undergraduate Medical Education	D. Rayner, M.D.
Associate Dean, Dentistry	N. Milos, M.D. (Acting)
Associate Dean, Postgraduate Medical Education	G. Elleker, M.D.
Associate Dean, Continuous Professional Learning	C. deGara, M.D.
Associate Dean, Research	J. Jhamandas, M.D., Ph.D.
Assistant Dean, Research	T. Krukoff, Ph.D.
Associate Dean, Faculty Development	B. Fisher, M.D.
Associate Dean, Rural and Regional Health	J. Konkin, M.D.
Associate Dean, Clinical Affairs	Vacant
Assistant Dean, Admissions	M. Moreau, M.D.
Assistant Dean, Student Affairs	L. Mereu, M.D. (Acting)
Assistant Dean, Clinical Education	P. Sagle, M.D.
Program Director, Undergraduate Medical Education	M. Diduck
Director, Communications	J. Nugent
Assistant Dean, External Relations	A. Grace
Assistant Dean, Health Informatics	R. Hayward
Assistant Dean, Global Health	G. Taylor
Director, Research	M. Taylor
Associate Dean, Equity	L. Breault, M.D.
Senior Associate Dean, Education	F. Brenneis, M.D.

Faculty Directors

Department and Division or Section Chairs

Anatomy	A. Walji, M.D., Ph.D.
Biochemistry	M. Michalak, Ph.D.
Biomedical Engineering	R. E. Burrell, Ph.D.
Cell Biology	R. Rachubinski, Ph.D.
Medical Laboratory Science	F. J. Bamforth, M.D.

Medical Microbiology and Immunology . . . . D. Evans, Ph.D.
Pharmacology . . . . S. Dunn, Ph.D.
Physiology . . . . K. Pearson, Ph.D. (Acting)

Clinical Sciences

Anesthesiology and Pain Medicine . . . . B. Finegan, M.D.
Critical Care Medicine. . . . . N. Gibney, M.D.
Dentistry . . . . N. Milos, Ph.D. (Acting)
Emergency Medicine . . . . B. Holroyd, M.D.
Laboratory Medicine and Pathology . . . . F. Bamforth, M.D.
Medical Genetics . . . . M. A. Walter, Ph.D.
Medicine. . . . . J. Meddings, M.D.
   Cardiology . . . . B. O'Neill, M.D.
   Clinical Hematology . . . . L. Larratt, M.D.
   Dermatology and Cutaneous Sciences . . . . T. Salopek, M.D.
   Endocrinology . . . . C. Chik, M.D.
   Gastroenterology . . . . S. VanZanten, M.D.
   General Internal Medicine . . . . N. Kassam, M.D. (Acting)
   Geriatrics. . . . . K. Lechelt, M.D.
   Immunology and Nephrology . . . . B. Ballerman, M.D.
   Infectious Diseases . . . . G. Taylor, M.D.
   Neurology . . . . T. Roberts, M.D.
   Pulmonary Medicine. . . . . I. Mayers, M.D.
   Rheumatology . . . . J. Homik, M.D.
Obstetrics and Gynecology . . . . D. Cumming, M.D. (Acting)
Oncology. . . . . A. McEwan, M.D.
Ophthalmology . . . . I. MacDonald, M.D.
Pediatrics . . . . L. Dibden, M.D. (Acting)
Physical and Rehabilitation Medicine . . . . N. Ashworth, M.B.,Ch.B.
Psychiatry . . . . P.J. White, Ph.D., D.Sc.
Radiology and Diagnostic Imaging . . . . R. Lambert, M.B.,B.Ch.
Surgery . . . . D. Hedden, M.D.
   Cardiac Surgery . . . . A. Koshal, M.D.
   General Surgery . . . . M. Chatenay, M.D.
   Neurosurgery . . . . K. Aronyk, M.D. (Acting)
   Orthopaedic Surgery . . . . D. D. Otto, M.D.
   Otolaryngology Surgery . . . . H. Seikaly, M.D.
   Pediatric Surgery . . . . D. Hedden, M.D.
   Plastic Surgery . . . . G. Wilkes, M.D.
   Surgical and Medical Research Group (Experimental) . . . . F. F. Tredget, M.D.
   Thoracic Surgery . . . . G. Todd, M.D. (Acting)
   Urology . . . . M. P. Chetner, M.D.

University of Calgary Faculty of Medicine

3330 Hospital Drive N.W.
Calgary, Alberta Canada T2N 4N1
403-220-4404; 220-6843 (dean's office); 283-4740 (fax)
E-mail: staylor@ucalgary.ca
Web site: http://faculty.med.ucalgary.ca

The University of Calgary Faculty of Medicine was initiated in 1966. Its first class of student physicians enrolled in September 1970 and graduated in 1973. The Calgary Health Sciences Centre is located on the Foothills Hospital site, approximately two kilometers from the main campus.

Type: public
2008-2009 total enrollment: 325
Clinical facilities: Foothills Provincial General Hospital, Peter Lougheed Centre, Rockyview General Hospital, University of Calgary Health Sciences Centre, Alberta Children's Hospital.

University Officials

President and Vice Chancellor . . . . H. P. Weingarten, Ph.D.
Provost and Vice President (Academic) . . . . A. Harrison, Ph.D.

Medical School Administrative Staff

Dean. . . . . T. E. Feasby, M.D.
Vice Dean . . . . R. B. Scott, MDCM
Senior Associate Dean, Education. . . . . B. Hallgrimsson, Ph.D.
Senior Associate Dean, Research . . . . R. Hawkes, Ph.D.
Associate Dean, Undergraduate Medical Education. . . . . B. J. Wright, M.D.
Associate Dean, Postgraduate Medical Education . . . . J. M. Todesco, M.D.
Associate Dean, Graduate Sciences Education. . . . . F. A. van der Hoorn, Ph.D.
Associate Dean, Clinical Affairs. . . . . R. Bridges
Associate Dean, Research. . . . . R. B. Hawkes, Ph.D.
Associate Dean, Continuing Medical Education. . . . . J. Lockyer, Ph.D.
Associate Dean, International Health . . . . T. Jadavji, M.D.
Associate Dean, Undergraduate Science Education . . . . Open
Associate Dean, Rural and Regional Affairs. D. L. Myhre, M.D.
Associate Dean, Basic Research. . . . . J. Reynolds
Associate Dean, Clinical Research. . . . . Open
Associate Dean, Equity and Teacher-Learner Relations . . . . J. de Groot, M.D.
Chief Financial Officer. . . . . G. Levy

Executive Director . . . . Open

Department and Division or Section Chairs

Basic Sciences

Cell Biology and Anatomy . . . . N. I. Syed, Ph.D.
Biochemistry and Molecular Biology . . . . L. W. Browder, Ph.D.
Microbiology and Infectious Diseases . . . . G. D. Armstrong, Ph.D.
Physiology and Biophysics . . . . G. W. Zamponi, Ph.D.
Pharmacology and Therapeutics . . . . D. L. Severson, Ph.D.

Clinical Sciences

Anaesthesia . . . . J. N. Armstrong, M.D.
Cardiac Sciences . . . . L. B. Mitchell, M.D.
Clinical Neurosciences . . . . J. G. Cairncross, M.D.
Community Health Sciences . . . . T. W. Noseworthy, M.D.
Critical Care Medicine . . . . P. J. E. Boiteau, M.D.
Family Medicine . . . . C. A. MacLean, M.D.
Medical Genetics . . . . O. Suchowersky, M.D.
Medicine . . . . J. M. Conly, M.D.
Obstetrics and Gynecology . . . . Open
Oncology . . . . P. S. Craighead, M.B.Ch.B. (Acting)
Paediatrics . . . . J. Kellner, M.D.
Pathology and Laboratory Medicine . . . . J. R. Wright, Jr., M.D., Ph.D.
Psychiatry . . . . G MacQueen, M.D.
Radiology . . . . R. J. Sevick, M.D.
Surgery . . . . J. B. Kortbeek, M.D.

*Specialty without organizational autonomy.

University of British Columbia Faculty of Medicine

317-2194 Health Sciences Mall
Vancouver, British Columbia Canada V6T 1Z3
604-822-2421 (dean's office); 822-6061 (fax)
Web site: www.med.ubc.ca

The faculty of medicine at the University of British Columbia was established in 1950. It is distributed to three university campuses, seven clinical academic campuses, and numerous affiliated teaching hospitals.

Type: public
2008-2009 total enrollment: 960
Clinical facilities: Vancouver Hospital and Health Sciences Centre, Children's and Women's Hospital and Health Centre, Providence Health Care Group, B.C. Cancer Agency, Prince George Regional Hospital, Royal Columbian Hospital, Victoria General Hospital, Royal Jubilee Hospital.

University Officials

President and Vice Chancellor . . . . Stephen Toope, Ph.D.
Vice President, Academic, and Provost . . . . David Farrar, Ph.D.
Vice President, Administration and Finance . . . . Vacant
Vice President, Development and Engagement . . . . Barbara Miles
Vice President, External, Legal, and Community
   Relations . . . . Stephen Owen, L.L.B., L.L.M., M.B.A.
Vice President, Research . . . . John Hepburn, Ph.D.
Vice President, Students. . . . . Brian Sullivan
Librarian protem. . . . . W. Peter Ward, Ph.D.
Associate Vice President, Enrollment Services and Registrar . . . . Brian Silzer

Medical School Administrative Staff

Dean. . . . . Gavin Stuart, M.D.
Senior Associate Dean, Education. . . . . Joanna Bates, M.D.
Associate Dean, M.D. Undergraduate Education-Admissions . . . . M. Clifford Fabian, M.D.
Associate Dean, M.D. Undergraduate Education-Student Affairs . . . . Sharon Salloum, M.D.
Associate Dean, M.D. Undergraduate Education-Curriculum . . . . Angela Towle, Ph.D.
Associate Dean, Postgraduate Education . . . . Kamal Rungta, M.D., and Kristin Sivertz, M.D.
Senior Associate Dean, Research . . . . Alison Buchan, Ph.D.
Associate Dean, Continuing Professional
   Development and Knowledge Translation . . . . Kendall Ho, M.D.
Senior Associate Dean, Faculty Affairs. . . . . Dorothy Shaw, M.B.Ch.B.
Special Advisor to the Dean on Clinical Faculty Affairs . . . . Katherine Paton, M.D.
Associate Dean, Island Medical Program. . . . . Oscar G. Casiro, M.D.
Associate Dean, Northern Medical Program . . . . David Snadden, M.B.Ch.B.
Associate Dean, Equity. . . . . Lori Charvat, J.D.
Special Advisor to the Dean on Planning . . . . David F. Hardwick, M.D.
Executive Director, Faculty Affairs . . . . Susan Langland
Executive Director, Resources and Operations . . . . Mark Vernon, CA, C.P.A.
Executive Director, Education and Strategic Projects. . . . . Jane Eibner, M.B.A., CMA

University of British Columbia Faculty of Medicine: BRITISH COLUMBIA

Department Heads and School Directors

Basic Sciences

Biochemistry and Molecular Biology . . . . Christopher Proud, Ph.D.
Cellular and Physiological Sciences . . . . Christian Naus, Ph.D.
Medical Genetics . . . . Robert McMaster, D.Phil.

Clinical Sciences

Anaesthesiology, Pharmacology, and Therapeutics . . . . Brian Warriner, M.D.
Dermatology and Skin Science . . . . Harvey Lui, M.D.
Family Practice . . . . Robert Woollard, M.D.
School of Population and Public Health . . . . Martin Schechter, M.D., Ph.D.
Medicine . . . . Graydon Meneilly, M.D.
Obstetrics and Gynaecology . . . . Robert Liston, M.B.Ch.B.
Occupational Sciences and Occupational Therapy . . . . Tal Jarus, Ph.D.
Ophthalmology and Visual Sciences . . . . Frederick Mikelberg, M.D.
Orthopaedics . . . . Bassam Masri, M.D.
Paediatrics . . . . Robert Armstrong, M.D, Ph.D.
Pathology and Laboratory Medicine . . . . Richard Hegele, M.D., Ph.D.
Physical Therapy . . . . Brenda Loveridge, Ph.D.
Psychiatry . . . . Trevor Young, M.D.
Radiology . . . . Nestor Müller, M.D., Ph.D.
Surgery . . . . Garth Warnock, M.D.
School of Audiology and Speech Sciences . . . . Valter Ciocca, Ph.D.
Urologic Sciences . . . . Larry Goldenberg, M.D.

University of Manitoba Faculty of Medicine
260 Brodie - 727 McDermot Avenue
Winnipeg, Manitoba Canada R3E 3P5
204-789-3557 (general office); 789-3485 (dean's office); 789-3928 (fax)
Web site: www.umanitoba.ca/faculties/medicine

Manitoba Medical College was established in 1883. In 1918, it ceased to exist as a separate institution and became known as the faculty of medicine of the University of Manitoba. It is located in Winnipeg near the health sciences centre, whereas the university proper is located in the suburb of Fort Garry, seven miles away.

Type: public
2008-2009 total enrollment: 280
Clinical facilities: Winnipeg Regional Health Authority (Health Sciences Centre, St. Boniface General Hospital, Deer Lodge Centre, Grace General Hospital, Seven Oaks General Hospital, Victoria General Hospital, Concordia Hospital, Misericordia Health Centre); Brandon General Hospital; Dauphin General Hospital; Thompson General Hospital.

University Officials

President . . . . Emőke Szathmáry, Ph.D.
Vice President (Administration) . . . . Deborah McCallum
Vice President (Academic) . . . . R. Kerr, Ph.D.
Director of Enrollment Services . . . . P. Dueck

Medical School Administrative Staff

Dean . . . . J. Dean Sandham, M.D.
Associate Dean (Academic) . . . . H. Dean, M.D.
Associate Dean (Research) . . . . P. Choy, M.D.
Associate Dean (Undergraduate Medical Education) . . . . B. Martin, M.D.
Associate Dean (Postgraduate Medical Education) . . . . I. Ripstein, M.D.
Associate to the Dean, Hospital Affairs (Health Sciences Centre) . . . . P. Gray, M.D.
Hospital Affairs (St. Boniface Hospital) . . . . Bruce Roe, M.D.
Associate Dean (Allied Health) . . . . E. Etcheverry, Ph.D.
Associate Dean (Student Affairs) . . . . L. Fraser-Roberts, M.D.
Assistant Dean (Admissions) . . . . F. Aoki, M.D.
Associate Dean (Continuing Medical Education) . . . . G. Bourgeois-Law, M.D.
Manager, Admissions and Student Affairs . . . . B. Jennings, B.Sc., M.Sc.

Department and Division or Section Chairs

Basic Sciences

Biochemistry and Medical Genetics .... L. Simard, Ph.D.
Community Health Sciences............................... L. Elliott, M.D. (Act. Head)
Human Anatomy and Cell Science............................. T. Klonisch, Ph.D.
Immunology .... R. Moqbel, Ph.D.
Medical Microbiology... J. Embree, M.D.
Pathology .... J. Gartner, M.D.
Pharmacology and Therapeutics................................. D. Sitar, Ph.D.
Physiology .... J. Dodd, Ph.D.

Clinical Sciences

Anesthesia... E. Jacobsohn, M.D.
Clinical Health Psychology....................................... R. McIlwraith, M.D.
Family Medicine .... J. Boyd, M.D. (Acting)
Internal Medicine .... D. Roberts, M.D.
  Acute Care.. B. Light, M.D.
  Cardiology... J. Ducas, M.D.
  Dermatology .... J. E. Toole, M.D.
  Endocrinology and Metabolism................................. L. Murphy, M.D.
  Gastroenterology .... C. Bernstein, M.D.
  General Medicine.. K. VanAmeyde, M.D.
  Gerontology.. E. Boustcha, M.D.
  Hematology and Oncology...................................... E. Bow, M.D.
  Hepatology .... G. Minuk, M.D.
  Immunology (Clinical)..................................... R. J. Warrington, M.D.
  Infectious Diseases .... P. Orr, M.D. (Acting)
  Nephrology .... D. Rush, M.D.
  Neurology .... B. Anderson, M.D.
  Pharmacology (Clinical)....................................... D. Sitar, M.D.
  Rehabilitation Medicine .... E. Boustcha, M.D.
  Respiratory.. S. Mink, M.D.
  Rheumatology .... H. El-Gabalawy, M.D.
Obstetrics, Gynecology, and Reproductive Sciences................. M. Morris, M.D.
Ophthalmology .... L. Bellan, Ph.D.
Otolaryngology .... B. Blakley, M.D.
Pediatrics and Child Health........................... C. Rockman-Greenberg, M.D.
Psychiatry .... M. Enns, M.D.
Radiology .... D. McClarty, M.D.
Surgery .... TBA
  Cardiac Surgery .... A. Menkis, M.D.
  Dental and Oral Surgery...................................... J. Curran, M.D.
  General Surgery.. J. Lipschitz, M.D.
  Neurosurgery... M. West, M.D.
  Orthopaedics.. P. Macdonald, M.D.
  Pediatric General Surgery.................................... B.J. Hancock, M.D.
  Plastic Surgery .... E. Buchel, M.D.
  Thoracic Surgery .... H. Unruh, M.D.
  Urology .... D. Hosking, M.D.
  Vascular Surgery.. R. Guzman, M.D.

Memorial University of Newfoundland Faculty of Medicine

Health Sciences Centre
300 Prince Philip Drive
St. John's, Newfoundland Canada A1B 3V6
709-777-6602 (dean's office); 777-6615 (admissions);
777-6669 (undergraduate medical educ.); 777-6680 (postgraduate medical stud.);
777-6746 (dean's office fax)
Web site: www.med.mun.ca/med

The faculty of medicine was founded in 1967 as part of a combined health sciences and life sciences complex on the campus of Memorial University. The first undergraduate class was admitted in September 1969. The medical school is part of the health sciences centre.

Type: public
2008-2009 total enrollment: 240
Clinical facilities: Health Care Corporation; St. John's; Western Regional Health Board (Corner Brook); Baie Verte Peninsula Health Centre (Baie Verte); Curtis Memorial Hospital (St. Anthony); Central Newfoundland Hospital (Grand Falls); Carbonear General Hospital (Carbonear); James Paton Memorial Hospital (Gander); Captain William Jackman Memorial Hospital (Labrador City); Notre Dame Bay Memorial Hospital (Twillingate); Green Bay Health Care Center (Springdale); G. B. Cross Memorial Hospital (Clarenville); Dr. Everett Chalmers Hospital (Fredericton).

University Officials

Chancellor . . . . General Rick Hillier
President and Vice Chancellor . . . . H. E. A. Campbell, Ph.D. (Acting)
Vice President (Academic) and Pro Vice Chancellor . . . . Michael Collins, Ph.D. (Acting)
Vice President (Administration and Finance) . . . . K. Decker
Vice President (Research) . . . . C. Loomis, Ph.D.
Registrar . . . . G. W. Collins

Medical School Administrative Staff

Dean of Medicine . . . . J. Rourke, M.D.
Vice Dean (Professional Development) . . . . S. Peters, M.D.
Associate Dean, BioMedical Sciences . . . . K. Mearow, Ph.D.
Associate Dean, Clinical Research . . . . P. Parfrey, M.D.
Associate Dean, Community Health and Humanities . . . . C. Donovan, M.D. (Acting)
Associate Dean, Research and Graduate Studies . . . . P. Moody-Corbett, Ph.D.
Assistant Dean, Admissions . . . . W. Parsons, M.D.
Assistant Dean, Postgraduate Medical Studies . . . . A. Samarasena, M.D.
Assistant Dean, Student Affairs . . . . J. Harris, Ph.D.
Assistant Dean, Undergraduate Medical Education . . . . G. Farrell, M.D.
Director of Animal Care . . . . L. Husa, M.V.Dr.
Manager of Medical School Laboratories . . . . E. Evelly
Associate University Librarian (Health Sciences) . . . . G. H. Beckett

Memorial University of Newfoundland Faculty of Medicine: NEWFOUNDLAND

Department and Division or Section Chairs

Clinical Sciences

Anesthesia* . . . . K. LeDez, M.D.
Family Medicine* . . . . R. Miller, M.D.
Medicine* . . . . A. Sclater, M.D.
Obstetrics and Gynecology* . . . . T. O'Grady, M.D.
Pathology* . . . . S. Avis, M.D.
Pediatrics* . . . . A. R. Cooper, M.D.
Psychiatry* . . . . T. Callanan, M.D.
Radiology* . . . . B. Cramer, M.D.
Surgery* . . . . W. Pollett, M.D.

Basic Sciences Resource People

Anatomy . . . . S. Chandra, Ph.D.
Biochemistry . . . . S. C. Vasdev, Ph.D.
Immunology . . . . M. Grant, Ph.D.
Neuroscience . . . . D. Corbett, Ph.D.
Physiology . . . . D. McKay, Ph.D.

*Specialty with partial organizational autonomy.

Dalhousie University Faculty of Medicine

Clinical Research Center
5849 University Avenue
Halifax, Nova Scotia Canada B3H 4H7
902-494-6592 (dean's office); 494-1874 (admissions office); 494-7119 (fax)
Web site: www.medicine.dal.ca

The faculty of medicine of Dalhousie University was organized in 1868, but the medical teaching was carried out by the independent Halifax Medical College from 1875 to 1911, when the faculty of medicine was reestablished by the university.

Type: public
2008-2009 total enrollment: 380
Clinical facilities: Queen Elizabeth II Health Sciences Centre (Victoria General Campus and Camp Hill Campus), IWK Health Centre; Archie McCullum Hospital (Department of National Defense); Nova Scotia Hospital; Sydney Community Health Centre; Queen Elizabeth Hospital; Prince County Hospital; Region 1 Hospital Corporation, South-East (Moncton, New Brunswick); Atlantic Health Sciences Corporation (Saint John, New Brunswick); Region 3 Hospital Corporation (Fredericton, New Brunswick); Region 7 Hospital Corporation (Miramichi, New Brunswick). A Clinical Skills Learning Centre is located at 5599 Fenwick Street, Halifax.

University Officials

President. . . . . T. Traves, Ph.D.
Vice President (Academic and Provost) . . . . A. Shaver, Ph.D.
Vice President (Finance and Administration) . . . . K. Burt
Vice President (Student Services) . . . . B. Neuman, Ph.D.
Vice President (External). . . . . F. Dykeman
Vice President (Research) . . . . M. Crago, Ph.D.

Medical School Administrative Staff

Dean. . . . . H. Cook, Ph.D.
Associate Dean, Postgraduate Medical Education . . . . M. Gardner, M.D.
Associate Dean, Undergraduate Medical Education. . . . . K. Blake, M.D.
Associate Dean, Research. . . . . G. C. Johnston, Ph.D.
Associate Dean, Continuing Medical Education. . . . . D. Sinclair, M.D.
Associate Dean Health Systems and Policy . . . . S. Spence Wach
Assistant Dean, Admissions and Student Affairs. . . . . E. Sutton, M.D.
Assistant Dean (New Brunswick). . . . . M. Raju, M.D.
Assistant Dean, Research (Clinical Departments) . . . . R. Brownstone, M.D.
Assistant Dean, Graduate and Postdoctoral Studies . . . . C. McMaster, Ph.D.
Secretary to the Faculty . . . . A. Weeden
Director, Health Law Institute . . . . W. Lahey
Director, Admissions and Student Affairs . . . . S. Graham
Director, Animal Care . . . . B. Hildebrand, D.V.M.
Head, Division of Medical Education . . . . B. Frank, Ph.D.
Director, Medical Informatics. . . . . D. Zitner, M.D.
Director, Finance. . . . . M. Radford
Director, Human Resources . . . . L. Power
Director, Administrative Services . . . . A. Weeden
Director, Communications . . . . C. Gaudet
Director of Information Technology. . . . . J. Robertson (Acting)
Health Sciences Librarian . . . . P. Ellis
Medical Alumni Affairs Coordinator . . . . K. Murphy

Department and Division or Section Chairs

Basic Sciences

Anatomy and Neurobiology . . . . R. Leslie, Ph.D.
Biochemistry and Molecular Biology. . . . . D. Byers, Ph.D.
Microbiology and Immunology. . . . . J. S. Marshall, Ph.D.
Pharmacology . . . . J. Sawynok, Ph.D.
Physiology and Biophysics . . . . P. R. Murphy, Ph.D.

Clinical Sciences

Anaesthesia . . . . M. Murphy, M.D.

Bioethics . . . . B. Frank, Ph.D.
Community Health and Epidemiology . . . . J. Guernsey, Ph.D. (Acting)
  Population Health Research Unit . . . . Open
Radiology . . . . C. Lo, M.D.
  Nuclear Medicine . . . . D. Barnes, M.D.
Emergency Medicine . . . . J. Ross, M.D.
Family Medicine . . . . P. Smith, M.D.
Medicine . . . . A. Purdy, M.D.
  Cardiology . . . . A. Quraishi, M.D. (Acting)
  Critical Care . . . . W. Patrick, M.D. (Acting)
  Palliative Care . . . . P. F. McIntyre, M.D.
  Dermatology . . . . L. Finlayson, M.D.
  Endocrinology and Metabolism . . . . S. Kaiser, M.D.
  Gastroenterology . . . . D. J. Leddin, M.D.
  General Medicine . . . . O. E. Mann, M.D.
  Geriatric Medicine . . . . L. Mallery, M.D.
  Hematology . . . . D. Anderson, M.D.
  Infectious Diseases . . . . B. L. Johston, M.D.
  Medical Oncology . . . . M. Doreen, M.D.
  Nephrology . . . . M. West, M.D.
  Neurology . . . . C. Maxner, M.D.
  Physical Medicine and Rehabilitation . . . . B. Joyce, M.D.
  Respirology . . . . G. Rocker, M.D. (Acting)
  Rheumatology . . . . E. Sutton, M.D.
Obstetrics and Gynaecology . . . . B. A. Armson, M.D.
  Gynaecology . . . . A. Bent, M.D.
  Maternal and Fetal Medicine . . . . M. Van den Hof, M.D.
  Oncology . . . . R. Grimshaw, M.D.
  Reproductive Endocrinology . . . . D. Young, M.D.
  Urolgynecology . . . . S. Farrell, M.D.
Ophthalmology and Visual Sciences . . . . A. Cruess, M.D.
Pathology and Laboratory Medicine . . . . G. Heathcote, Ph.D.
  Anatomical Pathology . . . . N. M. G. Walsh, M.D.
  Clinical Chemistry . . . . B. A. Nassar, Ph.D.
  Hematopathology . . . . I. Sadek, M.D.
  Medical Microbiology . . . . K. Forward, M.D.
  Molecular Pathology and Molecular Genetics . . . . D. Guernsey, Ph.D.
  Pediatric Pathology and Laboratory Medicine . . . . Open
Pediatrics . . . . J. Kronick, M.D., Ph.D., FRCPC
  Atlantic Research Centre . . . . N. Ridgway, Ph.D.
  Cardiology . . . . J. Finley, M.D., FRCPC
  Medical Genetics . . . . M. Ludman, M.D., FRCPC
  Developmental Pediatrics . . . . S. Shea, M.D.
  Endocrinology . . . . E. Cummings, M.D., FRCPC
  Gastroenterology and Nutrition . . . . A. Otley, M.D., FRCPC
  General Academic Pediatrics . . . . A. Larson, M.D., FRCPC
  Hematology/Oncology . . . . M. Bernstein, M.D.
  Immunology . . . . T. Issekutz, M.D., FRCPC
  Infectious Diseases . . . . S. Halperin, M.D., FRCPC
  Neonatal Pediatrics . . . . D. MacMillan, M.D., FRCPC
  Nephrology . . . . J. Crocker, M.D., FRCPC
  Neurology . . . . J. Dooley, M.D., FRCPC
  Palliative Care . . . . G. Frager, M.D., FRCPC
  Respirology . . . . W. Robinson, M.D.
  Rheumatology . . . . B. Lang, M.D., FRCPC
Psychiatry . . . . N. Delva, M.D.
Radiation Oncology . . . . C. T. Ago, M.D.
Surgery . . . . J. Bonjer, M.D.
  Cardiac . . . . G. Hirsch, M.D.
  General . . . . T. Topp, M.D.
  Neurosurgery . . . . I. Mendez, M.D.
  Orthopaedics . . . . D. Amirault, M.D.
  Otolaryngology . . . . D. Kirkpatrick, M.D.
  Pediatric . . . . M. Giacomantonio, M.D.
  Plastic . . . . Open
  Thoracic . . . . D. Bethune, M.D.
  Vascular . . . . G. MacKean, M.D.
Urology . . . . D. Bell, M.D. (Acting)

McMaster University Faculty of Health Sciences

1200 Main Street West
Hamilton, Ontario Canada L8N 3Z5
905-525-9140 Ext. 22141 (general info.); 546-0800 (fax)
Web site: www.fhs.mcmaster.ca

In 1967, the college of health sciences was formed as part of McMaster University. In 1969, in accordance with the McMaster Act of 1968-69, the structure was changed to the division of health sciences, incorporating the faculty of medicine and the school of nursing. The university structure was reorganized in 1974, at which time the division of health sciences became the faculty of health sciences. In 1989, the school of occupational therapy and physiotherapy was established. In 1993, a midwifery program was added.

Type: public
2008-2009 total enrollment: 434
Clinical facilities: Hamilton Health Sciences (Hamilton General Hospital, McMaster Children's Hospital, and the Hamilton Regional Cancer Centre), St. Joseph's Hospital, St. Peter's Hospital and various other community partners who provide clinical experience to the students.

University Officials

Chancellor . . . . L. Wilson
President and Vice Chancellor . . . . P. J. George, Ph.D., D.U, D. Hon. C., D. Litt (Hon.)
Provost and Vice President (Academic) . . . . Ilene Busch-Vishniac, Ph.D.
Vice President (Research and International Affairs) . . . . M. Elbestawi, Ph.D.
Dean and Vice President (Health Sciences) . . . . J. G. Kelton, M.D.
Vice President (Administration) . . . . K. S. Belaire
Vice President (University Advancement) . . . . R. Trull
Associate Vice President (Academic) . . . . F. A. Hall, Ph.D.
Associate Vice President (International Affairs) . . . . M. W. L. Chan, Ph.D.
Associate Vice President (Student Affairs) and Dean of Students . . . . P. E. Wood, Ph.D.
Registrar . . . . L. R. Ariano
University Librarian . . . . C. Stewart (Acting)
Principal of McMaster Divinity College . . . . S. E. Porter, Ph.D.
University Secretary and Secretary of the Board
   of Governors and the Senate . . . . W. B. Frank, Ph.D.
Assistant Vice President (Administration) . . . . L. M. Scime
Assistant Vice President (Human Resources) . . . . M. E. Haley

Michael G. DeGroote School of Medicine Administrative Staff

Dean and Vice President, Faculty of Health Sciences . . . . J. G. Kelton, M.D.
Associate Vice President, Academic and
   Associate Dean, Education . . . . S. D. Denburg, Ph.D., M.D.
Associate Dean (Research) . . . . S. Collins, M.D.
Associate Dean, Health Sciences (Nursing) . . . . C. H. Tompkins, Ph.D.
Associate Dean, Health Sciences (School of Rehabilitation Science) . . . . M. C. Law, Ph.D.
Assistant Dean, Bachelor of Health Sciences (Honours) Program . . . . D. G. Harnish, Ph.D.
Assistant Dean, Clinical Health Sciences (OT) Program . . . . D. A. Stewart, M.D.
Assistant Dean, Clinical Health Sciences (PT) Program . . . . L. R. Wishart, Ph.D.
Assistant Dean, Continuing Health Sciences Education Program . . . . G. O. Peachey, M.D.
Assistant Dean, Midwifery Education Program . . . . E. Hutton, Ph.D.
Postgraduate Medical Education Program . . . . J. M. Walton, M.D.
Assistant Dean, Program for Educational
   Research and Development . . . . G. R. Norman, Ph.D.
Assistant Dean, Program for Faculty Development . . . . A. E. Walsh, M.D.
Assistant Dean, Undergraduate Medical Education Program . . . . A. J. Neville, M.D.
Assistant Dean, Undergraduate Nursing Education Program . . . . J. Landeen, Ph.D.

Department and Division or Section Chairs

Basic Sciences

Biochemistry . . . . E. Brown, M.D.
Clinical Epidemiology and Biostatistics . . . . B. Haynes, M.D.
Pathology and Molecular Medicine. . . . . F. Smaill, Ph.D.

Clinical Sciences

Anaesthesia . . . . N. Buckley, M.D.
Family Medicine . . . . D. Price, M.D.
Medicine. . . . . P. O'Byrne, M.D.
Obstetrics and Gynecology. . . . . P. Mohide, M.D.
Paediatrics. . . . . P. Steer, M.D.
Psychiatry and Behavioural Neurosciences . . . . R. Zipursky, M.D.
Radiology . . . . D. Koff, M.D.
Surgery . . . . W. Orovan, M.D.

Queen's University Faculty of Health Sciences

Kingston, Ontario Canada K7L 3N6
613-533-2542 (medicine); 533-2668 (nursing); 533-6103 (rehabilitation therapy);
533-2544 (general); 533-6884 (fax)
Web site: http://meds.queensu.ca

Established in 1854, the faculty of health sciences of Queen's University is situated on the main campus. It was reorganized in 1866 as the Royal College of Physicians and Surgeons in affiliation with the university. In 1892, the original status was resumed. Effective July 1, 1997, Queen's University established the faculty of health sciences, integrating the schools of nursing, medicine, and rehabilitation therapy into a single academic unit.

Type: public
2008-2009 total enrollment: 1,119
Clinical facilities: Kingston General Hospital, Hotel Dieu Hospital, Providence Care (St. Mary's of the Lake Hospital and Mental Health Services sites), Cancer Centre of Southeastern Ontario, Ongwanada Hospital.

University Officials

Chancellor	David Dodge, L.L.D.
Principal and Vice Chancellor	Thomas R. Williams, Ph.D.

Health Sciences Administrative Staff

Dean	David M. C. Walker, M.D.
Director, School of Medicine	David M. C. Walker, M.D.
Associate Dean, Postgraduate Medical Education	Leslie V. Flynn, M.D.
Associate Dean, Academic	Kanji Nakatsu, Ph.D.
Associate Dean, Clinical	John F. Jeffrey, M.D.
Senior Associate Dean, Medical Education	Lewis L. Tomalty, Ph.D.
Director, Research	James F. Brien, Ph.D.
Associate Dean, Research	Roger G. Deeley, Ph.D.
Associate Dean, Undergraduate Medical Education	Anthony J. Sanfilippo, M.D.
Associate Dean, Health Institutions and Regional Liaison	Peter W. Munt, M.D.
Associate Dean, Health Sciences and Director, School of Nursing	Cynthia Baker, Ph.D.
Associate Dean, Health Sciences and Director, School of Rehabilitation Therapy	Elsie G. Culham, Ph.D.
Director, Student Affairs, Undergraduate Medical Education	Jennifer L. Carpenter, M.D.
Associate Dean, Continuing Professional Development	Lewis L. Tomalty, Ph.D.
Associate Dean, Life Sciences and Biochemistry	P. Ken Rose, Ph.D.
Secretary of the Faculty	David R. Edgar
Assistant Dean, Operations and Finance	David R. Edgar
Finance Manager	Joan Lee
Manager, Undergraduate Medical Education/Studies	Vacant
Education Coordinator, Continuing Medical Education	Patricia A. Payne
Manager, Postgraduate Medical Education	Nicholas Snider
Manager, Budgets and Administration	Jessie R. Griffin
Senior Staffing Officer	Gail L. Knutson

Department and Division or Section Chairs

Basic Sciences

Anatomy and Cell Biology	Charles H. Graham, Ph.D.
Biochemistry	Glenville Jones, Ph.D.
Community Health and Epidemiology	William J. Mackillop, Ch.B.
Microbiology and Immunology	R. Keith Poole, Ph.D.
Pharmacology and Toxicology	Thomas E. Massey, Ph.D.
Physiology	John T. Fisher, Ph.D.

Clinical Sciences

Anesthesiology. . . . . Joel Parlow, M.D.
Emergency Medicine . . . . Gordon R. Jones, M.D.
Family Medicine . . . . Glenn Brown, M.D.
Medicine. . . . . John L. McCans, M.D.
   Allergy and Immunology . . . . James H. Day, M.D.
   Cardiology. . . . . Christopher S. Simpson, M.D.
   Endocrinology . . . . Robert Hudson, M.D., Ph.D.
   Gastroenterology . . . . William G. Paterson, M.D.
   General Internal Medicine . . . . Daren K. Heyland, M.D.
   Geriatric Medicine . . . . John A. H. Puxty, M.D.
   Haematology and Oncology . . . . John H. Matthews, M.D.
   Infectious Diseases . . . . Dick E. Zoutman, M.D.
   Nephrology . . . . Edwin B. Toffelmire, M.D.
   Neurology . . . . Donald G. Brunet, M.D.
   Respiratory and Critical Care Medicine. . . . . Michael Fitzpatrick, M.D.
   Rheumatology . . . . Tassos P. Anastassiades, M.D.
Obstetrics and Gynaecology . . . . Michael M. J. McGrath, M.D.
Oncology. . . . . Anne M. Smith, M.D.
Ophthalmology . . . . Sherif El-Defrawy, M.D., Ph.D.
Otolaryngology . . . . Andre K. W. Tan, M.D.
Paediatrics. . . . . John F. Smythe, M.D. (Acting)
   Critical Care. . . . . Ellen Tsai, M.D.
   Hematology and Oncology . . . . Mariana Silva, M.D.
   Developmental Pediatrics . . . . Garth Smith, M.D.
   Neonatology. . . . . Michael P. Flavin, M.D.
Pathology and Molecular Medicine. . . . . Iain D. Young, M.D.
   Anatomical Pathology. . . . . Alexander H. Boag, M.D.
   Clinical Chemistry . . . . Christine P. Collier
   Genetics. . . . . Harriet E. Feilotter
   Hematological Pathology . . . . Dilys A. Rapson, M.B., Ch.B.
   Microbiology . . . . Dick E. Zoutman, M.D.
Psychiatry . . . . Roumen V. Milev, M.D., Ph.D.
   Adult Psychiatry . . . . Roumen V. Milev, M.D., Ph.D. (Acting)
   Adult Treatment and Rehabilitation Psychiatry . . . . Roumen V. Milev, M.D., Ph.D.
   Child and Adolescent Psychiatry . . . . John S. Leverette, M.D.
   Community Psychiatry . . . . J. Kenneth LeClair, M.D., and H. Joseph Burley, M.D.
   Consultant, Liaison Psychiatry. . . . . Louis van Zyl, M.D.
   Developmental Disabilities . . . . Bruce McCreary, M.D. (Acting)
   Forensic and Correctional Psychiatry. . . . . Julio Arboleda-Flórez, M.D.
   Geriatric Psychiatry. . . . . D.J. Kenneth LeClair, M.D.
   Neuropsychiatry . . . . L. Kola Oyewumi, MB.BS., D.Psych.
   Psychopharmacology. . . . . Amarenda N. Singh, M.D.
Diagnostic Radiology . . . . Annette McCallum, M.D. (Acting)
Physical Medicine and Rehabilitation . . . . Stephen D. Bagg, M.D.
Surgery . . . . C. Dale Mercer, M.D.
   Cardiac . . . . Andrew Hamilton, M.D.
   Thoracic . . . . Kenneth R. Reid, M.D.
   General Surgery. . . . . Paul J. Belliveau, M.D.
   Maxillofacial. . . . . Allan M. Rees, D.D.S.
   Neurosurgery. . . . . Ronald Pokrupa, M.D.
   Orthopaedics . . . . David R. Pichora, M.D.
   Plastic Surgery . . . . John S. D. Davidson, M.D.
   Vascular. . . . . David T. Zelt, M.D.
Urology. . . . . James W. L. Wilson, M.D.

University of Ottawa Faculty of Medicine

451 Smyth Road
Ottawa, Ontario Canada K1H 8M5
613-562-5800 x.8117 (dean's office); 562-5457 (fax)
E-mail: infomed@uottawa.ca
Web site: www.medicine.uottawa.ca

The faculty of medicine was established in 1945. Between 1978 and 1988, the school of medicine was regrouped into a faculty of health sciences along with the school of nursing and school of human kinetics. The faculty of medicine was reestablished as an entity in 1989.

Type: public
2008-2009 total enrollment: 156
Clinical facilities: The Ottawa Hospital, Royal Ottawa Health Care Group, Children's Hospital of Eastern Ontario, Montfort Hospital, Queensway Carleton Hospital, Sisters of Charity of Ottawa, Winchester District Memorial, Pembroke Regional Hospital.

University Officials

President. . . . . Allan Rock
Vice President (Academic and Provost) . . . . Robert Major, P.Eng.
Chief Negotiator and Liaison Officer . . . . Louise Pagé-Valin
Vice President (Resources). . . . . Victor Simon
Vice President (University Relations) . . . . Vacant
Vice President (Research) . . . . Mona Nemer, Ph.D.

Medical School Administrative Staff

Dean. . . . . Jacques Bradwejn, M.D.
Assistant Dean, Office of Francophone Affairs. . . . . Jean Roy, M.D.
Associate Dean, Postgraduate Medical Education . . . . Paul Bragg, M.D.
Director, Distributed Medical Education. . . . . Michael Hirsh, M.D.
Assistant Dean, Admissions. . . . . Richard Hébert, M.D.
Associate Dean, Undergraduate Medical Education. . . . . Geneviève Moineau, M.D.
Assistant Dean, Continuing Medical Education . . . . Paul Hendry, M.D.
Director, E-curriculum. . . . . Vacant
Associate Dean, Professional Affairs . . . . Rama C. Nair, Ph.D.
Assistant Dean, Academy for Innovation in
   Medical Education (AIME) . . . . Glenn Regehr, Ph.D. (Acting)
Director, Faculty Development. . . . . Jolanta Karpinski, M.D.
Director, Faculty Wellness Program . . . . Derek Puddester, M.D.
Director, Gender Equity Issues. . . . . Nahid Azad, M.D.
Vice Dean, Research . . . . Robert Haché, Ph.D.
Assistant Dean, Research . . . . Ken Dimock, Ph.D.
Assistant Dean, Graduate and Postdoctoral Studies . . . . Ruth Slack, Ph.D.
Associate Dean, Student Affairs . . . . Arlington F. Dungy, D.D.S.
Assistant Dean, Health and Hospital Services . . . . Sharon Whiting, M.D.
Director, Student Affairs . . . . Josée Taillefer
Director of Development . . . . Denyse Campeau
Secretary. . . . . Vasek Mezl, Ph.D.
Director, Animal Care Service . . . . Marilyn Keaney, D.V.M.
Director, Health Sciences Library. . . . . Dianne Kharouba
Chief Administrative Officer. . . . . Vanessa Sutton, F.C.I.S., C.M.A.
Operations Manager . . . . Linda Chenard
Assistant to the Dean. . . . . Gabrielle Galand, B.Sc.

University of Ottawa Faculty of Medicine: ONTARIO

Department and Division or Section Chairs

Basic Sciences

Biochemistry, Microbiology, and Immunology...................... Zemin Yao, Ph.D.
Cellular and Molecular Medicine .... Bernard Jasmin, Ph.D.
Epidemiology and Community Medicine .... Julian Little, Ph.D.

Clinical Sciences

Anaesthesia .... Homer Yang, M.D.
Emergency Medicine .... Ian Stiell, M.D.
Family Medicine .... Jacques Lemelin, M.D.
    Care of the Elderly... Vacant
Medicine.. Michele A. Turek, M.D. (Acting)
    Cardiology.. Terrence Ruddy, M.D.
    Clinical Epidemiology...................................... Jeremy Grimshaw, M.D.
    Critical Care.. Redouane Bouali, M.D.
    Dermatology .... James Walker, M.D.
    Endocrinology .... Alexander Sorisky, M.D.
    Gastroenterology .... Thomas Shaw-Stiffel, M.D.
    General Internal Medicine .... Anthony Weinberg, M.D.
    Geriatrics... Barbara Power, M.D.
    Hematology .... Philip Wells, M.D.
    Infectious Diseases .... Gary Garber, M.D.
    Medical Oncology .... Glenwood Goss, M.D.
    Nephrology .... Peter Magner, M.D.
    Neurology .... Antoine Hakim, M.D.
    Nuclear Medicine.. Terrence Ruddy, M.D.
    Palliative Care .... José Pereira, M.D.
    Rehabilitation Medicine .... Daniel DeForge, M.D.
    Respirology .... Shawn Aaron, M.D.
    Rheumatology .... Douglas Smith, M.D.
Obstetrics and Gynaecology.................................... Wylam Faught, M.D.
    Perinatology....................................... Lawrence Oppenheimer, M.D.
Ophthalmology .... Steven Gilberg, M.D. (Acting)
Otolaryngology .... Martin Corsten, M.D.
Paediatrics.. Joe Reisman, M.D.
Pathology and Laboratory Medicine .... Jean Michaud, M.D.
Psychiatry .... Katherine Gillis, M.D. (Acting)
    Addictions Psychiatry .... Allan Wilson, M.D., Ph.D.
    Child Psychiatry....................................... Simon Davidson, M.D.
    Forensic Psychiatry................................. John Bradford, M.B., Ch.B.
    Geriatric Psychiatry.......................... Marie-France Tourigny-Rivard, M.D.
Radiology .... Mark E. Schweitzer, M.D.
    Radiation Oncology .... Laval Grimard, M.D.
Surgery.. Éric Poulin, M.D.
    Cardiac Surgery .... Thierry Mesana, M.D.
    General Surgery.. Joseph Mamazza, M.D.
    Neurosurgery... Richard Moulton, M.D.
    Orthopaedic Surgery .... Geoffrey Dervin, M.D.
    Plastic Surgery .... Mario Jarmusk, M.D.
    Thoracic Surgery .... Sudhir Sundaresan, M.D.
    Urology .... Ron Gerridzen, M.D.
    Vascular Surgery....................................... Andrew Hill, M.D.

University of Toronto Faculty of Medicine

27 King's College Circle
Toronto, Ontario Canada M5S 1A1
416-978-6585 (dean's office); 416-978-1774 (fax)
Web site: www.facmed.utoronto.ca

The medical school was founded in 1843 as a part of King's College, which later became the University of Toronto. The faculty of medicine was established in 1888. The former school of hygiene merged with the faculty on July 1, 1975.

Type: public
2008-2009 total enrollment: 846
Clinical facilities: The University Health Network (includes the Toronto General Hospital, the Toronto Western Hospital, and Princess Margaret Hospital); Sunnybrook Health Sciences Centre; St. Michael's Hospital; Mount Sinai Hospital; Hospital for Sick Children; Centre for Addiction and Mental Health (includes the former Addiction Research Foundation, Clarke Institute of Psychiatry, Donwood Institute, Queen Street Mental Health Centre); Baycrest; Toronto Rehabilitation Institute; North York General Hospital; Toronto East General and Orthopaedic Hospital; St. Joseph's Health Centre-Toronto; Scarborough General Hospital; Bloorview MacMillan Centre; Hincks-Dellcrest Centre; Surrey Place Centre; George Hull Centre for Children and Families; Providence Centre; St. John's Rehab Hospital; West Park Healthcare Centre; Women's College Hospital; York Finch Hospital.

University Administration

President. . . . . C. David Naylor, M.D., D.Phil.
Vice President and Provost. . . . . C. Misak, Ph.D. (Interim)
Vice Provost, Academic . . . . E. Hillan, Ph.D.
Vice Provost, Relations with Health Care Institutions. . . . . C. Whiteside, M.D., Ph.D.
Vice President, Research and Associate Provost. . . . . T. McTiernan, Ph.D. (Interim)
Vice President and Chief Advancement Officer. . . . . D. Palmer, Ph.D.
Vice President, Business Affairs . . . . C. Riggall
Vice President, Human Resources and Equity. . . . . A. Hildyard, Ph.D.
Vice President, Government, Institutional and Community Relations. . . . . D. Atlin
Vice President and Principal, University of Toronto at Mississauga. . . . . I. Orchard, Ph.D.
Vice President and Principal, University of Toronto at Scarborough . . . . F. Vaccarino, Ph.D.
Deputy Provost . . . . C. Misak, Ph.D.
Vice Provost, Student Life . . . . L. Fromowitz

Faculty of Medicine Administrative Staff

Dean. . . . . C. Whiteside, M.D., Ph.D.
Deputy Dean. . . . . S. Verma, L.L.B, M.D.
Vice Dean, Research and International Relations . . . . P. Lewis, Ph.D.
Vice Dean, Continuing Education and Professional Development . . . . I. Silver, M.D.
Vice Dean, Graduate Affairs. . . . . A. Sass-Kortsak, Ph.D.
Vice Dean, Postgraduate Medical Education . . . . S. Verma, M.D.
Vice Dean, Undergraduate Medical Education . . . . J. Rosenfield, M.D., Ph.D.
Associate Vice Provost, Relations with Health Care Institutions . . . . L. Ferris, Ph.D., C. Psych.
Associate Dean, Health Professions Student Affairs . . . . A. Jarvis, M.D.
Associate Dean, Postgraduate Medical
   Education, Admissions, and Evaluations . . . . K. Imrie, M.D.
Associate Dean, Research and International Relations. G. Fantus, M.D.
Associate Dean, Undergraduate Medicine
   Admissions and Student Financial Services . . . . M. Shandling, M.D.
Chief Administrative Officer. . . . . T. Neff

Department and Division or Section Chairs

Basic Sciences

Banting and Best Department of Medical Research. . . . . B. Andrews, Ph.D.
Biochemistry . . . . R. Reithmeier, Ph.D.

Biomaterials and Biomedical Engineering, Institute of . . . . C. Yip, Ph.D. (Interim)
Immunology . . . . M. Ratcliffe, Ph.D.
Medical Biophysics. . . . . P. Burns, Ph.D.
Molecular Genetics . . . . H. Lipshitz, Ph.D.
Nutritional Sciences. . . . . M. Archer, Ph.D.
Pharmacology . . . . D. Grant, Ph.D.
Physiology . . . . S. Matthews, Ph.D. (Acting)

Clinical Sciences

Anesthesia. . . . . B. Kavanagh, M.D.
Family and Community Medicine. . . . . L. Wilson, M.D.
Laboratory Medicine and Pathobiology. . . . . A. Gotlieb, M.D.
Medical Imaging . . . . P. Babyn, M.D. (Acting)
Medical Science, Institute of . . . . O. Rotstein, M.D.
Medicine. . . . . W. Levinson, M.D.
Obstetrics and Gynaecology . . . . A. Bocking, M.D.
Ophthalmology and Vision Sciences . . . . J. Hurwitz, M.D.
Otolaryngology-Head and Neck Surgery . . . . P. Gullane, M.D.
Paediatrics. . . . . D. Daneman, M.D.
Psychiatry . . . . D. Wasylenki, M.D.
Radiation Oncology. . . . . M. Gospodarowicz, M.D.
Surgery . . . . R. Reznick, M.D.

Community Health

Health Policy, Management, and Evaluation . . . . L. Lemieux-Charles, Ph.D.
Public Health, Dalla Lana School of. . . . . M. Escobar, Ph.D. (Int. Dir.)

Rehabilitation Sciences

Occupational Science and Occupational Therapy . . . . B. Kirsh, Ph.D. (Interim)
Physical Therapy . . . . K. Berg, Ph.D.
Graduate Department of Rehabilitation Sciences. . . . . H. Polatajko, Ph.D.
Speech-Language Pathology. . . . . L. deNil, Ph.D.

*Specialty without organizational autonomy.

University of Western Ontario
Schulich School of Medicine & Dentistry

1151 Richmond Street North
London, Ontario Canada N6A 5C1
519-661-3744 (admissions); 661-3459 (dean's office); 661-3797 (fax)
Web site: www.schulich.uwo.ca

The faculty of medicine at Western was founded in 1881 and merged with the faculty of dentistry in 1997. In 2005, the faculty was named the Schulich School of Medicine & Dentistry in recognition of a landmark donation. The school is dedicated to preparing tomorrow's doctors, dentists, and health researchers to be outstanding leaders who will shape the future of health care. Beginning in 2008, 24 medical students will train full time in Windsor, Ontario, through a partnership between Western, the University of Windsor, and Windsor hospitals. The school receives more than $140 million in research funding annually and is home to 22 Canada research chairs and hundreds of world-class research teams and investigators

Type: public
2008-2009 total enrollment: 2,811
Clinical facilities: London Health Sciences Centre (including University Hospital, South Street Hospital, Victoria Hospital, Children's Hospital, London Regional Cancer Program), St. Joseph's Health Care, London (including St. Joseph's Hospital, Parkwood Hospital, Regional Mental Health Care/London and St. Thomas), Windsor Regional Hospital, Hotel Dieu-Grace Hospital, Child and Parent Resource Institute, Thames Valley Children's Centre.

University Officials

The Lieutenant Governor of Ontario
Chancellor . . . . Arthur Labatt
President and Vice Chancellor . . . . P. Davenport, Ph.D.
Vice President (Academic) and Provost . . . . Fred Longstaffe, Ph.D.
Vice President (Resources and Operations) . . . . Gitta P. Kulczycki
Vice Provost (Academic Planning, Policy, and Faculty) . . . . Alan C. Weedon, Ph.D.
Vice President, External . . . . T. Garrard
Vice President, Research and International Relations . . . . Ted Hewitt, Ph.D.
Vice Provost (Academic Programs and Students) [Registrar] . . . . R. M. Harris, Ph.D.
Director of Libraries . . . . Joyce Garnett

Medical School Administrative Staff

Dean . . . . C. P. Herbert, M.D.
Associate Dean, Admissions/Student Affairs . . . . Francis P. H. Chan, Ph.D.
Associate Dean, Basic Medical Sciences, Undergraduate Education . . . . Kem Rogers, Ph.D.
Associate Dean, Gender/Equity and Faculty Health . . . . Barbara Lent, M.D.
Associate Dean, Academic Affairs . . . . N. A. M. Paterson, M.D.
Associate Dean, Postgraduate Education . . . . Sal Spadafora, M.D.
Associate Dean, Research . . . . Victor Han, M.D., FRCPC, FRCP
Associate Dean and Interim Director, School of Dentistry . . . . Harinder S. Sandhu, D.D.S.
Associate Dean, Undergraduate Medical Education . . . . Margaretha Rebel, M.D.
Associate Dean, Windsor Southwestern Ontario Education Network . . . . Tom Scott, M.D.
Associate Dean, Continuing Medical Education . . . . Jatinder Takhar, M.D., FRCPC
Director of Administration . . . . Brian Jeffs
Chief of Finance . . . . Cindy Servos
Administrative Officer, Education . . . . John Ruicci
Administrative Officer, Admissions/Student and Equity Affairs . . . . Pam Bere
Administrative Officer, Office of Professional and Educational Development . . . . C. Blake
Administrative Officer, Postgraduate Education . . . . M. Morris
Administrative Officer, Research . . . . M. Hymowitz
Administrative Officer, Undergraduate Education . . . . Lesley DePauw
Assistant Dean, Research Institutes . . . . D. Hill, M.D.
Assistant Dean, Research (Clinical) . . . . James Lewis, M.D., FRCPC
Assistant Dean, Research (Graduate and
   Postdoctoral Studies, and Internationalization) . . . . Chris Elis, Ph.D.
Assistant Dean, External . . . . Kellie Leitch, M.D., FRCS(C)
Assistant Dean, Rural and Regional Medicine . . Thomas Lacroix, M.D., CM, FRCPC (Paediatric)

Assistant Dean, Southwestern Ontario Medical
  Education Network . . . . R. Cheung, M.D., SRCPC
Assistant Dean, Strategic Initiative . . . . Margaret Steel, M.D., FRCPC, M.Ed.

Department and Division or Section Chairs

Basic Sciences

Anatomy . . . . Michael Lehman, Ph.D.
Biochemistry . . . . David Litchfield, Ph.D.
  Clinical Biochemistry . . . . C. A. Rupar, M.D.
Epidemiology and Biostatistics . . . . K. Campbell, Ph.D.
History of Medicine and Science . . . . P. M. Potter, M.D.C.M., Ph.D.
Medical Biophysics. . . . . J. J. Battista, Ph.D.
Microbiology and Immunology. . . . . M. Valvano, M.D.
Pathology . . . . B. Garcia, Ph.D.
Physiology and Pharmocology . . . . Jane Rylett, Ph.D.

Clinical Sciences

Anesthesia. . . . . D. Cheng, M.D.
  Clinical Neurological Sciences . . . . M. J. Strong, M.D., and S. P. Lownie, M.D. (Co-Chairs)
Medical Imaging . . . . Rethy Chem, M.D., Ph.D., FRCPC
  Diagnostic Radiology . . . . Rethy Chem, M.D., Ph.D., FRCPC
  Imaging Sciences . . . . A. Fenster, Ph.D., FCCPM
  Nuclear Medicine. . . . . Jean-Luc Urbain, M.D, Ph.D., FRCPC
Family Medicine . . . . T. Freeman, M.D.
Medicine. . . . . D. J. Hollomby, M.D., FRCP[C; FACP, (FRCP) (GLASG)
  Cardiology . . . . Samuel Siu, M.D., SM, FRCPC, FACC
  Clinical Immunology and Allergy . . . . K. Payton, M.D.
  Clinical Pharmacology . . . . Richard B. Kim, M.D., FRCPC[C
  Critical Care Medicine . . . . F. Rutledge, M.D.
  Emergency Medicine . . . . G. Joubert, M.D.
  Endocrinology and Metabolism. . . . . I. Hramiak, M.D.
  Gastroenterology . . . . R. Reynolds, M.D.
  General Internal Medicine . . . . R. S. M. Eberhard, M.D., FRCPC, SACP
  Geriatric Medicine . . . . M. J. Borrie, M.B., Ch.B.
  Hematology and Oncology . . . . I. Chin-Yee, M.D.
  Infectious Disease. . . . . E. D. Ralph, M.D.
  Nephrology . . . . P. Blake, M.D.
  Respiratory Medicine . . . . G. George, M.B., B.S.
  Rheumatology . . . . J. Pope, M.D.
Obstetrics and Gynecology. . . . . Bryan Richardson, M.D., FRCSC
Oncology. . . . . Glenn Bauman, M.D.
  Experimental Oncology . . . . Gabriel E. DiMattia, Ph.D.
  Medical Oncology . . . . Scott Ernest, M.D., FRCPC
  Radiation Oncology . . . . Michael Lock, M.D., FRCPC
Ophthalmology. . . . . William Hodge, M.D.
Otolaryngology . . . . John Yoo, M.D., FRCSC, FACS
Paediatrics. . . . . Guido Filler, M.D., Ph.D., FRCPC
  Medical Genetics . . . . J. H. Jung, M.D.
Physical Medicine and Rehabilitation . . . . R. Teasell, M.D.
Psychiatry . . . . S. Fisman, M.D.
Surgery . . . . J. Denstedt, M.D.
  Cardiac . . . . R. J. Novick, M.D.
  General Surgery. . . . . Edward Davies, M.D., FRCSC
  Orthopaedic. . . . . R. B. Bourne, M.D.
  Paediatric. . . . . Kellie Leitch, M.D., FRCS[C
  Plastic and Reconstructive. . . . . D. Ross, M.D.
  Urology . . . . Hasan A. Razvi, M.D., FRCSC
  Vascular Surgery. . . . . Thomas Forbes, M.D., FRCSC, FACS
  Thoracic . . . . R. I. Inculet, M.D.

Laval University Faculty of Medicine

Pavillon Ferdinand-Vandry
Local 1219
Quebec City, Quebec Canada G1K 7P4
418-656-2301 (dean's office); 656-5062 (fax)
Web site: www.fmed.ulaval.ca

The present medical school was established in fall 1852, less than a year after the founding of Laval University. Before that time, there had been a medical school incorporated by the city of Quebec. The medical school is located on the campus of Laval University on the outskirts of Quebec City.

Type: private
2008-2009 total enrollment: 854
Clinical facilities: Centre hospitalier de l'Universite Laval, Hôtel-Dieu de Québec, Hôpital Laval, Hôpital du Saint-Sacrement, Hôpital de l'Enfant-Jésus, Hôpital Saint-Francois d'Assise, Hôtel-Dieu de Lévis.

University Officials

Rector . . . . Denis Brière, Ph.D.
Vice Rector (Teaching and International Development) . . . . Bernard Garnier
Vice Rector (Human Resources) . . . . Michel Beauchamp
Vice Rector (Research) . . . . Edwin Bourget
Vice Rector (Services Development) . . . . Diane Lachapelle
Secretary General . . . . Monique Richer
Executive Vice Rector (Executive Administration) . . . . Éric Bauce
Registrar . . . . Danielle Fleury

Medical School Administrative Staff

Dean . . . . Pierre J. Durand, M.D.
Associate Dean (Executive) . . . . Sylvie Marcoux, M.D., Ph.D.
Associate Dean (Research) . . . . Yvon Cormier, M.D.
Associate Dean (Relations and Development) . . . . Rénald Bergeron, M.D.
Associate Dean (Teaching) . . . . Joan Glenn, M.D.
Associate Dean (Clinical Affairs) . . . . Pierre LeBlanc, M.D.
Secretary of the Faculty . . . . Jean Talbot, M.D.
Director, Continuing Medical Education . . . . Michel Rouleau, M.D.
Assistant to the Dean (Student Affairs) . . . . Guy Pomerleau, M.D.
Administrative Assistant . . . . Carole Nadeau

Laval University Faculty of Medicine: QUEBEC

Department and Division or Section Chairs

Basic Sciences

Anatomy and Physiology . . . . Louis Larochelle, M.D., Ph.D.
Medical Biology. . . . . Denis Beauchamp, Ph.D.
   Clinical Biochemistry* . . . . Jean Talbot, M.D.
   Microbiology* . . . . Michel G. Bergeron, M.D., Ph.D.
   Pathology* . . . . Bernard Têtu, M.D.

Clinical Sciences

Anesthesiology. . . . . Martin Lessard, M.D.
Family Medicine . . . . Gilles Lortie, M.D.
Medicine. . . . . M.E.G. Louise Côté, M.D.
   Cardiology* . . . . Can Manh Nguyên, M.D.
   Dermatology*. . . . . Jimmy Alain, M.D.
   Gastroenterology . . . . Claude Parent, M.D.
   Geriatrics. . . . . Michel Dugas, M.D.
   Hematology* . . . . Pierre F. Leblond, M.D.
   Intensive Care . . . . François LeBlanc, M.D.
   Internal Medicine. . . . . Patrick Couture, M.D.
   Medical Microbiology and Infectious Diseases . . . . Louise Deschênes, M.D.
   Medical Oncology . . . . Danièle Marceau, M.D.
   Nephrology* . . . . Paul Isenring, M.D.
   Neurology* . . . . Steve Verreault, M.D.
   Palliative Care . . . . Johanne Côté, M.D.
   Physiatry . . . . Isabelle Côté, M.D.
   Pulmonary and Critical Care* . . . . Julie Plante, M.D.
   Radio-oncology. . . . . Isabelle Vallières, M.D.
   Rheumatology . . . . Louis Bessette, M.D.
Obstetrics and Gynecology. . . . . Normand Brassard, M.D.
Ophthalmology . . . . Nathalie Labrecque, M.D.
Otorhinolaryngology . . . . Denis Pouliot, M.D.
Pediatrics . . . . Bruno Piedboeuf, M.D.
Psychiatry . . . . Nathalie Gingras, M.D.
Radiology . . . . Marcel Dumont, M.D.
Rehabilitation . . . . Claude H. Côté, M.D.
Social and Preventive Medicine . . . . Philippe de Wals, M.D.
Surgery. . . . . Yvan Douville, M.D.
   General Surgery* . . . . Claude Thibault, M.D.
   Neurosurgery* . . . . Geneviève Milot, M.D.
   Orthopedics* . . . . Jean Lamontagne, M.D.
   Urology* . . . . Jean-François Audet, M.D.

*Specialty without organizational autonomy.

McGill University Faculty of Medicine

Room 600, 3655 Promenade Sir-William-Osler
Montreal, Quebec Canada H3G 1Y6
514-398-1768 (general information); 398-3595 (fax)
E-mail: recepmed@mcgill.ca, recept3605.med@mcgill.ca
Web site: www.med.mcgill.ca

The faculty of medicine of McGill University was established in 1829.

Type: public
2008-2009 total enrollment: 674
Clinical facilities: McGill University Health Centre (Montreal Children's Hospital, Montreal General Hospital, Montreal Neurological Hospital, Royal Victoria Hospital) Sir Mortimer B. Davis-Jewish General Hospital; Lakeshore General Hospital; Lasalle General Hospital; Montreal Chest Hospital; St. Mary's Hospital; Shriners Hospital; Douglas Mental Health University Institute.

University Officials

Principal and Vice Chancellor . . . . Heather Munroe-Blum, Ph.D.
Provost . . . . Anthony C. Masi, Ph.D.
Vice Principal (Administration and Finance) . . . . François Roy
Deputy Provost (Student Life and Learning). . . . . Morton J. Mendelson, Ph.D.
Vice Principal (Research and International Relations). . . . . Denis Therien, Ph.D.
Vice Principal (Development, Alumni, and University Relations) . . . . Marc Weinstein
Vice Principal (Public Affairs) . . . . Vaughan Dowie
Vice Principal (Health Affairs) . . . . Richard I. Levin, M.D.

Medical School Administrative Staff

Dean. . . . . Richard I. Levin, M.D.
Director (Administration and Operations) . . . . April Caluori
Director (Admissions) . . . . France Drolet
Associate Dean (Faculty Affairs) . . . . Mara Ludwig, M.D.
Associate Dean (Continuing Medical Education). . . . . Michael Rosengarten, M.D.
Associate Dean (Faculty Development) . . . . Yvonne Steinert, Ph.D.
Associate Vice Principal and Associate Dean (Interhospital Affairs) . . . . Sam Benaroya, M.D.
Associate Dean (Medical Education). . . . . Joyce L. Pickering, M.D.
Associate Dean (Postgraduate Medical Education
    and Professional Affairs) . . . . Sarkis Meterissian, M.D.
Assistant Dean (Research) . . . . Marianna Newkirk, M.D.
Director (Student Affairs) . . . . Pierre Tellier, M.D.
Director, Centre for Medical Education . . . . Yvonne Steinert, Ph.D.
Director, Animal Resources Centre. . . . . Jim Gourdon
Life Sciences Area Librarian. . . . . Jim Henderson

McGill University Faculty of Medicine: QUEBEC

Department and Division or Section Chairs

Basic Sciences

Anatomy and Cell Biology . . . . John J. Bergeron, Ph.D.
Biochemistry . . . . David Thomas, Ph.D.
Biomedical Engineering . . . . Henrietta Galiana, Ph.D.
Epidemiology, Biostatistics, and Occupational Health . . . . Rebecca Fuhrer, Ph.D.
Human Genetics . . . . David Rosenblatt, M.D.
Microbiology and Immunology . . . . Greg Matlashewski, Ph.D.
Pathology . . . . David Haegert, M.D.
Pharmacology and Therapeutics . . . . Hans Zingg, M.D.
Physiology . . . . John Orlowski, Ph.D.
Social Studies of Medicine . . . . Alberto Cambrosio, Ph.D.

Clinical Sciences

AIDS Research Centre* . . . . Mark Wainberg, Ph.D.
Anesthesia . . . . Steven Backman, M.D., Ph.D.
Artificial Cells and Organs Centre* . . . . T. M. S. Chang, M.D., Ph.D.
Biomedical Ethics* . . . . Kathleen Glass, Ph.D.
Centre for Host Resistance . . . . Emil Skamene, M.D., Ph.D.
Centre for Studies in Aging* . . . . Judes Poirier, Ph.D.
Experimental Medicine* . . . . Hugh Bennett, Ph.D.
Family Medicine . . . . Martin Dawes, M.D.
McGill Cancer Centre . . . . Michel Tremblay, Ph.D.
McGill Nutrition and Food Science Center* . . . . Errol B. Marliss, M.D.
Medical Physics Unit* . . . . Ervin Podgorsak, Ph.D.
Medicine . . . . David Eidelman, M.D.
Neurology and Neurosurgery . . . . Richard Riopelle, M.D.
Nonlinear Dynamics* . . . . Michael C. Mackey, Ph.D.
Obstetrics and Gynecology . . . . Seang L. Tan, M.D.
Oncology . . . . Gerald Batist, M.D.
Ophthalmology . . . . Miguel Burnier, M.D.
Otolaryngology . . . . Saul Frenkiel, M.D.
Pediatrics . . . . Harvey Guyda, M.D.
Psychiatry . . . . Mimi Israel, M.D.
Radiology (Diagnostic) . . . . Robert Lisbona, M.D.
Surgery . . . . Mostafa Elhilali, M.D.
Translational Research* . . . . Gerald Batist, M.D.

*Specialty without organizational autonomy.

Université de Montréal, Faculty of Medicine

2900 Boulevard Edouard-Montpetit
P.O. Box 6128, Succ. Centre-ville
Montreal, Quebec Canada H3C 3J7
514-343-6267; 343-6351 (dean's office); 343-5850 (fax)
E-mail: facmed@umontreal.ca
Web site: www.med.umontreal.ca

The faculty of medicine of the Université de Montréal can be traced back to a school established in Montreal in 1843 and incorporated in 1845 under the name of "Ecole de Médecine et de Chirurgie de Montréal." In 1891, this school merged with the faculty of medicine of the Montreal branch of Laval University, which had been founded in 1877. This agreement was approved by the Quebec legislature in the same year, and henceforth, the school of medicine and surgery of Montreal became the faculty of medicine of Laval University of Montreal. In 1920, by an act of the Quebec legislature, the Montreal branch of Laval University was granted its independence, and the school of medicine became known as the Université de Montréal Faculty of Medicine.

Type: private
2008-2009 total enrollment: 5,089
Clinical facilities: Centre Hospitalier de l'Université de Montréal, Hôpital Maisonneuve-Rosemont, Hôpital Rivière-des-Prairies, Hôpital du Sacré-Coeur de Montréal, Hôpital Louis-H. Lafontaine, Hôpital Sainte-Justine, Institut de Cardiologie de Montréal, Institut de Réadaptation de Montréal, Cité de la Santé de Laval, Institut Philippe-Pinel de Montréal, Institut Universitaire de Gériatrie de Montréal, Centre Hospitalier de Verdun, Institut de Recherches Cliniques de Montréal, Complexe Hospitalier de la Sagamie.

University Officials

Chancellor	Louise Roy (Interim)
Rector	Luc Vinet, Ph.D.
Provost and Vice Rector, Academic	Jacques Frémont, LL.M.
Vice Rector, Executive	Guy Breton, M.D.
Vice Provost and Vice Rector, Planification	Pierre Simonet, Ph.D. (Interim)
Vice Rector, Student Life and International	Open
Associate Vice Rector, Administration and Finances	Guy Breton, M.D.
Associate Vice Rector, Graduate Studies	Louise Béliveau, Ph.D.
Vice Rector, Research	Joseph Hubert, Ph.D.
Vice Rector, Development and Alumni Relations	Guy Berthiaume, Doctorat (3è cycle)
Secretary-General	Francine Verrier, LL.B.
Financial Officer	André Racette
Registrar	Pierre Chénard, Ph.D.

Medical School Administrative Staff

Dean	Jean L. Rouleau, M.D.
Vice Dean, Executive	François Lessard, M.D.
Vice Dean, Faculty Affairs	Serge Dubé, M.D.
Vice Dean, Research	Pierre Boyle, Ph.D.
Vice Dean, Graduate Studies	André Ferron, Ph.D.
Vice Dean, Undergraduate Studies	Raymond Lalande, M.D.
Vice Dean, Public Health, Health Sciences and International Relations	Christine Colin, M.D.
Vice Dean, Postgraduate Medical Studies	Guy Lalonde, M.D.
Secretary of the Faculty	Chantal Lambert, B.Pharm., Ph.D.
Associate Vice Dean, Research	Vincent Castellucci, Ph.D.
Assistant to the Dean Communications	Open
Assistants to the Vice Dean, Executive Physical Resources, Materials and Planning	Louise Bossé
Agreement and Special Projects	Anne-Marie Labrecque
Human Resources	Josée Veronneau
Responsible for Regional Training	Open
Financial Resources	Sylvie Monier

Coordinator of RUIS . . . . Richard Klein
Assistant to the Vice Dean, Postgraduate Medical Studies . . . . Lorraine Locas
Assistants to the Vice Dean, Undergraduate Studies
   Pregraduate Clerkship . . . . Martine Jolivet-Tremblay, M.D.
   Administrative Affairs . . . . Francyne Poulin
Assistant to the Vice Dean, Professoral Affairs
   Human Resources . . . . Line Ginchereau
Director of M.D. Program . . . . Marcel Julien, M.D.
Coordinators, Student Affairs . . . . Patricia Garel, M.D.
Director, Continuing Professional Development . Martin Labelle, M.D., and Ramsès Wassef, M.D.
President, Curriculum Committee . . . . Gilles Beauchamp, M.D.
President, Admission Committee . . . . Christian Bourdy, M.D.
Director, Medical Library . . . . Monique St-Jean

Department and Division or Section Chairs

Basic Sciences

Biochemistry . . . . Christian Baron, Ph.D.
Microbiology and Immunology . . . . Pierre Belhumeur, Ph.D.
Pathology and Cellular Biology . . . . Pierre Drapeau, Ph.D.
Pharmacology . . . . Patrick Du Souich, M.D., Ph.D.
Physiology . . . . Allan Smith, Ph.D.

Clinical Sciences

Anesthesia . . . . Pierre Drolet, M.D.
Family Medicine . . . . François Lehmann, M.D.
Medicine . . . . Denis Roy, M.D.
Obstetrics and Gynecology . . . . William Fraser, M.D.
Ophthalmology . . . . Jean-Daniel Arbour, M.D.
Pediatrics . . . . Marc Girard, M.D.
Psychiatry . . . . Jean Hébert, M.D.
Radiology, Radio-Oncology, and Nuclear Medicine . . . . Pierre Bourgouin, M.D.
Surgery . . . . Luc Valiquette, M.D.

Health Sciences

Nutrition . . . . Marielle LeDoux, M.D.
Rehabilitation . . . . Daniel Bourbonnais, Ph.D.
Speech Therapy and Audiology . . . . Louise Getty

Public Health Sciences

Environmental Health . . . . André Du Fresne, Ph.D.
Health Administration . . . . Renaldo Battista, Ph.D.
Social and Preventive Medicine . . . . Marie-France Raynault, M.D.

Université de Sherbrooke Faculty of Medicine and Health Sciences

3001 12th Avenue North
Sherbrooke, Quebec Canada J1H 5N4
819-564-5200; 564-5201 (dean's office); 564-5420 (fax)
Web site: www.usherbrooke.ca/medecine/

The faculty of medicine and health sciences of the Université de Sherbrooke was founded in March 1961. It is the last faculty of medicine to be organized in the province of Quebec since 1853. The first M.D. degrees were granted in 1970. The medical school is part of the Université de Sherbrooke.

Type: public
2008-2009 total enrollment: 560
Clinical facilities: In 1995, the merger of hospitals created a new 725-bed university hospital of acute care with large ambulatory care facilities, a new 400-bed chronic and long-term care university center, and a university-affiliated community care center. Five major regional hospitals are affiliated along with a number of private clinics.

University Officials

Chancellor . . . . His Excellency, and Monsignor André Gaumond, D.D.S.
Rector. . . . . Bruno-Marie Béchard, M.Sc.A., ing.
Executive Director. . . . . Jacques Viens
Vice Rector, Studies and Information Resources and Secretary . . . . Martin Buteau, D.Sc.
Vice Rector, International Relations . . . . Louis Marquis, Ph.D.
Vice Rector, Research . . . . Jacques Beauvais, Ph.D.
Vice Rector, Community . . . . Jean Desclos, Ph.D.
Rector Assistant, Vice Rector, Graduate Studies
    and Continuing Education . . . . Denis Marceau, Ph.D.
Vice Rector, Administration and Sustainable Development . . . . Alain Webster, M.Sc.
Registrar . . . . France Myette

Medical School Administrative Staff

Dean. . . . . Réjean Hébert, M.D.
Vice Dean, Executive . . . . Gilles Faust, M.D.
Vice Dean, Research . . . . Darel Hunting, Ph.D.
Vice Dean, Graduate Studies . . . . Claude Asselin, Ph.D.
Vice Dean, Undergraduate Medical Education . . . . Paul Grand'Maison, M.D.
Vice Dean, Postgraduate Medical Education . . . . François Lajoie, M.D.
Secretary and Vice Dean, Student Affairs . . . . Jocelyne Faucher, M.D.
Vice Dean, Nursing Sciences . . . . Luc Mathieu, D.B.A.
Vice Dean, Rehabilitation. . . . . Johanne Desrosiers, Ph.D.
Director, Continuing Education . . . . Gilles Voyer, M.D.
Director, Office of Medical Education . . . . Diane Clavet, M.D.
Chairperson of Admission Committee . . . . Daniel J. Côté, M.D.
Executive Director. . . . . Marc Lauzière
Administrative Director . . . . René Gagnon
Administrative Assistant for Undergraduate Medical Education . . . . Sylvie Lamarche
Medical Librarian . . . . Marthe Brideau
Director, Computer Science Office. . . . . David Serouge

Université de Sherbrooke Faculty of Medicine and Health Sciences: QUEBEC

Department and Division or Section Chairs

Basic Sciences

Anatomy and Cellular Biology . . . . Jean-François Beaulieu, Ph.D.
Biochemistry . . . . Jean-Pierre Perreault, Ph.D.
   Clinical Biochemistry . . . . Jean Dubé, Ph.D.
Microbiology and Infectiology . . . . Benoit Chabot, Ph.D.
Nuclear Medicine and Radiobiology . . . . Benoit Paquette, Ph.D.
Nursing Sciences . . . . Luc Mathieu, D.B.A.
Pharmacology . . . . Emanuel Escher, Ph.D.
Physiology and Biophysics . . . . Robert Dumaine, Ph.D.
Rehabilitation . . . . Johanne Desrosiers, Ph.D.
   Physiatry . . . . Anne Harvey, M.D.

Clinical Sciences

Anesthesia . . . . René Martin, M.D.
Community Health Sciences . . . . Maryse Guay, M.D.
   Drug Addiction . . . . Elise Roy, M.D.
Family Medicine . . . . Marie Giroux, M.D.
   Emergency . . . . Colette Bellavance, M.D.
Medicine . . . . Pierre Cossette, M.D.
   Cardiology . . . . Michel Nguyen, M.D.
   Dermatology . . . . Bruno Maynard, M.D.
   Endocrinology . . . . Patrice Perron, M.D.
   Gastroenterology . . . . Serge Langevin, M.D.
   Geriatrics . . . . Tamas Fülöp, M.D.
   Haematology . . . . Patrice Beauregard, M.D.
   Internal Medicine . . . . Luc Lanthier, M.D.
   Nephrology . . . . Paul Montambault, M.D.
   Neurology . . . . Jean Rivest, M.D.
   Respiratory Diseases . . . . Pierre Larivée, M.D.
   Rheumatology . . . . Artur De Brum Fernandes, M.D.
Microbiology and Infectiology (see Basic Sciences) . . . . Benoit Chabot, M.D.
   Infectiology . . . . Raymond Duperval, M.D.
Nuclear Medicine and Radiobiology (see Basic Sciences) . . . . Benoit Paquette, Ph.D.
   Nuclear Medicine . . . . Jean Verreault, M.D.
   Radio-Oncology . . . . Rachel Bujold, M.D.
Obstetrics and Gynaecology . . . . Jean-Marie Moutquin, M.D.
Pathology . . . . Bassem Sawan, M.D.
Pediatrics . . . . Hervé Walti, M.D.
   General Paediatrics . . . . Thérése Côté-Baileau, M.D.
   Immuno-Allergology . . . . Marek Rola-Pleszczynski, M.D.
   Neonatology . . . . Valérie Bertelle, M.D.
Psychiatry . . . . Pierre Beauséjour, M.D.
   Gerontopsychiatry . . . . Paule Hottin, M.D.
   Child Psychiatry . . . . Carmen Beauregard, M.D.
   Adult Psychiatry . . . . William Semann, M.D.
   Legal Psychiatry . . . . Pierre Gagné, M.D.
Radiology . . . . The-Bao Bui, M.D.
Surgery . . . . Gaétan Langlois, M.D.
   Cardiovascular . . . . David Greentree, M.D.
   General Surgery . . . . Francois Mosimann, M.D.
   Neurosurgery . . . . David Fortin, M.D.
   Ophthalmology . . . . Pierre Blondeau, M.D.
   Orthopedic Surgery . . . . Nicolas Patenaude, M.D.
   Ortorhinolaryngology . . . . Dominique Dorion, M.D.
   Urology . . . . Michel Carmel, M.D.
   Vascular . . . . Véronique Lapie, M.D.
   Thoracic . . . . Marco Sirois, M.D.

University of Saskatchewan College of Medicine

B103 Health Sciences Building
107 Wiggins Road
Saskatoon, Saskatchewan Canada S7N 5E5
306-966-2673 (dean's office); 966-6164 (fax); 966-6135 (admissions office);
966-2601 (fax)
Web site: www.usask.ca/medicine

The university began teaching medical students in 1926 when the school of medical sciences opened to provide the first two years of medical training. In 1953, the school became the college of medicine when a four-year term was instituted. The present program requires two years premedical university experience followed by a four-year program in the college of medicine.

Type: public
2008-2009 total enrollment: 238
Clinical facilities: Saskatoon Health Region: Royal University Hospital, St. Paul's Hospital, Saskatoon City Hospital. Regina Qu'Appelle Health Region: Regina General Hospital.

University Officials

President	P. MacKinnon, LL.B., LL.M.
Provost and Vice President, Academic	B. Fairbairn, Ph.D.
Vice President (Finance and Resources)	R. Florizone, Ph.D.
Vice Provost	Jim Germida, Ph.D.
Associate Vice President (Financial Services) and Controller	Laura Kennedy, CA
Associate Vice President Student and Enrollment Services	D. Hannah, Ph.D.

Medical School Administrative Staff

Dean	W. L. Albritton, M.D.
Associate Dean (Faculty Affairs)	TBA
Associate Dean (Medical Education)	S. R. Harding, M.D.
Associate Dean (Regina Programs)	G. White, M.D.
Associate Dean (Research and Graduate Studies)	J. Thornhill, Ph.D.
Associate Dean (Interdisciplinary Health Science Programs)	E. L. Harrison, Ph.D.
Associate Dean (Division of Biomedical Sciences)	N. Ovsenek, Ph.D.
Assistant Dean (Undergraduate Education)	L. F. Qualtiere, Ph.D.
Assistant Dean (Postgraduate Education)	K. McClean, M.D.
Director, School of Physical Therapy	A. Busch, Ph.D.
Director of Admissions and Student Affairs	B. Ziola, Ph.D.
Chief Financial Officer and Director of Administration	A.T. Schultz, CA
Director of the Physicians' Billing Office	V. Bennett, M.D.
Associate Director (Administration and Finance)	G. Melvin
Assistant Director (Administration and Finance)	C. Brooke
Director of Educational Support and Development	M. D'Eon, Ph.D.
Associate Director (Education Support and Development)	K. Premkumar
Director of CME and Professional Development	P. Davis, M.D.
Director of Information Technology Unit	J. Costa
Administrative Coordinator (Undergraduate)	R. Bourner
Administrative Coordinator (Postgraduate)	D. Spence
Administrative Coordinator (Postgraduate)	D. Toews
Administrative Coordinator (Integration and Assessment)	K. Mulligan
Administrative Coordinator (Admissions and Student Affairs)	H. Mandeville
Administrative Coordinator (Educational Support and Curriculum Evaluation)	L. Sibbald
Administrative Coordinator (Educational Support and Development, Community Faculty)	D. Bonnycastle
Administrative Coordinator (Animal Care)	C. Larson
Administrative Coordinator (Regina Programs)	R. Robertson
Administrative Coordinator (Graduate Programs)	J. Boyle
Administrative Coordinator (Research Groups)	D. Stumborg
Program Coordinator (Social Accountability)	D. Zaleschuk
Coordinator for Clinical Education	C. Yourk

University of Saskatchewan College of Medicine: SASKATCHEWAN

Librarian . . . . J. Bangma
Communications Officer (Alumni) . . . . A. Horvath
College Development Officer . . . . V. Moore-Wright
Career Development Officer (Undergraduate and Postgraduate) . . . . G. Mezo-Kricsfalsy
Administrative Coordinator (Clinical Sciences Education) . . . . S. Chernoff
Programs Manager (Postgraduate) . . . . S. Johnson

Department and Division or Section Chairs

Basic Sciences

Anatomy and Cell Biology . . . . R. Devon, Ph.D.
Biochemistry . . . . R. L. Khandelwal, Ph.D.
Community Health and Epidemiology . . . . N. Muhajarine, Ph.D.
Microbiology and Immunology . . . . W. Xiao, Ph.D.
Pharmacology . . . . V. Gopal, Ph.D.
Physiology . . . . W. Walz, Ph.D.

Clinical Sciences

Anaesthesia . . . . D. C. Campbell, M.D.
Family Medicine . . . . K. Ogle, M.D.
Medical Imaging . . . . S. Wiebe, M.D. (Acting)
Medicine . . . . T. W. Wilson, M.D.
Obstetrics, Gynecology, and Reproductive Sciences . . . . O. A. Olatunbosun, M.D.
Oncology . . . . D. R. Popkin, M.D.
Pathology . . . . J. Krahn, M.D.
Pediatrics . . . . W. T. Bingham, M.D.
Physical Medicine and Rehabilitation . . . . L. M. Rudachyk, M.D. (Acting)
Psychiatry . . . . R. Tempier, M.D.
Surgery . . . . A. G. Casson, M.D.

Provisional Affiliate School Member

2008–2009

Northern Ontario School of Medicine
East Campus, Laurentian University
935 Ramsey Lake Road
Sudbury, Ontario Canada P3E 2C6
705-675-4883; 675-4858 (fax)
Web site: www.nosm.ca

West Campus, Lakehead University
955 Oliver Road
Thunder Bay, Ontario Canada P7B 5E1
807-766-7300; 766-7370 (fax)
Web site: www.normed.ca

Founded in 2002, the Northern Ontario School of Medicine (NOSM) is a medical school for northern Ontario. NOSM is a joint initiative of Lakehead University in Thunder Bay and Laurentian University in Sudbury, aspiring to improve the health of the people of northern Ontario. The NOSM four-year M.D. program is organized around five themes: northern and rural health, personal and professional aspects of medical practice, social and population health, the foundations of medicine, and clinical skills in health care.

Type: public
2008-2009 total enrollment: 168
Clinical facilities: Sudbury Regional Hospital, Thunder Bay Regional Health Sciences Centre, other hospitals and health services throughout northern Ontario.

University Officials

President (Lakehead University).. Fred Gilbert, Ph.D.
President (Laurentian University)............................... Judith Woodsworth, Ph.D.

Medical School Administrative Staff

Founding Dean.. Roger Strasser, M.B.B.S., M.Cl.Sc.
Associate Dean, Community Engagement........................... Marc Blayney, M.D.
Associate Dean, Learner Affairs............................... Gerry Cooper, D.Ed.
Associate Dean, Faculty Affairs.................... William McCready, M.B., B.Ch., Ba.O.
Associate Dean, Continuing Health Professional Education.............. Wayne Bruce, Ph.D.
Associate Dean, Postgraduate Medical Education .... Maureen Topps, M.B.B.S.
Associate Dean, Undergraduate Medical Education................. Joel Lanphear, Ph.D.
Associate Dean, Administration .... Ken Adams
Associate Dean, Research.. Greg Ross, Ph.D.
Associate Dean, Informatics.................................. Robert Rubeck, Ph.D.
Assistant Dean, Admissions.................................... Blair Schoales
Assistant Dean, Informatics .... Rachel Ellaway
Director, Undergraduate Medical Education....................... Marie Matte
Director, Aboriginal Affairs .... Ian Peltier (Interim)
Director, E-Learning .... David Topps, M.B.B.S.
Director, Finance... Joe Lipinski
Director, Northern Ontario Health Information Network .... Patty Fink (Interim)
Director, Human Resources................................... Tina Vrbanac
Director, Technology....................................... Pasi Pinta
Director, Communications.................................... Kim Daynard

Department and Division or Section Chairs

Medical Sciences

Division Head, Medical Sciences................................. Garry Ferroni, Ph.D.
Biochemistry .... Hermann Falter, Ph.D., Tom Kovala, Ph.D., Amadeo Parissenti, Ph.D.,
and John Th'ng, Ph.D.
Cell and Molecular Biology ... Rob Lafrenie, Ph.D., Leslie Sutherland, Ph.D., Hoyun Lee, Ph.D.,
and Helga Duivenvoorden, Ph.D.
Haematology.. Dimitrios Vergidis, M.D.
Immunology .... Marina Ulanova, M.D., Ph.D., and Stacey Ritz, Ph.D.
Molecular Genetics .... Aseem Kumar, Ph.D., and Carita Lanner, Ph.D.
Pharmacology .... Miriam McDonald, Zacharias Suntres, Ph.D., and Brian Ross, Ph.D.
Physiology.................... David MacLean, Ph.D., and T. C. Tai, Ph.D.
Anatomy .... Donna Newhouse

Human Sciences

Division Head, Human Sciences..................................... Garry Ferroni, Ph.D.
Behavioral Medicine .... Patricia Smith, Ph.D.
Biostatistics .... Bruce Weaver
History of Medicine.. Geoff Hudson, Ph.D.
Medical Anthropology .... Kristen Jacklin, and Marion Maar, Ph.D.

Clinical Sciences

Division Head, Clinical Sciences................................ Thomas Szabo, M.D.
Anesthesia (East)... Wayne Lambert, M.D.
Anesthesia (West) .... Georg Doig, M.D.
Child and Adolescent Health (East).. Vacant
Child and Adolescent Health (West) .... Vacant
Clinical Education (East).. Joyce Helmer
Clinical Education (West) .... William Hettenhausen, D.D.S.
Diagnostic Radiology (East)..................................... Curtis Milner, M.D.
Diagnostic Radiology (West) .... John O'Brien, M.D.
Emergency Medicine (East)....................................... Lee Toner, M.D.
Emergency Medicine (West) .... Vacant
Family Medicine (East) .... Vacant
Family Medicine (West)... Vacant
Internal Medicine (East) .... Silvana Spadafora, M.D.
Internal Medicine (West)........................... Saleem Malik, M.B.B.S., Ph.D.
Lab Medicine and Clinical Pathology (East) .... Michel Bonin, M.D.
Lab Medicine and Clinical Pathology (West)..................... Nicholas Escott, M.D.
Psychiatry (East) .... Rayudu Koka, M.B.B.S.
Psychiatry (West)... Jack Haggarty, M.D.
Surgery (East).. Timothy Best, M.D.
Surgery (West) .... Barry Anderson, M.D.
Women's Health (East) .... Janice Willett, M.D.
Women's Health (West)....................................... Andrew Siren, M.D.

Council of Deans

2008–2009

Council of Deans Administrative Board, 2007-2008

Chair
H. David Wilson, M.D.*
University of North Dakota School of Medicine and Health Sciences

Chair-elect
E. Albert Reece, M.D., Ph.D., M.B.A.*
University of Maryland School of Medicine

Immediate Past Chair
Thomas J. Lawley, M.D.*
Emory University School of Medicine

Members

Barbara F. Atkinson, M.D.
University of Kansas School of Medicine

A. Lorris Betz, M.D., Ph.D.*
University of Utah School of Medicine

Betty M. Drees, M.D.
University of Missouri–Kansas City School of Medicine

Steven G. Gabbe, M.D., M.A.*
Vanderbilt University School of Medicine

Lois Margaret Nora, M.D., J.D.*
Northeastern Ohio Universities College of Medicine

Harold L. Paz, M.D.*
Pennsylvania State University College of Medicine

Philip A. Pizzo, M.D.*
Stanford University School of Medicine

John E. Prescott, M.D.
West Virginia University School of Medicine

Larry J. Shapiro, M.D.*
Washington University in St. Louis School of Medicine

* Denotes representative to AAMC Executive Council

307

Council of Deans

ALABAMA

University of Alabama School of Medicine
Robert R. Rich, M.D.

University of South Alabama
College of Medicine
Samuel J. Strada, Ph.D., M.S.

ARIZONA

University of Arizona College of Medicine
Steve Goldschmid, M.D.

ARKANSAS

University of Arkansas for Medical Sciences
College of Medicine
Debra H. Fiser, M.D.

CALIFORNIA

Keck School of Medicine of the
University of Southern California
Carmen A. Puliafito, M.D., M.B.A.

Loma Linda University School of Medicine
H. Roger Hadley, M.D.

Stanford University School of Medicine
Philip A. Pizzo, M.D.

University of California, Davis,
School of Medicine
Claire Pomeroy, M.D., M.B.A.

University of California, Irvine,
School of Medicine
David N. Bailey, M.D.

University of California, Los Angeles
David Geffen School of Medicine
Gerald S. Levey, M.D.

University of California, San Diego
School of Medicine
David A. Brenner, M.D.

University of California, San Francisco,
School of Medicine
Sam Hawgood, M.B,.B.S.

COLORADO

University of Colorado School of Medicine
Richard D. Krugman, M.D.

CONNECTICUT

University of Connecticut School of Medicine
Cato Laurencin, M.D., Ph.D.

Yale University School of Medicine
Robert J. Alpern, M.D.

DISTRICT OF COLUMBIA

George Washington University
School of Medicine and Health Sciences
James L. Scott, M.D.

Georgetown University School of Medicine
Stephen Ray Mitchell, M.D.

Howard University College of Medicine
Robert E. Taylor, M.D., Ph.D., M.S., F.A.C.P.

FLORIDA

Florida State University College of Medicine
John Fogarty, M.D.

University of Florida College of Medicine
Michael L. Good, M.D.

University of Miami Leonard M. Miller
School of Medicine
Pascal J. Goldschmidt, M.D.

University of South Florida
College of Medicine
Stephen Klasko, M.D., M.B.A.

GEORGIA

Emory University School of Medicine
Thomas J. Lawley, M.D.

Medical College of Georgia School of Medicine
D. Douglas Miller, M.D., C.M., M.B.A.

Mercer University School of Medicine
William F. Bina, M.D.

Morehouse School of Medicine
Eve J. Higginbotham, M.D.

HAWAII

University of Hawaii, John A. Burns
School of Medicine
Jerris Hedges, M.D., M.S., M.M.M.

ILLINOIS

Chicago Medical School at Rosalind Franklin
University of Medicine & Science
Arthur J. Ross III, M.D., M.B.A.

Loyola University Chicago
Stritch School of Medicine
John M. Lee, M.D., Ph.D.

Northwestern University
The Feinberg School of Medicine
J. Larry Jameson, M.D., Ph.D.

Rush Medical College of Rush University
Medical Center
Thomas A. Deutsch, M.D.

Southern Illinois University
School of Medicine
J. Kevin Dorsey, M.D., Ph.D.

University of Chicago
Division of the Biological Sciences
The Pritzker School of Medicine
James L. Madara, M.D.

University of Illinois College of Medicine
Joseph A. Flaherty, M.D.

INDIANA

Indiana University School of Medicine
D. Craig Brater, M.D.

IOWA

University of Iowa Roy J. and Lucille A. Carver
College of Medicine
Paul B. Rothman, M.D.

KANSAS

University of Kansas School of Medicine
Barbara F. Atkinson, M.D.

KENTUCKY

University of Kentucky College of Medicine
Jay A. Perman, M.D.

University of Louisville School of Medicine
Edward C. Halperin, M.D., M.A., F.A.C.R.

LOUISIANA

Louisiana State University
School of Medicine in New Orleans
Steve Nelson, M.D.

Louisiana State University
School of Medicine in Shreveport
John C. McDonald, M.D.

Tulane University School of Medicine
Benjamin P. Sachs, M.D.

MARYLAND

Johns Hopkins University School of Medicine
Edward D. Miller, M.D.

Uniformed Services University
of the Health Sciences
F. Edward Hebert School of Medicine
Larry W. Laughlin, M.D., Ph.D.

University of Maryland School of Medicine
E. Albert Reece, M.D., Ph.D., M.B.A.

MASSACHUSETTS

Boston University School of Medicine
Karen Antman, M.D.

Harvard Medical School
Jeffrey S. Flier, M.D.

Tufts University School of Medicine
Michael Rosenblatt, M.D.

University of Massachusetts Medical School
Terence R. Flotte, M.D.

MICHIGAN

Michigan State University
College of Human Medicine
Marsha Dawn Rappley, M.D.

University of Michigan Medical School
James O. Woolliscroft, M.D.

Wayne State University School of Medicine
Robert M. Mentzer, Jr., M.D.

MINNESOTA

Mayo Medical School
Keith D. Lindor, M.D.

University of Minnesota Medical School
Deborah E. Powell, M.D.

MISSISSIPPI

University of Mississippi School of Medicine
Daniel W. Jones, M.D.

Council of Deans

MISSOURI

Saint Louis University School of Medicine
Philip O. Alderson, M.D.

University of Missouri-Columbia
School of Medicine
William M. Crist, M.D.

University of Missouri-Kansas City
School of Medicine
Betty M. Drees, M.D., F.A.C.P.

Washington University in St. Louis
School of Medicine
Larry J. Shapiro, M.D.

NEBRASKA

Creighton University School of Medicine
Cecile Marie Zielinski, M.D.

University of Nebraska College of Medicine
John L. Gollan, M.D., Ph.D.

NEVADA

University of Nevada School of Medicine
Ole J. Thienhaus, M.D., M.B.A.

NEW HAMPSHIRE

Dartmouth Medical School
William R. Green, Ph.D.

NEW JERSEY

University of Medicine and Dentistry
of New Jersey-New Jersey Medical School
Robert L. Johnson, M.D., F.A.A.P.

University of Medicine and Dentistry
of New Jersey-Robert Wood Johnson
Medical School
Peter S. Amenta, M.D., Ph.D.

NEW MEXICO

University of New Mexico School of Medicine
Paul B. Roth, M.D.

NEW YORK

Albany Medical College
Vincent P. Verdile, M.D., M.S.

Albert Einstein College of Medicine
of Yeshiva University
Allen M. Spiegel, M.D.

Columbia University
College of Physicians and Surgeons
Lee Goldman, M.D., M.P.H.

Mount Sinai School of Medicine
of New York University
Dennis S. Charney, M.D.

New York Medical College
Ralph A. O'Connell, M.D.

New York University School of Medicine
Robert I. Grossman, M.D.

State University of New York
Downstate Medical Center College of Medicine
Ian L. Taylor, M.D., M.B.Ch.B., Ph.D.

State University of New York
Upstate Medical University
Steven J. Scheinman, M.D.

The School of Medicine
at Stony Brook University Medical Center
Richard N. Fine, M.D.

University at Buffalo
State University of New York
School of Medicine & Biomedical Sciences
Michael E. Cain, M.D.

University of Rochester
School of Medicine and Dentistry
David S. Guzick, M.D., Ph.D.

Weill Cornell Medical College
Antonio M. Gotto Jr., M.D.Ph.D., D.Phil.

NORTH CAROLINA

Brody School of Medicine
at East Carolina University
Phyllis Horns, R.N., D.S.N., F.A.A.N.

Duke University School of Medicine
Nancy C. Andrews, M.D., Ph.D., M.S.

University of North Carolina at Chapel Hill
School of Medicine
William L. Roper, M.D., M.P.H.

Wake Forest University School of Medicine
William B. Applegate, M.D., M.P.H.

NORTH DAKOTA

University of North Dakota
School of Medicine and Health Sciences
H. David Wilson, M.D.

OHIO

Case Western Reserve University
School of Medicine
Pamela B. Davis, M.D., Ph.D.

Northeastern Ohio Universities
Colleges of Medicine and Pharmacy
Lois M. Nora, M.D., J.D., M.B.A.

Ohio State University College of Medicine
Wiley Souba, M.D., D.Sc., M.B.A.

The University of Toledo College of Medicine
Jeffrey P. Gold, M.D.

University of Cincinnati College of Medicine
David M. Stern, M.D.

Wright State University
Boonshoft School of Medicine
Howard M. Part, M.D.

OKLAHOMA

University of Oklahoma College of Medicine
M. Dewayne Andrews, M.D.

OREGON

Oregon Health & Science University
School of Medicine
Mark A. Richardson, M.D., M.Sc.B,. M.B.A.

PENNSYLVANIA

Drexel University College of Medicine
Richard V. Homan, M.D.

Jefferson Medical College
of Thomas Jefferson University
Michael J. Vergare, M.D.

Pennsylvania State University
College of Medicine
Harold L. Paz, M.D., M.S.

Temple University School of Medicine
John Michael Daly, M.D.

University of Pennsylvania School of Medicine
Arthur H. Rubenstein, M.B.B.Ch.

University of Pittsburgh School of Medicine
Arthur S. Levine, M.D.

PUERTO RICO

Ponce School of Medicine
Raul A. Armstrong M.D.

San Juan Bautista School of Medicine
Yocasta Brugal Mena, M.D.

Universidad Central del Caribe
School of Medicine
Jose Ginel Rodriguez, M.D., M.B.B.Ch.

University of Puerto Rico School of Medicine
Walter Frontera, M.D., PhD

RHODE ISLAND

The Warren Alpert Medical School
of Brown University
Edward J. Wing, M.D.

SOUTH CAROLINA

Medical University of South Carolina
College of Medicine
Joseph G. Reves, M.D., M.S.

University of South Carolina
School of Medicine
Donald J. DiPette, M.D., F.A.C.P., F.A.H.A.

SOUTH DAKOTA

Sanford School of Medicine
of the University of South Dakota
Rodney R. Parry, M.D.

TENNESSEE

East Tennessee State University
James H. Quillen College of Medicine
Philip C. Bagnell, M.D.

Meharry Medical College
Valerie Montogomery Rice, M.D.

University of Tennessee Health Science Center
College of Medicine
Steven J. Schwab, M.D.

Vanderbilt University School of Medicine
Jeffrey Balser, M.D., Ph.D.

TEXAS

Baylor College of Medicine
Peter Traber, M.D.

Council of Deans

Texas A&M Health Science Center
College of Medicine
Christopher C. Colenda, M.D., M.P.H.

Texas Tech University Health Sciences Center
School of Medicine
Steven L. Berk, M.D.

University of Texas Medical Branch
School of Medicine
Garland D. Anderson, M.D.

University of Texas
Medical School at Houston
Giuseppe Colasurdo, M.D.

University of Texas
School of Medicine at San Antonio
William L. Henrich, M.D., M.A.C.P.

University of Texas
Southwestern Medical Center at Dallas
Southwestern Medical School
Alfred G. Gilman, M.D., Ph.D.

UTAH

University of Utah School of Medicine
A. Lorris Betz, M.D., Ph.D.

VERMONT

University of Vermont College of Medicine
Frederick C. Morin, III, M.D.

VIRGINIA

Eastern Virginia Medical School
Gerald J. Pepe, Ph.D.

University of Virginia School of Medicine
Steven T. DeKosky, M.D.

Virginia Commonwealth University
School of Medicine
Jerome F. Strauss, M.D., Ph.D.

WASHINGTON

University of Washington School of Medicine
Paul G. Ramsey, M.D.

WEST VIRGINIA

Joan C. Edwards School of Medicine
at Marshall University
Charles H. McKown, Jr., M.D.

West Virginia University School of Medicine
James E. Brick, M.D.

WISCONSIN

Medical College of Wisconsin
Jonathan Ravdin, M.D.

University of Wisconsin
School of Medicine and Public Health
Robert N. Golden, M.D.

Council of Academic Societies

2008–2009

Council of Academic Societies Administrative Board, 2007-2008

Chair
Joel A. Delisa, M.D., M.S.*
Association of Academic Physiatrists
Professor and Chair, Department of Physical
Medicine and Rehabilitation
UMDNJ-New Jersey Medical School

Chair-elect
Randall K. Holmes, M.D., Ph.D.*
*Association of Medical School Microbiology and
Immunology Chairs*
Professor and Chair, Department of Microbiology
University of Colorado Health Science Center
School of Medicine

Immediate Past Chair
Michael J. Friedlander, Ph.D.*
*Association of Medical School Neuroscience
Department Chairs*
Wilhelmina Robertson Professor and Chair
Director of Neuroscience Initiatives
Baylor College of Medicine

Board Members

James M. Crawford, M.D., Ph.D. *
Association of Pathology Chairs
Chair, Department of Pathology, Immunology, and
Laboratory Medicine
University of Florida College of Medicine

S. Edwards Dismuke, M.D., M.P.H.
Association for Prevention Teaching and Research
Dean and Professor, Department of Preventive
Medicine
University of Kansas Wichita Campus

Evelyn C. Granieri, M.D.
American Geriatric Society
Co-chair, Division of Geriatric Medicine and
Aging
Columbia University College of Physicians and
Surgeons

Mark C. Henry, M.D.
*Association of Academic Chairs of Emergency
Medicine*
Professor and Chair, Department of Emergency
Medicine
State University of New York, Stony Brook

Anthony A. Meyer, M.D., Ph.D.*
Society of Surgical Chairs
Professor and Chair, Department of Surgery
University of North Carolina at Chapel Hill
School of Medicine

Luis G. Navar, Ph.D.
Association of Chairs of Department of Physiology
Professor and Chair, Department of Physiology
Tulane University School of Medicine

Kathleen G. Nelson, M.D.*
Ambulatory Pediatric Association
Senior Associate Dean for Faculty Development
University of Alabama School of Medicine

Barbara L. Thompson, M.D.
Association of Departments of Family Medicine
Assistant Dean of Faculty
Practice and Hospital Clinics
University of Texas Medical Branch at Galveston

Thomas C. Westfall, Ph.D.
*Association of Medical School Pharmacology
Chairs*
Chair, Department of Pharmacological and
Physiological Science
St. Louis University School of Medicine

* Denotes representative to the AAMC Executive Council

Council of Academic Societies Representatives, 2007-2008

BASIC SCIENCES

ANATOMY AND CELL BIOLOGY

American Association of Anatomists

Richard D. Dey, Ph.D.
Professor and Chair, Department
Neurobiology & Anatomy
West Virginia University
School of Medicine
P.O. Box 9128
Morgantown, West Virginia 26506

Association of Anatomy, Cell Biology and Neurobiology Chairpersons

Richard D. Dey, Ph.D.
Professor and Chair, Department
Neurobiology & Anatomy
West Virginia University
School of Medicine
P.O. Box 9128
Morgantown, West Virginia 26506

Michael Shipley, Ph.D.
Chair, Department of Anatomy
and Neurobiology
University of Maryland
School of Medicine
20 Penn Street, HSFII, S251
Room 222
Baltimore, Maryland 21201

BIOCHEMISTRY

American Society for Biochemistry and Molecular Biology

William C. Merrick, Ph.D.
Professor
Case Western Reserve University
School of Medicine
10900 Euclid Avenue
Dept. of Biochemistry
Cleveland, Ohio 44106-4915

Thomas E. Smith, Ph.D.
Professor, Department of Biochemistry
Howard University
College of Medicine
520 W Street, N.W.
Washington, DC 20059

Association of Medical and Graduate Departments of Biochemistry

Yusuf A. Hannun, M.D.
Professor and Chairman
Department of Biochemistry and
Molecular Biology
Medical University of South Carolina
College of Medicine
96 Jonathan Lucas Street
P.O. Box 250617
Charleston, South Carolina 29425

ENDOCRINOLOGY

Endocrine Society

Melissa Thomas, M.D., Ph.D.
Assistant Professor
Department of Med/Lab of Molecular
Endocrinology
Harvard Medical School
50 Blossom Street, 320 Wellman Bldg
Boston, Massachusetts 02114

MICROBIOLOGY

American Society for Microbiology

Kenneth I. Berns, M.D., Ph.D.
Director, Genetics Institute
University of Florida
College of Medicine
1376 Mowry Road
PO Box 103610
Gainesville, Florida 32610-3610

Terrance G. Cooper, Ph.D.
Van Vleet Professor
Department of Microbiology
University of Tennessee
Health Science Center
College of Medicine
858 Madison Avenue
Memphis, Tennessee 38163

Association of Medical School Microbiology and Immunology Chairs

Randall Holmes, M.D.
Professor and Chairman
Department of Mircobiology
University of Colorado
School of Medicine
P.O. Box 6511
Mail Stop 8333
Aurora, Colorado 80045

NEUROSCIENCE

Association of Medical School Neuroscience Department Chairs

John H. Byme, Ph.D.
Professor and Chair
Department of Neurobiology & Anatomy
University of Texas
Medical School Houston
6431 Fannin Street
Houston, Texas 77030

Michael J. Friedlander, Ph.D.
Wilhelmina Robertson Professor and Chair
Department of Neuroscience,
Dir. Neuroscience Init.
Baylor College of Medicine
One Baylor Plaza
Suite S-740A
Houston, Texas 77030

Society for Neuroscience

Michael J. Friedlander, Ph.D.
Wilhelmina Robertson Professor and Chair
Department of Neuroscience,
Dir. Neuroscience Init.
Baylor College of Medicine
One Baylor Plaza
Suite S-740A
Houston, Texas 77030

M. Kerry O'Banion
Associate Professor of Neurobiology
Co-Director, MD/PhD Program
University of Rochester
School of Medicine & Dentistry
601 Elmwood Avenue
Box 7604
Rochester, New York 14534

PATHOLOGY

Academy of Clinical Laboratory Physicians and Scientists

Steven L. Spitalnik, M.D.
Department of Pathology
Columbia University
College of Physicians & Surgeons
630 West 168th Street
New York, New York 10032

American Society for Investigative Pathology, Inc.

Stephen Galli, M.D.
Professor & Chair, Department of
Pathology, Microbiol and Immunology
Stanford University
School of Medicine
300 Pasteur Drive
L-235
Stanford, California 94305-5324

Mark E. Sobel, M.D., Ph.D.
Managing Officer
American Society for Investigative
Pathology, Inc.
9650 Rockville Pike
Bethesda, Maryland 20814-3993

Association of Pathology Chairs, Inc.

James M. Crawford, M.D., Ph.D.
Chairman
Department Pathology, Immunology and
Lab. Medicine
University of Florida
College of Medicine
P.O. Box 100275
Gainesville, Florida 32610

Mark L. Tykocinski, M.D.
Professor and Chair
University of Pennsylvania
School of Medicine
3400 Spruce Street, 6 Gates
Philadelphia, Pennsylvania 19104-4283

PHARMACOLOGY - BASIC

American Society for Pharmacology and Experimental Therapeutics

Brian M. Cox, Ph.D.
Professor
Department of Pharmacology
Uniformed Services Hebert
School of Medicine
4301 Jones Bridge Road
Bethesda, Maryland 20814-4799

Gary O. Rankin, Ph.D.
Professor & Chair
Department of Pharm, Physio, &
Toxicology
Marshall University Edwards
School of Medicine
1542 Spring Valley Drive
Huntington, West Virginia 25704-9388

Association of Medical School Pharmacology Chairs

Joseph Haywood, Ph.D.
Professor and Chair, Department
Pharm. & Toxicology
Michigan State University
B440 Life Science Building
East Lansing, Michigan 48824

Thomas C Westfall, Ph.D.
Chairman, Department of Pharmacological
and Physiological Science
St Louis University
School of Medicine
1402 South Grand Boulevard
St. Louis, Missouri 63104

CAS Representatives

PHYSIOLOGY

American Physiological Society

Virginia Miller, Ph.D.
Professor
Mayo Medical School
200 First Street, S.W.
4-62A Medical Science Bldg.
Rochester, Minnesota 55905

Jeff M. Sands, M.D.
Emory University
School of Medicine
1639 Pierce Drive, NE
Renal Division, WMB Rm 338
Atlanta, Georgia 30322

Association of Chairs of Departments of Physiology

Luis Gabriel Navar, Ph.D.
Professor and Chairman
Department of Physiology
Tulane University
School of Medicine
1430 Tulane Avenue, SL-39
New Orleans, Louisiana 70112

William Spielman, Ph.D.
Professor
Department of Physiology
Michigan State University
College of Human Medicine
2201 Biomedical Physical Sciences
East Lansing, Michigan 48824

MULTISPECIALTY

International Association of Medical Science Educators

Giulia Bonaminio, Ph.D.
Associate Dean for Medical Education
University of Kansas
School of Medicine
3901 Rainbow Boulevard
3023 Murphy
Kansas City, Kansas 66160-7831

Aviad Haramati, Ph.D.
Director of Education
Department of Physiology and Biophysics
Georgetown University
School of Medicine
3900 Reservoir, N.W.
Washington, DC 20057

CLINICAL SCIENCES

ANESTHESIOLOGY

Association of Anesthesiology Program Directors

Jeffrey K. Kirsch, M.D.
Professor & Chair
Department of Anesthesiology
Oregon Health & Science
School of Medicine
3181 S.W. Sam Jackson Park Road
UHS 2
Portland, Oregon 97239

Kevin K. Tremper, M.D., Ph.D.
Professor and Chair
University of Michigan Medical Center
1500 E. Medical Center Drive
Ann Arbor, Michigan 48109-0048

Association of University Anesthesiologists

Steven J. Barker, M.D.
Professor & Head
Department of Anesthesiology
University of Arizona
College of Medicine
1501 N. Campbell
Tucson, Arizona 85724

Lee Fleisher
Professor and Chair of Anesthesiology
University of Pennsylvania
School of Medicine
680 Dulles Building, HUP
3400 Spruce Street
Philadelphia, Pennsylvania 19104

Society for Education in Anesthesia

Susan Cymbor, M.D.
Department of Anesthesia
Cleveland Clinic Foundation
9500 Euclid Avenue
Cleveland, Ohio 44195

Berend Mets, M.D.
Eric A. Walker Professor and Chair
Pennsylvania State University
College of Medicine
500 University Drive
Hershey, Pennsylvania 17033-0850

Society of Academic Anesthesiology Chairs

Roberta L. Hines, M.D.
Professor & Chair, Department of
Anesthesiology
Yale University
School of Medicine
333 Cedar Street, , TMP - 3
Post Office Box 20851
New Haven, Connecticut 06520-8055

W. Scott Jellish, M.D., Ph.D.
Prof & Chair, Anesthesiology
Loyola University Chicago Stritch
School of Medicine
2160 South First Avenue
Maywood, Illinois 60153

DERMATOLOGY

American Academy of Dermatology

Amit Pandya, M.D.
Professor
Department of Dermatology
University of Texas
Southwestern Medical School Dallas
5323 Harry Hines Boulevard
Dallas, Texas 75390-9190

Thomas Ray, M.D.
Professor
University of Iowa Hospital and Clinic
200 Hawkins Drive
Room W204
Iowa City, Iowa 52242

Association of Professors of Dermatology

Alice B. Gottlieb, M.D, Ph.D.
Chair and Dermatologist-in-Chief
Tufts-New England Medical Center
750 Washington Street, Box 114
Boston, Massachusetts 02111

Maria K. Hordinsky, M.D.
Chair, Department of Dermatology
University of Minnesota
Medical School
420 Delaware Street SE
Box 98 UMHC,
Minneapolis, Minnesota 55455

EMERGENCY MEDICINE

Association of Academic Chairs of Emergency Medicine

Mark C. Henry, M.D.
Professor and Chair
Department of Emergency Medicine
State University of New York-Stony Brook
University Hospital L-4, R-515
Stony Brook, New York 11794

Gabor Kelen, M.D.
Professor & Chair
Department of Emergency Medicine
Johns Hopkins University
School of Medicine
1830 East Monument Street
Suite 6-100
Baltimore, Maryland 21287

Council of Emergency Medicine Residency Directors

Hal Thomas, M.D.
Chief, Emergency Medicine
Council of Residency Directors
Oregon Health Science University
3181 SW Sam Jackson Park Rd.
UHN-52
Portland, Oregon 97201-3098

Society for Academic Emergency Medicine

Marcus L. Martin, M.D.
Vice President & Chief Officer for
Diversity and Equity
P.O. Box 800699
Charlottesville, Virginia 22908

David P. Sklar, M.D.
Associate Dean
University of New Mexico
School of Medicine
1 University of New Mexico
GME MSC 08 4770
Albuquerque, New Mexico 87131-0001

FAMILY MEDICINE

American Academy of Family Physicians

Samuel C. Matheny, M.D.
Chair, Department of Family Medicine
University of Kentucky
College of Medicine
K-312 Kentucky Clinic
Lexington, Kentucky 40536-0284

Perry A. Pugno, M.D.
Director
Division of Medical Education
American Academy of Family Physicians
11400 Tomahawk Creek Parkway
Leawood, Kansas 66211-2672

American Academy of Family Physicians Foundation

Roland Goertz, M.D.
President
Mclennan County Medical Education
1600 Providence Drive
Waco, Texas 76707

Samuel C. Matheny, M.D.
Chair, Department of Family Medicine
University of Kentucky
College of Medicine
K-312 Kentucky Clinic
Lexington, Kentucky 40536-0284

CAS Representatives

Association of Departments of Family Medicine

J. Lloyd Michener, M.D.
Chairman
Department of Community & Family
Medicine
Duke University
School of Medicine
319 Hanes House
Corner of Erwin Rd & Trent Drive
Durham, North Carolina 27705

Barbara L. Thompson, M.D.
Assistant Dean of Faculty
Practice and Hospital Clinics
University of Texas
Medical Branch Galveston
School of Medicine
301 University Boulevard
Galveston, Texas 77555-1123

Association of Family Medicine ResidencyDirectors

Edward T. Bope, M.D.
Residency Director
Riverside Family Practice Ctr
Ohio Health
697 Thomas Lane
Columbus, Ohio 43214

Penny Tenzer, M.D.
Department of Family Medicine and
Community Health
University of Miami Leonard M. Miller
School of Medicine
P.O. Box 016700 (R700)
Miami, Florida 33101

Society of Teachers of Family Medicine

Mark S. Johnson, M.D., M.P.H.
Chairman
Department of Family Medicine
UMDNJ-New Jersey Medical School
185 South Orange Avenue
MSB-B648
Newark, New Jersey 07103

Susan Skochelak, M.D., M.P.H
Sr. Associate Dean for Academic Affairs
University of Wisconsin
School of Medicine & Public Health
4121 Health Sciences Learning Center
750 Highland Avenue
Madison, Wisconsin 53705-2221

Society of Teachers of Family Medicine Foundation

Mark S. Johnson, M.D., M.P.H.
Chairman
Department of Family Medicine
UMDNJ-New Jersey Medical School
185 South Orange Avenue
MSB-B648
Newark, New Jersey 07103

Susan Skochelak, M.D., M.P.H
Sr. Associate Dean for Academic Affairs
University of Wisconsin
School of Medicine & Public Health
4121 Health Sciences Learning Center
750 Highland Avenue
Madison, Wisconsin 53705-2221

GENERAL SURGERY

American Surgical Association

L.D. Britt, M.D.
Chairman, Department of Surgery
Eastern Virginia Medical School
825 Fairfax Avenue
P.O. Box 1980
Norfolk, Virginia 23507

John Michael Daly, M.D.
Dean
Temple University
School of Medicine
3420 North Broad Street, MRB-Room 102
Philadelphia, Pennsylvania 19140

American Surgical Association Foundation

William G. Cioffi, M.D.
Surgeon-in-Chief
Rhode Island Hospital
593 Eddy Street
Surgery APS 432
Providence, Rhode Island 02903

Linda G. Phillips, M.D.
Senior Assoc Dean for Faculty Affairs
University of Texas
Medical Branch Galveston
School of Medicine
301 University Boulevard
Office of the Dean of Medicine
Galveston, Texas 77555-0133

Association for Academic Surgery

Ruth L. Bush, M.D.
Associate Professor of Surgery
Scott and White Memorial Hosp
2401 South 31st Street
Temple, Texas 76508

Kathrin L. Mayer, M.D.
Assistant Professor
University of California, Davis
Health System
2315 Stockton Boulevard
Sacramento, California 95817

Association for Surgical Education

Debra DaRosa, Ph.D.
Professor of Surgery
Vice Chair of Education
Northwestern University Feinberg
School of Medicine
251 East Huron St.,
Galter 3-150
Chicago, Illinois 60611

Merril Dayton, M.D.
Professor and Chair
Department of Surgery
University at Buffalo
School of Medicine
Buffalo General Hospital
100 High Street
Buffalo, New York 14202

Society of Surgical Chairs

Nancy Ascher, M.D., Ph.D.
Professor and Chair
Department of Surgery
University of California San Francisco
School of Medicine
513 Parnassus Avenue
Box 0104, S320
San Francisco, California 94143 0410

Anthony A. Meyer, M.D., Ph.D.
Professor and Chair, Department
of Surgery
University of North Carolina
School of Medicine
Campus Box 7050
Room 2115, Bioinformatics Bldg.
Chapel Hill, North Carolina 27599-7050

Anthony A. Meyer, M.D., Ph.D.
Professor and Chair, Department
of Surgery
University of North Carolina
School of Medicine
Campus Box 7050
Room 2115, Bioinformatics Bldg.
Chapel Hill, North Carolina 27599-7050

Society of University Surgeons

David A. Spain, M.D.
Profesor & Chief, Trauma & Surgical
Critical Care
Stanford University
School of Medicine
300 Pasteur Drive
Room H3680, MC: 5655
Stanford, California 94305

Mark A. Wilson, M.D.
Chief of Surgery-112U
VP of Surgical Service Line
VA Pittsburgh Health Care System
University Drive "C"
Pittsburgh, Pennsylvania 15240

GENETICS

American College of Medical Genetics

Charles J. Epstein, M.D.
Chair, Department of Pediatrics
University of California San Francisco
School of Medicine
Box 0748, U 585L
San Francisco, California 94143-0748

Michael S. Watson, Ph.D.
Executive Director
American College of Medical Genetics
9650 Rockville Pike
Bethesda, Maryland 20814

American College of Medical Genetics Foundation

Charles J. Epstein, M.D.
Chair, Department of Pediatrics
University of California San Francisco
School of Medicine
Box 0748, U 585L
San Francisco, California 94143-0748

Michael S. Watson, Ph.D.
Executive Director
American College of Medical Genetics
9650 Rockville Pike
Bethesda, Maryland 20814

American Society of Human Genetics

Louis J. Elsas II, M.D.
Professor and Director
Center for Medical Genetics
University of Miami Leonard M. Miller
School of Medicine
P.O. Box 016820 (D820)
Miami, Florida 33101

Huntington Willard, Ph.D.
Director, Institute for Genome Sciences
& Policy
Vice Chancellor for Genome Sciences
Duke University
School of Medicine
Box 3382
Durham, North Carolina 27710

CAS Representatives

Association of Professors of Human and Medical Genetics

Robert J. Desnick, M.D., Ph.D.
Professor and Chair
Department of Genetics and
Genomic Sciences
Mount Sinai School of Medicine
Fifth Avenue and 100th Street
New York, New York 10029-6574

Louis J. Elsas II, M.D.
Professor and Director
Center for Medical Genetics
University of Miami Leonard M. Miller
School of Medicine
P.O. Box 016820 (D820)
Miami, Florida 33101

HEALTH SERVICES RESEARCH

AcademyHealth

W. David Helms, Ph.D.
President and CEO
AcademyHealth
1150 17 Street, NW
Ste 600
Washington, DC 20036

Donald M. Steinwachs, Ph.D.
Professor and Director
Health Services Research and
Development Center
Johns Hopkins Bloomberg School
624 N Broadway
Room 482
Baltimore, Maryland 21205-1996

IMMUNOLOGY

American Academy of Allergy, Asthma and Immunology Training Program Directors

Amal Assaad, M.D.
Associate Professor of Clinical
Pediatrics
Children's Medical Center-Cincinnati
3333 Burnet Avenue
Cincinnati, Ohio 45229-3039

Richard D. deShazo, M.D.
Professor and Chair, Otolaryngology
University of Mississippi
School of Medicine
2500 North State Street
Jackson, Mississippi 39216-4505

INTERNAL MEDICINE

American Gastroenterological Association

David Katzka, M.D.
Director, GI Motility/Physiology Pgm.
Hospital of the University of
Pennsylvania
3400 Spruce Street
3 Dulles
Philadelphia, Pennsylvania 19104

Helen Shields
Assoc Prof
330 Brookline Avenue
Boston, Massachusetts 02215

American Society of Hematology

Scott D. Gitlin, M.D.
Associate Professor of Internal Medicine
University of Michigan Medical Center
1500 E. Medical Center Drive
C345 Med. Inn Building
Ann Arbor, Michigan 48109-0848

Elaine Muchmore, M.D.
Associate Chief of Staff for Education
VA San Diego Healthcare System
3350 La Jolla Village Drive
Mail Code 111E
San Diego, California 92161

Association of American Physicians

Harold Fallon, M.D.
Dean Emeritus
University of Alabama SOM
40 Marsh Edge Lane
Kiawah Island, South Carolina 29455

Association of Professors of Medicine

Esther A. Torres, M.D.
Professor and Chair of Medicine
University of Puerto Rico
School of Medicine
Medical Sciences Campus
P.O. Box 365067
San Juan, Puerto Rico 00936-5067

Association of Program Directors in Internal Medicine

Rosemarie L. Fisher, M.D.
Professor of Medicine
Director & Associate Dean GME
Yale University
School of Medicine
Yale-New Haven Hospital
20 York Street, T-236
New Haven, Connecticut 06504

Clerkship Directors in Internal Medicine

Steven J. Durning, M.D.
Associate Professor
Uniformed Services Hebert
School of Medicine
4301 Jones Bridge Road
Bethesda, Maryland 20814-4799

Shiphra Ginsburg
Assistant Professor, Department of
Medicine
Mount Sinai Hospital
600 University Avenue, #433
Toronto, Ontario 75G 1X5 Canada

Society of General Internal Medicine

Eugene C. Rich, M.D.
Senior Advisor, Office of Science Policy
National Institutes of Health
RKL1 - One Rockledge Center, Room 734
6705 Rockledge Drive
Bethesda, Maryland 20892

MULTISPECIALTY

American Academy of Sleep Medicine

Andrew L. Chesson, M.D.
Associate Dean for Academic Affairs
Lousiana State University
School of Medicine Shreveport
1501 Kings Highway
P.O. Box 33932
Shreveport, Louisiana 71130-3932

Michael Silber, M.B.Ch.B.
Associate Professor
Mayo Medical School
Mayo Clinic College of Medicine
200 First Street, S.W.
Rochester, Minnesota 55905

American Geriatrics Society

Evelyn Granieri, M.D., M.P.H.
Co-Chief, Division of Geriatric Medicine
Columbia University
College of Physicians & Surgeons
The Allen Pavilion 3-015
5141 Broadway
New York, New York 10034

American Medical Women's Association Foundation

Lynn Epstein, M.D., D.L.F.A.P.A., F.A.A.C.A.P.
Clinical Professor of Psychiatry
Tufts Medical Center
4 Longfellow Place, #2607
Boston, Massachusetts 02114

American Sleep Medicine Foundation

Andrew L. Chesson, M.D.
Associate Dean for Academic Affairs
Lousiana State University
1501 Kings Highway
P.O. Box 33932
Shreveport, Louisiana 71130-3932

Michael Silber, M.B.Ch.B.
Associate Professor
Mayo Medical School
Mayo Clinic College of Medicine
200 First Street, S.W.
Rochester, Minnesota 55905

NEUROLOGY

American Academy of Neurology

Deborah Joanne Lynn, M.D.
Department of Neurology
Ohio State University
College of Medicine & Public Health
1654 Upham Drive
451 Means Hall
Columbus, Ohio 43210

American Neurological Association

Richard T. Johnson, M.D.
Department of Neurology
Johns Hopkins University
School of Medicine
600 North Wolfe Street
Meyer 6-181
Baltimore, Maryland 21218

David Stumpf, M.D., Ph.D.
540 Judson Avenue
Evanston, Illinois 60202-3084

Association of University Professors of Neurology

James J. Corbett, M.D.
Professor and Chair
Department of Neurology
University of Mississippi
School of Medicine
2500 North State Street
Jackson, Mississippi 39216-4505

NEUROSURGERY

Society of Neurological Surgeons

Donald Quest, M.D.
Professor of Neurosurgery
Neurological Institute of New York
New York Presbyterian Hospital
710 W 168th St
New York, New York 10032

CAS Representatives

OBSTETRICS AND GYNECOLOGY

American College of Obstetricians and Gynecologists

Sharon T. Phelan, M.D.
Professor of Ob/GYN
Department of Ob/Gyn
University of New Mexico
School of Medicine
1 University of New Mexico
MSC 10 5580
Albuquerque, New Mexico 87131-0001

Robert J. Sokol, M.D.
Director for Human Growth and
Development
Wayne State University
School of Medicine
275 East Hancock Avenue
Detroit, Michigan 48201

American Society for Reproductive Medicine

PonJola Coney, M.D.
Sr. Assoc. Dean for Faculty Affairs
Virginia Commonwealth University
School of Medicine
Sanger Hall, Room 1022
Box 980565 1101 East Marshall Street
Richmond, Virginia 23298-0565

Association of Professors of Gynecology and Obstetrics

Alberto Manetta, M.D.
Senior Associate Dean for Educational
Affairs
University of California Irvine
College of Medicine
Medical Education Building 802
Irvine, California 92697-4089

Council of University Chairs of Obstetrics and Gynecology

Raul Artal, M.D.
Professor and Chair
Department of Ob/Gyn
Saint Louis University
6420 Clayton Road #290
St Louis, Missouri 63117-1811

William F. Rayburn, M.D., M.B.A.
Seligman Professor and Chair
Department of Obstetrics and Gynecology
University of New Mexico
School of Medicine
1 University of New Mexico
MSC 10 5580
Albuquerque, New Mexico 87131-0001

OPHTHALMOLOGY

American Academy of Ophthalmology

Linda Lippa, M.D.
Professor, Department
of Ophthalmology
University of California Irvine
College of Medicine
PO Box 16517
University of California
Irvine, California 92623-6517

Association of University Professors of Ophthalmology

Stuart L. Fine, M.D.
Professor of Ophthalmology
University of Pennsylvania
School of Medicine
51 North 39th Street
Philadelphia, Pennsylvania 19104

Robert E. Kalina, M.D.
Professor of Ophthalmology
University of Washington
School of Medicine
Box 356485
Seattle, Washington 98195

ORTHOPAEDICS

American Orthopaedic Association

Vincent D. Pellegrini Jr., M.D.
Professor and Chair
Department of Orthopaedics
University of Maryland
School of Medicine
22 S. Greene Street, Suite S11B
Room S11B
Baltimore, Maryland 21201

Eric L. Radin, M.D.
Professor, Orthopedic Surgery
Tufts University
School of Medicine
6 School Streets
Box 561
Marion, Massachusetts 02738-0010

OTOLARYNGOLOGY

Association of Academic Departments of Otolaryngology - Head and Neck Surgery

Lanny Garth Close, M.D.
Professor of Otolaryngology
Columbia University
College of Physicians & Surgeons
630 W. 168th Street., Box 21
Ph 11-131 STEM
New York, New York 10032

Scott Stringer, M.D.
Associate Vice Chancellor, Clinical
Affairs
Professor/Chair Otolaryngology
University of Mississippi
School of Medicine
2500 North State Street
Room L-216
Jackson, Mississippi 39216

Society of University Otolaryngologists/Head and Neck Surgeons

Mona Abaza
Department of Otolaryngology
University of Colorado
School of Medicine
12631 E. 17th Avenue, B-205
P.O. Box 6511
Aurora, Colorado 80045

PEDIATRICS

Academic Pediatric Association

Kathleen Nelson, M.D.
Sr. Assoc. Dean for Faculty Development
University of Alabama
School of Medicine
1530 3rd Ave South
SDB 102
Birmingham, Alabama 35294-0019

American Pediatric Society

Myron Genel, M.D.
Professor Emeritus of Pediatrics
Yale Child Health Research Ctr
Yale University
School of Medicine
333 Cedar Street, P.O. Box 208081
New Haven, Connecticut 06520-8081

Jimmy L. Simon, M.D.
Professor and Chairman Emeritus
Wake Forest University
School of Medicine
Medical Center Boulevard
Winston Salem, North Carolina 27157

Association of Medical School Pediatric Department Chairs

Jon S. Abramson, M.D.
Professor and Chair
Department of Pediatrics
Wake Forest University
School of Medicine
Medical Center Boulevard
Winston-Salem, North Carolina 27157

Russell W. Chesney, M.D.
Le Bonheur Professor and Chairman
Department of Pediatrics
University of Tennessee
Health Science Center
50 Dunlap Street
Memphis, Tennessee 38103

Society for Pediatric Research

Elena Fuentes-Afflick, M.D.
Professor of Pediatrics
University of California San Francisco
School of Medicine
1001 Potrero Avenue
Mail Stop 6E
San Francisco, California 94110

Thomas Green
Chair, Department of Pediatrics
Children's Memorial Hospital
2300 Children's Plaza
Chicago, Illinois 60614

PHARMACOLOGY - CLINICAL

American College of Neuropsychopharmacology

Eric Nestler, M.D.
Department of Psychiatry
University of Texas
Southwestern Medical School Dallas
5323 Harry Hines Boulevard
Dallas, Texas 75390-9070

Ronnie D. Wilkins, Ed.D.
Executive Director
American College of Neuropsychopharm
545 Mainstream Drive, Suite 110
Nashville, Tennessee 37228-1201

American College of Clinical Pharmacology

James F. Burris, M.D.
Chief Consultant for Geriatrics &
Extended Care
VAHS
810 Vermont Avenue NW (114)
Washington, DC 20420

Robert W. Piepho, Ph.D.
Dean, School of Pharmacy
University of Missouri Kansas City
5005 Rockhill Road
Kansas City, Missouri 64110-2499

American Society for Clinical Pharmacology and Therapeutics

Darrell Abernethy, M.D., Ph.D.
Chief Scientific Officer
U.S. Pharmacopeia
12601 Twinbrook Parkway
Rockville, Maryland 20852-1790

CAS Representatives

David W. Nierenberg, M.D.
Senior Associate Dean for Medical
Education
Dartmouth Medical School
DHMC, One Medical Center Drive
322 West, Borewell HB7506
Lebanon, New Hampshire 03756

PHYSICAL MEDICINE AND REHABILITATION

American Academy of Physical Medicine and Rehabilitation

Michael Boninger, M.D.
Professor and Research Director, PM&R
University of Pittsburgh
School of Medicine
3471 Fifth Avenue, Room 201
Kaufmann Medical Building
Pittsburgh, Pennsylvania 15261

Association of Academic Physiatrists

Ralph Buschbacher, M.D.
Chair, Department of PM&R
Indiana University
School of Medicine
Clinical Building Room 626
541 North Clinical Drive
Indianapolis, Indiana 46202-5111

Joel DeLisa, M.D., M.S.
Professor and Chair
Department of Physical Medicine and
Rehab.
UMDNJ-New Jersey Medical School
30 Bergen Street, Box 1709
Newark, New Jersey 07107-1709

PLASTIC SURGERY

American Association of Plastic Surgeons

Kenna S. Given, M.D.
Vice-Chairperson, Department of Surgery
Professor Emeritus
Medical College of Georgia
School of Medicine
1467 Harper Street
HB-5040
Augusta, Georgia 30912

Plastic Surgery Research Council

Matthew Klein
Associate Professor, Plastic Surgery
University of Washington
School of Medicine
Harborview Medical Center
Box 359796 - 325 9th Avenue
Seattle, Washington 98104

PREVENTIVE MEDICINE

Association for Prevention Teaching and Research

S. Edward Dismuke, M.D., MSPH
Dean and Professor
Department of Preventive Medicine
University of Kansas-Wichita
1010 N. Kansas Street
Wichita, Kansas 67214-3199

N. Lynn Eckhert, M.D., Dr.P.H.
Partners Harvard Medical International
Harvard Medical International
131 Dartmouth Street
Boston, Massachusetts 02116

PSYCHIATRY

American Association of Chairs of Departments of Psychiatry

Jed Magen, D.O.
Chair, Department of Psychiatry
Michigan State University
College of Human Medicine
A-222 East Fee Hall
East Lansing, Michigan 48824-1316

Michael J. Vergare, M.D.
Chair, Department Psychiatry & Human
Behavior Daniel Lieberman Professor
Jefferson Medical College
833 Chestnut East, Suite 210
Philadelphia, Pennsylvania 19107

American Association of Directors of Psychiatric Residency Training

Jed Magen, D.O.
Chair, Department of Psychiatry
Michigan State University
College of Human Medicine
A-222 East Fee Hall
East Lansing, Michigan 48824-1316

Sidney H. Weissman, M.D.
Professor of Psychiatry
Northwestern University Feinberg
School of Medicine
676 St. Clair Suite 1760
Chicago, Illinois 60611

American Psychiatric Association

Michael H. Ebert, M.D.
Associate Dean for Veterans Affairs
Yale University
School of Medicine
950 Campbell Avenue
West Haven, Connecticut 06516

Deborah J. Hales, M.D.
Director
Division of Education
American Psychiatric Association
1000 Wilson Blvd. Suite 1825
Arlington, Virginia 22209-3901

PSYCHOLOGY

Association of Psychologists in Academic Health Centers

Barry A. Hong, Ph.D.
Associate Professor of Psychiatry
and Medicine
Washington University in St Louis
School of Medicine
660 S. Euclid, Box 8134
St. Louis, Missouri 63110

Richard J. Seime, Ph.D.
Department of Psychiatry and
Psychology
Mayo Medical School
200 First Street, S.W.
GE M-W
Rochester, Minnesota 55905

RADIOLOGY

Association of University Radiologists

Jocelyn Deborah Chertoff, M.D.
Vice Chair
Assistant Dean for Clinical Affairs
Dartmouth Medical School
One Medical Center Drive
Lebanon, New Hampshire 03756-0001

Laurie L. Fajardo, M.D.
Professor and Chairman
Department of Radiology
University of Iowa Hospitals and Clinics
200 Hawkins Drive
Iowa City, Iowa 52242

Society of Chairs of Academic Radiology Departments

Laurie L. Fajardo, M.D.
Professor and Chairman
Department of Radiology
University of Iowa Hospitals and Clinics
200 Hawkins Drive
Iowa City, Iowa 52242

THORACIC SURGERY

American Association for Thoracic Surgery

Richard J. Shemin, M.D.
Chief, Div. of Cardiothoracic Surgery
University of California Los Angeles
Geffen School of Medicine
10833 Le Conte Avenue, 62-182 CHS
Los Angeles, California 90095

Graham Education and Research Foundation

Richard J. Shemin, M.D.
Chief, Div. of Cardiothoracic Surgery
University of California Los Angeles
Geffen School of Medicine
10833 Le Conte Avenue, 62-182 CHS
Los Angeles, California 90095

VASCULAR SURGERY

American Vascular Association Foundation

Caron Rockman, M.D.
Assistant Professor
New York University Medical Center
530 First Avenue #6F
New York, New York 10016

Society for Vascular Surgery

Caron Rockman, M.D.
Assistant Professor
New York University Medical Center
530 First Avenue #6F
New York, New York 10016

MULTISPECIALTY

American Headache Society

Alan Finkel, M.D.
Associate Professor of Neurology
University of North Carolina
School of Medicine
Clinical Sciences Building CB 7025
Chapel Hill, North Carolina 27599

Noah Rosen, M.D.
Director, NorthShore Headache Center
North Shore-Long Island Jewish
1554 Northern Boulevard, 4th Floor
Manhasset, New York 11030

American Medical Informatics Association

Paul N. Gorman, M.D.
Associate Professor
Medical Informatics and Clinical
Epidemiology
Oregon Health & Science
School of Medicine
3181 S.W. Sam Jackson Park Road
Portland, Oregon 97201-3098

American Medical Women's Association

Lynn Epstein, M.D., D.L.F.A.P.A., F.A.A.C.A.P.
Clinical Professor of Psychiatry
Tufts Medical Center
4 Longfellow Place, #2607
Boston, Massachusetts 02114

CAS Representatives

INTERDISCIPLINARY

American Society for Bioethics and Humanities

Joseph J. Fins, M.D., F.A.C.P.
Chief
Division of Medical Ethics
Weill Cornell Medical College
435 E 70 Street Ste 4J
New York, New York 10021

Association for the Behavioral Sciences and Medical Education

Lynn Epstein, M.D., D.L.F.A.P.A., F.A.A.C.A.P.
Clinical Professor of Psychiatry
Tufts Medical Center
4 Longfellow Place, #2607
Boston, Massachusetts 02114

Fredric W. Hafferty, Ph.D.
Professor
University of Minnesota
Medical School-Duluth
1035 University Drive
239 SMED
Duluth, Minnesota 55812

Association of Academic Health Sciences Libraries

Gary D. Byrd, Ph.D.
Director, Health Sciences Library
University at Buffalo
School of Medicine
3435 Main Street
Buffalo, New York 14214

Logan Ludwig, Ph.D.
Director, Media Development & Design
Health Science Library
Loyola University Medical Center
2160 South First Avenue
Bldg 101
Maywood, Illinois 60153

Society for Academic Continuing Medical Education

John R. Kues, Ph.D.
Assistant Dean for CME
University of Cincinnati
College of Medicine
P.O. Box 670582
College of Medicine
Cincinnati, Ohio 45267-0582

Stephen E. Willis, M.D.
Associate Dean, CME
East Carolina University Brody
School of Medicine
600 Moye Blvd., Venture Tower 210
Greenville, North Carolina 27834

Society of Directors of Research in Medical Education

LuAnn Wilkerson, Ed.D.
Senior Assoc Dean, Education
University of California Los Angeles
Geffen School of Medicine
10833 LeConte Avenue
Suite 60-048 CHS, Box 951722
Los Angeles, California 90095-1722

Council of Teaching Hospitals and Health Systems

2008–2009

Council of Teaching Hospitals and Health Systems Administrative Board, 2007-2008

Chair
Mark R. Laret*
University of California, San Francisco,
Medical Center
San Francisco, CA

Immediate Past Chair
Michael M.E. Johns, M.D.*
Emory University
Atlanta, GA

Chair-elect
Steve Lipstein*
BJC Healthcare
St. Louis, MO

Board Members

Gordon Alexander, M.D.
University of Minnesota Medical Center
Minneapolis, MN

Steven M. Altschuler, M.D.*
Children's Hospital of Philadelphia
Philadelphia, PA

Stanley Brezenoff
Continuum Health Partners, Inc.
New York, NY

Kenneth J. Clark
Department of Veterans Affairs VISN 22
Long Beach, CA

Deborah W. Davis
Virginia Commonwealth University
Medical Center
Richmond, VA

Dean M. Harrison*
Northwestern Memorial Hospital
Chicago, IL

Linda Hunt*
St. Joseph Hospital and Medical Center
Phoenix, AZ

Donna Katen-Bahensky
University of Iowa Hospitals and Clinics
Iowa City, IA

Robert J. Laskowski, M.D.
Christiana Care Health Services
Wilmington, DE

Marvin O'Quinn
Jackson Memorial Hospital
Miami, FL

Christopher Olivia, M.D.
Cooper University Hospital
Camden, NJ

Peter F. Rapp
Oregon Health & Science University
Portland, OR

Michael Riordan
Greenville Hospital System
Greenville, NC

Bruce Schroffell
University of Colorado Hospital
Aurora, CO

Karen H. Sexton, Ph.D.
University of Texas Medical Branch
Hospitals at Galveston
Galveston, TX

Kevin J. Sexton
Holy Cross Hospital
Silver Spring, MD

AHA Representative
James D. Bentley, Ph.D.
American Hospital Association
Washington, DC

* Representative to the AAMC Executive Council

331

MEMBER HOSPITALS

UNITED STATES

ALABAMA

Birmingham

Birmingham Veterans Affairs Medical Center
700 South 19th Street
Birmingham, Alabama 35233

Y. C. Parris, Chief Executive Officer	205/558-4726
Alan Tyler, Associate Director	
Mary Mitchell, Chief, Fiscal Service	205/933-4486
Susan J. Laing, Ph.D., Associate Chief of Staff for Education	205/933-8701
Donald Cox, Quality Management/Improvement Director	205/933-8101

Affiliation: University of Alabama School of Medicine

UAB Health System University of Alabama at Birmingham
500 22nd Street South
Suite #408
Birmingham, Alabama 35233-0500

David Hoidal, CEO, UAB Health System	205/975-5362
Mary Beth Briscoe, Chief Financial Officer	205/975-5413
Joan Hicks, Chief Information Officer	205/934-4724
Kathleen Kauffman, Legal Counsel	205/975-4844

Affiliation: University of Alabama School of Medicine

University of Alabama Hospital
619 South 19th Street
Birmingham, Alabama 35249-6505

Michael Waldrum, Chief Executive Officer	205/975-5138
Marybeth Briscoe, Chief Financial Officer	205/975-5413
Eli I. Capilouto, D.M.D., Provost	205/934-4720
Joan Hicks, Chief Information Officer	205/934-4724
W. John Daniel, University Counsel	205/934-3474
Deborah Grimes, Director of JCAHO/Regulartoy Compliance	205/975-3334

Affiliation: UAB Health System University of Alabama at Birmingham

Mobile

University of South Alabama Medical Center
2451 Fillingim Street
Mobile, Alabama 36617

Stan Hammack, V.P. Hospital Affairs	251/660-5595
A. Anderson, Chief Operating Officer	251/471-7110
William Bush, Chief Financial Officer	251/660-5596
Robert A. Kreisberg, M.D., Vice President, Medical Affairs Dean	251/460-7189
Susan Ankersen, Manager of Hospital Information Systems	251/434-3675
Sue Carney, Director, Quality Assurance	251/471-7418

Affiliation: University of South Alabama College of Medicine

ARIZONA

Phoenix

Banner Good Samaritan Medical Center
1111 East McDowell Road
Phoenix, Arizona 85062

Larry E. Volkmar, Chief Executive Officer 602/239-2716
Kathleen Kotin, Chief Financial Officer 602/239-4232
Alan I. Leibowitz, M.D., Chief Academic Officer 602/239-2296
Mike Warden, Senior Vice President Care Management &
   Quality 602/495-6353
David Bixby, Sr. VP/General Counsel 602/495-4130
John Hensing, M.D., Senior Vice President, Medical Affairs 602/747-4477
Anita Hancock, Director, QMS 602/239-6990
Affiliation: Bannerhealth

Bannerhealth
1441 North 12th Street
Phoenix, Arizona 85006

Peter Fine, President/CEO 623/327-4000
Affiliation: University of Arizona College of Medicine

Department of Veterans Affairs Veterans Integrated Service Network VISN 18
6590 East Williamsfield Road
Phoenix, Arizona 85212

Maricopa Medical Center
2601 East Roosevelt
Phoenix, Arizona 85008

Betsey Bayless, CEO 602/344-5566
Ann Thompson, Chief Operating Officer 602/239-4399
Ken Meinke, Vice President, Finance 305/585-7122
Phil Kelly, Interim Chief Information Officer 602/344-8576
Louis Gorman, County Counsel 602/506-8541
James Kennedy, M.D., Interim CEO Chief Medical Officer 602/344-5503
Affiliation: Mayo Medical School

Mayo Clinic Hospital~AZ
5777 East Mayo Boulevard
Phoenix, Arizona

Phoenix Children's Hospital
1919 East Thomas Street
Phoenix, Arizona

Robert Meyer, President and Chief Executive Officer 602/546-0400
Shane Brophy, Chief Financial Officer 602/546-0394
Affiliation: University of Arizona College of Medicine

St. Joseph's Hospital & Medical Center CHW Arizona-Nevada
350 West Thomas Road
Phoenix, Arizona 85013

Linda Hunt, President 602/406-6001
Patty White, R.N., Chief Operating Officer 602/406-3613
John Peters, VP / CFO 602/406-4618
Charles C. Daschbach, M.D., Director, Medical Education 602/406-3677
Joan Shapiro, Ph.D., VP Academic Affairs & Research 602/406-3499
Gayle V. Simkin, Chief Information Officer 602/307-2777
Sharon Lewis, CHWVP, Division General Counsel 602/406-3374
Robert Wilton Pryor, M.D., Chief Medical Officer 254/724-5359

Affiliation: Catholic Healthcare West

Scottsdale

Scottsdale Healthcare-Osborn
7400 East Osborn Road
Scottsdale, Arizona

Tucson

Southern Arizona Veterans Affairs Health Care System
Tucson, Arizona 85723

Jonathan H. Gardner, Chief Executive Officer 520/629-1821
Spencer Ralston, Chief Operating Officer 520/629-1821
Larry Korn, Financial Manager 520/629-1813
Jayendra H. Shah, M.D., Chief Medical Officer 520/629-1815

Affiliation: University of Arizona College of Medicine

University Medical Center~AZ
1501 N. Campbell
Tucson, Arizona 85724

Gregory A. Pivirotto, President/CEO 520/694-6148
Kevin Burns, Chief Financial Officer 520/694-4082
Sam Miller, Chief Information Officer 520/694-4790
James Richardson, In-House Counsel 520/694-6508
Andreas Theodorou, M.D., Medical Director 520/626-5485
Karin Toci, Director, Quality and Outcomes Management 520/694-2635

Affiliation: University Medical Center Health System; University of Arizona
College of Medicine

ARKANSAS

Little Rock

Arkansas Children's Hospital
800 Marshall Street
Little Rock, Arkansas 72202

Jonathan R. Bates, M.D., Chief Executive Officer/President 501/364-8000
Scott Gordon, Executive Vice President/COO 501/364-1414
Gena Wingfield, Senior Vice President/CFO 501/364-2555
Darrell Leonhardt, Senior Vice President/CIO 501/364-6002
Sherry Furr, Vice President, Legal Affairs 501/364-4862
Bonnie Taylor, M.D., Senior Vice President/Medical
Director 501/364-1401
Patti Higginbotham, R.N., Vice President, Quality
Management 501/364-4394
Affiliation: University of Arkansas for Medical Sciences College of Medicine

Central Arkansas Veterans Healthcare System
4300 W. 7th Street
Little Rock, Arkansas 72205

Michael Whinn, Medical Center Director 501/257-1000
Sallie Houser-Hanfelder, Associate Medical Center Director 501/257-5400
William D. White, M.D., Associate Chief of Staff for
Education 501/257-5300
Jim Hall, Acting Chief Information Officer 501/257-1522
Ronald H. Dooley, Regional Counsel 615/695-4622
Nicholas P. Lang, M.D., Chief Medical Officer 501/686-8111
Jennifer Purdy, Manager Quality Mangement 501/257-5314
Affiliation: University of Arkansas for Medical Sciences College of Medicine

University of Arkansas for Medical Sciences
4301 West Markham Street
Little Rock, Arkansas 72205

Richard A. Pierson, Vice Chancellor for Clinical Programs 501/686-5662
Melissa Fontaine, Chief Operating Officer 501/686-8955
Daniel Riley, Chief Financial Officer 504/686-8496
Kari L. Cassel, Chief Information Officer 501/686-6954
Robert Bishop, Vice Chancellor for Institutional Compliance 501/686-5699
Charles W. Smith, M.D., Executive Associate Dean UAMS
College of Medicine 501/686-8153
Barbara Warren, Project Specialist Quality Management
Department
Affiliation: University of Arkansas for Medical Sciences College of Medicine

CALIFORNIA

Bakersfield

Kern Medical Center
1830 Flower Street
Bakersfield, California 93305

Peter K. Bryan, Chief Executive Officer 661/326-2102
Fred Plane, Chief Financial Officer 661/326-2681
Jose A. Perez Jr., M.D., Director of Medical Education 661/326-2839
Karen Barnes, Deputy County Counsel 661/326-2029
Marvin Kolb, M.D., Medical Director 661/326-2217
Dianne McConnehey, Quality Improvement Manager 661/326-2696

Affiliation: University of California, Irvine, School of Medicine; University of
California, San Diego, School of Medicine; University of California,
Los Angeles, David Geffen School of Medicine

Duarte

City of Hope National Medical Center
1500 E. Duarte Road
Duarte, California

Michael A. Friedman, President and CEO 626/256-4673
Dennis Rusch, Chief Financial Officer 626/930-5445

Affiliation: University of California, Los Angeles, David Geffen School of
Medicine

Fresno

Community Regional Medical Center
2823 Fresno St.
Fresno, California

La Jolla

Scripps Green Hospital
10666 N. Torrey Pines Road
La Jolla, California 92037

Robin Brown, Administrator 858/554-3174
Linda Hodges, Associate Administrator 858/626-6398
John Armstrong, Regional Fiscal Director 858/626-7600
Stanley D. Freedman, M.D., Chair, Department of Graduate
Medical Education 858/459-5902
Robert Sarnoff, M.D., Chief of Staff 858/554-8862
Miriam Glendon, Director, PI/Risk Management 858/554-3600

Affiliation: Scripps Health

Loma Linda

Jerry L. Pettis Memorial Veterans Affair Medical Center
11201 Benton Street
Loma Linda, California 92357

Dean R. Stordahl, Director 909/583-6002
John M. Byrne, D.O., Assoc VP Med Aff for Education 909/583-6004
Shane Elliott, Chief Information Officer 909/583-6042
Jonathan Zirkle, J.D., Attorney, Regional Counsel 909/583-6297
Dwight Evans, M.D., Chief of Staff 909/583-6007
Patricia Zappia, R.N., HlthCare Quality Improv Coord 909/583-6171
Affiliation: Loma Linda University School of Medicine

Loma Linda University Medical Center
11234 Anderson Street
P.O. Box 2000
Loma Linda, California 92354

Ruthita Fike, Chief Executive Officer 909/558-4308
Kevin Lang, CFO and Treasurer 909/558-7570
Kent Hansen, General Counsel 909/558-2644
Daniel Giang, M.D., Associate Dean/Director of GME 909/558-8479
James Pappas, Vice President, Quality & Patient Safety 909/558-4637
Affiliation: Loma Linda University School of Medicine

Long Beach

Department of Veterans Affairs Veterans Integrated Service Network VISN 22
5901 E. Seventh Street
Long Beach, California 90822

Kenneth J. Clark, Network Director(10N22) 562/826-5968

Long Beach Memorial Medical Center
2801 Atlantic Avenue
Long Beach, California 90801

Byron Schweigert, CEO 562/933-1807
Ross Simmonds, Chief Operating Officer 562/933-1116
Wendy Dorchester, Senior Vice President/CFO 562/933-1900
Michael Nageotte, Executive Director for Medical Education 562/933-2738
J. Scott Joslyn, Senior Vice President/CIO 562/933-9419
Robert E. Siemer, J.D., General Counsel 562/933-9045
S. Gainer Pillsbury, M.D., Medical Director 562/933-1244
Casey Hudson, Executive Director Resource Management 562/933-0017
Affiliation: University of California, Irvine, School of Medicine

Members: CALIFORNIA

Veterans Affairs Long Beach Healthcare System
5901 E. 7th Street
Long Beach, California 90822

Ronald B. Norby, Medical Center Director 562/826-5400
Ada I. Neale, Associate Director 562/826-5401
Charles Feistman, Chief, Resources Health Care Group 562/826-5460
Kathleen Frechen, Acting Chief Academic Officer 562/826-5627
Michael Mitchell, Chief, Information Resource Management 562/826-5457
Sandor Szabo, M.D., Ph.D., Chief of Staff 562/826-5403
Susan Kulvinskas, Acting PI Coordinator 562/826-5419

Affiliation: University of California, Irvine, School of Medicine

Los Angeles

Cedars-Sinai Medical Center
8700 Beverly Boulevard
Los Angeles, California 90048

Thomas M. Priselac, President/CEO 310/423-5711
Mark Gavens, Senior VP/COO 310/423-6211
Edward Prunchunas, Senior Vice President/CFO 310/423-2312
Shlomo Melmed, M.D., Senior Vice President for Academic
    Affairs & Director of Burns and Allen 310/423-4691
Steve Reeves, Interim CIO 310/423-6642
Peter E. Braveman, Senior Vice President, Legal Affairs 310/423-5708
Michael L. Langberg, M.D., Senior Vice President, Medical
    Affairs/Chief Medical Officer 310/423-5147
Neil Romanoff, M.D., Vice President for Medical Affairs 310/423-3666

Affiliation: University of California, Los Angeles, David Geffen School of
    Medicine

LAC + USC Medical Center
1200 N. State Street
Los Angeles, California 90033

Pete Delgado, Chief Executive Officer 323/226-2800
Steve Matthews, Ph.D., Acting, Chief Operating Officer 323/226-5991
Henry Ornelas, Acting CEO 323/226-3162
Lawrence Opas, Associate Dean for GME Chief, Department
    of Pediatrics 323/226-3691
Stephanie L. Hall, M.D., Chief Medical Officer 323/226-6738

Affiliation: Keck School of Medicine of the University of Southern California

UCLA Healthcare
10833 LeConte Avenue
Los Angeles, California 90095

UCLA Medical Center

10833 Le Conte Avenue
Los Angeles, California 90095

Amir Rubin, Chief Operating Officer 310/206-9003
Paul Staton, CFO
J. Thomas Rosenthal, M.D., Chief Medical Officer 310/825-4686
Theodore Barry, Quality Management/Improvement
Director

Affiliation: UCLA Healthcare; University of California, Los Angeles, David
Geffen School of Medicine

USC University Hospital

1500 San Pablo Street
Los Angeles, California 90033

Debbie Walsh, Chief Executive Officer 323/442-8467
Strawn Steele, Chief Financial Officer 323/442-8444
Michael Jones, Medicaid Relationships Director/General
Counsel 714/428-6873
Steven Giannotta, M.D., Medical Director 323/442-8654
Mary Kingsley, Quality and Risk Management 323/442-8479

Affiliation: Keck School of Medicine of the University of Southern California;
Tenet Healthcare Corporation

Veterans Affairs Greater Los Angeles Health Care System

11301 Wilshire Boulevard
Los Angeles, California 90073

Donna M. Beiter, Director 310/268-3132
Arthur Friedlander, D.M.D., ACOS/Education 310/268-3155
Dean C. Norman, M.D., Chief of Staff, Based Services 310/268-3132

Affiliation: Keck School of Medicine of the University of Southern California;
University of California, Los Angeles, David Geffen School of
Medicine

Mare Island

VA Sierra Pacific Network (10N21) Department of Veterans Affairs VISN 21

201 Walnut Avenue
Mare Island, California 94592

Robert L. Wiebe, M.D., Network Director(10N21) 707/562-8350

Oakland

Kaiser Permanente Med Ctr Northern California

1950 Franklin Street, 20th Floor
Oakland, California

Gregory A. Adams, Northern CA President 510/987-3699
George Halvorson, Chief Financial Officer 510/271-5910

Members: CALIFORNIA

Orange

University of California, Irvine, Medical Center
101 The City Drive
Orange, California 92868

Maureen Zehntner, Interim Director 714/456-6922
Ron King, CFO 714/456-6885
Joy Grosser, Chief Information Officer Information Systems 714/456-5558
Eugene M. Spiritus, M.D., Medical Director 714/456-6844
Mary Owen, Director, Case Management 714/456-8964
Affiliation: University of California, Irvine, School of Medicine

Palo Alto

Veterans Affairs Palo Alto Health Care System
3801 Miranda Avenue
Palo Alto, California 94304

Elizabeth Joyce Freeman, Director 650/493-5000
John Sisty, Associate Director 650/493-5000
Melvin Niese, Chief, Fiscal Service 650/493-5000
John Pollard, M.D., Associate Chief of Staff for Education 650/493-5000
Peg Graham, Chief Information Officer 650/493-6000
Barbara A. Konno, Attorney at Law Office of Regional
Counsel 415/750-2288
Javaid I. Sheikh, Chief of Staff 650/493-5000
Affiliation: Stanford University School of Medicine

Pasadena

Huntington Memorial Hospital
100 West California Boulevard
Pasadena, California 91109-7013

Steve A. Ralph, President and CEO 626/397-5555
Bill Murin, VP, COO 626/397-5555
James Noble, VP, CFO 626/397-5555
Tim Kirk, Chief Information Officer 626/397-5300
Affiliation: Keck School of Medicine of the University of Southern California

Sacramento

University of California, Davis, Health System
2315 Stockton Boulevard
Sacramento, California 95817

Ann Rice, Chief Executive Officer 916/734-0751
William McGowan, Acting Chief Executive Officer 916/734-9129
Claire Pomeroy, M.D., M.B.A., Vice Chancellor for Human
Health Sciences and Dean 916/734-7131
Guy Koppel, Assoc Dir/Chief Information Officer 916/734-3866
Anna Orlowski, Hospital Counsel 916/734-2288
Allan Siefkin, M.D., Medical Director, UC Davis Medical Ctr 916/734-1166
Affiliation: University of California, Davis, School of Medicine

San Diego

Scripps Health
4275 Campus Point Drive
Suite 220
San Diego, California 92121
    Chris Van Gorder, Chief Executive Officer 858/678-7200
    Richard Sheridan, General Counsel 858/678-7226
Affiliation: University of California, San Diego, School of Medicine

UCSD Healthcare
200 West Arbor Drive, MC 8986
San Diego, California 92103-8986
    Richard J. Liekweg, Chief Executive Officer 619/543-6654
Affiliation: University of California, San Diego, School of Medicine

University of California, San Diego, Medical Center
200 West Arbor Drive
San Diego, California 92103-8970
    Richard J. Liekweg, Chief Executive Officer 619/543-6654
    Mona Sonnenshein, Chief Operating Officer
    Robert Hogan, Chief Financial Officer 619/543-6060
    Tom McAfee, M.D., Dean of Clinical Affairs 619/543-5338
    Edward Babakanian, Director, Information Systems 619/543-6880
    Angela Scioscia, Medical Director 619/543-2699
    Andrea Snyder, Director, PIPS 619/543-6475
Affiliation: UCSD Healthcare

Veterans Affairs San Diego Healthcare System
3350 La Jolla Village Drive
San Diego, California 92161
    Gary Rossio, Director 858/552-8585
    Debra Dyer, Chief Information Officer 858/552-8585
    Eric Lazare, General Counsel 619/400-5240
    Jacqueline G. Parthemore, M.D., Chief of Staff 858/552-8585
    Janet Tremblay, R.N., Chief, Performance Improvement
    Management 858/552-8585
Affiliation: University of California, San Diego, School of Medicine

San Francisco

California Pacific Medical Center
P. O. Box 7999
San Francisco, California 94120
    Martin Brotman, M.D., President/CEO 415/600-3575
    Jack Bailey, Executive Vice President/COO 415/923-3339
    John Gates, Chief Financial Officer 415/600-6519
    Jerry Padavano, Chief Information Officer 415/750-6405
Affiliation: University of California, San Francisco, School of Medicine

Members: CALIFORNIA

Catholic Healthcare West
185 Berry Street, Suite 300
San Francisco, California 94111

Lloyd Dean, President/CEO 415/438-5500
Michael Erne, Chief Operating Officer, Catholic Health Care
West/CEO, St. Joseph's Hospital and Medical 602/406-3101
Michael Blaszyk, CFO 415/438-5500
Affiliation: University of Arizona College of Medicine; University of California,
San Francisco, School of Medicine

Community Health Network
2789 25th Street
Second Floor
San Francisco, California 94110

San Francisco General Hospital and Medical Center
1001 Potrero Avenue
San Francisco, California 94110

Gene O'Connell, Executive Administrator 415/206-3517
Ken Jensen, Chief Financial Officer 415/206-7848
Philip Hopewell, M.D., Associate Dean 415/206-8509
Robert Brody, M.D., Chief Information Officer 415/206-8267
Kathy Murphy, Legal Counsel 415/206-2380
Affiliation: Community Health Network; University of California, San Francisco,
School of Medicine

UCSF Medical Center
500 Parnassus Avenue
San Francisco, California 94143-0296

Mark R. Laret, Chief Executive Officer 415/353-2733
Tomi S. Ryba, Chief Operating Officer 415/353-2735
Kenneth Jones, Chief Financial Officer 415/353-2742
Larry Lotenero, Chief Information Officer 415/353-4273
Marcia Canning, Chief Campus Counsel 415/476-5003
Ernest Ring, Chief Medical Officer 415/353-2760
Betsy Stone, M.P.H., Mr.P.H., Director, Quality
Improvement 415/353-3017
Affiliation: University of California, San Francisco, School of Medicine

San Jose

Santa Clara Valley Health and Hospital Systems
751 South Bascom Avenue
San Jose, California 95128

Robin Roche, Acting Director 408/885-4004
Kim Roberts, Chief Financial Officer 408/885-6868
David Kerns, M.D., Chief Medical Officer 408/885-4001
Robert Feldman, Chief Information Officer 408/885-5356
Dolly Goel, M.D., Medical Director 408/885-5105
Carolyn Brown, Director, Performance and Outcomes Mgmt. 408/885-5105
Affiliation: Santa Clara Valley Health Hospital System

Santa Barbara

Tenet Healthcare Corporation
3820 State Street
Santa Barbara, California 93105

Trevor Fetter, Chief Executive Officer 469/893-6175
Reynold Jennings, Chief Operating Officer 469/893-2790
Bob Smith, SVP, Regional Operations 469/893-2200
W. Randolph Smith, Senior Vice President, Central and
Northeast Divisions 215/255-7408
Affiliation: Creighton University School of Medicine; Louisiana State University
School of Medicine in New Orleans; Keck School of Medicine of
the University of Southern California; Drexel University College of
Medicine

Stanford

Stanford Hospital and Clinics
300 Pasteur Drive
Stanford, California 94305

Martha H. Marsh, President and CEO Hospital and Clinics 650/723-8542
Michael J. Peterson, Chief Operating Officer 650/723-8542
Eugene A. Bauer, M.D., President/CEO 650/723-5708
Carolyn Byerly, Chief Information Officer 650/723-3992
Peter Gregory, M.D., Senior Associate Dean for Clinical
Affairs 650/723-9673
Larry Shuer, Chief of Staff 650/725-3038
Kim Purdini Kiely, R.N., Director Quality Improvment &
Patient Safety 650/736-2191
Affiliation: Stanford University School of Medicine

Torrance

Harbor-UCLA Medical Center
1000 W Carson Box 27 PO Box 2910
Torrance, California 90509

Miguel Ortiz-Marroquin, Interim Chief Executive Officer 210/222-2101
Jody Nakasuji, Chief Financial Officer 210/222-3004
Affiliation: University of California, Los Angeles, David Geffen School of
Medicine

COLORADO

Denver

Children's Hospital~CO
1056 East 19th Avenue, Box 020
Denver, Colorado 80218

Jim Shmerling, President/CEO 720/777-6091
Dick Argys, Executive Vice President/COO 303/861-6822
David Kirschner, Chief Financial Officer 617/355-6881
M. Douglas Jones, M.D., Chief Academic Officer
    Pediatrician-in-Chief 303/837-2766
Jim Turnbull, Chief Information Officer 303/861-6822
Peter Durante, M.D., J.D., Senior Vice President, Medical
    and Legal Affairs 303/861-6654
Affiliation: University of Colorado School of Medicine

University of Colorado Hospital
13001 East 17th Place
PO Box 6508
Mail Stop F417
Denver, Colorado 80010

Bruce Schroffel, President and CEO 720/848-7833
Forrest Cason, Senior Vice President, Finance/CFO 303/724-5209
Gregory Stiegmann, M.D., Vice President, Clinical Affairs 303/315-5526
Stephen P. Clark, Ph.D., Vice President, Information
    Services 303/724-5100
Allen W. Staver, Esq., Vice President and General Counsel/
    Secretary to the Board of Directors 303/724-5295
Steven P. Ringel, M.D., President, Medical Staff 303/315-7221
Affiliation: University of Colorado School of Medicine

Veterans Affairs Eastern Colorado Health Care System
1055 Clermont Street
Denver, Colorado 80220

Lynette Ross, Medical Center Director 303/393-2800
Eliott Vanderstek, Director, Business Office 303/331-5976
Thomas Meyer, M.D., Associate Chief of Staff, Academic
    Affiliations 303/393-2880
Leigh Anderson, Chief of Staff 303/393-2820
Jan Kemp, R.N., Acting Quality Management Coordinator 303/393-4650
Affiliation: University of Colorado School of Medicine

Glendale

Department of Veterans Affairs Veterans Integrated Service Network VISN 19
Mountain Towers, Suite 510
4100 E. Mississippi Avenue
Glendale, Colorado 80222

CONNECTICUT

Bridgeport

Bridgeport Hospital
267 Grant Street
Bridgeport, Connecticut 06610

Robert J. Trefry, President/CEO 203/384-3478
Hope Juckel Regan, Executive Vice President/COO 203/384-3338
Patrick McCabe, Senior Vice President, Finance 203/384-3775
Karen Anne Hutchinson, M.D., Director, Medical Education 203/384-3446
Mark Tepping, Acting Chief Information Officer 203/384-3619
Bruce M. McDonald, M.D., Senior Vice President, Medical
Affairs 203/384-3717

Affiliation: Yale University School of Medicine; Yale-New Haven Health System

Danbury

Danbury Hospital
24 Hospital Avenue
Danbury, Connecticut 06810

Frank J. Kelly, President/CEO 203/797-7403
Ronald Sperling, Chief Financial Officer 203/797-7403
Gerard D. Robilotti, Executive Vice President 203/797-7414
Peter Courtway, Chief Information Officer 203/730-5200
Michael Eisner, General Counsel, Wiggin & Dana 203/797-7110
Matthew Miller, M.D., Vice President, Medical Affairs 203/797-7966
Dawn Myles, Chief Quality Officer 203/797-7668

Affiliation: New York Medical College; University of Connecticut School of
Medicine; Yale University School of Medicine

Farmington

Univ of Connecticut Health Center/John Dempsey Hospital
263 Farmington Avenue
Farmington, Connecticut 06030-3802

Jim Thornton, Director, John Dempsey Hospital 860/679-2222
Daniel Upton, Chief Financial Officer 860/679-1145
Sandra Armstrong, Chief Information Officer 860/679-3855
William N. Kleinman, Esq., Assistant Attorney General 860/679-1114
Richard Simon, Professor of Surgery Division of
Neurosurgery 860/679-3533
Rhea Sanford, Quality Management Director 860/679-3519

Affiliation: University of Connecticut School of Medicine

Hartford

Hartford Hospital
80 Seymour Street
P. O. Box 5037
Hartford, Connecticut 06102.5037

John J. Meehan, President/CEO 860/545-2100
Kevin Hannifan, Executive Vice President/COO 860/545-2349
Elliott Joseph, President/CEO 860/696-6253
Neil S. Yeston, M.D., Vice President, Academic Affairs 860/545-2036
Stephan O'Neill, Chief Information Officer 860/545-3972
Joseph Klimek, Vice President, Medical Affairs 860/545-3501
Affiliation: University of Connecticut School of Medicine

Saint Francis Care
114 Woodland Street
Hartford, Connecticut 06105

Christopher M. Dadlez, President and CEO 860/714-5541
Affiliation: University of Connecticut School of Medicine

Saint Francis Hospital and Medical Center
114 Woodland Street
Hartford, Connecticut 06105

Christopher M. Dadlez, President and CEO 860/714-5541
Steven Rosenberg, Sr VP Finance/CFO for Finance/CFO 860/714-4812
Susan Freeman, M.D., Senior Vice President for Medical
Affairs 860/714-4361
David C. Stone, J.D., Director, Legal Services 860/714-4656
Michael Laurent Therrien, M.D., Director of Quality
Outcomes 860/714-4572
Affiliation: Saint Francis Care

New Britain

Central Connecticut Health Alliance Inc.
100 Grand Street
New Britain, Connecticut 06050

Laurence A. Tanner, President/CEO 860/224-5666
Affiliation: University of Connecticut School of Medicine

New Haven

Hospital of St. Raphael
1450 Chapel Street
New Haven, Connecticut 06511

David W. Benfer, President & CEO 203/789-3020
Lawrence McMannis, Vice President, Finance & CFO 203/789-3000
Charles E. Riordan, M.D., Vice President, Medical Affairs 203/789-4196
Gary R. Davidson, Chief Information Officer 203/789-5921
J.C. Lubin-Szafranski, Vice President/General Counsel
Corporate Compliance Officer 203/789-3336
Affiliation: Yale University School of Medicine

Yale-New Haven Health System
789 Howard Avenue
New Haven, Connecticut 06504

Marna P. Borgstrom, President and Chief Executive Officer 203/688-2608
Affiliation: Yale University School of Medicine

Yale-New Haven Hospital
20 York Street
New Haven, Connecticut 06504

Marna P. Borgstrom, President and Chief Executive Officer 203/688-2608
Richard Aquila, Executive Vice President & Chief Operating
Officer 203/688-2606
Steve Allegretto, Chief Financial Officer 203/688-5593
Peter Herbert, M.D., Senior Vice President, Medical Affairs 203/688-2604
Mark Andersen, Senior Vice President, Information Services 203/688-2100
Sarah D. Cohn, J.D., Executive Director, Legal Services 203/688-2291
Peter Herbert, M.D., Senior Vice President, Medical Affairs 203/688-2604
William Crede, M.D., Med Dir/CQI/Co-Director 203/688-2252
Affiliation: Yale University School of Medicine; Yale-New Haven Health System

Norwalk

Norwalk Hospital
Norwalk, Connecticut 06856

Geoffrey Cole, Chief Executive Officer 203/852-2211
Paul E. Nurick, Chief Operating Officer 203/852-3327
Daniel Debarba, Vice President of Finance/CFO 203/852-2000
Lynda Nemeth, R.N., Director, Quality Assurance 203/852-2732
Affiliation: Chicago Medical School at Rosalind Franklin University of Medicine
& Science

Stamford

Stamford Health System
P. O. Box 9317
Stamford, Connecticut 06904

Brian G. Grissler, President/CEO 203/325-5555
Affiliation: Columbia University College of Physicians and Surgeons

Stamford Hospital
Shelburne Road & West Broad Street
P.O. Box 9317
Stamford, Connecticut 06904

Brian G. Grissler, President/CEO 203/325-5555
Kathleen A. Silard, Senior Vice President, Operations 203/325-7505
John Ansorge, Sr. Vice President - Finance Chief Financial
Officer 203/276-7463
Noel I. Robin, M.D., Physician-in-Chief 203/276-7485
Affiliation: Columbia University College of Physicians and Surgeons; Stamford
Health System

West Haven

Veterans Affairs Connecticut Health Care System
950 Campbell Avenue
West Haven, Connecticut 06516

Roger L. Johnson, Director 203/937-3888
Karen Waghorn, Chief Operating Officer 203/937-3889
Jeffrey Lustman, M.D., Associate Chief of Staff 203/937-3827
Joseph Erdos, M.D., Chief Information Officer 203/932-5711
Michael Ebert, M.D., Chief of Staff 203/937-3825

Affiliation: Yale University School of Medicine

DELAWARE

Newark

Christiana Care Health System
P.O. Box 1668
Newark, Delaware 19899

Robert J. Laskowski, M.D., President and Chief Executive
Officer 302/428-2570
Gary W. Ferguson, M.P.H., Chief Operating Officer 302/733-1321
Thomas Corrigan, Senior VP, Finance/Managed Care and
CFO 302/623-7205
Brian W. Little, M.D., Ph.D., VP, Academic Affairs/Research 302/733-1042
Steve Hess, Senior VP, Information Services/CIO 302/324-3628
Brenda K. Pierce, J.D., R.N., Corporate Counsel, Legal
Affairs 302/428-4568
Jim H. Newman, Chief Medical Officer 302/733-1049
Sharon Anderson, R.N., Senior VP, PI and Care
Management 302/733-1203

Affiliation: Jefferson Medical College of Thomas Jefferson University

Wilmington

Veterans Affairs Medical and Regional Office Center
1601 Kirkwood Highway
Wilmington, Delaware 19805

Richard S. Citron, Medical Center Director 302/633-5201
Loci Barbanel, Chief Financial Officer/Resource 302/633-5432
Tom Tierney, Chief Information Officer 302/633-5496
Morris D. Kerstein, M.D., Chief of Staff 302/633-5203

Affiliation: Jefferson Medical College of Thomas Jefferson University; University
of Maryland School of Medicine

DISTRICT OF COLUMBIA

Washington

Children's National Medical Center
111 Michigan Avenue, N.W.
Washington, District of Columbia 20010

Edwin K. Zechman Jr., President/CEO 202/884-5402
Jody M. Burdell, Vice President & Cheif Operating Officer 202/884-3924
Mark L. Batshaw, M.D., Chief Academic Officer/Chairman
of Pediatrics 202/884-4007
Kelly Styles, Chief Information Officer 202/884-3792
Raymond S. Sczudlo, Vice President & Chief Legal Officer 202/884-4502
Peter Holbrook, M.D., Chief Medical Officer 202/884-3256
Kathleen Chavanu, Director, Performance Improvement and
Case Management 202/884-4750
Affiliation: George Washington University School of Medicine and Health
Sciences

George Washington University Hospital
2131 K Street, NW
Washington, District of Columbia 20037

Richard J. Becker, M.D., Chief Executive Officer 202/715-4006
Trent Crable, Chief Operating Officer 202/715-4016
Richard Davis, Chief Financial Officer 202/715-4006
John F. Williams Jr., M.D., Provost and Vice President for
Health Affairs School of Medicine & Health Sciences 202/994-3727
Gretchen Tegethoff, Chief Information Officer 202/715-4440
Bruce Gilbert, General Counsel 800/347-7750
Carlos Silva, Medical Director 202/715-4016
Affiliation: George Washington University School of Medicine and Health
Sciences; Universal Health Services, Inc. George Washington
University Hospital

Georgetown University Hospital
3800 Reservoir Road, N.W.
Washington, District of Columbia 20007
Affiliation: Georgetown University School of Medicine; MedStar Health

Howard University Hospital
2041 Georgia Avenue, N.W.
Washington, District of Columbia 20060

Larry Warren, Chief Executive Officer 202/865-6660
John Grish, Chief Financial Officer 202/865-6660
Alem Moges, Interim Director, Management Services Interim
Director, Management Services 202/865-6781
Natasha Mckenzie, Senior Associate General Counsel for
Health Affair 202/806-8650
Thomas E. Gaiter, M.D., Medical Director/Associate Dean
for Clinical Affairs 202/865-6698
Linda Robertson, Director, Quality Management 202/865-6704
Affiliation: Howard University College of Medicine

Universal Health Services, Inc. George Washington University Hospital

901 23rd Street, NW
Washington, District of Columbia 20037

Alan B. Miller, President/Chairman of the Board 800/347-7750

Affiliation: George Washington University School of Medicine and Health
Sciences

Veterans Affairs Medical Center

50 Irving Street, NW
Washington, District of Columbia

Veterans Affairs Office of Academic Affiliations (144)

1800 G Street, NW, Room 872
Washington, District of Columbia

Malcolm Cox, M.D., Chief Academic Affiliations Officer 202/357-4010

Washington DC Veterans Affairs Medical Center

50 Irving Street, N.W.
Washington, District of Columbia 20422

Sanford M. Garfunkel, Medical Center Director 202/745-8100
Nancy A. Thompson, Ph.D., Associate Director, VHA Office
of Special Projects 202/745-2200
Richard Pasquale, Chief, Resource Management 202/745-8229
Galen L. Barbour, M.D., Director, Planning, Education and
Performance Improvement Services 202/745-8416
F. Joseph Dagher, M.D., Chief of Staff 202/745-8225

Affiliation: George Washington University School of Medicine and Health
Sciences

Washington Hospital Center

110 Irving Street, N.W.
Washington, District of Columbia 20010

James F. Caldas, President 202/877-6102
Daniel Macksood, Chief Financial Officer 202/877-6147
James Howard, M.D., Vice President for Academic Affairs 202/877-5285
Kenda Tavakoli, Chief Information Officer
Robert Ryan, General Counsel/CCO MedStar Health 410/772-6833
Janis M. Orlowski, M.D., Senior Vice President/Chief Med.
Officer 202/877-5284
Christina M. Emrich, R.N., Quality Resource Coordinator 202/877-2085

Affiliation: George Washington University School of Medicine and Health
Sciences; Howard University College of Medicine; MedStar Health

FLORIDA

Bay Pines

Department of Veterans Affairs Veterans Integrated Service Network VISN 8

10000 Bay Pine Road
Building 24-Room 305
Bay Pines, Florida 33744

Michela Zbogar, Network Director 727/319-1126

Gainesville

North Florida/South Georgia Veterans Health Care System-Malcom Randall VA Medical Center
1601 SW Archer Road
Gainesville, Florida 32608

Thomas A. Cappello, Director, FACHE 404/728-7601
Thomas J. Sutton, Associate Director 352/374-6012
Wendy Daughter, Chief Financial Officer 352/337-2330
Craig Kitchens, Associate Chief of Staff for Education 352/376-1611
Deborah Michel-Ogborn, Chief Information Officer 352/376-1611
Ann Barnett, Attorney, Office of Regional Counsel 352/376-1611
Bradley S. Bender, M.D., Chief of Staff 352/374-6018
Richard E. Walker, Chief, Performance Improvement 352/379-4071
Affiliation: University of Florida College of Medicine

Shands Healthcare
1600 S.W. Archer Road
P.O. Box 100326
Gainesville, Florida 32610

Timothy M. Goldfarb, Chief Executive Officer 352/265-8929
Jodi J. Mansfield, Executive Vice President/COO 352/265-0440
William Robinson, Sr VP/Treasurer 352/265-0429
Timothy C. Flynn, M.D., Interim Sr Assoc Dean-Clinical
Affairs 352/273-7520
Joan Hovhanesian, Sr. VP/Chief Information Officer 352/265 8317
Paul M. Rosenberg, Senior Vice President/General Counsel 352/265-6995
Nicholas J. Cassisi, M.D., Senior Associate Dean for Clinical
Affai 352/265-0429
Debbie Lynn, Director, Quality and Accreditation Shands
Healthcare 352/265-0002
Affiliation: University of Florida College of Medicine

Jacksonville

Mayo Clinic Hospital~FL
4500 San Pablo Road
Jacksonville, Florida

Shands Jacksonville Medical Center
655 W. 8th Street
Jacksonville, Florida 32209

Jim Burkhart, President & Administrator 904/244 3002
Scott Metheny, Chief Financial Officer 904/244-1828
Guy Benrubi, Chief Academic Officer 904/244-3112
Bill Hastede, Director of Information Services 904/244-4846
Mary J. Berger, J.D., Senior Attorney 904/244-1281
David Vukich, Chief Medical Officer & Vice President 904/244-6340
Joni Lourcey, Dir Quality/Risk Managment 904/244-3477
Affiliation: University of Florida College of Medicine

Members: FLORIDA

St. Luke's Hospital~FL
4201 Belfort Road
Jacksonville, Florida 32216

Robert M. Walters, Chair, Department of Administration 904/296-3700
Hilary Mathews, R.N., Administrator 904/296-3796
Mary Hoffman, Chief Financial Officer 904/953-2171
Anthony Windebank, Keith D. Lindor 507/284-3268
Cheryl Croft, Director, Information Sevices 904/953-0447
Stephen Nelson, General Counsel 904/953-2827
Charles Burger, Medical Director 904/296-3713

Affiliation: Florida State University College of Medicine; Mayo Medical School

Miami

Jackson Memorial Hospital
1611 N.W. 12th Avenue
Miami, Florida 33136

Marvin O'Quinn, President and Chief Executive Officer 305/585-6754
Steven M. Klein, Executive Vice President/Chief Operating
Officer 305/585-1111
Frank Barrett, Executive Vice President/CFO 305/585-7137
James S. Phillips, Senior Vice President/CIO 305/585-7137
Eugene Shy, Assistant County Attorney 305/585-1313
Alan Livingstone, M.D., Professor & Chairman DeWitt
Daughtry Family Dept. of Surgery 305/585-1284

Affiliation: University of Miami Leonard M. Miller School of Medicine

Miami Veterans Affairs Medical Center
1201 N.W. 16th Street
Miami, Florida 33125

Mary D. Berrocal, Director 305/324-4455
Paul D. Magalian, Associate Director 305/575-3203
Sandra Cole, Chief Financial Officer 305/575-3115
Gwendolyn Findley, Ph.D., Acting Chief, IRMS 305/324-4455
John R. Vara, M.D., Chief of Staff 305/575-3157
Kathleen Coniglio, Chief, QMPI 305/324-4289

Affiliation: University of Miami Leonard M. Miller School of Medicine

Miami Beach

Mount Sinai Medical Center
4300 Alton Road
Miami Beach, Florida 33140

Steven D. Sonenreich, Chief Executive Officer 305/674-2223
Amy Perry, Senior Vice President & Chief Operating Officer 305/674-2520
Alex Mendez, Sr. VP and Chief Financial Officer Officer 305/674-2089
Paul Katz, M.D., VP, Academic Affairs and Research 305/674-2633
Tom Gilette, Vice President and Chief Information Officer 305/674-5445
Arnold Jaffee, General Counsel 305/674-2444
Kenneth Ratzan, M.D., Director, Medical Services 305/674-2766
Natasha Oyarzun, Director, Performance Improvement 305/674-2484

Affiliation: University of Miami Leonard M. Miller School of Medicine;
University of South Florida College of Medicine

Orlando

Florida Hospital Orlando
601 East Rollins Street
Orlando, Florida

Lars Houmann, President and CEO 407/303-1531
Affiliation: Florida State University

Orlando Health
1414 Kuhl Avenue
MP 56
Orlando, Florida 32806

John Hillenmeyer, President/CEO 321/841-5203
Sherrie Sitarik, Executive Vice President 321/841-5111
Bob Miles, Vice President, Financial Planning Budge 321/843-1046
Jay L. Falk, M.D., Chief Academic Medical Officer 407/237-6324
Rick Schooler, Vice President and CIO 321/841-5233
Timothy Bullard, M.D., Chief Medical Officer 321/848-4242
Stephan J. Harr, Senior Vice President 407/481-7256
Affiliation: Florida State University College of Medicine

St. Petersburg

All Children's Hospital
801 Sixth Street South
St. Petersburg, Florida 33701

Gary Carnes, President/CEO 727/767-4474
Arnold Stenberg, Senior Vice President, Finance 727/898-7451
Joel Momberg, Senior Vice President, Marketing and
Community Relations 813/892-4193
Jack Hutto, M.D., Senior Vice President, Medical Affairs 813/892-8656
Affiliation: University of South Florida College of Medicine

Tampa

H. Lee Moffitt Cancer Center and Research Institute
12902 Magnolia Drive
Tampa, Florida 33612

William Dalton, M.D., Director/CEO 813/615-4261
Nicolas C. Porter, Associate Center Director for
Administration 813/745-7277
Jack Kolosky, EVP Planning & Finance/CFO Finance/CFO 813/979-7222
S. C. Schold, Assoc. Dir. Clinical Affairs 813/745-7424
Edward Martinez, Chief Information Officer
W. Michael Alberts, M.D., Chief Medical Officer 813/979-7236
Affiliation: University of South Florida College of Medicine

Tampa General Hospital

P.O. Box 1289
Tampa, Florida 33601

Ronald A. Hytoff, President/CEO 813/844-7662
Steve Short, Exec VP, Finance and Administration 813/253-4805
J. Thomas Danzi, M.D., Senior V.P., Chief Medical Officer 813/844-7218
Ginger Oliver, VP, Chief Information Officer 813/844-4845
Jim Kennedy, Attorney 813/222-8185
Chuck Bombard, Director of Quality Improvement 813/844-4097

Affiliation: University of South Florida College of Medicine

Veterans Affairs Medical Center James A. Haley Veterans Hospital

13000 Bruce B. Downs Boulevard
Tampa, Florida 33612

Stephen M. Lucas, Medical Center Director 813/972-7536
Steven W. Young, Associate Director 813/972-7626
Ariel Rodriguez, M.D., Associate Chief of Staff for Education 813/972-7649
Carolyn Clark, Public Affairs Officer 813/979-3645
Thomas E. Bowen, M.D., Chief of Staff 813/972-7537
Janet Webb, Chief, Quality Management 813/972-7695

Affiliation: University of South Florida College of Medicine

GEORGIA

Atlanta

Atlanta Medical Center

303 Parkway Drive, N.E.
Atlanta, Georgia 30312

William T. Moore, Chief Executive Officer 404/265-6155
Kem M. Mullins, Chief Operating Officer 404/265-4857
William Masterton, Chief Financial Officer 404/265-4301
Steven L. Saltzman, M.D., Sr. Vice President and Medical
    Director 404/265-4600
Maryland McCarty, Director, Information Systems 404/265-6034
Lea Gardner, Director, Quality/Risk Management 404/265-3762

Affiliation: Medical College of Georgia School of Medicine; Tenet Healthcare
    Corporation

Children's Healthcare of Atlanta

1600 Tullie Circle
Atlanta, Georgia 30329

Donna Hyland, Senior Vice President/COO 404/785-6000
Jay E. Berkelhamer, M.D., Senior Vice President Medical
    Affairs 404/785-7007

Affiliation: Emory University School of Medicine

Children's Healthcare of Atlanta (Includes Egleston and Scottish Rite)
1405 Clifton Road, N.E.
Atlanta, Georgia 30322

Donna Hyland, Senior Vice President/COO 404/785-6000
Beth Howell, Senior Vice President Academic Medicine 404/785-7526
Ruth Fowler, Senior Vice President/CFO 404/250-5437
Jay E. Berkelhamer, M.D., Senior Vice President Medical
Affairs 404/785-7007
Jack Storey, Chief Information Officer 404/929-8737
Dale Hetzler, Vice President General Counsel 404/785-7522
Affiliation: Children's Healthcare of Atlanta

Crawford Long Hospital of Emory University
550 Peachtree Street, N.E.
Atlanta, Georgia 30365-2225

John T. Fox, President and Chief Executive Officer 404/778-4432
Albert K. Blackwelder, COO, Emory Crawford Long Hospital 404/686-2450
Dee Cantrell, Chief Information Officer 404/727-3604
Jane Jordan, Deputy General Counsel Chief Health Counsel 404/712-1512
Harold S. Ramos, M.D., Medical Director 404/686-8111
William A. Bornstein, M.D., Chief Quality Officer 404/686-2821
Affiliation: Emory Healthcare

Department of Veterans Affairs Veterans Integrated Service Network VISN 7
2200 Century Parkway, NE-Suite 260
Atlanta, Georgia 30345

Emory Healthcare
1440 Clifton Road NE
Atlanta, Georgia 30722

Fred Sanfilippo, M.D., Ph.D., Executive VP for Health
Affairs and CEO Woodruff Health Sciences Center 404/778-3500
Jimmy Hatcher, Chief Financial Officer of Emory Healthcare 404/686-7529
Affiliation: Emory University School of Medicine

Emory University Hospital
1364 Clifton Road, N.E.
Atlanta, Georgia 30322

John T. Fox, President and Chief Executive Officer 404/778-4432
Robert J. Bachman, Chief Operating Officer 404/686-8500
Mark Aycock, Director, Financial Services Chief Financial
Officer 404/686-7519
Dee Cantrell, Chief Information Officer 404/727-3604
Jane Jordan, Deputy General Counsel Chief Health Counsel 404/712-1512
Robert B. Smith III, M.D., Medical Director 404/712-7371
William A. Bornstein, M.D., Chief Quality Officer 404/686-2821
Affiliation: Emory Healthcare

Members: GEORGIA

Grady Memorial Hospital-Atlanta, GA
80 Jesse Hill Jr Drive, S.E.
Atlanta, Georgia 30335

Michael A. Young, President & Chief Executive Officer 404/616-1000
Timothy Jefferson, Executive Vice President/COO 404/616-6162
Michael Ayers, Chief Financial Officer/Vice President 404/616-7104
Richard Hergert, Chief Information Officer/Vice President 909/558-3995
Curtis A. Lewis, Senior Vice President for Medical Affairs 404/616-4261
Judy Molette, Dir Quality/Utilization Mgmt 404/616-7751

Affiliation: Emory University School of Medicine; Morehouse School of
Medicine

Augusta

Augusta Veterans Affairs Medical Center
One Freedom Way
Augusta, Georgia 30904-6285

Rebbecca Wiley, Director 706/733-0188
Ralph R. Angelo, Associate Director 706/823-2225
Walter Hitch, Chief, Fiscal Department 706/733-0188
Elizabeth Northington, Augusta Informatics Manager 706/733-0188
Thomas W. Kiernan, M.D., Chief of Staff 706/733-0188
Ellen W. Harbeson, Quality Management Coordinator 706/733-0188

Affiliation: Medical College of Georgia School of Medicine

MCG Health, Inc.
1120 15th Street
Augusta, Georgia 30912

Donald F. Snell, President/CEO 706/721-6569
Patricia K. Sodomka, Executive Vice President/COO 706/721-3924
Dennis Romer, Senior Vice President/CFO 706/721-3929
Daniel W. Rahn, M.D., President 706/721-2301

Affiliation: Medical College of Georgia School of Medicine

Medical College of Georgia Hospital and Clinics
1120 15th Street
Augusta, Georgia 30912

Donald F. Snell, President/CEO 706/721-6569
Dennis Romer, Senior Vice President/CFO 706/721-3929
Barry D. Goldstein, Ph.D., Provost 706/721-4014
Hal Scott, Vice President/CIO 703/721-9674
Virginia Roddy, General Counsel 706/721-5709
Ralph John Caruana, M.D., Sr. Vice President/CMO 706/721-7348
Patricia Sodomka, SVP Patient Family Centered Care 706/721-3924

Affiliation: MCG Health, Inc.

Decatur

Veterans Affairs Medical Center (Atlanta)
1670 Clairmont Road
Decatur, Georgia 30033

James A. Clark, Chief Operating Officer 404/728-7602
Vince Covington, Acting Chief Financial Officer 404/728-7685
Norberto Fas, Chief Academic Officer 404/321-6111
Antonia Mohamed, Chief Information Officer 404/321-6111
David Bower, M.D., Chief of Staff 404/728-7604
Gladys Felan, Quality Managerment/Improvement Director 404/321-6111
Affiliation: Emory University School of Medicine

Macon

Central Georgia Health Systems
691 Cherry Street
Macon, Georgia 31201

A. Don Faulk, President/CEO 478/633-1450
Affiliation: Mercer University School of Medicine

Medical Center of Central Georgia
777 Hemlock Street
PO Box 6000
Macon, Georgia 31208-6000

A. Don Faulk, President/CEO 478/633-1450
Michael Gilstrap, Executive Vice President/COO 478/633-1152
Rhonda Perry, Senior Vice President 478/633-1452
Madison O. Mock, Vice President and CIO Adminsitration 478/633-2473
Ken Banks, General Counsel 478/633-6980
Louis W. Goolsby, M.D., Senior Vice President/Associate
  Dean 478/633-1115
Steve Barry, PI/RM 478/633-7932
Affiliation: Central Georgia Health Systems; Mercer University School of
  Medicine

Savannah

Memorial Health University Medical Center
4700 Waters Avenue
Savannah, Georgia 31404

Margaret M.C. Gill, Senior Vice President, Operations 912/350-8515
Jeff Treasure, Sr Vice President and CFO 608/782-7300
Edward E. Abrams, D.Ed., Exec Dir & Associate Dean 912/350-8302
Steven Stanic, VP, Information Services & CIO 912/350-8081
Joseph Ross, Esq., Senior VP Corporate Legal Counsel 912/350-5159
Ramon Meguiar, M.D., Sr V.P. & Chief Medical Officer 912/350-9456
Affiliation: Emory University School of Medicine; Medical College of Georgia
  School of Medicine; Mercer University School of Medicine;
  Memorial Health, Inc.

Members: GEORGIA-ILLINOIS

Memorial Health, Inc.
4700 Waters Avenue
Savannah, Georgia 31404

Affiliation: Emory University School of Medicine; Medical College of Georgia
School of Medicine; Mercer University School of Medicine

ILLINOIS

Chicago

Advocate Illinois Masonic Medical Center
836 Wellington Ave
Chicago, Illinois 60657

Susan Nordstrom Lopez, President 773/296-7081
Larry Wrobel, Vice President Operations 773/296-7004
Jack Gilbert, Vice President Finance 773/296-7809
William Werner, M.D., Designated Institutional Officer 773/296-5888
Adem Arslani, Director, Information Systems 773/296-8022
Michael E. Kerns, Vice President, Legal Counsel 630/990-5026

Affiliation: Advocate Health Care; Chicago Medical School at Rosalind Franklin
University of Medicine & Science

Children's Memorial Hospital
2300 Children's Plaza
Chicago, Illinois 60614

Patrick Magoon, M.A., President & CEO 773/880-4008
Gordon Bass, Chief Operating Officer 773/880-4010
Paula Noble, Treasurer/CFO 773/880-3978
Sharon M. Unti, M.D., Asst Prof, Res Prog Dir 773/880-4302
Stanley B. Krok, Chief Information Officer 773/880-4939
Donna Wetzler, General Counsel 773/880-3934
Edward Ogata, M.D., Chief Medical Officer 773/880-4012

Affiliation: Northwestern University The Feinberg School of Medicine

John H. Stroger Jr. Hospital of Cook County
1835 West Harrison Street
Chicago, Illinois 60612

Johnny Brown, Chief Operating Officer 312/864-5500
Michael Bernard, Chief Financial Officer 312/864-6000
Mike Sommers, Chief Information Officer 312/864-8060
Bradley Langer, M.D., Interim Medical Director 312/864-5100
Susan Klein, Director, Quality Assurance 312/864-0800

Affiliation: Loyola University Chicago Stritch School of Medicine

Mount Sinai Hospital~IL
California & 15th Streets
Chicago, Illinois 60608

> **Karen Teitelbaum,** Chief Executive Officer Executive Vice
> President/COO 773/257-5322
> **Charles Weis,** Chief Financial Officer 773/257-6642
> **Maurice A. Schwartz, M.D.,** Vice President, Medical Affairs 773/257-6971
> **Peter Ingram,** Vice President, Strategy and Information
> Systems 773/257-6541
> *Affiliation:* Chicago Medical School at Rosalind Franklin University of Medicine
> & Science

Northwestern Memorial Hospital
251 East Huron Street
Chicago, Illinois 60611

> **Dean M. Harrison,** President/CEO 312/926-3007
> **Dennis Murphy,** Executive Vice President 312/926-0882
> **Doug Young,** Chief Financial Officer 312/926-6953
> **Charles W. Watts, M.D.,** Senior Vice President, Medical
> Affairs 312/926-4774
> **Timothy Zoph,** Vice President, Information Services 312/926-3040
> **Rachel Dvorken,** Deputy Gernal Counsel 312/926-2236
> **Cynthia Barnard,** Director, Quality Strategies 312/926-4822
> *Affiliation:* Northwestern University The Feinberg School of Medicine

Rush System for Health
1653 W. Congress Parkway
Chicago, Illinois 60612

> **Larry J. Goodman, M.D.,** President and CEO 312/942-7073
> *Affiliation:* Rush Medical College of Rush University Medical Center

Rush University Medical Center
1653 W. Congress Parkway
Chicago, Illinois 60612

> **Larry J. Goodman, M.D.,** President and CEO 312/942-7073
> **Peter W. Butler,** Executive VP and Chief Operating Officer 312/942-8801
> **Catherine Jacobson,** Chief Financial Officer 312/942-5600
> **Thomas A. Deutsch, M.D.,** Dean, Rush Medical College,
> Provost, Rush Univ Senior VP, Medical Affairs, Rush Univ
> Med Ctr 312/942-5567
> **Luc Van Tran,** Senior Vice President/CIO 312/942-3400
> **Max Brown,** Vice President-Legal Affairs/General Co
> Counsel 312/942-6886
> **Marcia Hargreaves,** Assistant V. P., Quality Improvement 312/942-7116
> *Affiliation:* Rush Medical College of Rush University Medical Center; Rush
> System for Health

University of Chicago Hospitals and Health System
5841 South Maryland, MC1114
Chicago, Illinois 60637

University of Chicago Medical Center
5841 South Maryland, MC1114
Chicago, Illinois 60637

David Hefner, President & CEO 773/702-6240
Kenneth Kates, Chief Executive Officer 319/356-4752
Lawrence Furnstahl, Chief Financial Officer 773/834-5354
Eric Yablonka, Chief Information Officer 773/702-9665
Susan S. Sher, J.D., VP Legal/Governmental Affairs 773/834-2659
Christopher Clardy, Quality Management/Improvement
Director 773/702-6412

Affiliation: University of Chicago Division of the Biological Sciences The
Pritzker School of Medicine; University of Chicago Hospitals and
Health System

University of Illinois at Chicago Medical Center
1740 West Taylor Street
Chicago, Illinois 60612

John J. DeNardo, Executive Director 312/413-8202
Bernadette Biskup, Acting Medical Center Director 312/996-3909
William Devoney, Chief Financial Officer 312/996-3620
William H. Chamberlin, Chief Medical Officer 312/996-3893
Thomas R. Bearrows, University Counsel 312/996-7762
Maureen T. Perry, Director, Quality and Accreditation 312/996-7788

Affiliation: University of Illinois College of Medicine

Veterans Affairs Chicago Health Care System
333 East Huron Street
Chicago, Illinois

Richard S. Citron, Medical Center Director 302/633-5201
Richard Rooney, Acting Associate Director for
Administration 312/469-2240
Kalpana Mehta, Chief Fiscal Officer 708/202-2480
Howard Loewenstein, Chief, Information Resources
Management Service 312/569-6511
Brian Schmitt, M.D., Chief of Staff Lakeside Division 312/469-2101

Affiliation: Northwestern University The Feinberg School of Medicine

Evanston

Evanston Northwestern Healthcare
1301 Central Street
Evanston, Illinois 60201

Mark R. Neaman, President/CEO 847/570-5005
Jeff Hillebrand, Chief Operating Officer 847/570-5151
Thomas Hodges, Ex VP, Finance and Treasurer 847/570-5445
Ruric Anderson, M.D., GME Program Director 847/570-2509
Tom Smith, CIO, Information Services 847/570-5421
Janardan D. Khandekar, M.D., Chairman, Dept of Medicine 847/570-2510
Chyna Wilcoxson, Manager, Clinical Decision Support 847/570-1647

Affiliation: Northwestern University The Feinberg School of Medicine

Hines

Department of Veterans Affairs Veterans Integrated Service Network VISN 12
Fifth Avenue & Roosevelt Road
P.O.Box 5000, Building 18
Hines, Illinois 60141-5000

Edward Hines, Jr. Hospital Department of Veterans Affairs
P. O. Box 5000
Hines, Illinois 60141

Jack G. Hetrick, Director 708/202-2153
Jeff Gering, Associate Director 708/202-5637
Kalpana Mehta, Chief Fiscal Officer 708/202-2480
Barbara K. Temeck, M.D., Chief of Staff 708/202-2154
Gordon Brown, Chief, Information Resources Management 708/202-2432
Earl Parsons, Regional Counsel 708/202-2216
Affiliation: Loyola University Chicago Stritch School of Medicine

Maywood

Loyola University Health System
2160 South First Avenue
Maywood, Illinois 60153

Loyola University Medical Center
2160 South First Avenue
Maywood, Illinois 60153

Paul K. Whelton, M.D., M.B.Ch.B., BAO, MSc, President &
CEO 708/216-3215
Martin Massiello, Executive Vice President 708/216-9000
Sabrina Olsen, Chief Financial Officer 708/216-3404
Arthur J. Krumrey, VP and Chief Information Officer 708/216-8190
Charles E. Reiter III, Vice President/General Counsel,
Loyola University Health System 708/216-4220
William Cannon, Chief of Staff and Associate Dean, GME 708/216-4400
Affiliation: Loyola University Chicago Stritch School of Medicine; Loyola
University Health System

Oak Lawn

Advocate Christ Medical Center
4440 West 95th Street
Oak Lawn, Illinois 60453

Robert Pekofske, VP, Finance 708/346-5133
Robert N. Stein, M.D., Vice President, Medical Management 708/346-5007
Ann Sayvetz, General Counsel 630/990-5089
Leticia Losurdo, Manager, Performance Improvement 708/684-3036
Affiliation: Advocate Health Care

Oakbrook

Advocate Health Care
2025 Windsor Drive
Oakbrook, Illinois 60523

James H. Skogsbergh, President/CEO 630/572-9393
Tina Esposito, Manager, Business Analytics Center for
Health Information Services 630/990-5658
Affiliation: Chicago Medical School at Rosalind Franklin University of Medicine
& Science

Park Ridge

Advocate Lutheran General Hospital
1775 Dempster Street
Park Ridge, Illinois 60068

Bruce C. Campbell, Dr.P.H., President 847/723-8446
Julie W. Schaffner, R.N., Chief Operating Officer/Chief
Nurse Exec 847/723-6004
Susan Nibbe, Vice President, Finance 503/273-8020
Kris Narasimhan, M.D., Vice President, Medical Management 847/723-3024
Richard Erspamer, Director, Information Systems 847/723-2014
Michael E. Kerns, Vice President, Legal Counsel 630/990-5026
Affiliation: Advocate Health Care; Chicago Medical School at Rosalind Franklin
University of Medicine & Science

Peoria

OSF HealthCare System
800 NE Glen Oak Avenue
Peoria, Illinois 61637

James Moore, Chief Executive Officer 309/655-2039
Affiliation: University of Illinois College of Medicine

OSF Saint Francis Medical Center
530 NE Glen Oak Avenue
Peoria, Illinois 61637

Keith Steffen, Administrator 309/655-2439
Sue Wozniak, Chief Operating Officer 309/655-2668
Ken Harbaugh, Chief Financial Officer 309/671-4398
Tim Miller, M.D., Director of Academic and Medical Affairs 309/655-2244
Affiliation: OSF HealthCare System

Springfield

Hospital Sisters Health System
Sangamon Avenue
PO Box 19456
Springfield, Illinois 62769

Memorial Health System
701 N. First Street
Springfield, Illinois 62781

Memorial Medical Center
701 North First Street
Springfield, Illinois 62781

Edgar J. Curtis, President and CEO 217/788-3181
Robert Kay, Senior Vice President/CFO 217/788-3198
Kerra L. Guffey, Senior VP and Chief Information Officer 217/788-4083
Robert Vautrain, M.D., Medical Director 217/788-3135
James Bente, Vice President Quality Resources 217/788-3685
Affiliation: Memorial Health System

St. John's Hospital
800 East Carpenter Street
Springfield, Illinois 62769

Richard Carlson, Executive Vice President 217/544-6464
Greg Weller, Interim Chief Financial Officer 217/544-6464
Gordon Lashmett, Director, Information Systems 217/544-6464
Rick Wilderson, General Counsel 217/523-4569
Ronald Deering, M.D., Medical Director 217/544-6464
Michelle McCarthy, R.N., Division Director, Quality Resource
Management 217/544-6464
Affiliation: Hospital Sisters Health System

INDIANA

Indianapolis

Clarian Health Partners, Inc.
I-65 at 21st Street
P.O. Box 1367
Indianapolis, Indiana 46206

Daniel F. Evans Jr., President/CEO 317/962-5900
Samuel L. Odle, Chief Operating Officer 317/929-8641
Marvin Pember, Executive Vice President/CFO 317/962-3005
Eric Williams, M.D., Exec. Vice President-Academic Affairs 317/962-0551
Rich Johnson, VP/CIO 317/962-8796
Norman Tabler, Senior Vice President/General Counsel 317/962-3306
Richard Graffis, M.D., Executive Vice President and CMO 317/962-8258
Susan McAlister, Director, Nurs Quality and Reg Comp 317/278-6925
Affiliation: Indiana University School of Medicine

Members: INDIANA

Richard L. Roudebush Veterans Affairs Medical Center
1481 W. 10th Street
Indianapolis, Indiana 46202

Susan P. Bowers, Acting Medical Center Director/CEO 317/554-0000
Thomas Mattice, Associate Medical Center Director 317/554-0128
Paul Pessagno, Chief, Fiscal Service 317/554-0000
Diane Wiesenthal, Ed.D., Chief Education Officer, Education
Service 317/554-0000
John Burke, Chief Information Officer, Information
Management Services 317/554-0000
John Houff, District Counsel 317/226-7876
Kenneth Klotz, M.D., Chief of Staff 317/554-0412
Mary Ann Payne, Chief, Quality Management 317/554-0000
Affiliation: Indiana University School of Medicine

St. Vincent Hospitals and Health Services, Inc.
2001 W. 8th Street
Indianapolis, Indiana 46240

Vincent C. Caponi, Chief Executive Officer 317/338-7000
Lynne O'Day, Senior Vice President, Delivery Systems 317/338-2882
Ian Worden, Chief Financial Officer 317/338-7074
Robert M. Lubitz, M.D., Director of Medical Education 317/338-6386
Hall Render Killian, Hospital Legal Counsel 317/338-3218
Daniel LeGrand, M.D., President Medical Staff 317/338-2161
Carol Fridlin, Director, Quality Review 317/338-3957
Affiliation: Indiana University School of Medicine

Wishard Health Services
1001 West 10th Street
Indianapolis, Indiana 46202

Lisa E. Harris, M.D., Chief Executive Officer and Medical
Director 317/630-7033
Jim N. Hayman, Chief Operating Officer 317/630-6785
Lee Livin, EVP and Chief Financial Officer 317/630-7033
David J. Shaw, Chief Information Officer 317/630-2487
Jessica Barth, Chief Counsel 317/630-6425
Affiliation: Indiana University School of Medicine

Muncie

Cardinal Health System, Inc.
2401 West University Avenue
Muncie, Indiana 47303

Kelly Stanley, President and Chief Executive Officer 765/747-3393
Robert Gildersleeve, Executive VP/Chief Financial Officer 765/747-3205
Thomas Powers, Vice President Information Systems 765/751-5065
Michael J. Hawkins, J.D., Director Risk Management &
Corporate Compliance 765/751-5000
Affiliation: Indiana University School of Medicine

IOWA

Des Moines

Iowa Health - Des Moines
1200 Pleasant Street
Des Moines, Iowa 50308

Eric Crowell, President & CEO 515/241-6396
David Stark, Executive VP and COO 515/253-3501
Joseph Corfits, Senior VP and CFO 515/241-6507
Douglas B. Dorner, M.D., Senior VP, Med Ed and Research 515/241-5901
Sid Ramsey, Vice President, Business Development 515/263-5375
David Burlage, Associate Counsel 515/241-4651
Mark Purtle, VP of Medical Affairs 515/241-5100
Kathie Nessa, Director of Quality 515/263-5448
Affiliation: University of Iowa Roy J. and Lucille A. Carver College of Medicine

Iowa City

Iowa City Veterans Affairs Medical Center
601 Highway 6 West
Iowa City, Iowa 52246

Barry Sharp, Director 319/338-0581
Gary Million, Quality Management Officer 319/338-0581
Terri Schuchard, Chief Financial Officer 319/338-0581
Steve Breese, Chief Academic Officer 319/338-0581
Nancy Johnson, Staff Attorney/Office of Regional Counsel 515/284-4092
Kevin Dellsperger, Medical Director
Andrea Moen, Quality Management/Improvement Director 319/339-7173
Affiliation: University of Iowa Roy J. and Lucille A. Carver College of Medicine

University of Iowa Hospitals and Clinics
200 Hawkins Drive, 1353 JCP
Iowa City, Iowa 52242

Gordon D. Williams, Interim CEO 319/356-3155
Ann Madden Rice, Chief Executive Officer 916/734-3096
Ken Fisher, Associate Vice President for Finance 319/384-2844
Jean E. Robillard, M.D., Vice President for Medical Affairs 319/335-8064
Lee T. Carmen, Director, Health Care Information Systems 319/356-4445
William Hesson, Associate Director/ Legal Counsel 319/356-4009
Charles M. Helms, M.D., Ph.D., Chief of Staff 319/356-1570
Affiliation: University of Iowa Roy J. and Lucille A. Carver College of Medicine

KANSAS

Westwood

University of Kansas Hospital
2330 Shawnee Mission Parkway, Suite 308
Westwood, Kansas 66160
Bob Page-Adams, President and Chief Executive Officer 913/588-1270
Scott Glasrud, Senior Vice President/CFO 913/945-5464
H. William Barkman, M.D., Chief of Staff 913/588-1200
Affiliation: University of Kansas School of Medicine

KENTUCKY

Lexington

Lexington Veterans Affairs Medical Center
2250 Leestown Road
Lexington, Kentucky 40511
Forest Farley, Hospital Director 813/972-7536
Walter Zawisza, Acting Chief Fiscal Service 859/233-4511
James R. McCormick, M.D., Associate Chief of Staff for
Education 859/281-4914
June Heligrath, Chief Information Management Service 606/281-5985
Daniel Reese, Chief of Staff 606/281-4902
Linda Cranfill, Quality Management and Improvement
Coordinator 606/281-4901
Affiliation: University of Kentucky College of Medicine

University of Kentucky Hospital
800 Rose Street
Lexington, Kentucky 40536
Murray Clark, AVP Opertions 859/323-5470
Sergio Melgar, Chief Financial Officer 859/323-0053
Zed Day, Chief Information Officer 859/257-1114
Edmund J. Benson, J.D., Associate Counsel 859/323-1161
A. Bryon Young, Medical Director 859/257-6467
Louise White, Quality Management Director 859/323-8062
Affiliation: University of Kentucky College of Medicine

Louisville

Jewish Hospital and St. Mary's Healthcare System
217 E. Chestnut Street
Louisville, Kentucky 40202
Robert Shircliff, President and Chief Executive Officer 502/587-4310
Affiliation: University of Louisville School of Medicine

Louisville Veterans Affairs Medical Center

800 Zorn Avenue
Louisville, Kentucky 40206

Michael R. Winn, Associate Director 318/424-6088
Babs Roberts, Chief, Fiscal Service 502/287-6256
Stephanie Mayfield, Associate Chief of Staff for Education 502/287-6871
Augustine M. Bittner, Chief Information Officer 502/287-6977
David Busse, J.D., District Counsel 502/287-6122
Marylee Rothschild, Acting Chief of Staff 502/287-6200

Affiliation: University of Louisville School of Medicine

U of L Health Care University Hospital

530 S. Jackson Street
Louisville, Kentucky 40202

James Taylor, President/CEO 502/562-4002
Robert Barbier, CFO 502/562-4004
Troy May, CIO, Information Systems 502/562-3637
John Johnson, General Counsel 502/587-3400
Kay Lloyd, Vice President, Operations Improvement 502/562-4584

Affiliation: University of Louisville School of Medicine

LOUISIANA

Baton Rouge

Baton Rouge General Medical Center

3600 Florida Boulevard
Baton Rouge, Louisiana 70806

William Holman, President/CEO 225/387-7767
Dionne Viator, Senior Vice President and CFO 225/763-4040
Floyd J. Roberts Jr., M.D., Chief Medical Officer 225/387-7767
Lisa Lejeune, Chief Information Officer 225/387-7000
Catherine Nobile, General Counsel
Cindy Munn, Admin Director Quality Mgmt 225/387-7767

Affiliation: General Health System; Tulane University School of Medicine

General Health System

3600 Florida Boulevard
Baton Rouge, Louisiana 70806

William Holman, President/CEO 225/387-7767

Affiliation: Louisiana State University School of Medicine in New Orleans;
Tulane University School of Medicine

Our Lady of The Lake Regional Medical Center

5000 Hennessy Boulevard
Baton Rouge, Louisiana

K. Scott Wester, Chief Executive Officer 225/765-8866
Robert Ramsey, CFO 225/765-6306
John Clifford, Medical Director, GME 225/765-1955

Members: LOUISIANA

Kenner

Kenner Regional Medical Center
180 West Esplanade Avenue
Kenner, Louisiana 70065

Paolo Zambito, Chief Executive Officer 504/464-8065
Mark Eckert, Chief Financial Officer 504/464-8065
Affiliation: Tenet Healthcare Corporation

New Orleans

Medical Center of Louisiana at New Orleans
2021 Perdido Street
New Orleans, Louisiana 70112

Colleen Colligan, Chief Financial Officer 504/903-1012
Wayne Wilbright, M.D., Head, Medical Informatics &
    Telemedicine 504/903-3985
Cathi Fontenot, M.D., Medical Director
Affiliation: Louisiana State University School of Medicine in New Orleans;
    Tulane University School of Medicine

Ochsner Clinic Foundation
1514 Jefferson Highway
New Orleans, Louisiana 70121

Patrick J. Quinlan, M.D., Chief Executive Officer 504/842-4051
Warner Thomas, Executive Vice President Chief Operating
    Officer 504/842-4598
Scott Posecai, Executive Vice President Chief Financial
    Officer 504/842-4097
William W. Pinsky, M.D., Chief Academic Officer 504/842-6120
Lynn R. Witherspoon, M.D., Vice President Chief
    Information Officer 504/842-3582
Cristina Wheat, Counsel , Leg Aff/Risk Mgmt 504/842-4003
Affiliation: Louisiana State University School of Medicine in New Orleans;
    Tulane University School of Medicine

Southeast Louisiana Veterans Health Care System
1601 Perdido Street
New Orleans, Louisiana 70112-1262

Julia Calvalier, President 504/556-7218
Fernando O. Rivera, Associate Medical Center Director 504/589-5238
Patricia Smith, Chief Financial Officer 504/412-3700
Paul S. Rosenfeld, M.D., Chief of Staff 504/589-5214
Karen Merrill, Director, Clinical Information Mgmt. S/L 504/619-4083
Andree' Boudreaux, District Counsel 504/619-4541
Harry Pigman, M.D., Associate COS for Performance Imp. 504/589-5241
Affiliation: Louisiana State University School of Medicine in New Orleans;
    Tulane University School of Medicine

Touro Infirmary

1401 Foucher Street
New Orleans, Louisiana 70115

Leslie Hirsch, President and CEO 504/897-8246
Robert Ficken, Chief Financial Officer 504/897-8344
Peter Dougherty, Director, Information Services 504/897-8297
Kevin T. Jordan, Director of Medical Affairs ED Medical
Director 504/897-8392
Michelle Delatte, Director, Quality Assurance & Utilization
Review 504/897-8779

Affiliation: Louisiana State University School of Medicine in New Orleans;
Tulane University School of Medicine

Tulane University Hospital & Clinic

1415 Tulane Avenue
New Orleans, Louisiana 70112

Robert Lynch, CEO 504/988-1595
Andre duPlessis, Chief Operating Officer 504/988-1902
Robert Hatcher, Chief Financial Officer 504/988-6606
Sue Rachuig, Director, Information Services 504/988-2884
Tammy Friloux, Associate Vice President 504/988-5410

Affiliation: Tulane University School of Medicine

Shreveport

Overton Brooks Veterans Affairs Medical Center

510 E. Stoner Avenue
Shreveport, Louisiana 71101

George Moore, Medical Center Director 318/424-6037
Kimberly Lane, Fiscal Officer 318/221-8411
John Leavitt, Ph.D., Chief, Education and Training 318/424-6119
Michael Vesta, Chief, Information Resources Management 311/424-6155
Patrick Keen, Staff Attorney 318/424-6196
Lloyd G. Phillips, M.D., Ph.D., Chief of Staff 318/424-6089
Kathryn L. Brooks, Chief, Performance Improvement 318/424-6141

Affiliation: Louisiana State University School of Medicine in Shreveport

MAINE

Portland

Maine Medical Center

22 Bramhall Street
Portland, Maine 04102

Richard W. Petersen, President and Chief Executive Officer 207/662-4466
John Heye, Vice President for Finance 207/662-2654
George Higgins III, M.D., Assoc Dean Maine Affairs & CMO 207/662-2776
Paul Gray, Vice President, Planning 207/662-2451
Donald E. Quigley, J.D., General Counsel 207/725-7010
Deb Tollotson, Director of Center for Performance
Improvement (CRI) 207/662-4681

Affiliation: University of Vermont College of Medicine

MARYLAND

Baltimore

Franklin Square Hospital
9000 Franklin Square Drive
Baltimore, Maryland 21237

Carl J. Schindelar, President 443/777-7000
Eric L. Conley, Vice President, Operations 443/777-7115
Robert Lally, Chief Financial Officer 443/777-7248
Anthony Sclama, Vice President, Medical Affairs 443/777-7298
Patricia Norstrand, Senior Director Department of Quality,
Risk and Safety 443/777-7039
Affiliation: Georgetown University School of Medicine; Johns Hopkins
University School of Medicine; MedStar Health

Johns Hopkins Bayview Medical Center
4940 Eastern Avenue
Baltimore, Maryland 21224

Gregory Schaffer, President 410/550-0123
Richard Bennett, Executive Vice President/COO 410/550-0781
Carl Francioli, Chief Financial Officer 410/550-0909
David B. Hellmann, M.D., Vice Dean, Bayview Campus 410/550-0516
Stephanie Reel, Chief Information Officer
Joanne E. Pollak, Vice President & General Counsel, JHM 410/614-3322
Dana Anderson, M.D., Chairman, Medical Board 410/550-2821
Janet M. McIntyre, Director, Quality Management 410/550-7674
Affiliation: Johns Hopkins Health System

Johns Hopkins Health System
600 North Wolfe Street
Baltimore, Maryland 21287

Ronald R. Peterson, President 410/955-9540
Affiliation: Johns Hopkins University School of Medicine

Johns Hopkins Hospital
600 North Wolfe Street
Baltimore, Maryland 21287

Ronald R. Peterson, President 410/955-9540
Judy A. Reitz, Sc.D., Executive Vice President/COO 410/614-2953
Ronald Werthman, Vice President, Finance/Treasurer 410/955-6552
Stephanie Reel, Vice Provost for Information Technology
CIO 410/735-7333
Joanne E. Pollak, Vice President & General Counsel, JHM 410/614-3322
Beryl J. Rosenstein, M.D., Vice President Medical Affairs 410/955-0620
Affiliation: Johns Hopkins Health System

LifeBridge Health, Inc.
2401 West Belvedere Avenue
Baltimore, Maryland 21215

Warren Green, President/CEO, LifeBridge Health, Inc. 410/601-5134
Affiliation: Johns Hopkins University School of Medicine; University of
Maryland School of Medicine

Mercy Medical Center
301 St. Paul Place
Baltimore, Maryland 21202

Thomas R. Mullen, President/CEO 410/332-9202
John Topper, Sr VP/CFO Financie & Syste s and Systems 410/332-4313
Grant Shackelford, Vice President/CIO Information Systems 410/332-9805
Scott A. Spier, Senior Vice President Medical Affairs 410/332-9070

University of Maryland Medical Center
22 South Greene Street
Baltimore, Maryland 21201

Jeffrey A. Rivest, President and Chief Executive Officer 410/328-0313
Herbert Buchanan, Senior Vice President and COO 410/328-3788
Henry Franey, Senior Vice President/CFO 410/328-3276
Michael N. Minear, Chief Information Officer 916/703-5511
Megan Arthur, Sr. Vice President/General Counsel 410/328-1635
Sherry Perkins, Ph.D., Vice President, Clinical Effectiveness 410/328-1704
Affiliation: University of Maryland Medical System

University of Maryland Medical System
250 W. Pratt Street, Suite 880
Baltimore, Maryland 21201

Edmond F. Notebaert, President/CEO 410/328-7555
Affiliation: University of Maryland School of Medicine

Veterans Affairs Maryland Health Care System
10 N. Greene Street
Baltimore, Maryland 21201-1524

Dennis H. Smith, Director, VA Maryland Health Care System
   (VAMHCS) 410/605-7016
Kathy Lockhart, R.N., Associate Director, Operations 410/642-1012
Thomas Scheffler, Chief, Fiscal Service 410/642-2411
Dorothy A. Snow, M.D., Associate Chief of Staff Performance
   Improvement and Education 410/605-7121
Sharon Zielinski, Chief, Information Resource Service 410/605-7083
Frank Giorno, Regional Counsel 410/605-7600
Chuck Swindell, Director, Performance Assessment
   Management Accreditation 410/605-7009
Affiliation: Johns Hopkins University School of Medicine; University of
    Maryland School of Medicine

Members: MARYLAND

Bethesda

The National Institutes of Health (NIH) Clinical Center
10 Center Drive
Room 2C146
Bethesda, Maryland 20892-1504

John I. Gallin, M.D., Director, Clinical Center 301/496-4114
Maureen E. Gormley, Chief Operating Officer 301/496-2897
Jon Mckerby, Chief Information Officer
Patricia Kvochak, General Counsel 301/496-6043
David K. Henderson, M.D., Deputy Director for Clinical
Care 301/496-3515

Affiliation: Georgetown University School of Medicine; Uniformed Services
University of the Health Sciences F. Edward Hebert School of
Medicine

Columbia

MedStar Health
5565 Sterret Place-Fifth Floor
Columbia, Maryland 21044

Kenneth A. Samet, Executive Vice President/CEO 410/772-6500
William L. Thomas, M.D., Executive Vice President for
Medical Affairs 410/772-6544

Affiliation: George Washington University School of Medicine and Health
Sciences; Howard University College of Medicine; Johns Hopkins
University School of Medicine

Linthicum

Department of Veterans Affairs Veterans Integrated Service Network VISN 5
849 International Drive, Suite 275
Linthicum, Maryland 15215

Silver Spring

Holy Cross Hospital
1500 Forest Glen Road
Silver Spring, Maryland 20910

Kevin J. Sexton, Chief Executive Officer 301/754-7010
Gary Vogan, SVP, Financial 301/754-7035
Kevin Orndorff, Vice President, Information Resources 301/754-7190
Sarah Shulman, Hospital Attorney 301/754-7438
Blair Eig, Vice President, Medical Affairs 301/754-7060
Brooks Sutton, Chief Operating Officer 301/754-7474

Affiliation: George Washington University School of Medicine and Health
Sciences

MASSACHUSETTS

Bedford

Department of Veterans Affairs Veterans Integrated Service Network VISN 1
200 Spring Road
Building 61
Bedford, Massachusetts 01730

Jeannette Chirico-Post, M.D., Network Director (10N1) VISN
1 Network Office, Bldg. 61 .... 781/687-3400

Boston

Beth Israel Deaconess Medical Center
330 Brookline Avenue
Boston, Massachusetts 02215

Paul F. Levy, Chief Executive Officer 617/667-0270
Eric Buehrens, Chief Operating Officer 617/667-4609
Steven Fischer, Chief Financial Officer 617/667-1961
John D. Halamka, M.D., Chief Information Officer 617/754-8002
Patricia McGovern, General Counsel & SVP Corp/Comm
Affairs 617/667-7323
Kenneth Sands, M.D., Vice President/Healthcare Quality 617/667-1325
Affiliation: CareGroup, Inc.

Boston Medical Center
1 Boston Medical Center Place
Boston, Massachusetts 02118

Elaine S. Ullian, President/CEO 617/638-6900
Ronald Bartlett, Vice President/CFO 617/638-7402
Meg Aranow, Vice President/CIO 617/638-8505
Edward J. Christiansen, General Counsel 617/638-7928
William Barron, Vice President Quality and Patient Safety
Chief Quality Officer
Affiliation: Boston University School of Medicine

Brigham and Women's Hospital
75 Francis Street
Boston, Massachusetts 02115

Gary Gottlieb, President 617/732-5537
Kate Walsh, Executive Vice President 617/525-7990
Michael Reney, Chief Financial Officer 617/732-7899
Sue Schade, Chief Information Officer 617/525-6050
Joan Stoddard, General Counsel 617/726-4244
Anthony Whittemore, M.D., Chief Medical Officer 617/732-8515
Michael Gustafson, VP, Center for Clinical Excellence 617/732-8894
Affiliation: Harvard Medical School; Partners HealthCare System, Inc.

CareGroup, Inc.
330 Brookline Avenue
Boston, Massachusetts 02215

Paul F. Levy, Chief Executive Officer 617/667-0270
Affiliation: Harvard Medical School

Members: MASSACHUSETTS

Caritas Christi Health Care System
736 Cambridge Street
Boston, Massachusetts 02135

    Ralph delaTorre, President/CEO 617/789-2500
Affiliation: Tufts University School of Medicine

Caritas St. Elizabeth's Medical Center of Boston
736 Cambridge Street
Boston, Massachusetts 02135

    Christopher O'Connor, President Interim Cheif Executive
    Officer 617/789-2262
    William Sullivan, Chief Financial Officer 617/789-2366
    William Garvin, M.D., Director of Medical Education 617/789-2384
    John P. Burke, Chief Information Officer 617/789-2282
    Wilson D. Rogers Jr., J.D., Legal Counsel 617/723-1100
    H. David Mitcheson, M.D., President, Medical Staff 617/782-1200
Affiliation: Caritas Christi Health Care System

Children's Hospital~MA
300 Longwood Avenue
Boston, Massachusetts 02115

    James Mandel, M.D., President and CEO 617/355-8555
    Sandra L. Fenwick, Chief Operating Officer 617/355-7272
    David Kirshner, Senior Vice President/CFO 617/355-6881
    Orah Platt, Dean, Academic Affairs 617/355-6347
    Daniel Nigrin, M.D., Acting Vice President, Information
    Systems 617/355-8977
    Stuart Novick, Senior Vice President/General Counsel 617/355-6108
    John E. Mayer, M.D., Special Assistant to the President 617/355-8258
    Nina A. Rauscher, Executive Director Program for Patient
    Safety and Quality 617/355-7742
Affiliation: Harvard Medical School

Faulkner Hospital
1153 Centre Street
Boston, Massachusetts 02130

    David J. Trull, President/CEO 617/983-7400
    Michael Conklin, Senior Vice President for Finance 617/983-7159
Affiliation: Tufts University School of Medicine

Massachusetts General Hospital
Fruit Street
Boston, Massachusetts 02114

    Peter Lawrence Slavin, M.D., President 617/724-9300
    Cindy Aiena, Chief Financial Officer 617/726-7814
    Debra F. Weinstein, M.D., Vice President of Graduate
    Medical Education Education 617/726-3616
    James W. Noga, Chief Information Officer 617/726-7709
    Christopher Clark, Legal Counsel Partners Health Care
    System 617/724-8079
    Britain Nicholson, M.D., Chief Medical Officer 617/726-8283
    Cyrus Hopkins, M.D., Office of Quality & Patient Safety 617/726-4304
Affiliation: Harvard Medical School; Partners HealthCare System, Inc.

Partners HealthCare System, Inc.
800 Bolyston Street
Suite 1150
Boston, Massachusetts

James J. Mongan, M.D., President 617/278-1004
Thomas P. Glynn, Ph.D., Chief Operating Officer 617/278-1005
Peter Markell, Chief Financial Officer 617/724-4537
George Thibault, M.D., Vice President for Clinical Affairs 617/278-1003
Linda Shaughnessy, Project Manager, Office of Clinical
Affairs 781/433-3685

Affiliation: Harvard Medical School

Tufts Medical Center
750 Washington Street
Boston, Massachusetts 02111

Ellen Zane, CEO 617/636-9589
Edward M. Schottland, Executive Vice President/COO 617/636-8700
Michael Burke, Chief Financial Officer 617/636-7767
William Shickolovich, VP IS, CIO 617/636-5899
Jeffrey Weinstein, General Counsel 617/636-2815
David Fairchild, M.D., M.P.H., Chief Medical Officer 617/636-1166

Affiliation: Tufts University School of Medicine

Veterans Affairs Boston Healthcare System
150 S. Huntington Avenue
Boston, Massachusetts 02130

Michael M. Lawson, Director 617/323-7700
Joseph Costa, Chief, Fiscal Service 617/232-9500
Frederick Kanter, M.D., Associate Chief of Staff/ Education 857/364-4141
David Goodman, Ph.D., Chief, Information Officer 617/232-9500
Edward Lukey, Regional Counsel 781/687-3600

Affiliation: Boston University School of Medicine; Tufts University School of
Medicine

Brockton

Veterans Affairs Medical Center (West Roxbury/Brockton)
940 Belmont Street
Brockton, Massachusetts 02401

Michael M. Lawson, Director 617/323-7700
Susan MacKenzie, Associate Director 617/323-7700
Joseph Costa, Chief, Fiscal Service 617/232-9500
Edward Lukey, Regional Counsel 781/687-3600
Michael Charness, Assoc Prof

Affiliation: Boston University School of Medicine; Harvard Medical School;
Tufts University School of Medicine; University of Massachusetts
Medical School

Members: MASSACHUSETTS

Burlington

Lahey Clinic Medical Center
41 Mall Road
Burlington, Massachusetts 01805

David M. Barrett, M.D., Chief Executive Officer 781/744-5796
Sanford R. Kurtz, M.D., Chief Operating Officer 781/744-8623
Timothy O'Connor, Chief Financial Officer 781/744-8134
David J. Schoetz, M.D., Chairman, Department of Medical
Education Professor of Surgery, Tufts University 781/744-8889
Nelson Gagnon, Chief Information Officer 781/744-2922
Donna Cameron, General Counsel 781/744-8408
Affiliation: Harvard Medical School; Tufts University School of Medicine

Cambridge

Cambridge Health Alliance~MA3
1493 Cambridge Street
Cambridge, Massachusetts 02139

Dennis Keefe, Chief Executive Officer 617/665-1448
Gordon Boudrow, Chief Financial Officer 781/306-8861

Cambridge Health Alliance~MA6
1496 Cambridge Street
Cambridge, Massachusetts
Affiliation: Cambridge Health Alliance

Mount Auburn Hospital
330 Mount Auburn Street
Cambridge, Massachusetts 02138

Jeanette G. Clough, President & CEO 617/499-5700
Nicholas DiIeso, Chief Operating Officer 617/499-5642
Peter Semenza, Chief Financial Officer 617/499-5021
Charles J. Hatem, M.D., Director of Medical Education 617/499-5140
Robert Todd, Director of Information Systems 617/599-5606
Leslie A. Joseph, J.D., General Counsel 617/499-5752
Eileen Dillon, R.N., Executive Director, Quality & Safety 617/499-5073
Affiliation: CareGroup, Inc.

Pittsfield

Berkshire Medical Center
725 North Street
Pittsfield, Massachusetts 01201

David Phelps, President/CEO 413/447-2743
Helen Downey, COO 413/395-7999
Darlene Rodowicz, Chief Financial Officer 413/447-2994
Henry Tulgan, M.D., Director, Medical Education/Associate
Dean 413/447-2715
Charles Podesta, Director, Information Services 413/447-2956
John Rogers, Vice President & Coporate Counsel 413/445-9528
Mark Pettus, Chief of Staff
Diane E. Kelly, VP, Quality Management 413/447-2316
Affiliation: University of Massachusetts Medical School

Springfield

Baystate Health System
280 Chestnut Street
Springfield, Massachusetts 01199

Mark R. Tolosky, President and Chief Executive Officer 413/794-5890
Affiliation: Tufts University School of Medicine

Baystate Medical Center
759 Chestnut Street
Springfield, Massachusetts 1199

Mark R. Tolosky, President and Chief Executive Officer 413/794-5890
Trish Hannon, Senior Vice President/COO 413/794-5516
Dennis Chalke, Vice President, Finance, Healthcare
Operations 413/794-3290
Hal B. Jenson, M.D., M.B.A., Chief Academic Officer 413/794-5588
Mark Gorrell, Vice President/CIO 413/794-3230
Loring S. Flint, M.D., Senior Vice President, Medical Affairs 413/794-5612
Evan M. Benjamin, M.D., Medical Director, Divsion of
Healthcare Quality 413/794-2527
Affiliation: Baystate Health System; Tufts University School of Medicine

Worcester

UMass Memorial Health Care
One Biotech Park
Worcester, Massachusetts 01605

John G. O'Brien, President and CEO 508/334-0100
Wendy Warring, Executive Vice President 508/334-0258
Therese Day, Chief Financial Officer 508/856-2848
Pamela Arora, Senior Vice President, Chief Information
Officer 508/334-0414
Douglas Brown, General Counsel 508/334-0424
Stephen E. Tosi, M.D., Chief Medical Officer 508/334-7746
Affiliation: University of Massachusetts Medical School

MICHIGAN

Ann Arbor

Department of Veterans Affairs Veterans Integrated Service Network VISN 11
40 Frank Lloyd Wright Drive
Lobby L, Third Floor
Ann Arbor, Michigan 48105
Linda W. Belton, Network Director, VISN 11 VISN 11
Network Office 734/930-5950

St. Joseph Mercy Hospital
PO Box 995
Ann Arbor, Michigan 48106
Garry C. Faja, Chief Executive Officer 734/712-4986
Julie McDonald, COO/Patient Care Services 734/712-2887
Charles Hoffman, VP Financial Services/CFO 734/712-2887
Bruce Deighton, Chief Academic Affairs Officer 734/712-5359
Rolland Mambourg, M.D., Vice President, Physician Services 734/712-7358
Mark E. Cowen, M.D., Medical Director, Quality Institute 734/887-0470
Affiliation: Trinity Health

University of Michigan Health System
1500 E. Medical Center Dr
Ann Arbor, Michigan 48109-0474
Jocelyn DeWitt, Chief Information Officer 734/764-4262
Affiliation: University of Michigan Medical School

University of Michigan Medical Center
1500 E. Medical Center Drive
Ann Arbor, Michigan 48109-0474
Douglas Strong, Director & CEO 734/764-1505
T. A. Denton, COO 734/647-6623
David Morlock, Chief Financial Officer 734/615-0574
Jocelyn DeWitt, Ph.D., Chief Information Officer 734/764-4262
Edward B. Goldman, Esq., Health System Attorney 734/764-2178
Darrell A. Campbell, M.D., Medical Director 734/936-5814
Deb Guglielmo, Director, Quality Improvement Operations 734/615-5378
Affiliation: University of Michigan Health System

Veterans Affairs Ann Arbor Healthcare System
2215 Fuller Road
Ann Arbor, Michigan 48105
James W. Roseborough, Medical Center Director 734/761-5458
Karen Ruedel, Chief, Resource Officer 734/761-7972
Mary K. East, M.D., Associate Chief of Staff for Education 734/761-7901
Shannon Rhodes, Chief Information Officer 734/769-7100
Eric Young, M.D., Chief of Staff 734/769-7100
Debra Crouch, Performance Improvement Coordinator 734/769-7100
Affiliation: University of Michigan Medical School

Dearborn

Oakwood Healthcare System
One Parklane Boulevard, Suite 1000E
Dearborn, Michigan 48126

Brian C. Connolly, President & Chief Executive Officer 313/253-6050
Affiliation: University of Michigan Medical School; Wayne State University
School of Medicine

Oakwood Hospital and Medical Center
1 Parklane Blvd
Dearborn, Michigan 48124

Michael Geheb, Division President 313/593-7125
Ronald Britt, Chief Financial Officer 313/593-7853
Paula Smith, Chief Information Officer 313/724-4506
Mark Lezotte, Corporate Director, Legal Affairs 313/791-1730
Malcolm Henoch, M.D., SVP & Chief Medical Officer 313/253-6009
Sara Atwell, Corporate Director Quality and Care Mgmt 313/791-4620
Affiliation: Oakwood Healthcare System

Detroit

Detroit Medical Center
3663 Woodward Avenue
Detroit, Michigan 48201-2403

Michael Duggan, President and Chief Executive Officer 313/745-5192
Jay Rising, CFO 313/966-4166
Conrad L. Mallett Jr., President 313/966-3300
Affiliation: Wayne State University School of Medicine

Henry Ford Hospital
One Ford Place
Detroit, Michigan 48202

Anthony Armada, President and CEO 313/916-8058
James Connelly, Senior Vice President/CFO 313/876-8714
Arthur A. Gross, Chief Information Officer 313/874-9878
Mark Kelley, M.D., Executive Vice President-Chief Medical
Officer/CEO Henry Ford Medical Group 313/876-8701
Affiliation: Michigan State University College of Osteopathic Medicine; The
University of Toledo College of Medicine

John D. Dingell VA Medical Center
4646 John R.
Detroit, Michigan 48201

Michael K. Wheeler, Medical Center Director 313/576-3234
Leslie Wiggins, Associate Director 313/576-4421
Patricia Kelly, Chief, Finiancial and Budget Service 313/576-1000
Robert C. Johnson, M.B.A., Chief, Business Practice 313/576-3750
Basim Dubaybo, Chief of Staff 313/576-3327
Tarynne Bolden, R.N., Quality Manager 313/576-4644
Affiliation: Wayne State University School of Medicine

Members: MICHIGAN

Sinai-Grace Hospital
6071 W. Outer Drive
Detroit, Michigan 48235

Conrad L. Mallett Jr., President 313/966-3300
Vernell Williams, Vice President, Operations 313/966-4681
Ken Lipan, Vice President, Finance 313/966-1920
Donald Ragan, Ph.D., Chief Information Officer 313/578-2223
John Haapaniemi, D.O., Chief of Staff 313/966-3224
Affiliation: Detroit Medical Center; Wayne State University School of Medicine

St. John Hospital and Medical Center
22101 Moross
Detroit, Michigan
Affiliation: St. John Health System

Farmington Hills

Trinity Health
34605 Twelve Mile Road
Farmington Hills, Michigan 48331

Joseph Swedish, President and Chief Executive Officer 248/489-6000
Affiliation: University of Michigan Medical School

Flint

Hurley Medical Center
One Hurley Plaza
Flint, Michigan 48502

Patrick Wardell, Cheif Executive Officer 810/257-9237
Kevin Murphy, Chief Financial Officer 810/257-9396
Daniel Coffield, Executive Vice President and Chief
Financial Officer 810/257-9844
Patrick Milostan, Chief Information Officer 810/257-9642
Michael Boucree, M.D., Vice President for Medical Affairs 810/257-9544
Chris Surratt, R.N., Director, Quality Management/
Improvement 810/762-6336
Affiliation: Michigan State University College of Human Medicine

McLaren Regional Healthcare Corporation
401 S. Ballenger Highway
Flint, Michigan 48532

Philip A. Incarnati, President/CEO 810/342-2443
Affiliation: Michigan State University College of Human Medicine

McLaren Regional Medical Center
401 S. Ballenger Highway
Flint, Michigan 48532

Donald C. Kooy, President/CEO 810/342-2446
David Senchak, Vice President of Ancillary/Support Services 810/342-4407
Rick Wyles, Chief Financial Officer 810/342-2516
Paul M. Romanelli, Ph.D., Director of Medical Education 810/342-2321
Richard Sardelli, Director of Legal Affairs/Risk Management 810/342-2427
Edwin H. Gullekson, M.D., Chief Medical Officer 810/342-2450
Affiliation: McLaren Regional Healthcare Corporation

Grand Rapids

Spectrum Health
100 Michigan Street, NE
Grand Rapids, Michigan 49503

Matthew Van Vranken, President 616/391-1285
Bruce P. Hagen, Executive Vice President, Hospitals/COO 616/391-1285
Michael Freed, Executive Vice President, ... 616/391-2774
Patrick O'Hare, SVP, Chief Information Officer 616/391-2774
Bridget Tucker Gonder, Vice President, Risk & Compliance
Administration 616/391-2762
Lowell Bursch, M.D., Executive Vice President for Medical
Affairs 616/391-6321
John Byrnes, SVP, System Quality 616/391-1245
Affiliation: Michigan State University College of Human Medicine; Spectrum
Health

Kalamazoo

Bronson Methodist Hospital
601 John Street
Kalamazoo, Michigan 49007

Frank J. Sardone, President and Chief Executive Officer 269/341-6000
Kenneth Taft, CFO 269/341-6000
Milton McClurkan Jr , Vice President, Information
Technology/CIO 269/341-6000
James B. Falahee Jr., J.D., General Counsel 269/341-6000
Jane Janssen, Director 269/341-8539
Affiliation: Michigan State University College of Human Medicine

Lansing

Ingham Regional Medical Center
401 W. Greenlawn Ave
Lansing, Michigan 48910

Paula Reichle, Chief Financial Officer & Sr VP 517/975-7558
Earl J. Reisdorff, M.D., Director, Medical Education 517/334-2195
Geoffrey M. Linz, M.D., Chief Medical Officer 517/334-2576
Jeanie Taylor, Director, Quality Improvement 517/334-2896
Affiliation: Michigan State University College of Human Medicine

Royal Oak

William Beaumont Hospital
3601 W. Thirteen Mile Road
Royal Oak, Michigan 48073

Kenneth J. Matzick, President and CEO 248/551-0680
Dennis Herrick, Senior Vice President/CFO 248/551-0676
John R. Musich, M.D., Vice President and Director, Medical
   Education DIO 248/551-0427
Paul S. Peabody, Vice President/Chief Information Officer 248/597-2800
Thomas McAskin, Vice President and Chief Legal Officer 248/551-0572
Steven Winokur, M.D., Medical Director of Quality
   Improvement 248/551-0431
Affiliation: University of Michigan Medical School; Wayne State University
   School of Medicine; William Beaumont Hospital System

William Beaumont Hospital System
3601 West 13 Mile Road
Royal Oak, Michigan 48073

Ted D. Wasson, President/CEO 248/551-0680
Affiliation: University of Michigan Medical School; Wayne State University
   School of Medicine

MINNESOTA

Bloomington

HealthPartners, Inc.
8100 34th Avenue South
PO Box 1309
Bloomington, Minnesota 55440-1309

Mary Brainerd, President/CEO 952/883-6000
Affiliation: University of Minnesota Medical School

Minneapolis

Abbott Northwestern Hospital
800 East 28th Street
Minneapolis, Minnesota 55407

Richard Pettingill, CEO 612/262-0601
Michael McAnder, Chief Financial Officer 612/262-0622
Virginia Reed, Chief Information Officer 612/863-3003
Richard Sturgeon, Medical Director 612/863-8279
Affiliation: Allina Hospitals and Clinics

Allina Hospitals and Clinics
710 East 24th Street
PEI Medical Office Building
Minneapolis, Minnesota 55405

Department of Veterans Affairs Veterans Integrated Service Network VISN 23
5445 Minnehaha Avenue South
Minneapolis, Minnesota 55417

Robert A. Petzel, M.D., Network Director(10N23) 612/725-1968

Fairview Health Services
2450 Riverside Avenue
Minneapolis, Minnesota 55454

Mark A. Eustis, President 612/672-6161
Affiliation: University of Minnesota Medical School

Hennepin County Medical Center
701 Park Avenue South
Minneapolis, Minnesota 55415

Lynn Abrahamsen, Chief Executive Officer 612/873-2352
Larry Kryzaniak, Chief Financial Officer 612/873-3040
Andy Mitchell, Assistant County Attorney 512/873-3195
Michael B. Belzer, M.D., Medical Director 612/873-2979
Affiliation: University of Minnesota Medical School

Minneapolis Veterans Affairs Medical Center
One Veterans Drive
Minneapolis, Minnesota 55417

Steven P. Kleinglass, Medical Center Director 612/725-2101
Paul Resel, Chief, Fiscal Service 612/725-2150
Kent B. Crossley, M.D., Associate Chief of Staff, Education
Service 612/725-2031
Douglas Ball, Chief Information Management Service 612/725-2070
John Dryden, Chief of Staff
Jack Drucker, Chief of Staff 612/725-2105
Linda B. Duffy, Director, Continuous Improvement and
Public Relations 612/725-2102
Affiliation: University of Minnesota Medical School

Univ of Minnesota Med Ctr, Fairview
2450 Riverside Avenue
Minneapolis, Minnesota 55455

Gordon Alexander, M.D., President 612/273-6150
Steve Hill, Vice President, Finance 612/273-6575
William Showalter, Chief Information Officer Information
Mgmt Svcs. 612/672-6900
Paul Torgerson, Senior Vice President, General Counsel 612/672-6217
Affiliation: Fairview Health Services

Rochester

Mayo Health System
Rochester, Minnesota 55901

Glenn Forbes, President and CEO 507/255-5123
Denis Cortese, M.D., President & CEO 507/284-2663
Affiliation: Florida State University College of Medicine; Mayo Medical School

Saint Mary's Hospital
1216 Second Street, S.W.
Rochester, Minnesota 55902

Hugh Smith, Chair, Board of Governers 507/255-5123
Jeff Korsmo, Chief Operating Officer 507/255-5123
Lee Hecht, Chief Financial Officer 507/255-3550
Anthony Windebank, Keith D. Lindor 507/284-3268
Chris Gade, Chair Division of External Relations 507/284-2430
Sherry L. Hubert, J.D., Legal Counsel 507/284-0787
Affiliation: Mayo Health System

St. Paul

Regions Hospital
640 Jackson Street
St. Paul, Minnesota 55101

Brock Nelson, President and CEO 651/254-2189
Gregory Klugherz, Vice President/CFO 651/254-0933
Carl A. Patow, M.D., Assoc. Dean, Medical Education 952/883-7185
Alan Abramson, Senior Vice President/CIO Information
   Systems 952/883-7883
Barbara Tretheway, Senior Vice President, General Counsel 952/883-5137
Michael Trangle, Vice President, Medical Affairs 651/254-2734
Affiliation: HealthPartners, Inc.

MISSISSIPPI

Jackson

Department of Veterans Affairs Veterans Integrated Service Network VISN 16
VISN 16
Jackson, Mississippi 39216

Robert Lynch, CEO 504/988-1595

G. V. (Sonny) Montgomery Veterans Affairs Medical Center
1500 East Woodrow Wilson Drive
Jackson, Mississippi 39216

Richard J. Baltz, Medical Center Director 601/364-1201
Rebecca Wiley, Chief-Fiscal Service 601/364-1204
Joy Willis, Chief Financial Officer 601/364-1283
Kent Kirchner, M.D., Chief of Staff 601/364-1207
Robert Wolak, Chief, Information Resource Management 601/364-1260
Mary E. Barrett, Regional Counsel 601/364-1261
Chief Library Service (142D), Chief, Library Service (142D) 601/364-5378
Janet C. Autry, Director, Office of Quality Assessment 601/364-1219
Affiliation: University of Mississippi School of Medicine

Methodist Rehabilitation Center
1350 East Woodrow Wilson Blvd
Jackson, Mississippi

Mark A. Adams, President/CEO 601/364-3462
Joseph Morette, Executive Vice President & COO
Gary Armstrong, Executive Vice President & CFO
Dobrivoje (Boba) Stokic, M.D., Administrative Director of
Research 601/364-3314
Tammy Voynik, Vice President, Legal Services 601/364-3360
Samuel Grissom, Medical Director 601/364-3425
Marcia King, Quality Management/Improvement Director 601/364-3359
Affiliation: University of Mississippi School of Medicine

University Hospitals and Clinics/University of Mississippi Medical Center
2500 North State Street
Jackson, Mississippi 39216

David Putt, Interim CEO 601/984-4107
Jenny Walker, Director, Finance 601/984-4113
A. Wallace Conerly, M.D., Dean Emeritus 601/984-1010
Robert Jenkins, Staff Attorney 601/984-1776
Margaret Davis, Director of Admissions 601/984-5010
Judy Stump, Director of Performance Improvement 601/984-4100
Affiliation: University of Mississippi School of Medicine

MISSOURI

Columbia

University of Missouri Health Care
One Hospital Drive
Columbia, Missouri 65212

James Ross, Chief Executive Officer 573/884-4174
Sharon Yaeger, Chief Financial Officer 573/882-1184
George Carr, Chief Information Officer 573/884-6117
William F. Arnet, Counsel 573/882-3211
Joseph Giangiacomo, Chief of Staff 573/882-4913
Kay Davis, Director, Patient Financial Services 573/882-7183
Affiliation: University of Missouri-Columbia School of Medicine

Kansas City

Children's Mercy Hospital
2401 Gillham Road
Kansas City, Missouri 64108

Randall L. O'Donnell, Ph.D., President/CEO 816/234-3650
Jo Stueve, Senior VP, Administrative Services 816/234-3623
Sandra Lawrence, Executive Vice President/CFO 816/234-3205
Joanne Kennedy, M.D., Director, Medical Education 816/234-3371
Jean Ann Breedlove, Chief Information Officer Information
Systems 816/234-3000
Sally Surridge, Vice President/General Counsel 816/234-3653
V. Fred Burry, M.D., Executive Medical Director 816/234-3780
Affiliation: University of Missouri-Kansas City School of Medicine

Department of Veterans Affairs Veterans Integrated Service Network VISN 15
1201 Walnut Street
Suite 800
Kansas City, Missouri 64128

Peter Almenoff, Network Director (10N15) 816/922-2908
James Sanders, Chief Medical Officer 816/922-2926

Saint Luke's Hospital of Kansas City
Wornall Road at Forty-Fourth
Kansas City, Missouri 64111

G. Richard Hastings, Chief Executive Officer 816/932-2101
Mark S. McPhee, M.D., Chief Operating Officer 816/932-3601
Jama Johnson, CFO 816/932-2589
John Wade, Chief Information Officer 816/932-2514
E. E. Fibuch, M.D., Associate Director, Medical Affairs 816/932-5132

Affiliation: Saint Luke's Shawnee Mission Health System

Saint Luke's Shawnee Mission Health System
Wornall Road at Forty Fourth
Kansas City, Missouri 64111

G. Richard Hastings, Chief Executive Officer 816/932-2101

Affiliation: University of Kansas School of Medicine; University of Missouri-
Kansas City School of Medicine

Truman Medical Center Hospital Hill
2301 Holmes Street
Kansas City, Missouri 64108

John W. Bluford, Chief Executive Officer 816/404-3500
Catherine Disch, Chief Operating Officer 816/554-3500
Allen Johnson, Chief Financial Officer 816/404-3500
Mark Steele, M.D., Chief Medical Officer Associate Dean 816/404-5300
Tom Pagano, Chief Information Officer 816/404-2000
Lewis Popper, General Counsel 816/404-3625

Affiliation: University of Missouri-Kansas City School of Medicine

Saint Louis

Barnes-Jewish Hospital
One Barnes Jewish Plaza
Saint Louis, Missouri 63110

Andrew Ziskind, President 314/362-5400
Sharon L. O'Keefe, Vice President and Chief Operating
Officer 314/454-7000
Mark Krieger, VP & Chief Financial Officer
Keith Segraves, Director, Information Systems 314/362-7770
James P. Crane, M.D., Associate Vice Chancellor for Clinical
Affairs/Chief Executive Officer, ... 314/362-6249
Missy Bax, Quality Management-Improvement Director 314/362-5581

Affiliation: BJC HealthCare

St. Louis

BJC HealthCare
4444 Forest Park Avenue
Suite 500
St. Louis, Missouri 63108

Steve Lipstein, President/CEO 314/286-2024
Kevin Roberts, Vice President and CFO 314/286-2002
David A. Weiss, Vice President and Chief Information
Officer 314/286-2008
Michael DeHaven, Senior Vice President and General
Counsel 314/286-2010
Clay Dunagan, M.D., Vice President, Center for Healthcare
Quality and Effectiveness 314/286-2164
Belinda Ireland, M.D., M.S., Adj Assistant Professor 636/458-5394
Affiliation: Washington University in St. Louis School of Medicine

Saint Louis University Hospital
3635 Vista at Grand Boulevard
St. Louis, Missouri 63110

Crystal Haynes, Chief Executive Officer 314/577-8004
Raymond Alvey, Chief Financial Officer 314/577-8005
Dawn Anuszkiewicz, Cheif Operating Officer 314/577-8103
Beckie Patrick, Chief Information Officer 314/268-7396
Sue Monaco, Managing Senior Counsel 469/893-2429
Karen B. Webb, M.D., Chief Medical Officer 314/577-8008
Nancy Noedel, Director, Clinical Quality Improvement 314/577-8807
Affiliation: Saint Louis University School of Medicine; Tenet Healthcare
Corporation

St. John's Mercy Medical Center
615 South New Ballas Road
St. Louis, Missouri 63141

Denny DeNarvaez, President and Chief Executive Officer 314/251-1952
Mark Stauder, COO 314/251-1953
Randy Combs, Chief Financial Officer 314/364-3308
Christopher Veremakis, M.D., Chairman, Graduate Medical
Education 314/251-1375
Mark Hutson, Chief Information Officer 314/251-1918
John S. Howard, Director of Legal Services 314/364-3388
Paul Hintze, M.D., Vice President of Medical Affairs 314/251-1955
Mike Moonier, Director, Quality Management 314/569-6544
Affiliation: Saint Louis University School of Medicine

St. Louis Children's Hospital
One Children's Place
St. Louis, Missouri 63110

Lee F. Fetter, President & Senior Executive Officer 314/454-6009
Doug Vanderslice, Chief Financial Officer 314/454-4275
Gary R. LaBlance, Ph.D., Vice President, Quality Service &
Information Services 314/454-2850
Affiliation: BJC HealthCare

St. Mary's Health Center
6420 Clayton Road
St. Louis, Missouri 63117

William Jennings, President Chief Operating Officer 314/768-8075
Mary Sue Embertson, Chief Financial Officer 314/989-2000
Howard Podosky, Medical Director 314/768-8057
Shelly Pierce, Quality Management Director 314/768-8868

Affiliation: Saint Louis University School of Medicine

NEBRASKA

Lincoln

Department of Veterans Affairs Veterans Integrated Service Network VISN 14
600 S. 70th Street-Building 5
Lincoln, Nebraska 68510-2451

Omaha

The Nebraska Medical Center
987400 Nebraska Medical Center
Omaha, Nebraska 68198-7400

Glenn A. Fosdick, President/CEO 402/552-3452
Joe B. Graham, Chief Operating Officer 402/552-3485
William Dinsmoor, Chief Financial Officer 402/552-3202
Lianne O. Stevens, Executive Director, Information
Technolo 402/552-2480
Stephen B. Smith, Chief Medical Officer 402/552-2290

Affiliation: University of Nebraska College of Medicine

Saint Joseph Hospital
601 North 30th Street
Omaha, Nebraska 68131

J. Richard Stanko, President/CEO 402/449-5990
Robert Beehler, Chief Operating Officer 402/449-5295
Andrea Heffelfinger, Vice President/Chief Financial Officer 402/449-5371
Stephen J. Lanspa, M.D., Sr. Assc Dean, Academic and
Clinical 402/280-3792
Pat Hoidal, Quality Manager 402/449-4013

Affiliation: Creighton University School of Medicine; Tenet Healthcare
Corporation

VA Nebraska-Western Iowa Health Care System-Omaha Division
4101 Woolworth Avenue
Omaha, Nebraska 68105

Albert B. Washko, Director 402/346-0600
Nancy Gregory, Acting Associate Director 402/346-8800
Kirk Kai, Chief Financial Officer 402/346-8800
William F. Gust, M.D., Associate Chief of Staff, Education 402/346-8800
Kenneth R. Huibregtse, Chief Information Officer 402/346-8800
Paul L. Pullum, St. Louis Regional Counsel Omaha Office 402/346-8800
Rowen K. Zetterman, Acting Chief of Staff 402/346-8800
Shirley Simons, Chief Quality Officer 402/346-8800
Affiliation: Creighton University School of Medicine; University of Nebraska
College of Medicine

NEW HAMPSHIRE

Lebanon

Dartmouth Hitchcock Alliance
One Medical Center Drive
Lebanon, New Hampshire

Dartmouth-Hitchcock Medical Center
One Medical Center Drive
Lebanon, New Hampshire 03756

Nancy A. Formella, R.N., President 603/650-7422
Stephan J. LeBlanc, COO 603/650-5340
Steve LeBlanc, COO 603/650-5340
Dan Jantzen, Chief Financial Officer 603/653-1100
William R. Green, Ph.D., Dean, Chair and Professor of
Microbiology and Immunology 603/650-1200
Peter A. Johnson, Vice President, Information Systems 603/650-8811
John Butterly, Executive Medical Director 603/650-5606
Polly Campion, Director, Clinical Improvement Director,
Office of Patient Safety 603/653-1056
Affiliation: Dartmouth Hitchcock Alliance

NEW JERSEY

Camden

Cooper University Hospital
One Cooper Plaza
Camden, New Jersey 08103

John P. Sheridan, President and Chief Executive Officer 856/968-7481
Jeffrey N. Yarmel, Chief Operating Officer 856/342-2443
Dennis Pettigrew, Chief Financial Officer 856/342-2121
Carolyn E. Bekes, M.D., Chief Academic Officer 856/342-2940
Karen Graham, Director, Information Technology 856/968-7135
John Newsome, Chief Legal Officer 856/968-7380
Raymond Baraldi, Acting Chief Medical Officer 856/968-7397
Affiliation: University of Medicine and Dentistry of New Jersey-Robert Wood
Johnson Medical School

Members: NEW JERSEY

East Orange

Department of Veterans Affairs New Jersey Health Care System
385 Tremont Avenue
East Orange, New Jersey 07018

Kenneth Mizrach, Director 973/676-1000
Philip C. Moschitta, Associate Director, East Orange 973/676-1000
Tyrone Taylor, Chief, Fiscal Service 973/676-1771
Marilyn A. Miller, Associate Chief of Staff for Education 973/676-1000
Beverly Erhardt, Chief, Information Resources Management
Services 973/676-1000
Max Shemtob, Regional Counsel 973/676-1000
Linda Mowad, Office of Performance Measurement &
Improvement Coordinator 973/676-1000

Affiliation: University of Medicine and Dentistry of New Jersey-New Jersey
Medical School; University of Medicine and Dentistry of New Jersey-
Robert Wood Johnson Medical School

Florham Park

Atlantic Health System
325 Columbia Turnpike
Florham Park, New Jersey 07902

Joseph A. Trunfio, President & CEO 973/660-3270
Kevin Shanley, Vice President, Finance/CFO 973/660-3166
Linda Reed, Chief Information Officer
Stephen Sepaniak, Vice President Legal Affairs-General
Counsel 973/660-3169

Affiliation: Columbia University College of Physicians and Surgeons; Mount
Sinai School of Medicine of New York University; Drexel University
College of Medicine

Hackensack

Hackensack University Medical Center
30 Prospect Avenue
Hackensack, New Jersey 07601

John P. Ferguson, President/CEO 201/996-2002
Robert Garrett, Vice President/COO 201/996-2004
Robert Glenning, Sr. VP Finance/CFO 201/996-3371
William Black, M.D., Vice President, Medical Academic
Affairs 201/996-2794
Lex Ferrauiola, Vice President, Information Technology 201/996-3662
Audrey Murphy, Vice President, General Counsel 201/996-3771

Affiliation: University of Medicine and Dentistry of New Jersey-New Jersey
Medical School

Hoboken

Hoboken University Medical Center
308 Willow Avenue
Hoboken, New Jersey

Harvey Holzberg, Consulting Director/CEO 201/418-1002
Affiliation: University of Medicine and Dentistry of New Jersey-New Jersey
Medical School

Livingston

Saint Barnabas Medical Center
94 Old Short Hills Road
Livingston, New Jersey 07039

John F. Bonamo, M.D., Executive Director 973/322-5502
Patrick Ahearn, Chief Financial Officer/VP of Finance 973/322-2721
Henry Rosenberg, M.D., Director, Department of Medical 973/322-5777
David Mebane, SBHCS Corporate Counsel 973/322-4042
Pamela Micchelli, Director of Standards, Performance
Improvement and Quality 973/322-2614
Affiliation: Mount Sinai School of Medicine of New York University; Saint
Barnabas Health Care System

Long Branch

Monmouth Medical Center
300 Second Avenue
Long Branch, New Jersey 07740

Frank Vozos, M.D., Executive Director 732/923-7502
Gerald Tofani, Senior Vice President, Finance 732/923-0180
Joseph Jaegar, Assoc. VP Academics 732/923-6781
Rich Wheatley, Chief Information Officer 732/923-7566
Eric Burkett, Medical Director
Pat Keating, Administrative Director, Performance
Improvement 732/923-6620
Affiliation: Drexel University College of Medicine; Saint Barnabas Health Care
System

Morristown

Morristown Memorial Hospital
100 Madison Avenue
P.O. Box 1956
Morristown, New Jersey 07962-1956

Kevin Shanley, Vice President, Finance/CFO 973/660-3166
Don Casey, Vice President for Quality Chief Medical Officer 973/660-3556
Affiliation: Atlantic Health System

Neptune

Jersey Shore University Medical Center
1945 Route 33
Neptune, New Jersey 07754

Steve Littleson, President 732/776-4900
John Gantner, Executive Vice President /CFO Finance 732/751-7520
Rebecca Weber, Director, Information Systems 732/776-4186
Ann Gavzy, Vice President Legal Affairs and General
Counsel 732/751-7550
Richard Nobile, D.D.S., Medical Staff President 732/776-4250
Lori Christensen, M.D., Chair, Outcomes Management
Committee 732/776-4747
Affiliation: Meridian Health System

Meridian Health System
Monmouth Shores Corporate Park
1350 Campus Parkway
Neptune, New Jersey 07753

John K. Lloyd, President/CEO 732/751-7510
Marc H. Lory, Executive Vice President 732/751-7512
Affiliation: University of Medicine and Dentistry of New Jersey-Robert Wood
Johnson Medical School

New Brunswick

Robert Wood Johnson Health System
One Robert Wood Johnson Place
New Brunswick, New Jersey

Robert Wood Johnson University Hospital
One Robert Wood Johnson Place
New Brunswick, New Jersey 08901

Stephen K. Jones, Interim President and CEO 732/937-8902
Carl O'Brien, Treasurer 732/937-8910
Robert Irwin, Vice President
Peter S. Amenta, M.D., Ph.D., Dean 732/235-6300
Affiliation: Robert Wood Johnson Health System; University of Medicine and
Dentistry of New Jersey-Robert Wood Johnson Medical School

Saint Peter's University Hospital
254 Easton Avenue
New Brunswick, New Jersey 08903-0591

Alfred Glover, President/CEO 732/745-7944
Garrick Stoldt, Senior Vice President, Finance & CFO 732/745-8600
Affiliation: Drexel University College of Medicine

Newark

Newark Beth Israel Medical Center
201 Lyons Avenue
Newark, New Jersey 07112

John A. Brennan, Vice President for Medical Affairs 973/322-4074
Kenneth L. Tyson, Senior Vice President, Operations 973/926-7851
Veronica Zeichner, Chief Financial Officer 973/926-7849
Joshua Rosenblatt, M.D., Director, Medical Education 973/926-3233
Murray E. Belsky, M.D., Vice President, Medical Affairs 973/926-7411
Margo Malaspina, R.N., Director, Quality Management 973/926-7822
Affiliation: Mount Sinai School of Medicine of New York University; Saint
   Barnabas Health Care System

University of Medicine and Dentistry of New Jersey-University Hospital
150 Bergen Street
Newark, New Jersey 07103

Darlene Cox, President and CEO 973/972-5658
Robin Wittenstein, Chief Operating Officer 973/972-0871
Thomas Daly, Chief Financial Officer 973/972-3721
Robert A. Saporito, Senior Vice President for Academic
 Affairs 973/972-3645
Susan Mettlen, Vice President of Information Technology 973/972-3800
Vivian Sanks-King, J.D., Vice President of Legal Management............. 973/972-4705
Catherine T. Marino, M.D., Medical Director 973/972-0440
Maryann Sakmyster, Director, Quality Assurance &
 Performance Improvement 973/972-1353
Affiliation: University of Medicine and Dentistry of New Jersey-New Jersey
   Medical School

West Orange

Saint Barnabas Health Care System
95 Old Short Hills Road
West Orange, New Jersey 07039

Ronald J. Del Mauro, President/CEO 973/322-4002
Mark Pilla, Executive Vice President of Operations 973/322-4069
Affiliation: Drexel University College of Medicine

NEW MEXICO

Albuquerque

New Mexico Veterans Affairs Health Care System
1501 San Pedro SE
Albuquerque, New Mexico 87108

George Marnell, Director 505/265-1711
Jerald D. Molnar, Associate Director 505/265-1711
Michael McNeill, Chief, Fiscal Service 505/265-1711
Curtis O. Kapsner, M.D., Associate Director Academic &
 Research A 505/265-1711
Renee Lameka, Quality Manager 505/265-1711
Affiliation: University of New Mexico School of Medicine

University of New Mexico Hospital

2211 Lomas Boulevard, N.E.
Albuquerque, New Mexico 87106

Stephen W. McKernan, CEO/Assoc. VP, UNMHSC Clinical
Operations 505/272-2121
Jody Harris, Chief Financial Officer 505/272-3335
Paul B. Roth, M.D., Executive Vice President for Health
Sciences and Dean 505/272-5849
Ronald Margolis, Chief Information Officer 505/272-2121
Saundra Brown-Savoy, General Counsel 505/272-2377
Robert Bailey, MD 505/272-5002

Affiliation: University of New Mexico School of Medicine

NEW YORK

Albany

Albany Medical Center Hospital

43 New Scotland Avenue
Albany, New York 12208

James J. Barba, President/CEO/Chairman of the Board 518/262-3830
Gary J. Kochem, Chief Operating Officer 518/262-3028
William Hasselbarth, Executive Vice President/CFO 518/262-8795
Vincent P. Verdile, M.D., M.S., Executive Vice President
Albany Medical Center Dean 518/262-6008
Dennis DeLisle, Vice President Information Technology 518/262-8006
Arthur Gross, Senior Vice President/CIO Albany Medical
Center Hospital 518/262-8006
Lee R. Hessberg, Senior Vice President/General Counsel 518/262-3808
Karen Houston, R.N., Director, Quality Management 518/262-3796

Affiliation: Albany Medical College

Albany Veterans Affairs Medical Center

113 Holland Avenue
Albany, New York 12208

Mary-Ellen Piche, Medical Center Director 518/626-6731
Douglas Erickson, M.H.A., Chief Operating Officer
Martha Farber, M.D., Associate Chief of Staff for Education 518/626-6885
Mullahey Michael, Program Mgr., Information Resource
Mgmt. 518/462-3311
Kevin Thiemann, District Counsel Attorney 518/462-3311
Eina Fishman, M.D., M.S., Physician Executive 518/462-3311

Affiliation: Albany Medical College

Department of Veterans Affairs Veterans Integrated Service Network VISN 2

VA Healthcare Network Upstate New York
113 Holland Avenue, Building 7
Albany, New York 12208

Binghamton

United Health Services Hospitals
33-57 Harrison Street
Binghamton, New York 13790

Matthew J. Salanger, President/CEO 607/763-6130
Robert Gomulka, Vice President, Finance 607/762-3011
Don Carlin, General Counsel 607/762-3366
Rajesh Dave, M.D., M.B.A., Vice President for Medical
Affairs and Medical Education 607/763-6690
Affiliation: State University of New York Upstate Medical University

Bronx

Bronx Lebanon Hospital Center
1276 Fulton Avenue
Bronx, New York 10456

Miguel A. Fuentes Jr., President/CEO 718/590-1800
Steven Anderman, Senior Vice President of Operations/
COO 718/588-5586
Victor De Marco, Senior Vice President/CFO 718/901-8600
Fred Miller, General Counsel Garfunkel, Wild & Travis PC 516/393-2250
Milton A. Gumbs, M.D., Associate Dean for Minority Student
Affairs Associate Professor, Dept of Surgery 718/430-3091
Affiliation: Albert Einstein College of Medicine of Yeshiva University

Bronx Veterans Affairs Medical Center
130 West Kingsbridge Road
Bronx, New York 10468

Mary Ann Musumeci, Medical Center Director 718/584-9000
Roger Johnson, Associate Director 631/261-2747
Edward Ronan, Ph.D., Director, Education Program 718/584-9000
Linda Bund, Director, Education & Information Mgmt. 718/584-9000
Max Shemtob, Regional Counsel 973/676-1000
Jack Hirschowitz, M.D., Mb.Bs., Chief of Staff 718/584-9000
Affiliation: Mount Sinai School of Medicine of New York University

Department of Veterans Affairs Veterans Integrated Service Network VISN 3
130 W. Kingsbridge Road-Building 16
Bronx, New York 10468

James J. Farsetta, Network Director(10N3) VISN 3 Network
Office, Bldg 16 .... 718/741-4110

Members: NEW YORK

Jacobi Medical Center
Pelham Parkway S. and Eastchester Road
Bronx, New York 10461

William P. Walsh, Senior Vice President/Executive Director 718/918-8141
Arthur Wagner, Chief Operating Officer 718/918-4648
Kathy Garramone, Chief Operating Officer 718/918-3677
Diane Carr, Chief Information Officer 718/918-3690
Joseph Skarzynski, M.D., Medical Director 718/918-4606
Anne Iasiello, Associate Executive Director 718/918-5320

Affiliation: Albert Einstein College of Medicine of Yeshiva University; NYC
Health and Hospitals Corporation

Lincoln Medical and Mental Health Center
234 Eugenio Maria de Hostos
Boulevard (149th Street)
Bronx, New York

Victor Bekker, Network CFO 718/579-5788
Suzanne Monique Carter, Chief Information Officer 212/423-7230
Alan Aviles, President 212/788-3321
Melissa Schori, M.D., Medical Director 718/579-5235
Sara Shahim, Senior Associate Executive Director 718/579-4945

Affiliation: NYC Health and Hospitals Corporation

Montefiore Medical Center
111 East 210 Street
Bronx, New York 10467

Steven M. Safyer, M.D., President/CEO 718/920-2001
Robert B. Conaty, Executive Vice President, Operations 718/920-4131
Joel Perlman, Chief Financial Officer 718/920-9501
Dominick P. Purpura, M.D., Professor of Neuroscience Dean
Emeritus 718/430-3617
Jack Wolf, Vice President, Management Information Systems...................... 718/405-4311
Stanley Jacobson, Senior Vice President/General Counsel 718/920-8500

Affiliation: Albert Einstein College of Medicine of Yeshiva University

North Central Bronx
3424 Kossuth Avenue
Bronx, New York

Peter Wolf, COO 718/918-8141
Arthur Wagner, Chief Operating Officer 718/918-4648
Kathy Garramone, Chief Operating Officer 718/918-3677
Diane Carr, Chief Information Officer 718/918-3690
Joseph Skarzynski, M.D., Medical Director 718/918-4606
Anne Iasiello, Associate Executive Director 718/918-5320

Affiliation: Albert Einstein College of Medicine of Yeshiva University; NYC
Health and Hospitals Corporation

Our Lady of Mercy Healthcare System
600 East 233rd Street
Bronx, New York 10466

Gary S. Horan, President/CEO 718/920-9501

Affiliation: New York Medical College

Our Lady of Mercy Medical Center

600 East 233rd Street
Bronx, New York 10466

Richard Celiberti, President and Chief Executive Officer 718/920-9501
Gerard Villucci, Chief Operating Officer
Joel Perlman, Chief Financial Officer 718/920-9501
Barbara Oddo, On-Site Attorney 718/920-9910
Maquid Megalli, M.D., Executive Vice President for Medical
Aff 718/920-9501

Affiliation: New York Medical College; Our Lady of Mercy Healthcare System

Brooklyn

Brooklyn Hospital Center

121 DeKalb Avenue
Brooklyn, New York 11201

Samuel Lehrfeld, CEO 718/250-8005
Paul Albertson, Sr. VP Hosp Operations/Ambulatory Care 718/250-8176
Joseph Guarracino, Chief Financial Officer 718/488-3755
Romulo Genato, Institutional Director for GME 718/250-6920
Irene Farrelly, Vice President, Information Systems 718/250-8330

Affiliation: New York-Presbyterian Healthcare System

Coney Island Hospital

2601 Ocean Parkway
Brooklyn, New York

Peter Wolf, Chief Operating Officer 718/616-4100
Silvana Dixon, Chief Information Officer 718/616-5340
Laura Battaglia, Quality Management/ Improvement
Director 718/616-5420

Affiliation: NYC Health and Hospitals Corporation; State University of New
York Downstate Medical Center College of Medicine

Kings County Hospital Center

451 Clarkson Avenue
Brooklyn, New York 11203

Jean G. Leon, Senior Vice President/CEO 718/245-3900
George Proctor, Chief Financial Officer/Chief Operating
Officer 718/245-3919
Julian John, Chief Financial Officer 718/245-2984
Dino Civan, Acting Chief Information Officer 718/245-3919
Kathie Rones, M.D., Medical Director/Associate Dean 718/245-3921

Affiliation: NYC Health and Hospitals Corporation; State University of New
York Downstate Medical Center College of Medicine

Long Island College Hospital
339 Hicks Street
Brooklyn, New York 11201

Rita Battles, President & CEO 718/780-4651
John Byne, Chief Operating Officer 718/283-8004
Frank E. Lucente, M.D., Vice Dean, GME 718/270-4188
Marc Milstein, Corp. Chief Information Officer 212/523-8448
Jill Clayton, Hospital Counsel 718/780-2927
Edmund Giegerich, M.D., Senior Vice President, Medical
    Affairs 718/780-4797
Margaret Casey, Director of Admissions 902/494-1847

Affiliation: Continuum Health Partners, Inc.

Maimonides Medical Center
4802 10th Avenue
Brooklyn, New York 11219

Pamela S. Brier, President 718/283-7025
Robert Naldi, Senior Vice President/CFO, Finance 718/283-3900
Kathryn M. Lane, Ed.D., Vice President, Academic Affairs 718/283-8245
Walter Fahey, Chief Information Officer 718/283-1800
Joyce A. Leahy, Vice President/General Counsel 718/283-7441
Samuel Kopel, M.D., Medical Director 718/283-7088
Sheila Namm, Associate Vice President, ... 718/283-6839

Affiliation: Mount Sinai School of Medicine of New York University

MediSys
One Brookdale Plaza
Brooklyn, New York

David P. Rosen, President/CEO 718/240-5212

Affiliation: State University of New York Downstate Medical Center College of
    Medicine

New York Methodist Hospital
506 Sixth Street
Brooklyn, New York 11215

Mark J. Mundy, President/CEO 718/780-3101
Edward Zaidberg, Senior Vice President, Finance 718/780-3031
Stanley Sherbell, M.D., Executive Vice President/Medical
    Affairs 718/780-3284
Grethel Marks, Director of Medical Records 718/780-3385

Affiliation: New York-Presbyterian Healthcare System; State University of New
    York Downstate Medical Center College of Medicine

SUNY Downstate Medical Center/University Hospital of Brooklyn
445 Lenox Road
Box 75
Brooklyn, New York 11203

Debra D. Carey, Chief Executive Officer 718/270-4293
Gerry Dantis, Director of Hospital Finance 718/826-4901
Eugene B. Feigelson, M.D., Senior Vice President for
Biomedical Education and Research and Dean (Until 8/
31/06) 718/270-3776
Bert Robles, Interim Chief Information Officer 718/270-2335
Kevin O'Mara, Associate University Counsel 718/270-4762
Torrance Akinsanya, Sr. Assoc Administrator/Quality Mgmt 718/270-4762
Affiliation: State University of New York Downstate Medical Center College of
Medicine

Veterans Affairs New York Harbor Health Care System-Brooklyn Campus
800 Poly Place
Brooklyn, New York 11209

John J. Donnellan Jr., Medical Center Director 718/630-3521
Robert Valenti, Chief, Fiscal Service 718/836-6600
Andrew J. Adler, M.D., Vice Chief of Staff 718/630-3653
Charles Desanno, Chief, Information Resources Management.............. 718/630-2850
Affiliation: State University of New York Downstate Medical Center College of
Medicine

Woodhull Medical & Mental Health Center
760 Broadway
Brooklyn, New York

Iris Jimenez-Hernandez, Senior Vice President 718/963-8101
K. Candis Best, Chief Operating Officer 718/963-8105
Milton Nunez, Chief Financial Officer 718/963-8125
Edward Fishkin, Medical Director 718/963-8569
Affiliation: NYC Health and Hospitals Corporation; State University of New
York Downstate Medical Center College of Medicine

Buffalo

Kaleida Health
100 High Street
Buffalo, New York 14203

James Kaskie, Chief Executive Officer 716/859-2732
Joseph Kissler, Senior Vice President, Finance/CFO 716/859-5600
Francis Meyer, Vice President, Information Systems &
Technology 718/588-6921
Linda J. Nenni, Vice President/General Counsel 718/588-6921
Cynthia Ann Ambres, M.D., Chief Medical Officer/Executive
Vice President 718/588-6921
C.J. Urlaub, Vice President, Process Improvement 718/588-6921
Affiliation: Kaleida Health/Buffalo General Hospital; University at Buffalo State
University of New York School of Medicine & Biomedical Sciences

Members: NEW YORK

Kaleida Health/Buffalo General Hospital
The Buffalo General Hospital
100 High Street
Buffalo, New York 14203

Robert Lovell, President 716/859-5600
Joseph Kissler, Senior Vice President, Finance/CFO 716/859-5600

Affiliation: Kaleida Health; University at Buffalo State University of New York
School of Medicine & Biomedical Sciences

Roswell Park Cancer Institute
Elm and Carlton Streets
Buffalo, New York 14263

Donald Trump, President and CEO 716/845-4062
Gregory McDonald, Chief Financial Officer
Arthur M. Michalek, Ph.D., Dean/Senior Vice President,
Acad Affair 716/845-2339
JoAnne Ruh, Vice President of Information Technology 716/845-3033
Michael Sexton, J.D., General Counsel 716/845-8717
Judy Smith, M.D., Medical Director 716/845-7724
Dana Fox-Jenkins, Assistant Vice President Organizational
Performance Improvement 716/845-8921

Affiliation: University at Buffalo State University of New York School of
Medicine & Biomedical Sciences

Veterans Affairs Western New York Healthcare System
Buffalo, New York

Michael Finegan, Medical Center Director 518/626-7300
Dennis D. Heberling, Facility Manager 716/862-8526
Royce Calhoun, Business Manager 716/862-8503
Patricia Widzinski, R.N., Facility Education Coordinator 716/862-6085
Margaret Owczarzak, Information Systems Manager 716/862-3254
Avery Ellis, M.D., Physician Executive 716/862-8530

Affiliation: University at Buffalo State University of New York School of
Medicine & Biomedical Sciences

Cooperstown

Bassett Healthcare
One Atwell Road
Cooperstown, New York 13326

William F. Streck, M.D., President/CEO 607/547-3100

Affiliation: Columbia University College of Physicians and Surgeons; University
of Rochester School of Medicine and Dentistry

Mary Imogene Bassett Hospital
One Atwell Road
Cooperstown, New York 13326

William F. Streck, M.D., President/CEO 607/547-3100
Bertine C. McKenna, Ph.D., Executive Vice President/COO 607/547-3100
Nicholas Nicoletta, Corporate Vice President/CFO 607/547-3635
James T. Dalton, M.D., Director of Medical Education 607/547-3764
Kenneth Deans, VP, Information Services and CIO 607/547-3094
L. Andrew Rauscher, Medical Director 607/547-3779
Ronette Kinzelman, Director, Organizational Quality
    Program 607/547-6609
Affiliation: Bassett Healthcare

Elmhurst

Elmhurst Hospital Center
79-01 Broadway
Elmhurst, New York 11373

Chris D. Constantino, Executive Director 718/334-1638
Julius Wool, Chief Finanical Officer 718/334-4900
Alfred Marino, Chief Information Officer 718/334-2401
Carolyn Adderley, Associate Executive Director 718/334-3692
Affiliation: Mount Sinai School of Medicine of New York University

Queens Hospital Center
79-01 Broadway
Elmhurst, New York

Antonio Martin, Executive Director 718/334-4900
Julius Wool, Chief Finanical Officer 718/334-4900
Alfred Marino, Chief Information Officer 718/334-2401
Terry Flexer, Senior Associate Executive Director 718/883-2222
Affiliation: Mount Sinai School of Medicine of New York University

Great Neck

North Shore-Long Island Jewish Health System
145 Community Drive
Great Neck, New York 11021

Michael Dowling, Chief Executive Officer 516/465-8003
Mark Solazzo, Chief
R. Shapiro, Sr VP Finance/CFO 516/465-8162
David Battinelli, M.D., Chief Academic Officer 516/465-3174
Charles M. Trunz III, Acting Chief Information Officer 516/465-8836
Keith C. Thompson, Sr VP Legal Affairs 516/465-8333
Lawrence Smith, Chief Medical Officer 516/465-3194
Joseph Conte, Sr. Vice President Quality Management 516/465-8313
Affiliation: Albert Einstein College of Medicine of Yeshiva University; State
    University of New York Downstate Medical Center College of
    Medicine; New York University School of Medicine; The School of
    Medicine at Stony Brook University Medical Center

Members: NEW YORK

Manhasset

North Shore University Hospital
300 Community Drive
Manhasset, New York 11030

Charles M. Trunz III, Acting Chief Information Officer 516/465-8836
R. Shapiro, Sr VP Finance/CFO 516/465-8162
Richard P. McGrail, Vice President,, CIO 516/734-3333
Keith C. Thompson, Sr VP Legal Affairs 516/465-8333
Paul Gitman, M.D., Vice President, Clinical Care and
Medical Director 718/470-7606
Yosef Dlugacz, Ph.D., Sr VP, Quality Management 516/465-2686
Affiliation: Albert Einstein College of Medicine of Yeshiva University; New York
University School of Medicine; North Shore-Long Island Jewish
Health System

Melville

Winthrop South Nassau University Health System, Inc.
100 Huntington Quadrangle
Suite 1C14
Melville, New York 11747

Deborah A. Gray, Executive Vice President 631/420-6711
Affiliation: The School of Medicine at Stony Brook University Medical Center

Mineola

Winthrop-University Hospital
259 First Street
Mineola, New York 11501

Daniel P. Walsh, President/CEO 516/663-2200
John Collins, Vice President for Finance 516/663-2311
John F. Aloia, M.D., Chief Academic Officer 516/663-2442
Nicholas A. Casabona, Director of Information Technology 516/663-2370
Joseph Greensher, M.D., Medical Director 516/663-2288
James Flaherty, Associate Administrator 718/470-7646
Affiliation: The School of Medicine at Stony Brook University Medical Center;
Winthrop South Nassau University Health System, Inc.

New Hyde Park

Long Island Jewish Medical Center
270-05 76th Avenue
New Hyde Park, New York 11040

Dennis Dowling, Executive Director 718/470-7764
R. Shapiro, Sr VP Finance/CFO 516/465-8162
Charles M. Trunz III, Acting Chief Information Officer 516/465-8836
Keith C. Thompson, Sr VP Legal Affairs 516/465-8333
Paul Gitman, M.D., Vice President, Clinical Care and
Medical Director 718/470-7606
Yosef Dlugacz, Ph.D., Sr VP, Quality Management 516/465-2686
Affiliation: Albert Einstein College of Medicine of Yeshiva University; North
Shore-Long Island Jewish Health System

New Rochelle

Sound Shore Health System
16 Gion Place
New Rochelle, New York

John R. Spicer, President/CEO 914/637-1100
Affiliation: New York Medical College

Sound Shore Medical Center of Westchester
16 Guion Place
New Rochelle, New York 10802

John R. Spicer, President/CEO 914/637-1100
Douglas O. Landy, Executive Vice President/COO 914/637-1100
Thomas Poccia, Acting Senior Vice President/CFO 914/637-1508
Jeffrey Brensilver, M.D., Chief Academic Offcer 914/637-1681
Barbara J. Cooke, Director, Hospital Information Systems 914/637-1525
Nancy Markey, In-House Labor Counsel 914/632-5000
Jeffrey S. Stier, M.D., Medical Director 914/637-1186
Affiliation: New York Medical College

New York

Bellevue Hospital Center
27th and First Avenue
New York, New York 10016

Lynda D. Curtis, CEO 212/562-1000
Mary E. Thompson, Chief Operating Officer 212/562-3757
Aaron Cohen, CFO 212/562-4372
Robert M. Glickman, M.D., Professor 212/263-5372
Mary McKenna, Chief Information Officer 212/562-3391
Alan Aviles, President 212/788-3321
Eric Manheimer, M.D., Medical Director 212/562-4743
Emily Mescon, Quality Management/ Improvement Director 212/562-3718
Affiliation: New York University School of Medicine

Beth Israel Medical Center
First Avenue at 16th Street
New York, New York 10003

David Shulkin, M.D., President & Chief Executive Officer 212/420-2873
Richard Freeman, Chief Operating Officer
John Collura, Sr. VP and Chief Financial Officer
Harris M. Nagler, M.D., Chairman, Department of Urology
    Director, Continuing Medical Education 212/844-8920
Marc Milstein, Corp. Chief Information Officer 212/523-8448
Kathryn C. Meyer, J.D., Senior Vice President, Legal Affairs 212/523-2162
David Bernard, Chief Medical Officer 212/420-2140
Donna Wilson, R.N., Director, Quality Improvement 212/420-4596
Affiliation: Albert Einstein College of Medicine of Yeshiva University;
    Continuum Health Partners, Inc.

Continuum Health Partners, Inc.
555 West 57th Street
19th Floor
New York, New York 10019

Stanley Brezenoff, President 212/523-8130
Brendan Loughlin, Sr. VP and Chief Financial Officer 212/523-2912
Harris M. Nagler, M.D., Chairman, Department of Urology
Director, Continuing Medical Education 212/844-8920
Affiliation: Albert Einstein College of Medicine of Yeshiva University; State
University of New York Downstate Medical Center College of
Medicine; New York University School of Medicine

Harlem Hospital Center
506 Lenox Avenue
New York, New York 10037

John M. Palmer, Ph.D., Executive Director/Network Chief
Operating Officer 212/939-1340
Stephen Lawrence, Ph.D., Chief Operating Officer 212/939-1398
Rick Walker, Chief Financial Officer 212/939-2027
Gerald Edmund Thomson, M.D., Senior Associate Dean 212/939-1375
Suzanne Monique Carter, Chief Information Officer 212/423-7230
Alan Aviles, President 212/788-3321
Glendon Henry, M.D., Medical Director 212/939-3872
Emma Beveridge, Senior Associate Director, Quality
Management 212/939-1287
Affiliation: Columbia University College of Physicians and Surgeons; NYC
Health and Hospitals Corporation

Hospital for Joint Diseases Orthopaedic Institute
301 East 17th Street
New York, New York 10003

David A. Dibner, FACHE, Senior Vice President/Site
Administrator 212/598-6534
Gerald Ferlisi, Vice President of Finance and CFO 212/404-4161
Joseph D. Zuckerman, M.D., Chairman of Orthopaedic
Surgery 212/598-6674
Annette Johnson, Senior Vice Pres.- & Senior General
Counsel 212/263-7921
H. Michael Belmont, M.D., Chief Medical Officer 212/598-6518
Maureen Keyes, Director of Regulatory Affairs 212/460-0118
Affiliation: New York University School of Medicine; NYU Medical Center

Hospital for Special Surgery
535 East 70th Street
New York, New York 10021

John R. Reynolds, President/CEO 212/606-1444
Lisa Goldstein, Vice President/COO 212/606-1236
Stacey Malakoff, Chief Financial Officer 212/606-1239
Thomas P. Sculco, M.D., Executive Assistant to the Surgeon-in-Chief 212/606-1475
John Cox, M.D., Chief Information Officer 212/606-1554
Constance Margolin, Vice President Legal Affairs 212/606-1153
Russell F. Warren, M.D., Surgeon-in-Chief/Medical Director 212/606-1178
Marion Hare, Associate Director, Administration and Quality Management 212/606-1236
Affiliation: Weill Cornell Medical College

Lenox Hill Healthcare Network
100 East 77th Street
New York, New York 10021

Gladys George, President/CEO 212/434-2010
Affiliation: New York University School of Medicine

Lenox Hill Hospital
100 East 77th Street
New York, New York 10021

Gladys George, President/CEO 212/434-2010
Terence M. O'Brien, Executive Vice President/COO 212/434-2010
Michael Breslin, Vice President/CFO 212/434-2040
Louis Ajamy, Vice President/CIO 212/434-2180
Terri Gillette, Director of Performance Improvement and Patient Sa 212/434-2434
Affiliation: Lenox Hill Healthcare Network

Memorial Sloan-Kettering Cancer Center
1275 York Avenue
New York, New York 10021

Harold Varmus, M.D., President/CEO 212/639-6561
John R. Gunn, Executive Vice President 212/639-6017
Michael Gutnick, Senior Vice President, Finance 646/227-3413
Patricia Skarulis, Chief Information Officer 646/227-3315
Roger N. Parker, Senior Vice President and General Counsel 212/639-5800
Affiliation: Weill Cornell Medical College

Metropolitan Hospital Center
1901 First Avenue
New York, New York 10029

Jose R. Sanchez, Senior Vice President, Metropolitan Hospital Center/Executive Director 212/423-6501
John M. Palmer, Ph.D., Executive Director/Network Chief Operating Officer 212/939-1340
Elizabeth Guzman, Chief Financial Officer 212/423-7722
Suzanne Monique Carter, Chief Information Officer 212/423-7230
Alan Aviles, President 212/788-3321
Sara Shahim, Senior Associate Executive Director 718/579-4945
Affiliation: New York Medical College

Mount Sinai Hospital~NY

One Gustave L. Levy Place
New York, New York 10029

Burton Drayer, President 212/241-7001
Donald Scanlon, Chief Financial Officer 212/731-3534
Nathan G. Kase, M.D., Interim CEO/President, Mt. Sinai
Medical Center/Interim Dean, Mt. Sinai School 212/241-8888
Michael G. MacDonald, Senior Vice President/General
Counsel 212/263-7291
Arthur Figur, M.D., Medical Director 212/241-6500

Affiliation: Mount Sinai School of Medicine of New York University; Sinai
Health System

New York-Presbyterian Healthcare System

525 East 68th Street
New York, New York 10021

Herbert Pardes, Chief Executive Officer 212/305-8000
Arthur A. Klein, M.D., Senior Vice President/COO 212/746-3577

Affiliation: Columbia University College of Physicians and Surgeons; Weill
Cornell Medical College; State University of New York Downstate
Medical Center College of Medicine

NewYork-Presbyterian Hospital The University Hospital of Columbia and Cornell

525 E. 68th Street
New York, New York 10021

Herbert Pardes, Chief Executive Officer 212/305-8000
Richard Aquila, Executive Vice President & Chief Operating
Officer 203/688-2606
Phyllis Lantos, Chief Financial Officer 212/305-6845
Walter Zerrenner, Senior VP/CIO 212/305-0090
Maxine Fass, Esq., Sr. VP, Chief Legal Officer 212/746-6500
Steven Corwin, M.D., Senior VP/Chief Medical Officer 212/305-0075

Affiliation: Columbia University College of Physicians and Surgeons; Weill
Cornell Medical College; New York-Presbyterian Healthcare System

NYC Health and Hospitals Corporation

125 Worth Street
New York, New York

Alan Aviles, President 212/788-3321

Affiliation: Albert Einstein College of Medicine of Yeshiva University; New York
Medical College; Mount Sinai School of Medicine of New York
University

NYU Hospitals Center
550 First Avenue
New York, New York 10016

Robert I. Grossman, M.D., The Saul J. Farber Dean Chief
Executive Officer, NYU Hospitals Center 212/263-3269
John P. Harney, Executive Vice President/COO 212/263-5505
Richard Baum, Controller 212/404-4121
Annette Johnson, Senior Vice Pres.- & Senior General
Counsel 212/263-7921
Max Cohen, Medical Director 212/263-2680
Edwina Thompson, Director of Quality Assessment and
Improvement 212/263-6601
Affiliation: New York University School of Medicine; NYU Medical Center

NYU Medical Center
1425 Madison Avenue
New York, New York 10029

St. Luke's-Roosevelt Hospital Center
1000 Tenth Avenue
New York, New York 10025

Frank Cracolici, President/CEO 212/523-5100
Anthony Pramberger, Senior Associate Dean 212/305-2311
Brendan Loughlin, Sr. VP and Chief Financial Officer 212/523-2912
Richard P. McGrail, Vice President,, CIO 516/734-3333
Palmer Delasandro, Vice President, Information Technology 212/523-4597
Kathryn C. Meyer, J.D., Senior Vice President, Legal Affairs 212/523-2162
Timothy Day, Vice President, Quality Initiatives 212/523-3718
Affiliation: Columbia University College of Physicians and Surgeons;
Continuum Health Partners, Inc.

Veterans Affairs New York Harbor Health Care System-New York Campus
423 East 23rd Street
New York, New York 10010

John J. Donnellan Jr., Medical Center Director 718/630-3521
D. Max Lewis, Associate Director 212/686-7500
Daniel Downey, Chief, Fiscal Service 212/686-7500
M. Joyce Rico, M.D., Associate Chief of Staff for Education 212/686-7500
M. Joyce Rico, M.D., Associate Chief of Staff for Education 212/686-7500
Peter J. Juliano, Chief, Medical Administration Service 212/686-7500
Michael S. Simberkoff, M.D., Chief of Staff 212/686-7500
Joann Flannery, Special Assistant Director, Quality
Management 212/686-7500
Affiliation: New York University School of Medicine

Northport

Northport Veterans Affairs Medical Center
79 Middleville Road
Northport, New York 11768

Gerald Culliton, Director 631/261-4400
Maria Favale, Associate Director 631/261-2741
Robert Ziskin, Chief, Information Resource Management
   Service 631/261-4400
Edward J. Mack, M.D., Chief of Staff 631/261-4400
Affiliation: The School of Medicine at Stony Brook University Medical Center

Rochester

Strong Health System
601 Elmwood Avenue
Rochester, New York 14642

Leo P. Brideau, Vice President, Regional Network and
   Managed Care Contracting 585/275-5534
Michael Goonan, VP, Finance/CFO 585/275-3300
Steven I. Goldstein, Vice President, Acute Care,Health
   System General Director/CEO, Strong Memorial 585/275-7685
Jerome Powell, Director of Information Systems 585/784-6118
Jeanine Arden Ornt, General Counsel, URMC/Strong Health............................ 585/275-8571
Peter G. Robinson, VP, Strategic Planning, Marketing &
   Operations 585/275-4036
Affiliation: University of Rochester School of Medicine and Dentistry

Strong Memorial Hospital
601 Elmwood Avenue
Rochester, New York 14642

Steven I. Goldstein, General Director/CEO, Strong
   Memorial Hospital, Vice President for Acute Care 585/275-7685
Kathleen M. Parrinello, R.N., Senior Director/COO 585/275-4605
Leonard Shute, Sr Dir, Finance/CFO Memorial and
   Highland Hospitals 585/275-3033
Richard Irving Burton, M.D., Senior Associate Dean,
   Academic Affairs 585/275-2747
Jerome Powell, Director of Information Systems 585/784-6118
Jeanine Arden Ornt, General Counsel, URMC/Strong Health............................ 585/275-8571
Robert J. Panzer, M.D., Director, OCPE/Chief Quality
   Officer 585/273-4438
Affiliation: Strong Health System

Staten Island

Staten Island University Hospital
475 Seaview Avenue
Staten Island, New York 10305

Anthony Ferreri, President and CEO 718/226-9034
Al Glover, Chief Operating Officer 718/226-1950
Tom Reca, Chief Financial Officer
Frank DiSanzo, Chief Information Officer 718/226-1075
Mark Jarrett, Chief Medical Director 718/226-1944
Joseph Conte, Sr. Vice President Quality Management 516/465-8313
Affiliation: North Shore-Long Island Jewish Health System

Stony Brook

University Hospital, SUNY Health Science Center, Stony Brook
HSC, Level 4, Suite 215
Stony Brook, New York 11794

Steven L. Strongwater, M.D., CEO 631/444-2701
Amir Rubin, Chief Operating Officer 631/444-2836
Dennis Mitchell, Chief Financial Officer 631/444-4100
N.H. Edelman, M.D., VP, Health Sciences Center/Dean
Dennis L. Proul, Chief Information Officer 631/444-7994
Susan Blum, J.D., Associate Counsel 631/444-8250
Thomas M. Biancaniello, M.D., Chief Medical Officer
   Associate Dean of Medical Affairs 631/444-8067
William H. Greene, M.D., Associate Director of Medical and
   Regulatory Affairs 631/444-2721
Affiliation: The School of Medicine at Stony Brook University Medical Center

Syracuse

Syracuse Veterans Affairs Medical Center
800 Irving Avenue
Syracuse, New York 13210

James Cody, Medical Center Director 315/425-4892
Robert Alsheimer, Chief Financial Officer 315/425-4400
Michael W. Valerio, Ph.D., Associate Chief of Staff for
   Education 315/425-4639
Michael LeRoy, Director Information Services 315/425-4400
David Altieri, Legal Counsel 315/425-4839
E. Jackson Allison Jr., M.D., Associate Dean & Professor of
   Emergency Medicine 315/425-4888
John LeBeau, Patient Safety Manager 315/425-2430
Affiliation: State University of New York Upstate Medical University

University Hospital, SUNY Upstate Medical University
750 E. Adams Street
Syracuse, New York 13210

Phillip S. Schaengold, J.D., CEO 315/464-4223
Ann Sedore, Ph.D., Chief Operating Officer 315/464-6138
Stuart Wright, Chief Financial Officer 315/464-6530
Terry Wagner, Chief Information Officer University Hospital 315/464-4252
Patricia Numann, M.D., Medical Director 315/464-4603
Affiliation: State University of New York Upstate Medical University

Valhalla

Westchester Medical Center
Valhalla, New York 10595

Michael D. Israel, President/CEO 914/493-7018
Gary Burnicke, Executive Vice President, Business 914/493-2816
David Steele, M.B.A., Senior Vice President, Westchester
County HealthCare Corporation 914/493-1540
Marilyn Slaatten, Esq., Executive Vice President 914/493-2800
George Reed, M.D., Medical Director/Vice Dean 914/493-8781
Affiliation: New York Medical College

NORTH CAROLINA

Chapel Hill

UNC Health Care System
101 Manning Drive
Chapel Hill, North Carolina 27514

William L. Roper, M.D., M.P.H., Dean, School of Medicine
VC, Medical Affairs & CEO, UNC Hlth Care System 919/966-4161
Affiliation: University of North Carolina at Chapel Hill School of Medicine

University of North Carolina Hospitals
101 Manning Drive
Chapel Hill, North Carolina 27514

Gary L. Park, President 919/966-5111
Todd L. Peterson, Executive Vice President & COO, UNC
Hospitals 919/966-5111
John Lewis, Senior Vice President & CFO 919/966-3530
J. Kichak, Vice President & CIO 919/966-2320
Benjamin I. Gilbert, Senior Vice President, Legal Services 919/966-6285
Brian Goldstein, Executive Associate Dean for Clinical
Affairs/Chief of Staff 919/966-8622
Stanley R. Mandel, M.D., Chief of Staff Emeritus 919/966-4131
Martha Shackelford, Clinical Compliance Manager
Performance Improvement/Patient Safety
Affiliation: UNC Health Care System

Charlotte

Carolinas HealthCare System
1000 Blythe Boulevard
Charlotte, North Carolina 28203
    Michael C. Tarwater, President/CEO 704/355-3216
Affiliation: University of North Carolina at Chapel Hill School of Medicine

Carolinas Medical Center
1000 Blythe Boulevard
P.O. Box 32861
Charlotte, North Carolina 28232-2861
    Suzanne H. Freeman, R.N., President 704/355-3344
    Phyllis Wingate-Jones, Senior Vice President, Operations 704/355-5073
    Greg Gombar, EVP Administrative Services, CFO-CHS 704/355-2154
    James McDeavitt, M.D., Senior VP, Education & Research 704/355-3146
    John J. Knox, Senior VP/Chief Information Officer 704/355-1116
    Keith Smith, Senior Vice President & General Counsel 704/355-3858
    Pat Taylor, Vice President, Administration 704/355-8050
Affiliation: Carolinas HealthCare System

Durham

Department of Veterans Affairs Veterans Integrated Service Network VISN 6
300 Morgan Street-Suite 1402
Durham, North Carolina 27701
    Daniel F. Hoffmann, Network Director(10N6) 919/956-5541
    Albert Brese, Chief Financial Officer 919/956-5541
    Milton Harrison, Chief Information Officer 919/956-5541
    Mark Shelhorse, M.D., Chief Medical Officer 919/956-5541

Duke University Health System
Box 3701
Durham, North Carolina 27710
    Victor Dzau, Chancellor for Health Affairs & President and
    CEO 919/684-2255
    Mark Miller, Chief Financial Officer 919/613-8924
Affiliation: Duke University School of Medicine

Duke University Hospital
Box 3708
Durham, North Carolina 27710
    William J. Fulkerson, M.D., VP & Chief Executive Officer 919/684-8076
    Kevin Sowers, Chief Operating Officer 919/681-6624
    Mark Miller, Chief Financial Officer 919/613-8924
    Asif Ahmad, M.D., Chief Information Officer 919/286-6324
    Gail Shulby, Compliance Officer 919/681-8176
Affiliation: Duke University Health System

Members: NORTH CAROLINA

Durham Veterans Affairs Medical Center
508 Fulton Street
Durham, North Carolina 27705

Ralph Gigliotti, Medical Center Director 919/286-6904
Phyllis Smith, Associate Director 919/286-6904
David Kuboushek, Chief Financial Manager 919/286-6914
Catherine Kaminetzky, Associate Chief of Staff for Education............................... 919/286-6909
Toby Dickerson, Chief, Information Resources Management
John D. Shelburne, M.D., Ph.D., Chief of Staff 919/286-6907
Jane Penny, Chief, Quality Management 919/286-6905
Affiliation: Brody School of Medicine at East Carolina University

Greenville

Pitt County Memorial Hospital
2100 Stantonsburg Road
Greenville, North Carolina 27835

Jim Carter, Chief Medical Officer E. Carolina 252/847-4398
Jack Holsten, Chief Financial Officer 252/847-4582
Edward L. McFall, Chief Information Officer 252/847-4976
Nancy B. Aycock, General Counsel 252/847-6300
Ernest Larkin, M.D., Chief Medical Officer 252/847-5345
Affiliation: Brody School of Medicine at East Carolina University; University
Health System of Eastern Carolina, Inc.

University Health System of Eastern Carolina, Inc.
2100 Stantonsburg Road
Greenville, North Carolina 27835

Dave C. McRae, Chief Executive Officer 252/847-4583
Jack Holsten, Chief Financial Officer 252/847-4582
Edward L. McFall, Chief Information Officer 252/847-4976
Nancy B. Aycock, General Counsel 252/847-6300
Affiliation: Brody School of Medicine at East Carolina University

Winston-Salem

North Carolina Baptist Hospital
Medical Center Boulevard
Winston-Salem, North Carolina 27157

Donny C. Lambeth, Interim President and Chief Operating
Officer 336/716-3003
Gina Ramsey, Vice President, Financial Serv 336/716-3005
Paul M. Lorusso, Vice President, Information Services/Chief
Information Officer 336/716-3781
J. McLain Wallace Jr., Vice President, Legal Affairs 336/716-2817
Patricia L. Adams, M.D., Chief of Professional Services 336/716-9592
Ronald H. Small, Vice President, Quality Outcomes 336/713-3406
Affiliation: Wake Forest University School of Medicine

NORTH DAKOTA

Fargo

MeritCare Hospital
PO Box MC
Fargo, North Dakota 58122

Roger L. Gilbertson, M.D., President/CEO, MeritCare
Health System 701/234-6960
John Doherty, Senior Executive, Chief Financial Officer 701/234-6952
Lisa Carlson, CFO 701/234-4811
Bruce Pitts, M.D., Assoc Dean, Med Educ Ctr 701/293-4108
Craig Hewitt, Executive Partner, Information Systems
Paul Richard, General Legal Counsel 701/234-6919
Gregory Post, M.D., Chief of Staff
Rhonda Ketterling, Quality Management/Improvement
Director

Affiliation: University of North Dakota School of Medicine and Health Sciences

OHIO

Akron

Akron General Medical Center
400 Wabash Ave.
Akron, Ohio 44307

Alan J. Bleyer, President 330/344-7679
Cathy Ceccio, COO 330/344-1019
Deborah Gorbach, Interim Chief Financial Officer 330/444-6000
James Dougherty, M.D., Chairman, Med. Educ. 330/344-6050
Richard J. Streck, M.D., Senior Vice President, Medical
Affairs 330/344-6789

Affiliation: Northeastern Ohio Universities Colleges of Medicine and Pharmacy

Children's Hospital Medical Center of Akron
One Perkins Square
Akron, Ohio 44308-1062

William H. Considine, President 330/543-8293
John P. Stoner, Executive Vice President/Treasurer 203/276-7463
Dennis Jancsy, Chief Financial Officer 330/543-8384
John McBride, M.D., Vice Chairman, Department of
Pediatrics 330/543-8142
Jeffrey J. Hale, Vice President, Information Services 330/543-8280
Keith R. Powell, M.D., Vice President for Clinical Services
and Chairman, Department of Pediatrics 330/543-8906

Affiliation: Northeastern Ohio Universities Colleges of Medicine and Pharmacy

Members: OHIO

Summa Health System Hospitals
525 East Market Street
P. O. Box 2090
Akron, Ohio 44309-2090

Thomas Strauss, President/CEO 330/375-3000
Robert Harrigan, Executive Vice President/COO 330/375-3000
Michael Rutherford, Chief Financial Officer 330/375-3196
Joseph Zarconi, M.D., Vice President, Medical Education and
    Research 330/375-3106
Charles Ross, M.D., Chief Information Officer/Vice
    President, Information and Technical 330/996-8544
William Powell, Vice President Legal Services 330/375-3954
Dale Murphy, M.D., Vice President Medical Affairs 330/375-3314
Don Jackovitz, Director, Quality & Resource Management 330/375-3880
Affiliation: Northeastern Ohio Universities Colleges of Medicine and Pharmacy

Canton

Aultman Hospital
2600 Sixth Street, S.W.
Canton, Ohio 44710

Edward Roth, President/CEO 330/363-6241
Mark Wright, CFO 330/363-6093
Tim Oberschlake, Associate Vice President Information
    System 330/363-3448
Affiliation: Northeastern Ohio Universities Colleges of Medicine and Pharmacy

Cincinnati

Cincinnati Children's Hospital Medical Center
3333 Burnet Avenue
Cincinnati, Ohio 45229-3039

James M. Anderson, President/CEO 513/636-4000
Scott Hamlin, Senior Vice President, Finance 513/636-7454
Thomas F. Boat, M.D., Professor and Chair 513/636-4588
Elizabeth A. Stautberg, Vice Presdient, General Counsel 513/636-4069
Michael K. Farrell, M.D., Chief of Staff 513/636-6717
Affiliation: University of Cincinnati College of Medicine

Cincinnati Veterans Affairs Medical Center
3200 Vine Street
Cincinnati, Ohio 45220

Linda Smith, M.P.A., Medical Center Director 513/475-6300
Thomas P. Pishioneri, Associate Medical Center Director 513/475-6301
Mary Oden, Assistant Medical Center Director for Education............................... 513/475-6517
Debra Luttjohann, Chief, Information Resource Management
    Service 513/475-6314
Mary Garcia, Regional Counselor 513/475-6421
Creighton Wright, Chief of Staff 513/475-6302
Affiliation: University of Cincinnati College of Medicine

Department of Veterans Affairs Veterans Integrated Service Network VISN 10
11500 Northlake Drive, Suite 200
Cincinnati, Ohio 45249

Good Samaritan Hospital
375 Dixmyth Avenue
Cincinnati, Ohio 45220

John Prout, President/CEO 513/569-6141
Claus von Zychlin, Executive Vice President/COO 513/563-6149
Craig Rucker, Chief Financial Officer 513/569-6107
Thomas A. Saladin, M.D., Vice President of Academic Affairs 513/872-2778
Rick Moore, Vice President Chief Information Officer 513/569-6800
Donna Nienaber, Vice President, Corporate Counsel 513/569-6062
Larry Johnstal, Director, Clinical Improvement & Medical
Staff Administration 513/569-6160
Affiliation: University of Cincinnati College of Medicine

Health Alliance of Greater Cincinnati
3200 Burnet Avenue
Cincinnati, Ohio 45229

Kenneth Hanover, President/CEO 513/585-8708
Dorman Fawley, Executive Vice President/COO 513/585-8702
Gary R. Harris, Esq., General Counsel 513/585-6452
Affiliation: University of Cincinnati College of Medicine

University Hospital
234 Goodman Street
Cincinnati, Ohio 45219

Lee Ann Liska, Executive Director 513/584-4742
Rick Hinds, Vice President, Financial Services 513/584-2135
Andrew Filak, M.D., Senior Associate Dean for Academic
Affairs 513/558-7342
Alex Rodriguez, Vice President, Information Technology 513/585-8883
Kathleen Beal, Director, Quality Management 513/584-5721
Affiliation: Health Alliance of Greater Cincinnati

Cleveland

Cleveland Clinic Health System
9500 Euclid Avenue
Cleveland, Ohio 44195

Louis Stokes Veterans Affairs Medical Center
10701 East Boulevard
Cleveland, Ohio 44106

William D. Montague, M.S., Medical Center Director 216/791-3800
Gene DeAngelas, Chief, Fiscal Service 216/526-3030
Murray Altose, M.D., Chief of Staff (WP) 216/421-3030
Michael Hickman, Chief, Information Resources 216/838-6096
Peter F. Goyer, M.D., Chief of Staff 216/526-3030
Affiliation: Case Western Reserve University School of Medicine

Members: OHIO

MetroHealth System
2500 MetroHealth Drive
Cleveland, Ohio 44109

John Sideras, CEO 216/778-5700
Bill Reniff, Vice President and Chief Financial Officer 216/778-5716
Ben Brouhard, Executive Vice President Chief of Staff 216/778-4900
Vince Miller, Vice Presdient/CIO 216/778-5007
William G. West, General Counsel 216/778-5723
Christopher Brandt, President of Medical Staff 216/778-4797
Gloria Letostak, Manager Accreditation Readiness Quality
Management Department 216/778-3135

Affiliation: Case Western Reserve University School of Medicine; MetroHealth
System

University Case Medical Center
11100 Euclid Avenue
Cleveland, Ohio 44106-5000

Fred Craig Rothstein, M.D., President 216/844-6217
Michael Szubski, Senior Vice President/CFO 216/844-3500
Jerry Mark Shuck, M.D., D.Sc., Director of GME 216/844-3871
Mary Alice Annecharico, Senior Vice President and CIO 216/767-8655
Janet L. Miller, Senior Vice President and General 216/844-3817
Michael Anderson, Interim Chief Medical Officer 216/983-5633
Randy Harmatz, VP Quality Outcomes/Clinical DecisionSup 216/844-7015

Affiliation: Case Western Reserve University School of Medicine; University
Hospitals Heatlh System

University Hospitals HeatlhSystem
11100 Euclid Avenue
Cleveland, Ohio 44106-5000

Thomas F. Zenty III, President/CEO 216/844-7565
Michael Szubski, Senior Vice President/CFO 216/844-1000

Affiliation: Case Western Reserve University School of Medicine

Columbus

Arthur G. James Cancer Hospital and Richard J. Solove Research Institute
300 West 10th Avenue, Suite 519
Columbus, Ohio 43210

David E. Schuller, M.D., Director 614/293-5485
Dennis J. Smith, Director of Administration 614/293-3300
Julian Bell, Administrator of Financial Services 614/293-3300
Maxine J. Moehring, Director of Information Systems 614/293-3300
Colleen Allen, R.N., M.B.A., Director of Clinical Quality &
Resource Management 614/293-3300

Affiliation: Ohio State University College of Medicine

Grant-Riverside Methodist Hospitals, Grant Medical Center Campus
111 S. Grant Avenue
Columbus, Ohio 43215

> **Dave Bloom,** Chief Operating Officer 614/566-9900
> **Edsel Cotter,** Senior Operations Officer 614/566-9164
> **Vinson Yates,** Financial Controller 614/566-5759
> **Bruce T. Vanderhoff, M.D.,** Director, Medical Education 614/566-9294
> **Fred T. Nobrega, M.D.,** Vice President, Medical Affairs 614/566-9971
> *Affiliation:* Ohio State University College of Medicine; OhioHealth

Grant-Riverside Methodist Hospitals, Riverside Campus
3535 Olentangy River Road
Columbus, Ohio 43214

> **Bruce Hagen,** President 614/566-3602
> **Michael Louge,** Chief Financial Officer 614/566-4757
> *Affiliation:* Ohio State University College of Medicine; OhioHealth

Nationwide Children's Hospital, Inc.
700 Children's Drive
Columbus, Ohio 43205

> **Rick Miller,** President/CEO 614/722-2259
> **Tim Robinson,** Chief Financial Officer 614/722-5972
> *Affiliation:* Ohio State University College of Medicine

Ohio State University Health System
410 West Tenth Avenue
Columbus, Ohio 43210

> **Peter Geier,** CEO 614/292-2635
> *Affiliation:* Ohio State University College of Medicine

Ohio State University Hospitals
410 West Tenth Avenue
Columbus, Ohio 43210

> **Larry A. Anstine,** Executive Director 614/293-9700
> **Eric Kunz,** Associate VP Facilities/Materiel Mgt 614/247-8328
> **John Stone,** Administrator 614/293-2130
> **Hagop Mekhjian, M.D.,** Assoc. Dean/Medical Director 614/293-8158
> **Asif Ahmad, M.D.,** Chief Information Officer 919/286-6324
> **Hagop Mekhjian, M.D.,** Assoc. Dean/Medical Director 614/293-8158
> **Gail Marsh,** Chief Strategy Officer 614/247-8314
> *Affiliation:* Ohio State University College of Medicine; Ohio State University
> Health System

OhioHealth
3555 Olentangy River Road
Columbus, Ohio 43214

> **David P. Blom,** President-OhioHealth 614/544-4412
> *Affiliation:* Ohio State University College of Medicine

Dayton

Children's Medical Center
One Children's Plaza
Dayton, Ohio 45404

David Kinsaul, President/CEO 937/641-3445
David Miller, Vice President/CFO 937/641-3000
Elizabeth Fredette, CIO/Director/Information Services 937/641-3000
Thomas F. Murphy, M.D., Vice President, Medical Affairs 937/641-5871
Carol Wise, Director Quality Resource Mgmt 937/641-3000
Affiliation: Wright State University Boonshoft School of Medicine

Dayton Veterans Affairs Medical Center
4100 West Third Street
Dayton, Ohio 45428

Guy Richardson, Medical Center Director 937/262-2114
Joe Battle, Associate Medical Center 937/262-2166
Lawrence Andrews, Chief, Fiscal Service 937/268-6511
Melissa Miller, Staff Attorney 937/268-6511
Steven M. Cohen, M.D., Chief of Staff 937/262-2106
Lisa Durham, R.N., Chief, Quality Management Service 937/268-6511
Affiliation: Wright State University Boonshoft School of Medicine

Miami Valley Hospital
One Wyoming Street
Dayton, Ohio 45409

Mary H. Boosalis, President & CEO 937/208-2701
Tom Duncan, Executive Vice President/CFO 937/208-8000
Gary Collier, VPMA/CMO
Nikkie Clancy, Chief Information Officer
Dale Creech, General Counsel
David Uddin, Ph.D., Vice Chair, Medical Education Director,
    Clinical Research Center 937/208-2239
Tim Collins, Vice President, Quality Management 937/208-6047
Affiliation: Wright State University Boonshoft School of Medicine

Independence

Cleveland Clinic Foundation
6801 Brecksville Rd, RK45
Independence, Ohio 44195

Delos M. Cosgrove, M.D., Chief Executive Officer 216/444-6733
Michael P. O'Boyle, Chief Operating Officer 216/444-0603
Steven Glass, Chief Fianancial Officer 216/444-2575
Eric Topol, M.D., Chief Academic Officer 216/445-9490
C. Martin Harris, M.D., Chief Information Officer 216/444-4246
David W. Rowan, General Counsel 216/444-2340
J. Michael Henderson, Director, Quality Insititute 216/445-0318
Affiliation: Case Western Reserve University School of Medicine; Cleveland
    Clinic Health System

Kettering

Kettering Medical Center
3535 Southern Boulevard
Kettering, Ohio 45429

Fred Manchur, President 937/395-8165
Brett Spenst, VP, Finance and Operations 937/395-8520
Charles Scriven, Chief Academic Officer 937/395-8618
Frank Engler, Manager, Community Affairs & Institutional
  Advancement 937/395-8866
Gregory R. Wise, M.D., VP, Medical Affairs 937/395-8658
Stephen House, M.D., Director, Clinical Management 937/395-8856
Affiliation: Loma Linda University School of Medicine; Wright State University
  Boonshoft School of Medicine

Toledo

University of Toledo Medical Center
3000 Arlington Avenue
Toledo, Ohio 43614

Lloyd Jacobs, President 419/530-2211
Scott Scarborough, Senior VP, Finance & Administration 419/383-6866
Roland Skeel, M.D., Interim Dean 419/383-4242
Melodie Rufener, M.B.A., Admn Director of Information
  Systems 419/383-4587
Margaret McFadden, Adm. Dir. Qual. Management 419/383-4977
Affiliation: The University of Toledo College of Medicine

Youngstown

Forum Health
3530 Belmont Avenue
Youngstown, Ohio 44505

Forum Health-Western Reserve Care System
500 Gypsy Lane
Youngstown, Ohio 44501

Kevin Spiegel, Chief Executive Officer 901/516-2600
Roxia B. Boykin, R.N., Executive Vice President & COO 330/884-5858
Chuck Lane, Chief Financial Officer 901/516-2193
Mark Kishel, Chief Medical Officer 330/884-5089
Tim Roe, Chief Information Officer 330/884-1365
Eugene Mowed, M.D., Director of Medical Ecucation 330/884-3951
Affiliation: Forum Health; Northeastern Ohio Universities Colleges of Medicine
  and Pharmacy

St. Elizabeth Health Center

1044 Belmont Avenue
P.O. Box 1790
Youngstown, Ohio 445011790

Robert Shroder, President & CEO 330/480-3570
Donald Kline, Chief Financial Officer 330/884-7055
Kenneth P. Heaps, M.D., Sr. Vice President, Medical Affairs 330/480-3279
Chuck Folkwein, M.B.A., Sr. VP/Chief Information Officer 330/746-1010
Joseph Shoaff, Legal Counsel 330/480-3847
Mary Bigowsky, R.N., M.S.N., Director Case Mgmt/Quality
Improvement 330/480-3298

Affiliation: Northeastern Ohio Universities Colleges of Medicine and Pharmacy

OKLAHOMA

Oklahoma City

Oklahoma City Veterans Affairs Medical Center

921 N.E. 13th Street
Oklahoma City, Oklahoma 73104

David Wood, Medical Center Director 405/456-1000
Kathleen Fogarty, Associate Director 405/270-5134
Haze McDougal, Chief Fiscal Service 405/290-1807
Steven R. Orwig, M.D., Associate Chief of Staff for
Education 405/270-5199
Leigh Mulanax, Chief, Information Managment Service 405/270-5172
Stephanie Darr, Staff Attorney 405/270-5177
D. Robert McCaffree, M.D., Chief of Staff, Associate Dean,
College of Medicine 405/270-5135
Donna DeLise, Director, Quality Management 405/270-5194

Affiliation: University of Oklahoma College of Medicine

OU Medical Center

P. O. Box 26307
1200 Everett Drive, Everett Tower
Oklahoma City, Oklahoma 73104

Cole C. Eslyn, President and Chief Executive Officer 405/271-5911
Becki Benoit, Chief Operating Officer, Adult Services 405/271-5911
Jim Watson, Chief Financial Officer 405/271-5911
Larry Forsyth, Director, Information Systems 405/271-5559
J. Andy Sullivan, M.D., Chief Medical Officer 405/271-5911
Kathy Jost, Quality Management-Improvement Director 405/271-6310

Affiliation: University of Oklahoma College of Medicine

OREGON

Portland

Oregon Health & Science University
3181 SW Sam Jackson Park Road
Portland, Oregon 97201

Peter F. Rapp, VP and Executive Director 503/494-4036
Diana Gernhart, Director of Fiscal Services Chief Financial
Officer 503/494-1283
Lesley M. Hallick, Ph.D., Vice President/Provost 503/494-4460
John Jay Kenagy, Chief Information Officer 503/494-8341
Ronald W. Schumacher, Chief Information Officer 503/494-4420
Steve Stadum, General Counsel 503/494-5222
A. Roy Magnusson, M.D., Director, Medical/Clinical Services 503/494-6020
Christine Slusarenko, Director, Quality Management 503/494-6459
Affiliation: Oregon Health & Science University School of Medicine

Portland Veterans Affairs Medical Center
PO Box 1034
Portland, Oregon 97207

James Tuchschmidt, M.D., Medical Center Director 503/273-5247
Kathleen Chapman, R.N., Deputy Director/AD for Patient
Care Svcs 503/273-5001
Susan Heublein, AD for Finance & Support Services 503/273-5278
David Douglas, AD for Information Management 503/220-8262
Michael McCarthy, Regional Counsel 503/326-2441
Susan Gilbert, Chief, Quality & Performance Service 503/220-8262
Affiliation: Oregon Health & Science University School of Medicine

PENNSYLVANIA

Allentown

Lehigh Valley Hospital
P.O. Box 7017,
17th & Chew Streets
Allentown, Pennsylvania 18105

Elliot J. Sussman, M.D., President/CEO 610/402-7505
Louis L. Liebhaber, Chief Operating Officer 610/402-7516
Vaughn Gower, Senior Vice President, Finance 610/402-7535
Sara S. Viessman, Director, Division of Education 610/402-2501
Harry F. Lukens, Sr VP Information Services/CIO 610/402-1406
Glenn Guanowsky, Legal Counsel 610/402-2776
Ronald Swinfard, Chief Medical Officer 610/402-7502
Robert Murphy, Senior VP, Quality and Care Management 610/402-1770
Affiliation: Drexel University College of Medicine

Members: PENNSYLVANIA

Bethlehem

St. Luke's Hospital~PA
801 Ostrum Street
Bethlehem, Pennsylvania 18015

Richard A. Anderson, President & CEO 610/954-4000
Thomas Lichten Walner, Senior Vice President, Finance 610/954-3100
Joel C. Rosenfeld, M.D., Director, Medical Education 610/954-2255
Cynthia Jones, Chief Information Officer 610/954-3331
Seymour Traub, Vice President/General Counsel 610/954-4114
Charles D. Saunders, M.D., Senior Vice President Medical
and Academic Affairs 610/954-4654
Donna Sabol, Assistant Vice President Network Performance
Improvement 610/954-4102
Affiliation: Philadelphia College of Osteopathic Medicine

Danville

Geisinger Health System
100 N. Academy Avenue
Danville, Pennsylvania 17822

Glenn D. Steele Jr., M.D., Ph.D., President/CEO 570/271-6168
Frank J. Trembulak, Executive Vice President/COO 570/271-6467
Kevin Brennan, Vice President, Finance 570/271-6211
Linda M. Famiglio, M.D., Chief Academic Officer Assistant
Dean, Temple University SOM 570/271-6114
Kristen Beech, General Counsel
Howard Grant, Chief Medical Officer 570/271-6832
Albert Bothe Jr., M.D., Chief Quality Officer 570/271-7936
Affiliation: Temple University School of Medicine

Erie

Hamot Medical Center
201 State Street
Erie, Pennsylvania 16550

John T. Malone, President/CEO 814/877-2431
James Pepicello, Chief Operating Officer 814/877-3210
Steve Danch, CFO 814/877-6162
Joseph Butler, Chief Information Officer 814/877-2432
James Donnelly, Quality Management/Improvement Director 814/877-4143
Affiliation: Drexel University College of Medicine

Harrisburg

Pinnacle Health Hospitals
409 South Second Street
P.O. Box 8700
Harrisburg, Pennsylvania

Roger Longenderfer, President & CEO 717/231-8200
William Pugh, Chief Financial Officer 717/782-3131

Hershey

The Milton S. Hershey Medical Center
500 University Drive
P.O. Box 850
Hershey, Pennsylvania 17033

A. Craig Hillemeier, Vice Dean for Clinical Affairs 717/531-6700
Kevin J. Haley, Director of Finance Chief Financial Officer 717/531-6614
Kenneth Blythe, Chief Information Officer The Milton S.
Hershey Medical Center 717/531-1083
R. Mark Faulkner, Esq., General Counsel 814/238-4926
Michael R. Weitekamp, M.D., Medical Director 717/531-8803
Affiliation: Pennsylvania State University College of Medicine

Philadelphia

Albert Einstein Medical Center (Albert Einstein Healthcare Network)
5501 Old York Road
Philadelphia, Pennsylvania 19141

Barry R. Freedman, President and CEO 215/456-7010
A. Susan Bernini, Chief Operating Officer 215/456-6010
Brian Derrick, Chief Financial Officer 215/456-7030
Douglas McGee, Chief Academic Officer 215/456-7056
Kenneth D. Levitan, Chief Information Officer 215/456-8131
Penny Rezet, Esq., General Counsel 215/456 7993
Richard Greenberg, M.D., President Medical Staff 215/457-4444
Jeffrey Cohn, M.D., Chief Quality Officer 215/456-8914
Affiliation: Jefferson Medical College of Thomas Jefferson University

Children's Hospital of Philadelphia
34th and Civic Center Boulevard
Philadelphia, Pennsylvania 19104

Steven M. Altschuler, M.D., President and Chief Executive
Officer 267/426-6142
Gavin Kerr, Executive Vice President & COO 267/426-6981
Thomas Todorow, Sr. Vice President, Finance 267/426 6957
Charles Enicks, SVP and Chief Information Officer 267/426-6939
Bonnie S. Brier, J.D., General Counsel 267/426-6131
James Steven, M.D., Sr Vice President, Medical Affairs
Affiliation: University of Pennsylvania School of Medicine

Fox Chase Cancer Center
333 Cottman Avenue
Philadelphia, Pennsylvania 19111

Robert C. Young, M.D., President 215/728-2781
R. Donald Leedy, Executive Vice President 215/728-2453
Joseph Hediger, Chief Financial Officer 215/728-6900
Robert F. Ozols, M.D., Senior Vice President, Medical
Science Division 215/728-2673
Delinda Pendleton, R.N., Director, Quality Management &
Infection Control 215/728-2660
Affiliation: Temple University School of Medicine

Hospital of the University of Pennsylvania
3400 Spruce Street
Philadelphia, Pennsylvania 19104

Ralph W. Muller, Chief Executive Officer 215/662-2203
Garry L. Scheib, Chief Operating Officer 215/662-3227
Keith Casper, Chief Financial Officer 215/662-2792
Lee J. Dobkin, Chief Counsel, UPHS 215/746-5220
Bernett L. Johnson Jr., M.D., Senior Medical Officer, HUP 215/662-6153
Patrick J. Brennan, M.D., Chief Medical Officer and Senior
Vice President 215/615-0668

Affiliation: University of Pennsylvania Health System

Philadelphia Veterans Affairs Medical Center
University and Woodland Avenues
Philadelphia, Pennsylvania 19104

Michael J. Sullivan, Medical Center Director 215/823-5857
Margaret O'Shea Caplan, Chief Operating Officer 215/823-5858
Vinh Tran, Chief Financial Officer 215/823-6005
Laura Veet, M.D., ACOS Medical Center Education 215/823-5998
Jose Lopez, Regional Counsel 215/823-7811
Martin F. Heyworth, M.D., Chief of Staff 215/823-5859
Michael Neiman, Quality Management Director 215/823-5836

Affiliation: University of Pennsylvania School of Medicine

St. Christopher's Hospital for Children
Erie Avenue at Front Street
Philadelphia, Pennsylvania 19134-1095

Bernadette Mangan, Chief Executive Officer 215/427-5146
Jill Tillman, M.S.N., M.B.A., Chief Operating Officer/Acting
CEO 215/427-5146
Gil Cottle, Chief Financial Officer 215/427-4828
Daniel V. Schidlow, M.D., Physician-in-Chief/Chief Medical
Officer 215/427-4801
Angelo Giardino, Associate Physician-in-Chief 215/427-8872

Affiliation: Drexel University College of Medicine

Temple University Health System
Broad and Ontario Streets
Philadelphia, Pennsylvania 19140

Joseph W. Marshall III, President & CEO 215/707-0900

Affiliation: Temple University School of Medicine

Temple University Hospital
Broad and Ontario Streets
Philadelphia, Pennsylvania 19140

Joseph W. Marshall III, President & CEO 215/707-0900
Robert Pezzoli, President & COO 215/707-5776
Robert Lux, Vice President & CFO 215/707-3802
John Michael Daly, M.D., Dean 215/707-8773
Arthur Papacostas, Ph.D., Chief Information Officer 215/707-2000
Beth C. Koob, J.D., Chief Counsel 215/707-5605
Howard Grant, Chief Medical Officer 570/271-6832
Susan L. Freeman, Chief Medical Officer 215/707-0766
Affiliation: Temple University Health System

Tenet Health System, Hahnemann University Hospital
Broad and Vine Streets-MS #300
Philadelphia, Pennsylvania 19102

Michael P. Halter, CEO 215/762-7167
James Burke, COO
Brian Rielly, Chief Financial Officer 215/762-3180
Paula Hudson, Chief Information Officer 215/255-3302
Barbara Zurzolo, Senoir Managing Counsel 215/255-7413
George Amrom, M.D., Vice President of Medical Affairs 215/762-3209
Joann Lucas, Quality Improvement Director 215/762-4783
Affiliation: Drexel University College of Medicine

Thomas Jefferson University Hospital
11th and Walnut Streets
Philadelphia, Pennsylvania 19107

Thomas J. Lewis, President/CEO 215/955-7018
Neil Lubarsky, Sr. VP/CFO 202/476-3000
Stephen Tranquillo, Chief Information Officer 215/955-2790
Stacey Meadows, J.D., Vice President and General Counsel 215/955-0765
Geno Merli, SVP for Clincal Affairs and CMO 215/955-8433
Patrice Miller, VP, Clinical Resource Systems 215/955-1349
Affiliation: Jefferson Health System

University of Pennsylvania Health System
3400 Spruce Street
Philadelphia, Pennsylvania 19104

Ralph W. Muller, Chief Executive Officer 215/662-2203
Garry L. Scheib, Chief Operating Officer 215/662-3227
Keith Casper, Chief Financial Officer 215/662-2792
Arthur H. Rubenstein, M.B.B.Ch., Executive Vice President,
   UPenn Health System and Dean 215/898-6796
Lee J. Dobkin, Chief Counsel, UPHS 215/746-5220
Patrick J. Brennan, M.D., Chief Medical Officer and Senior
   Vice President 215/615-0668
Affiliation: University of Pennsylvania School of Medicine

Pittsburgh

Allegheny General Hospital
420 East North Avenue,
Ste. 420
Pittsburgh, Pennsylvania 15212

Christopher Olivia, President Chief Executive Officer 412/359-8588
Augstine Lopez, Vice President/Finance 412/359-8550
Richard P. Shannon, M.D., Director, Medical Education 412/359-3022
Nick Valadja, Vice President/CIO 412/359-1793
Judith Hlafscak, Senior Legal Counsel 412/359-4932
Duke Rupert, Vice President, Performance Improvement 412/359-4631
Affiliation: Drexel University College of Medicine; West Penn Allegheny Health
    System

Department of Veterans Affairs Veterans Integrated Service Network VISN 4
Delafield Road-Building 32, 2nd Floor
Pittsburgh, Pennsylvania 15215

Magee-Womens Hospital
300 Halket Street
Pittsburgh, Pennsylvania 15213

Leslie C. Davis, President 412/641-4010
William L. Cook, Vice President of Operations 412/641-8746
Eileen Simmons, Chief Financial Officer 412/641-4460
Allen Hogge, Chairman, OB/GYN Reproductive Services 412/641-4212
Bruce Haviland, Chief Information Officer 412/641-2880
Affiliation: University of Pittsburgh School of Medicine

Mercy Hospital of Pittsburgh
1400 Locust Street
Pittsburgh, Pennsylvania 15219

Kenneth Eshak, President & CEO 412/232-7510
Jack Gaenzle, Chief Operating Officer 412/232-7107
Ed Karlovich, Chief Financial Officer 412/232-5792
Irving Freeman, Ph.D., Executive Director, Academic Affairs 412/232-5522
Stephen D. Adams, Vice President, IT, & CIO 412/232-7544
Rebecca C. O'Connor, J.D., General Counsel 412/232-7977
JoAnn V. Narduzzi, M.D., Vice President, Academic Affairs 412/232-7601
Mary Menegazzi, Director, Quality/Clinical Applications 412/232-8371
Affiliation: Jefferson Medical College of Thomas Jefferson University;
    Pittsburgh Mercy Health System, Inc.

Pittsburgh Mercy Health System, Inc.
1400 Locust Street
Pittsburgh, Pennsylvania 15219

Kenneth Eshak, President & CEO 412/232-7510
Ed Karlovich, Chief Financial Officer 412/232-5792
Stephen D. Adams, Vice President, IT, & CIO 412/232-7544
Affiliation: Jefferson Medical College of Thomas Jefferson University

UPMC

200 Lothrop Street
Pittsburgh, Pennsylvania 15213

Jeffrey A. Romoff, President 412/647-4800
John W. Paul, Executive Vice President/CFO 412/642-4820
Loren H. Roth, M.D., Sr VP Medical Services and Chief
Medical Officer 412/647-4860
Daniel Drawbaugh, Chief Information Officer 412/647-2411
Jeannine Konzier, Administrative Director, Institute for
Performance Improvement 412/647-5676
Affiliation: University of Pittsburgh School of Medicine

UPMC Presbyterian Shadyside

200 Lothrop Street
Pittsburgh, Pennsylvania 15213

John Innocenti, President 412/647-5286
Edward Karlovich, Senior Vice President of Finance 412/647-8328
W. Dennis Zerega, Ed.D., Vice President, Office of Graduate
Medical Education 412/647-6340
Richard L. Simmons, M.D., Medical Director 412/648-1823
Lyda Dye, Director, Clinical Information & Program 412/647-9276
Affiliation: University of Pittsburgh School of Medicine

Veterans Affairs Pittsburgh Healthcare System

University Drive
Pittsburgh, Pennsylvania 15240

Michael E. Moreland, Director 412/688-6100
Robert Callahan, Associate Director for Site Operations
James Baker, Chief Fiscal Officer 412/822-1055
Mary Lou Zemaitis, Director of Education 412/365-5723
Angelo Baiocchi, Vice President, Information Management 412/688-6476
Rajiv Jain, Chief of Staff
Barbara Reichbaum, R.N., Quality & Performance
Management Coord. 412/784-3777
Affiliation: University of Pittsburgh School of Medicine

West Penn Allegheny Health System

1800 Friendship Avenue
Pittsburgh, Pennsylvania 15224

Christopher Olivia, President Chief Executive Officer 412/359-8588
Affiliation: Drexel University College of Medicine

Members: PENNSYLVANIA

Western Pennsylvania Hospital
4800 Friendship Avenue
Pittsburgh, Pennsylvania 15224

Edward M. Klaman, President and CEO 412/578-3878
Augustine Lopez, Chief Financial Officer 412/578-6907
Elliot Goldberg, M.D., Director Medical Education Vice
    Chairman Dept. of Medicine 412/578-6929
Christina Middlemiss, Senior Director, Information Services 412/578-1088
Robert B. Templin Jr., Chief Legal Counsel 412/578-5883
Marian R. Block, M.D., Chief Quality Officer 412/578-7227
Holly M. Hampe, Dir., Quality & Risk Mgmt, Regulatory Af 412/578-7479

Affiliation: Temple University School of Medicine; West Penn Allegheny
    Health System

Radnor

Jefferson Health System
259 Radnor Chester Road, Suite 290
Radnor, Pennsylvania 19087-5261

Joseph Sabastianelli, President/CEO 610/225-6238

Affiliation: Jefferson Medical College of Thomas Jefferson University

Reading

Reading Hospital and Medical Center
Sixth Avenue and Spruce Street
Reading, Pennsylvania

Springfield

Crozer-Keystone Health System
Healthplex Pavilion II
100 W. Sproul Road
Springfield, Pennsylvania 19064

Gerald Miller, President/CEO 610/338-8211
Joan K. Richards, President 610/338-8278
Richard Bennett, Senior Vice President/CFO 610/338-8225
Robert E. Wilson, V.P. & Chief Information 610/338-8237
Rebecca Davis Prince, Esq., Vice President, Legal Services 610/338-8214

Affiliation: Temple University School of Medicine

Upland

Crozer-Chester Medical Center
One Medical Center Boulevard
Upland, Pennsylvania 19013

Joan K. Richards, President 610/338-8278
Joseph H. Saunders, Vice President, Operations 610/447-2000
Phillip Ryan, Chief Financial Officer 610/338-8278
Marc Edelman, Vice President, Quality Improvement and
Utilization Management 610/447-2380
Affiliation: Crozer-Keystone Health System

Wynnewood

Lankenau Hospital
100 Lancaster Avenue
Wynnewood, Pennsylvania 19096

Joel Fagerstrom, Hospital CEO - Full Member 215/762-7000
Robert Kauffman, VP Finance and Budget 610/526-8482
Karen Thomas, Sr. VP and Chief Information Officer 610/993-2322
Affiliation: Jefferson Medical College of Thomas Jefferson University

Main Line Health
100 Lancaster Ave
Wynnewood, Pennsylvania

John Lynch, Chief Executive Officer 610/526-3010
Michael Buongiorno, Chief Financial Officer 610/526-8481
Brian Corbett, Sr. VP and Chief Counsel 610/526-3814
Affiliation: Lankenau Hospital

York

Wellspan Health
45 Monument Road
Suite 200
York, Pennsylvania 17405

Bruce M. Bartels, President 717/851-2124
Affiliation: Pennsylvania State University College of Medicine

York Hospital
YH-1001 S. George St.
York, Pennsylvania 17403

Richard L. Seim, President-York Hospital Sr. Vice President-
WellSpan Health 717/851-2650
Raymond Rosen, Vice President, Operations 717/851-2122
Michael O'Connor, Senior Vice President, Finance 717/851-2123
Peter M. Hartmann, M.D., Vice President, Medical Affairs 717/851-2224
William J. Gillespie, Vice President/CIO 717/851-2447
Glen D. Moffett, Vice President/General Counsel 717/851-4413
Affiliation: Pennsylvania State University College of Medicine; Wellspan Health

PUERTO RICO

San Juan

San Juan Veterans Affairs Medical Center
10 Casia Street
San Juan, Puerto Rico 00921-3201

Rafael Ramirez, Medical Center Director	787/641-7582
Jeanette Diaz, Associate Center Director	787/641-3668
Ricardo Ochoa, Financial Manager	787/641-7582
David Kitterman, Chief, Health Administration and Informatics Service	787/641-2974
John Thompson, Acting General Counsel	202/273-6666
Marta Vazquez-Pares, M.A., Compliance Officer	787/641-3665

Affiliation: Ponce School of Medicine

RHODE ISLAND

Pawtucket

Memorial Hospital of Rhode Island
111 Brewster Street
Pawtucket, Rhode Island 02860

Francis R. Dietz, President	401/729-2130
Shelley MacDonald, R.N., Senior Vice President, Operations/Chief of Nursing	401/729-2341
Michael Ryan, Sr. VP, Finance	401/729-2260
Elizabeth Girard, Senior Vice President, Administration	401/729-2130
Raymond Ortelt, Director, Information Services	401/729-2993

Affiliation: The Warren Alpert Medical School of Brown University

Providence

Care New England Health System
45 Willard Avenue
Providence, Rhode Island

John J. Hynes, President/CEO	401/453-7900

Affiliation: The Warren Alpert Medical School of Brown University

Lifespan, Inc.
Coro Building
167 Point Street
Providence, Rhode Island 02903

George A. Vecchione, President/CEO	401/444-6699
Mamie Wakefield, SR. VP of Finance	401/444-7914
Carole M. Cotter, Senior Vice President/CIO	401/444-6404

Affiliation: The Warren Alpert Medical School of Brown University

Miriam Hospital
164 Summit Avenue
Providence, Rhode Island 02906

Kathleen Hittner, M.D., President/CEO 401/793-2002
Sandra Coletta, Chief Operating Officer 401/793-2002
Mary Wakefield, Vice President, Finance 401/444-7914
Boyd P. King, M.D., Senior Vice President, Medical Affairs 401/444-5074
Carole M. Cotter, Senior Vice President/CIO 401/444-6404
Kenneth E. Arnold, Senior Vice President/General Counsel 401/444-6627
Diana Wantoch, Director, Quality Management 401/793-2015
Affiliation: Lifespan, Inc.

Rhode Island Hospital
593 Eddy Street
Providence, Rhode Island 02903

Joseph F. Amaral, M.D., President/CEO 401/444-5131
Mary Wakefield, Vice President, Finance 401/444-7914
Carole M. Cotter, Senior Vice President/CIO 401/444-6404
Kenneth E. Arnold, Senior Vice President/General Counsel 401/444-6627
Affiliation: Lifespan, Inc.

Roger Williams Hospital
825 Chalkstone Avenue
Providence, Rhode Island 02908

Addy Kane, Senior Vice President, CFO 401/456-2476
Alan B. Weitberg, M.D., Chairman, Department of Medicine 401/456-2070
Susan Cerrone Abely, Vice President, CIO 401/456-6750
Kimberly A. O'connell, Vice President and General Counsel 401/456-2498
Thomas DeNucci, M.D., President, Medical Staff 401/456-2000
Nancy Fogarty, Director of Quality 401/456-2043
Affiliation: Boston University School of Medicine

Women and Infants Hospital of Rhode Island
101 Dudley Street
Providence, Rhode Island 02905

Constance A. Howes, Chief Executive Officer 401/274-1100
Debra Paul, Vice President for Fianance 401/274-1122
Donald R. Coustan, M.D., Obstetrician & Gynecologist-in-
Chief 401/274-1100
Bruce Reirden, Vice President, Information Services 401/921-2711
Thomas R. Courage, Esq., Vice President/General Counsel 401/274-1100
Denise Henry, Directory, Quality Management 401/274-1122
Affiliation: Care New England Health System

SOUTH CAROLINA

Charleston

Medical University of South Carolina Medical Center
169 Ashley Avenue
Charleston, South Carolina 29425

W. Stuart Smith, Vice President/Executive Director 843/792-4000
Lisa Montgomery, Admin for Financial Services 843/792-4775
John Raymond, M.D., VP for Academic Affairs & Provost 843/792-3031
David J. Northrup, Director, Healthcare Computing Services 843/792-6675
Annette Drachman, Director, Legal Affairs 843/792-3864
John E. Heffner, M.D., Executive Medical Director 843/792-9537
Rosemary Ellis, Quality Director 843/792-0855

Affiliation: Medical University of South Carolina College of Medicine

Ralph H. Johnson Veterans Affairs Medical Center
109 Bee Street
Charleston, South Carolina 29401

John E. Barilich, Director 843/789-7200
Nancy P. Campbell, M.S.W., Associate Director 843/789-7500
Joseph John, ACOS for Education 843/789-7942
Tonya C. Lobbestael, Public Affairs Officer 843/789-7699
Florence N. Hutchison, M.D., Chief of Staff 843/577-5011
Shirley Cooper, M.S.N., R.N., Quality Management
Coordinator 843/789-7303

Affiliation: Medical University of South Carolina College of Medicine

Columbia

Palmetto Health
1301 Taylor Street, Suite 9A
PO Box 2266
Columbia, South Carolina 29203

Charles D. Beaman, President/CEO 803/296-5042
John Singlering, Chief Operating Officer 803/434-2819
Paul Duane, Chief Financial Officer 803/296-2112
James I. Raymond, M.D., Sr VP for Quality, Med Educ &
Research 803/296-2152
Dave Garrett, Sr. VP and Chief Information Officer 803/434-4949
Howard West, Senior Vice President/General Counsel 803/296-2100
Fran King, Director of Outcomes - Risk Management 803/434-3122

Affiliation: Palmetto Health Alliance

Palmetto Health Alliance
PO Box 2266
Columbia, South Carolina 29202-2266

Charles D. Beaman, President/CEO 803/296-5042

Affiliation: University of South Carolina School of Medicine

Greenville

Greenville Hospital System
701 Grove Road
Greenville, South Carolina 29605

Michael C. Riordan, President/CEO 864/455-7978
Gregory J. Rusnak, Chief Operating Officer 864/455-6146
Susan Bichel, VP Financial Services 864/455-8978
Jerry R. Youkey, M.D., VP Medical and Academic Services 864/455-7880
Doran A. Dunaway, VP Information&Technological
Innovation 864/455-4707
Joseph Blake, VP Legal Affairs and General Counsel 864/455-8780
John R. Sanders, M.D., Chief Medical Staff Officer 864/455-8771
Affiliation: Medical University of South Carolina College of Medicine;
University of South Carolina School of Medicine

SOUTH DAKOTA

Sioux Falls

Avera McKennan Hospital and University
800 East 21st Street
Sioux Falls, South Dakota

Fred Slunecka, Regional President 605/322-7808
Ronald Farr, Sr. V.P. Finance 605/322-7818
Matthew J. Michels, Legal Counsel 605/322-7013
Mary Leedom, Medical Support Services Director 605/322-7975
Affiliation: Sanford School of Medicine of the University of South Dakota

Sanford USD Medical Center
1305 West 18th Street
Sioux Falls, South Dakota 57117-5039

Charles P. O'Brien, President and CEO 605/333-6437
Randy Bury, Chief Administrative Officer 605/333-7177
Jeffrey Sandene, Chief Financial Officer 605/333-6450
David Rossing, Senior VP Sioux Valley Clinic 605/328-6943
Arlyn Broekhuis, Director of Information Systems 605/333-7329
Kim Patrick, Corporate Counsel 605/357-2904
Ken Aspaas, Chief Medical Officer 605/333-6426
Jenn Wagenaar, Quality Management Coordinator 605/328-7876
Affiliation: Sanford School of Medicine of the University of South Dakota;
Sioux Valley Hospitals and Health System

Sioux Valley Hospitals and Health System
1305 W. 18th Street
Sioux Falls, South Dakota 57117-5039

TENNESSEE

Chattanooga

Erlanger Health System
975 East Third St.
Chattanooga, Tennessee

Members: TENNESSEE

Erlanger Medical Center
975 East Third Street
Chattanooga, Tennessee 37403

Johnson City

Johnson City Medical Center Hospital, Inc.
400 North State of Franklin Road
Johnson City, Tennessee 37604
Dennis Vonderfecht, President/CEO 423/431-1040
Candace Jennings, Vice President/COO Washington County
Operations 423/431-1061
Marvin Eichorn, Senior Vice President/CFO 423/461-1017
Richard Eshbach, Chief Information Officer 423/431-1662
Affiliation: East Tennessee State University James H. Quillen College of
Medicine; Mountain States Health Alliance

Mountain States Health Alliance
701 N. State of Franklin Rd., Suite 1
Johnson City, Tennessee 37604
Dennis Vonderfecht, President/CEO 423/431-1040
Marvin Eichorn, Senior Vice President/CFO 423/461-1017
Affiliation: East Tennessee State University James H. Quillen College of
Medicine

Knoxville

University of Tennessee Medical Center
1924 Alcoa Highway
Knoxville, Tennessee
Joseph R. Landsman Jr., President and Chief Executive
Officer 865/305-9430
Thomas Fisher, Chief Financial Officer 865/305-6097
Affiliation: University of Tennessee Health Science Center College of Medicine

Memphis

Methodist Healthcare-University Hospital
1265 Union Avenue
Memphis, Tennessee
Chris McLean, Chief Financial Officer 901/516-7000
Affiliation: University of Tennessee Health Science Center College of Medicine

Regional Medical Center at Memphis
877 Jefferson Avenue
Memphis, Tennessee 38103

Skip Reeder, CEO 901/575-7928
Brenita Crawford, Chief Operating Officer 901/545-6916
Peggie Allen, Chief Financial Officer 901/545-7676
Wayne McDaniel, Chief Information Officer 904/545-7479
Mary Whitaker, J.D., Vice President, Corporate Legal 901/545-8223
Stuart M. Polly, M.D., Chief Medical Officer/Senior Vice
President, Clinical Affairs 901/575-7676
Affiliation: University of Tennessee Health Science Center College of Medicine

Veterans Affairs Medical Center, Memphis, Tennessee
1030 Jefferson Avenue
Memphis, Tennessee 38104

Patricia O. Pittman, Medical Center Director 901/577-7200
Patrick Coney, Chief, Fiscal Service 901/523-8990
James B. Dale, M.D., Associate Chief of Staff for Education 901/577-7207
Charles D. Sternberg, Chief Information Officer 901/577-7209
Ronald H. Dooley, Regional Counsel 615/695-4622
Margarethe Hagemann, M.D. 901/577-7202
Mary Jean Erwin, Director, Quality and Management 901/577-7489
Affiliation: University of Tennessee Health Science Center College of Medicine

Mountain Home

James H. Quillen Veterans Affairs Medical Center
PO Box 4000
Mountain Home, Tennessee 37684

Charlene Ehret, Medical Center Director 423/926-1171
John W. McFadden, Associate Medical Center Director 423/926-1171
Brian Fuchs, Chief, Fiscal Service 901/523-8990
Felix A. Sarubbi, M.D., Interim Chair 423/439-6282
Karen Presnell, Chief Information Resources Management 423/926-1171
Louis A. Cancellaro, Ph.D., M.D., Chief of Staff 423/926-1171
Norma Swanson, R.N., Chief, Quality Management &
Improvement Service 423/926-1171
Affiliation: East Tennessee State University James H. Quillen College of
Medicine

Nashville

Department of Veterans Affairs Veterans Integrated Service Network VISN 9
1801 West End Ave
Suite 1100
Nashville, Tennessee 37212

John Dandridge Jr., Network Director Department of
Veterans Affairs 615/340-2380

Vanderbilt University Hospital

1161 21st Avenue, South
Nashville, Tennessee 37232-2102

Larry Goldberg, Executive Director and Chief Executive
Officer 615/343-4501
Warren E. Beck, Director, Finance - Hospital Chief Financial
Officer 615/322-0084
William W. Stead, M.D., Associate Vice Chancellor 615/936-1424
Julia Caldwell Morris, Associate General Counsel 615/936-0323
C. Wright Pinson, Associate Vice-Chancellor for Clinical
Affairs Chief Medical Officer 615/343-9324
Affiliation: Vanderbilt University School of Medicine

Vanguard Health System

20 Burton Hills Blvd
Suite 100
Nashville, Tennessee

Charles N. Martin, Chairman and CEO 615/665-6000

Veterans Affairs Tennessee Valley Health Care System

1310 24th Avenue South
Nashville, Tennessee 37212

Juan Marales, Chief Executive Officer 615/327-5334
Tony Bennett, Associate Director for Operations 615/327-5334
Terry Simmons, Chief Financial Officer 615/867-6004
Mark J. Koury, M.D., Associate Chief of Staff for Education 615/327-6169
Bernice G. Burchfield, Chief, Information Resources
Management 901/577-7209
Ronald H. Dooley, Regional Counsel 615/695-4622
Dolores Kaplan, Chief Quality Management 615/327-5609
Affiliation: Meharry Medical College; Vanderbilt University School of Medicine

TEXAS

Dallas

Baylor University Medical Center

3500 Gaston Avenue
Dallas, Texas 75246

John McWhorter, President 214/820-4140
Janie Wade, VP-Finance 214/820-1933
Brad Gahm, Interim-General Counsel 214/820-3924
David J. Ballard, M.D., Ph.D., Senior Vice President
Healthcare Research & Improvement 214/820-7986
Affiliation: University of Texas Southwestern Medical Center at Dallas
Southwestern Medical School

Children's Medical Center of Dallas
1935 Motor Street
Dallas, Texas 75235

Christopher J. Durovich, President/CEO 214/456-7890
Ray Dziesinski, Sr. Vice President and CFO 214/456-2960
Thomas Zellers, M.D., Interim Chief Medical Officer 214/456-2933
Richard Duncan, Chief Information Officer 214/456-6000
Anne Long, J.D., VP of Legal Affairs 214/456-2099

Affiliation: University of Texas Southwestern Medical Center at Dallas
Southwestern Medical School

Dallas County Hospital District, Parkland Health & Hospital System
5201 Harry Hines Boulevard
Dallas, Texas 75235

Ron J. Anderson, M.D., President/CEO 214/590-8076
Samuel Lee Ross Jr., M.D., Chief Medical Officer
John Dragovits, Chief Financial Officer 214/590-8097
Les Clonch, Senior Vice President/CIO 214/590-4786
Tom L. Cox, Director of Legal Affairs 214/590-4575
Kirk A. Calhoun, M.D., President 903/877-7750

Affiliation: University of Texas Southwestern Medical Center at Dallas
Southwestern Medical School

Methodist Dallas Medical Center
1441 N. Beckley Avenue
Dallas, Texas 75203

Stephen Mansfield, Chief Executive Officer 214/947-8181
Michael Schaefer, Executive Vice President/CFO 214/947-4510
Pamela G. McNutt, Senior Vice President/CIO 214/947-4530
Mickey Price, Senior Vice President-Legal Affairs 214/947-4515
Virginia Davis, Vice President 214/947-2524

Affiliation: University of Texas Southwestern Medical Center at Dallas
Southwestern Medical School

UT Southwestern Medical Center
5151 Harry Hines Boulevard
Dallas, Texas 75235

Kern Wildenthal, M.D., President 214/648-2508
John McConnell, M.D., Exec VP for Health System Affairs 214/648-2800
Jim Wentz, Chief Financial Officer 214/645-5480
Kirk A. Kirksey, VP for Information Resources 214/648-6252
Leah A. Hurley, J.D., Vice President for Legal Affairs 214/648-7986

Affiliation: University of Texas Southwestern Medical Center at Dallas
Southwestern Medical School

Veterans Affairs North Texas Health Care System

4500 South Lancaster Road
Dallas, Texas 75216

Alan G. Harper, Medical Center Director 214/857-1166
William E. Cox, M.S., Associate Director 214/857-1143
Val Martin, Chief, Fiscal Service 214/857-1181
Gail Bentley, Ph.D., Associate Chief of Staff for Education 214/857-1152
Herbert Doller, Ph.D. 214/857-0512
Catherine Rich, Office of Regional Counsel 214/857-1156
Robert Cronin, M.D., Chief of Staff 214/857-1150
Michael George, Chief, Quality Management Service 214/857-0480

Affiliation: University of Texas Southwestern Medical Center at Dallas
Southwestern Medical School

El Paso

Thomason Hospital

4815 Alameda
El Paso, Texas

James N. Valenti, President, CEO and Chief Financial
Officer 915/521-7600

Fort Worth

John Peter Smith Hospital (Tarrant County Hospital District)

1500 South Main
Fort Worth, Texas 76104

David Cecero, President and CEO 817/927-1230
Dee Chaisson, Chief Financial Officer 817/920-6895

Galveston

University of Texas Medical Branch Hospitals at Galveston

301 University Boulevard
Galveston, Texas 77555

Karen Sexton, R.N., Ph.D., C.H.E., Vice President and Chief
Executive Officer 409/772-6116
David Connaughton, Quarterly Benchmark Report Recipient
Chief Financial Officer
Charles H. Christiansen, Ed.D., Dean, School of Allied
Health Sciences
Richard S. Moore, Vice President for Business and
Administration 409/772-6454
Crillon C. Payne, Director of Legal Affairs 409/772-4898
Jennifer Baer, Director Quality & Healthcare Safety
Management 409/772-5098

Affiliation: University of Texas Medical Branch School of Medicine

Grand Prairie

Department of Veterans Affairs Veterans Integrated Service Network VISN 17
1901 N. Highway 360, Suite 350
Grand Prairie, Texas 75050

    Thomas J. Stranova, Network Director(10N17) Department
of Veterans Affairs 817/652-1111

Houston

Baylor Clinic & Hospital Baylor of Medicine
One Baylor Plaze, Suite 191A
Houston, Texas

Harris County Hospital District
2525 Holly Hall
P.O. Box 66769
Houston, Texas 77054

    David S. Lopez, Chief Operating Officer 713/873-2300
    George Masi, Chief Operating Officer 713/873-2300
    Gwendolyn Huskey, Interim Senior Vice President/CFO 713/566-6746
    Tim Tindle, Chief Information Officer 713/566-6034
    Mercedes Leal, Div Chief Harris Co Attny Off 713/566-6550
    Wayne J. Riley, M.D., M.P.H., Office of the President 713/798-9188
    Constance Ferguson, Director, Quality Assurance 713/566-6413
Affiliation: Baylor College of Medicine

Memorial Hermann Healthcare System
6411 Fannin
Houston, Texas 77030

    Juanita Romans, Senior Vice President/CEO 713/704-6614
    Greg Harb, Chief Operating Officer 713/704-5076
    Barrie Strickland, Vice President/CFO 713/704-5292
    David F. Bradshaw, Chief Information Officer 713/776-4042
    Randy Gleason, General Counsel 713/704-4000
    Craig Cordola, Interim Medical Director 713/704-3700
Affiliation: University of Texas Medical School at Houston

Methodist Health Care System
6565 Fannin Street
Houston, Texas 77030

    Ronald G. Girotto, President/CEO 713/790-3366
Affiliation: Baylor College of Medicine

Methodist Hospital
6565 Fannin Street
Houston, Texas 77030

Ronald G. Girotto, President/CEO 713/790-3366
Marc Boom, M.D., Executive Vice President 713/441-2671
John Hagale, Executive VP, Chief Financial Officer 713/441-4340
H. Dirk Sostman, M.D., EVP and Chief Medical Officer 713/441-3455
Jerry Vuchak, Director, Information Technology 832/667-5433
Ramon Cantu, J.D., Senior VP, Chief Legal Officer 713/441-4182
Michael J. Reardon, M.D., Business Practices Medical Center............................... 713/441-6566
Affiliation: Methodist Health Care System

Michael E. DeBakey Veterans Affairs Medical Center
2002 Holcombe Boulevard
Houston, Texas 77030

Edgar L. Tucker, Medical Center Director 713/794-7100
Jim Eddins, Business Office Service Line Executive 713/794-7104
Travis Courville, Education Service Line Executive 713/794-7141
Francisco Vazquez, Information Management Service Line
Exec 713/794-7148
Logan Slaughter, General Counsel 713/794-3656
Thomas B. Horvath, M.D., Chief of Staff 713/794-7011
Betty McDuffie, Quality Management Improvement Director............................... 713/794-7504
Affiliation: Baylor College of Medicine

St. Luke's Episcopal Health System
PO Box 20269
Houston, Texas 77225

David Fine, Chief Executive Officer 832/355-7661
David Koontz, Chief Financial Officer 832/355-8100
Affiliation: Baylor College of Medicine

St. Luke's Episcopal Hospital
6720 Bertner
Houston, Texas 77030

David C. Pate, M.D., Senior Vice President & Chief
Executive Officer 832/355-2300
Steve Pickett, Chief Finanical Officer 832/355-8701
Kay Carr, Senior Vice President, Information Services 832/355-6352
Affiliation: Baylor College of Medicine

Texas Children's Hospital
6621 Fannin
Houston, Texas 77030

Mark A. Wallace, President/CEO 832/824-1160
Benjamin Melson, CFO/Executive VP 832/825-1120
Affiliation: Baylor College of Medicine

University of Texas M. D. Anderson Cancer Center
1515 Holcombe Boulevard
Houston, Texas 77030

John Mendelsohn, M.D., President 713/792-6000
Leon J. Leach, Executive Vice President 713/745-1076
Dwain, VP and CFO 713/794-5162
Lynn Vogel, VP & Chief Information Officer
Matt Masek, VP & Chief Legal Officer 713/745-6633
Thomas W. Burke, M.D., EVP & Physician-In-Chief 713/745-3825
Affiliation: Baylor College of Medicine

Lubbock

University Medical Center Health System
602 Indi
Lubbock, Texas

University Medical Center~TX
602 Indiana Avenue
Lubbock, Texas 79415

David Allison, Chief Executive Officer 806/775-8517
Mark Funderburk, Chief Operating Officer 806/775-8511
Jeff Dane, Chief Financial Officer 806/775-8505
Bill Eubanks, Vice President and CIO 806/775-9055
Lois Wischkaemper, Legal Counsel 806/740-0474
Vernon Farthing, M.D., Vice President of Medical Staff
Affairs 806/762-8461
Michelle Sturgill, Performance Improvement Project
Manager 806/775-9270
Affiliation: Texas Tech University Health Sciences Center School of Medicine

Odessa

Medical Center Hospital
500 W. 4th Street
Odessa, Texas

William Webster, Chief Executive Officer 432/640-2404
Scott Taylor, Chief Operating Officer
Robert Abernethy, Chief Financial Officer
Gary Barnes, Chief Information Officer
Bruce Becker, Medical Director
Sherrill Rhodes, Director of Performance Improvement 432/640-1175
Affiliation: Texas Tech University Health Sciences Center School of Medicine

Members: TEXAS

San Antonio

University Health System
4502 Medical Drive
San Antonio, Texas 78229

George B. Hernandez Jr., President/CEO Administrator		210/358-2005
Greg Rufe, Administrator		210/358-2022
Peggy Deming, Executive Vice President/CFO		210/358-2101
Jim Rogers, M.D., Vice President, Quality and Cost Improvement		210/358-4543
John Blandford, Vice President, Information Services		210/358-4300
Joseph Naples, Prof & Chair		

Affiliation: University of Texas School of Medicine at San Antonio

Veterans Affairs South Texas Health Care System
7400 Merton Minter Boulevard
San Antonio, Texas 78229

Jose R. Coronado, FACHE, Director		210/617-5253
Charles E. Sepich, C.H.E., Acting Associate Director		210/617-5141
I. Rachal, Chief, Fiscal Service		210/617-5124
Raymond Chung, M.D., Assoc. Chief of Staff for Education		210/617-5109
Simon Willett, Chief, Office of Information Technology		210/617-5126
Richard Bauer, M.D., Chief of Staff		210/617-5176
Gary Anziani, Chief, Quality Management		210/617-5300

Affiliation: University of Texas School of Medicine at San Antonio

Temple

Central Texas Veterans Health Care Sys
1901 Veterans Memorial Drive
Temple, Texas

Bruce Gordon, Director		254/743-2306

Affiliation: Texas A&M Health Science Center College of Medicine

Scott and White Memorial Hospital
2401 South 31st Street
Temple, Texas 76508

Alfred B. Knight, M.D., President/CEO		254/724-1912
Patricia Currie, Chief of Hospital Services		254/724-4537
Donny Sequin, Chief Operating Officer		254/724-5359
Dennis Laraway, Chief Financial Officer		254/724-4482
Donald Wesson, Vice Dean-Temple Campus		254/724-2368
William McCombs, Chief Information Officer		254/724-7439
Jimmy Carroll, J.D., General Counsel		254/724-2543
David Lindzey, M.D., Hospital Medical Director		254/724-2111
Robert Wilton Pryor, M.D., Chief Medical Officer		254/724-5359

Affiliation: Texas A&M Health Science Center College of Medicine

UTAH

Salt Lake City

University of Utah Health System
50 North Medical Drive
Salt Lake City, Utah 84132

A. Lorris Betz, M.D., Ph.D., Sr VP for Hlth Sciences, Executive Dean SOM CEO, University of Utah Health System 801/581-7480
Affiliation: University of Utah School of Medicine

University of Utah Hospital
50 North Medical Drive
Salt Lake City, Utah 84132

David Entwistle, Chief Executive Officer 801/587-3572
Gordon Crabtree, Interim Executive Director Chief Financial Officer 801/587-3572
Pierre Pincetl, M.D., Asst. VP, Information Technology Service 801/585-9568
Mo Mulligan, R.N., J.D., Director, Performance Monitoring & Improvement 801/585-1336
Affiliation: University of Utah Health System

VERMONT

Burlington

Fletcher Allen Health Care
111 Colchester Avenue (Burgess 1)
Burlington, Vermont 05401

Melinda L. Estes, M.D., CEO 802/847-5959
Angeline Marano, COO 802/847-5040
Roger Deshares, Chief Financial Officer 617/732-5500
John K. Evans, Chief Technology Officer 802/847-8100
Spencer Knapp, General Counsel
Norman Ward, M.D., Vice President Medical Affairs
Anna Noonan, R.N., VP, Quality & Care Management 802/847-2468
Affiliation: University of Vermont College of Medicine

White River Junction

Veterans Affairs Medical and Regional Office Center
215 North Main Street
White River Junction, Vermont 05009

Gary M. De Gasta, Medical Center Director 802/295-9363
Christopher Ellington, Chief Financial Officer 802/295-9363
Dennis Shanley, Chief Information Officer 802/295-9363
Neil Nulty, J.D., Regional Counsel Attorney 802/296-5116
Arthur Sauvigne, M.D., Chief of Staff 802/295-9363
Joanne Puckett, R.N., E.D.M., Quality Manager 802/295-9363
Affiliation: Dartmouth Medical School; University of Vermont College of Medicine

VIRGINIA

Charlottesville

University of Virginia Medical Center
Jefferson Park Avenue
Charlottesville, Virginia 22908

R. Edward Howell, VP/CEO 434/243-9308
Margaret M. Van Bree, Ph.D., Chief Operations Officer 434/243-6637
Larry Fitzgerald, Chief Financial Officer 434/924-5426
Arthur Garson Jr., M.D., Executive Vice President and
Provost 434/924-5118
Barbara Baldwin, Chief Information Officer 434/982-1022
Sally Nan Barber, Senior Assistant to the CEO, Medical Cen 434/243-5788
Thomas A. Massaro, M.D., Ph.D., Associate Dean for GME 434/924-2411
Stacy Crowell, Director, Quality & Performance
Improvement 434/924-5120

Affiliation: University of Virginia School of Medicine

Falls Church

INOVA Fairfax Hospital
3300 Gallows Road
Falls Church, Virginia 22046

Rubin Pasternak, CEO 703/698-1110
Candice Saunders, COO, INOVA Heartt & Vascular Institute
Ron Ewald, Chief Financial Officer 703/698-2711
Russell Seneca, VP Academic Affairs, IHS Associ Adm &
Chmn. Surgery IFH/IFHC 703/698-3563
Nanci Little-Gosnell, Vice President, Information Systems,
Inova Health System 703/205-2352
Shannon Sinclair, Vice President, General Counsel 703/289-2028
Joseph Hallal, President, Medical Staff 703/560-7799
Adrienne Barton, Director Quality Leadership 703/698-2741

Affiliation: George Washington University School of Medicine and Health
Sciences; INOVA Health System

INOVA Health System
3300 Gallows Road
Falls Church, Virginia 22046

J. Knox Singleton, President 703/321-4213

Affiliation: George Washington University School of Medicine and Health
Sciences

Norfolk

Sentara Norfolk General Hospitals
600 Gresham Drive
Norfolk, Virginia 23507

Robert Broermann, Vice President of Finance	757/455-7020
Bert Reese, Vice President	757/857-8110
Gail P. Heagen, Lawyer	757/455-7114
Gary Yates, Medical Director	757/668-4852
Gene Burke, M.D., VPMA	757/668-3288

Affiliation: Eastern Virginia Medical School

Richmond

Hunter Holmes McGuire Veterans Affairs Medical Center
1201 Broad Rock Boulevard
Richmond, Virginia 23249

Michael B. Phaup, Medical Center Director	804/675-5500
Thomas Vergne, Chief, Fiscal Service	804/675-5004
Katherine Gianola, M.D., Chief Information Officer	804/675-5000
Judy L. Brannen, M.D., Chief of Staff	804/675-5511
Rose Polatty, Interim, Chief of Quality Management	804/675-5000

Affiliation: Virginia Commonwealth University School of Medicine

Medical College of Virginia Hospitals
P.O. Box 980510
Richmond, Virginia 23298

Deborah W. Davis, Chief Operating Officer MCV Hospitals	804/628-7565
Linda Pearson, Senior VP of Finance	804/828-7076
Carl F. Gattuso, Senior Vice President Chief Information Officer	804/828-4638
Jean F. Reed, J.D., General Counsel	804/828-9010
Ron Clark, M.D., Chief Medical Officer, Clinical Enterprise	804/828-4654

Affiliation: Virginia Commonwealth University School of Medicine

Roanoke

Carilion Medical Center
1906 Belleview Avenue
Roanoke, Virginia 24018

Edward Murphy, President and CEO	540/981-7893
Donald Lorton, Chief Financial Operator	540/985-5125

Affiliation: University of Virginia School of Medicine

Members: VIRGINIA-WASHINGTON

Salem

Salem Veterans Affairs Medical Center
1970 Roanoke Boulevard
Salem, Virginia 24153

John Patrick, Director	540/983-1046
Carolyn Adams, Associatiate Medical Director	540/983-1046
Richard Schroeder, Chief, Resources Support Service	540/982-2463
Maureen F. McCarthy, M.D., Associate Chief of Staff/ Education	540/982-2463
John R. Miller, Chief, Information Management Service	540/982-2463
Kathleen K. Oddo, Regional Counsel	540/857-2162
Carol S. Carlson, Quality Manager	540/982-2463

Affiliation: Edward Via Virginia College of Osteopathic Medicine; University of Virginia School of Medicine

WASHINGTON

Seattle

Children's Hospital and Regional Medical Center
4800 Sand Point Way, N.E.
Seattle, Washington 98105

Thomas N. Hansen, M.D., Chief Executive Officer	206/987-2001
Patrick J. Hagan, Executive Vice President	206/526-2003
Kelly Wallace, Vice President/CFO	206/526-2003
Fielding Stapleton, Chairman, Department of Pediatrics	206/897-2150
John Dwight, Director, Information Services	206/526-2002
Jeffrey M. Sconyers, J.D., Vice President/General Counsel	206/987-2044
Richard A. Molteni, M.D., Medical Director	206/987-2005
Cara Bailey, Administrator, Systems & Logistics	206/526-2012

Affiliation: University of Washington School of Medicine

Harborview Medical Center University of Washington Hospitals
325 Ninth Avenue, #359717
Seattle, Washington 98104

Johnese Spisso, Interim Executive Director	206/731-5020
Lori Mitchell, Chief Financial Officer	206/744-9280
Tom M. Martin, Director of UW Medicine	206/543-3155
Scott Barnhart, M.D., Medical Director/Associate Dean	206/731-3134

Affiliation: University of Washington Academic Medical Center

University of Washington Academic Medical Center
1959 NE Pacific Street, Box 356151
Seattle, Washington 98195

Paul G. Ramsey, M.D., CEO, UW Medicine Exec Vice President for Medical Affairs and Dean	206/543-7718

Affiliation: University of Washington School of Medicine

University of Washington Medical Center
1959 NE Pacific Street, Box 356429
Seattle, Washington 98195-6151

Stephen Zieniewicz, Executive Director 206/598-6364
Preston Simmons, Senior Operating Officer 206/598-6301
Paul Ishizuka, Chief Financial Officer 206/598-6305
Tom M. Martin, Director of UW Medicine 206/543-3155
Dina Yunker, Assistant Attorney General 206/543-9220
Edward A. Walker, M.D., Medical Director 206/598-6600
Julie Duncan, Director, Quality Assessment and Improvement 206/598-6168
Affiliation: University of Washington Academic Medical Center

Veterans Affairs Puget Sound Health Care System
1660 South Columbian Way
Seattle, Washington 98108

Timothy B. Williams, Director 206/764-2299
Sandy J. Nielsen, Deputy Director 206/764-2299
Kenneth Hudson, Chief Financial Officer 206/764-2666
Phillip G. Rakestraw, Ph.D., Executive Director Center for
Education & Development 206/764-2596
Glen Zwinger, Service Line Manager Information Systems
Service 206/764-2221
Gordon Starkebaum, Chief of Staff 206/764-2260
Affiliation: University of Washington School of Medicine

Vancouver

Department of Veterans Affairs Veterans Integrated Service Network VISN 20
1601 E. Fourth Plain Boulevard
Vancouver, Washington 98661

WEST VIRGINIA

Charleston

CAMC Health System
501 Morris Street
PO Box 1547
Charleston, West Virginia 25326

Charleston Area Medical Center
501 Morris Street
P.O. Box 1547
Charleston, West Virginia 25326

David L. Ramsey, President/CEO 304/348-7627
Glenn Crotty, Executive Vice President/COO 304/348-7438
Larry Hudson, Executive Vice President/CFO 304/388-7629
Lynn Pettry Brookshire, Vice President for Information
Services 304/348-9705
Marshall McMullen, General Counsel 304/348-6710
Elizabeth Spangler, Chief Medical Officer 304/388-7177
Affiliation: CAMC Health System

Members: WEST VIRGINIA-WISCONSIN

Fairmont

West Virginia United Health System
1000 Technology Drive, Suite 2320
Fairmont, West Virginia 26554
   J. Thomas Jones, President/CEO 304/368-2700
Affiliation: West Virginia University School of Medicine

Morgantown

West Virginia University Hospitals, Inc.
Morgantown, West Virginia 26506
   Bruce McClymonds, President & CEO 304/598-4355
   John H. Yoder, Chief Operating Officer 304/598-4057
   David Salsberry, Chief Financial Officer 304/598-4554
   Cindy Klein, Vice President, Human Resources 304/598-4188
   Mike Blassone, Vice President, Information Technology 304/598-4133
   Robert Royston, General Counsel 304/598-4070
   Kevin Halbritter, M.D., Vice President, Medical Affairs 304/598-4156
Affiliation: West Virginia United Health System

WISCONSIN

LaCrosse

Gundersen Lutheran Health Care System
1910 South Avenue
LaCrosse, Wisconsin 54601
   Jeffrey E. Thompson, Chief Executive Director 608/782-7300
Affiliation: University of Wisconsin School of Medicine and Public Health

Lutheran Hospital-LaCrosse
1910 South Avenue
LaCrosse, Wisconsin 54601
   Jeffrey E. Thompson, Chief Executive Director 608/782-7300
   David Chestnut, M.D., Director of Medical Education
   Professor of Anesthesiology 608/775-2081
   Charles Schauberger, M.D., Medical Director, Quality
   Improvement 608/782-7300
Affiliation: Gundersen Lutheran Health Care System

Madison

University of Wisconsin Hospital and Clinics
600 Highland Avenue
Madison, Wisconsin 53792
   Donna Katen-Bahensky, President & CEO 608/263-8025
   Gary Eiler, Chief Financial Officer 608/263-7877
   James Roberts, General Counsel 608/261-0025
   Carl J. Getto, M.D., Senior Vice President, Medical Affairs 608/264-9145
   Judy Wanless, Quality Improvement Analyst 608/203-4618
Affiliation: University of Wisconsin School of Medicine and Public Health

Milwaukee

Aurora Health Care
3000 W. Montana Street
Milwaukee, Wisconsin 53215

Nick Turkal, President/CEO 414/647-3130
Affiliation: Medical College of Wisconsin; University of Wisconsin School of
Medicine and Public Health

Children's Hospital of Wisconsin
9000 West Wisconsin Avenue
Milwaukee, Wisconsin 53226

Jon E. Vice, President 414/266-3032
Cinthia Christensen, Executive Vice President/COO 414/266-3010
Timothy Birkenstock, Treasurer/CFO 414/266-6220
Michael L. Jones, M.B.A., Corp. Vice President/CIO 414/266-6412
Sheila Reynolds, Corporate Vice President/General Counsel 414/266-3469
Robert Miller, M.D., Vice President, Medical Affairs 414/266-3002
Affiliation: Medical College of Wisconsin

Froedtert Hospital and Health System
9200 West Wisconsin Avenue
Milwaukee, Wisconsin 53226

William D. Petasnick, President 414/805-2606
Blaine O'Connell, Vice President, Finance 414/805-4291
Rodney C. Dykehouse, Vice President, Information Systems 414/805-4041
Andrew J. Norton, M.D., Chief Medical Officer, SVP of
Medical Affairs Associate Dean for GME 414/805-3060
John A. Paudl, Director, Quality Improvement 414/259-3600
Affiliation: Medical College of Wisconsin

Sinai Samaritan Medical Center,
945 N. 12th Street
P. O. Box 342
Milwaukee, Wisconsin 53201-0342

George Hinton, Vice President and Chief Administrative
Officer 414/647-3000
Leonard Wilk, Site Administrator 414/219-7293
David Eager, Senior Vice President, Systems Finance 414/647-3139
Jack Steinman, Vice President Information Services 414/345-3400
Diane Beaudry, Director, Quality Management 414/649-7152
Affiliation: Aurora Health Care

St. Luke's Medical Center
2900 W. Oklahoma Avenue
Milwaukee, Wisconsin 53215

Mary O'Brien, Vice President and Chief Administrative
Officer 414/647-3000
Mark Wiener, Site Administrator 414/649-7500
David Eager, Senior Vice President, Systems Finance 414/647-3139
Jack Steinman, Vice President Information Services 414/345-3400
Cathy Ptak, Director, Clinical Information Services 414/649-7288
Affiliation: Aurora Health Care

CORRESPONDING MEMBER HOSPITALS

CALIFORNIA

Martinez

Veterans Affairs Northern California Health Care System
150 Muir Road
Martinez, California 94553

Brian O'Neil, Director 916/843-9058
Lawrence H. Carroll, Associate Director/East Bay Division 925/372-2015
Alice M. Defriese, Ph.D., Associate Chief of Staff for
  Education 916/843-7334
Elizabeth Blohm, Chief, Benefits & Data Management Svc. 925/370-4558
Lucille W. Swanson, Medical Director 925/372-2010
Affiliation: University of California, Davis, School of Medicine

COLORADO

Denver

National Jewish Medical and Research Center
1400 Jackson Street
Denver, Colorado 80206

Michael Salem, President & CEO 303/398-1031
Christine Forkner, Comptroller/CFO 303/398-1031
Richard Johnston, Executive Vice President Academic Affair 303/398-1774
Jim Harbin, Director, Information Systems 303/398-1950
Gary Cott, M.D., Executive Vice President, Medical and
  Clinical Services 303/398-1084
Affiliation: University of Colorado School of Medicine

CONNECTICUT

Greenwich

Greenwich Hospital
Five Perryridge Road
Greenwich, Connecticut 06830-4697

Frank A. Corvino, President/CEO 203/863-3900
Quinton Friesen, Chief Operating Officer 203/863-3905
Eugene Colucci, Chief Financial Officer 203/863-3006
James Weeks, Chief Information Officer 203/863-3422
Charles B. Seelig, M.D., Director of Medical Education 203/863-3913
Affiliation: Yale University School of Medicine; Yale-New Haven Health System

IDAHO

Boise

Boise Veterans Affairs Medical Center
500 W. Fort Street
Boise, Idaho 83702

Wayne C. Tippets, Medical Center Director 208/422-1100
Jim Sola, Associate Director 208/422-1104
Ronald Blanton, Chief, Fiscal Service 208/422-1200
David K. Lee, M.D., Chief of Staff 208/422-1102
Mark Cecil, Chief, Information Resource Management
Service 208/422-1183
Affiliation: University of Washington School of Medicine

ILLINOIS

Berwyn

MacNeal Hospital
3249 South Oak Park Avenue
Berwyn, Illinois 60402

Brian Lemon, President 708/783-3380
Gary Wainer, D.O., Vice President 708/783-3406
Ken Kuhn, Chief Financial Officer
Affiliation: University of Chicago Division of the Biological Sciences The
Pritzker School of Medicine; Vanguard Health System

Chicago

Rehabilitation Institute of Chicago
345 East Superior Street
Suite 1507
Chicago, Illinois 60611

Joanne C. Smith, M.D., Senior Vice President and Chief
Operating Officer 312/238-0838
Chris Frommelt, Director/Information Systems 312/238-5194
Nancy E. Paridy, J.D., Senior Vice President/General
Counsel & GRR General Counsel 312/238-6208
Elliot J. Roth, M.D., Senior Vice President/Medical Director 312/238-4864
Jean Deddo, Manager, Quality Improvement Accreditation 312/238-2877
Affiliation: Northwestern University The Feinberg School of Medicine

North Chicago

Veterans Affairs Chicago Health Care System
3001 Green Bay Road
North Chicago, Illinois 60064

Patrick L. Sullivan, Medical Center Director 847/578-3727
Sant P. Singh, M.D., Associate Chief of Staff for Academic
  Affairs 847/578-3700
Brad Nystrom, Chief, Informatics 847/578-3815
Tariq Hassan, Chief of Staff 847/578-3701
Affiliation: Chicago Medical School at Rosalind Franklin University of Medicine
  & Science

INDIANA

Muncie

Ball Memorial Hospital, Inc.
2401 University Avenue
Muncie, Indiana 47303

Thomas K. Gardiner, M.D., Executive VP Clinical
  Development 765/747-3205
Robert Gildersleeve, Executive VP/Chief Financial Officer 765/747-3205
Thomas Powers, Vice President Information Systems 765/751-5065
Michelle R. Altobella, Director of Risk Management 765/751-5000
Michael J. Hawkins, J.D., Director Risk Management &
  Corporate Compliance 765/751-5000
Douglas A. Triplett, M.D., Vice President, Medical Education 765/747-3246
Claire Lee, R.N., Director, Quality Management 765/747-4284
Affiliation: Cardinal Health System, Inc.

MASSACHUSETTS

Boston

Dana-Farber Cancer Institute
44 Binney Street
Boston, Massachusetts 02115

Edward J. Benz Jr., M.D., President & CEO 617/632-4266
Janet E. Porter, Ph.D., Executive VP & COO 617/632-4602
Dorothy Puhy, Executive VP/CFO 617/632-5244
Jeffrey R. Kessler, Vice President Information Services 617/632-3316
Richard Boskey, General Counsel 617/632-3606
Lawrence Shulman, M.D., Senior VP for Medical Affairs
  Chief Medical Officer 617/632-2277
Maureen Connor, R.N., Director for Quality Improvement
  Interim Director 617/632-4263
Affiliation: Harvard Medical School

MICHIGAN

Kalamazoo

Michigan State University Kalamazoo Center for Medical Studies
1000 Oakland Drive
Kalamazoo, Michigan 49008-1282

Robert P. Carter, M.D., Chief Executive Officer 269/337-4415
Thomas Zavitz, Chief Operating Officer 269/337-4404
Amy Smitchols, Controller/Dir. Finance & Acct Accounting 269/337-4411
Harriet Roelof, M.D., Director, Medical Education 269/337-4601
Carol Heinicke, Manager, Information Systems 269/337-4405
Mark Loehrke, Assistant Professor of Medicine Program
Director, Internal Medicine 616/337-6356
Affiliation: Michigan State University College of Human Medicine

TEXAS

Tyler

University of Texas Health Center at Tyler
11937 U.S. Highway 271
Tyler, Texas 75708

Kirk A. Calhoun, M.D., President 903/877-7750
Vernon Moore, Chief Business and Finance Officer 903/877-2831
Affiliation: University of Texas Southwestern Medical Center at Dallas
Southwestern Medical School

WEST VIRGINIA

Huntington

Cabell Huntington Hospital
1340 Hal Greer Boulevard
Huntington, West Virginia 25701

Brent A. Marsteller, Executive Director 304/526-2052
Robert Hickman, Vice President, Administration 304/526-2052
David Ward, Senior Vice President/CFO 304/526-2052
Paul English Smith, J.D., General Counsel Legal Services and
Risk Management 304/526-2057
Hoyt J. Burdick, M.D., Vice President, Medical Affairs 304/526-2064
Valerie Smith, Director, Quality and Resource Management
Management 304/526-2396
Affiliation: Joan C. Edwards School of Medicine at Marshall University

Steering Committees of AAMC Groups

2008–2009

Steering Committees of AAMC Groups

Government Relations Representatives (GRR) Steering Committee

Chair
Stacey T. Cyphert, Ph.D.
University of Iowa Hospitals and Clinics

Chair-elect
Heidi L. Gartland
University Hospitals of Cleveland

Immediate Past Chair
Ross A. Frommer
Columbia University College of Physicians and Surgeons

Robert D. Bartee
University of Nebraska College of Medicine

Steven Bristow
Parkland Health and Hospital System
Dallas County Hospital District-Parkland

Theresa Alberghini DiPalma
Fletcher Allen Health Care

Beth Felder
Johns Hopkins University

Angela Godby
University of Texas System

Stephen P. Johnson
Cornell University

Lynne Lyons
University of Colorado School of Medicine

Fred H. Salzinger
Creighton University

Jonathan Sender
University of Wisconsin Medical School

Group on Graduate Research, Education, and Training (GREAT) Steering Committee

Chair
Allan Yates, M.D., Ph.D.
Ohio State University College of Medicine

Chair-elect
Henry H. Wortis, M.D.
Tufts University School of Medicine

Immediate Past Chair
Nancy B. Schwartz, Ph.D.
University of Chicago, The Pritzker School of Medicine

C. Gita Bosch, Ph.D., M.B.A.
Sloan-Kettering Institute, Memorial Sloan-Kettering Cancer Center

Roger Chalkley, Ph.D., D.Phil., M.A.
Vanderbilt University School of Medicine

Philip S. Clifford, Ph.D.
Medical College of Wisconsin

Perry V. Halushka, M.D., Ph.D.
Medical University of South Carolina College of Medicine

Susan R. Ross, Ph.D.
University of Pennsylvania School of Medicine

Nancy E. Street, Ph.D.
University of Texas Southwestern Medical Center

Thomas Yorio, Ph.D.
University of North Texas, Health Science Center

MD-PhD Section Officers

Chair
David M. Engman, M.D., Ph.D.
Northwestern University, The Feinberg School of Medicine

Chair-elect
Clayton A. Wiley, M.D., D.Phil.
University of Pittsburgh School of Medicine

Immediate Past Chair
Skip Brass, M.D., Ph.D.
University of Pennsylvania School of Medicine

Postdoctorate Leaders Section Officers

Chair
Phillip S. Clifford, Ph.D.
Medical College of Wisconsin

Chair-elect
Joan M. Lakoski, Ph.D.
University of Pittsburgh School of Medicine

Steering Committees

Group on Graduate Research, Education, and Training (GREAT) Steering Committee, *(con't)*

Immediate Past Chair
John. H. Russell, Ph.D.
Washington University in St. Louis School of Medicine

CAS Liaison
Michael J. Friedlander, Ph.D.
Baylor College of Medicine

COD Liaison
E. Albert Reece, M.D., Ph.D., M.B.A.
University of Maryland School of Medicine

Ex Officio
Charlotte V. Kuh, Ph.D.
National Research Council

Executive Secretary
Jodi B. Lubetsky, Ph.D.
AAMC

Group on Educational Affairs (GEA) Steering Committee

Chair
Karen V. Mann, Ph.D.
Dalhousie University

Chair-Elect
Suzanne Rose, M.D.
Mt. Sinai Medical School

Past Chair and COD Liaison
Lois Margaret Nora, M.D., J.D. , M.P.H.
Northeastern Ohio Universities College of Medicine

Central Chair
Kristi J. Ferguson, Ph.D. , M.S.W.
University of Iowa Carver College of Medicine

Northeast Chair
Karen Richardson-Nassif, Ph.D.
University of Vermont College of Medicine

Southern Chair
Karen E. Szauter, M.D.
University of Texas Medical Branch at Galveston

Western Chair
Carol S. Kamin, Ed.D.
University of Colorado School of Medicine

ORR Liaison to GEA
Kelli Harding, M.D.
New York Presbyterian Hospital, Columbia University

OSR Liaison to GEA
Diane C. Reis
University of Wisconsin School of Medicine

Research In Medical Education (RIME)
Section Leader
Kyle E. Rarey, Ph.D.
University of Florida College of Medicine

Undergraduate Medical Education (UGME)
Section Leader
Lynn M. Cleary, M.D.
State University of New York Upstate

Graduate Medical Education (GME)
Section Leader
Franklin J. Medio, Ph.D.

Continuing Medical Education (CME)
Section Leader
Nancy Ryan Lowitt, M.D., M.Ed
University of Maryland School of Medicine

Executive Secretary
M. Brownell Anderson, M.Ed.
AAMC

Group on Faculty Affairs (GFA) Steering Committee

Chair
Valerie N. Williams, Ph.D., M.P.A.
University of Oklahoma Health Sciences Center

Chair-elect
Kevin Grigsby, D.S.W.
Pennsylvania State University
College of Medicine

Mary M. Moran, M.D.
Drexel University College of Medicine

Karen Novielli, M.D.
Jefferson Medical College

Vivian M. Reznik, M.D., M.P.H.
University of California, San Diego,
School of Medicine

Laura Schweitzer, Ph.D.
Bassett Healthcare

Jeannette M. Shorey, M.D.
University of Arkansas for Medical Sciences
College of Medicine

Henry W. Strobel, Ph.D.
University of Texas Medical School at Houston

Kathleen Nelson, M.D.
University of Alabama School of Medicine

ORR Liaison
Adina Knight, M.D.
University of Alabama at Birmingham

COD Liaison
A. Lorris Betz, M.D., Ph.D.
University of Utah School of Medicine

AAMC Staff
Diane Magrane, M.D.
Valarie Clark, M.P.A.

Group on Faculty Practice (GFP) Steering Committee

Chair
Jane T. Schumaker
University of Chicago,
The Pritzker School of Medicine

Chair-Elect
Lisa Anastos
Northwestern University,
The Feinberg School of Medicine

Immediate Past Chair
David A. Spahlinger, M.D.
University of Michigan Medical School

At-Large Members

Michael J. Duncan
Columbia University College of Physicians and
Surgeons

Richard P. Lofgren, M.D.
University of Kentucky College of Medicine

James J. Potyraj
Virginia Commonwealth University

Cory D. Shaw
Nebraska Medical Center

Curt M. Steinhart M.D.
Medical College of Georgia

Paul A. Taheri, M.D.
University of Vermont College of Medicine

COD Liaison
Vacant

Steering Committees

Group on Information Resources (GIR) Steering Committee

Chair
Kari L. Cassel
University of Arkansas for Medical Science

Chair-elect
Vincent Sheehan
Indiana University School of Medicine

Immediate Past Chair
Lynn Kasner Morgan, M.L.S.
Mount Sinai Medical Center

Members, term ends spring 2009

Robert McAuley
University of Illinois College of Medicine

Arnold J. Smolen, Ph.D.
Drexel University College of Medicine

Members, term ends spring 2010

Joy Grosser
University of California Irvine
College of Medicine

Michael Phillips
Texas Tech University Health Sciences Center

Members, term ends spring 2011

Barbara Baldwin
University of Virginia Health System

Barbara Epstein
University of Pittsburgh School of Medicine

Group on Institutional Advancement (GIA) Steering Committee

Chair
Tom H. Fortner
University of Mississippi Medical Center

Chair-elect
Larry Schafer
Cornell University
Joan & Sanford I. Weill Medical College

Immediate Past Chair
Kathleen Kane
City of Hope National Medical Center

Vice Chair, Marketing, Public Relations and
Public Affairs
Dale Triber Tate
UCLA Health Sciences and
UCLA Medical Center

Vice Chair, Alumni and Development
Karen D. Skiba
Mayo Clinic

Development Chair
Candler Gibson
Johns Hopkins Heart and Vascular Institute

Alumni Chair
Gwendolyn Smith-Johnson
Baylor College of Medicine

Public Relations Chair
Richard Puff
University of Cincinnati College of Medicine

Public Affairs Chair
Jonathan Sender
University of Wisconsin School of Medicine

Marketing Chair
Sue Jablonski
OhioHealth

Development Representative
Jancy Houck
Yale University School of Medicine

Alumni Representative
Patricia Comey
Drexel University College of Medicine

Public Relations Representative
Joni Westerhouse
Washington University School of Medicine in St. Louis

Public Affairs Representative
Michael E. Knecht
University of Medicine and Dentistry of Jew Jersey

Marketing Representative
Janet M. Caldwell
Meharry Medical College

Executive Secretary-Treasurer
Chris Tucker
AAMC

Administrative Support
Sandra Dunmore
AAMC

Group on Institutional Planning (GIP) Steering Committee

Chair
David H. Browdy
Northwestern University,
The Feinberg School of Medicine

Chair-elect
Robert Marriott
University of North Carolina School of Medicine

Immediate Past Chair
Thomas B. Higerd, Ph.D.
Medical University of South Carolina College of Medicine

Member-at-Large (2007–2009)
Angie Souza
University of Arizona College of Medicine

Member-at-Large (2007–2009)
Donna K. Gissen
Medical College of Wisconsin

Member-at-Large (2007–2009)
Vicky Zickmund
Wake Forest University School of Medicine

Member-at-Large (2008–2010)
Rhonice Burnett
Johns Hopkins Medicine

Member-at-Large (2008–2010)
Sean Ossont
University of Rochester School of Medicine and Dentistry

Member-at-Large (2008–2010)
Lynette Seebohm
University of Utah Health Science Center

Steering Committees

Group on Regional Medical Campuses (GRMC) Steering Committee

Chair
John B. Molidor, Ph.D.
Michigan State University–Flint

Chair-elect
Gerard P. Clancy, M.D.
University of Oklahoma–Tulsa

Vice Chair
S. Edwards Dismuke, M.D.
University of Kansas–Wichita

Secretary
Michael L. Friedland, M.D.
University of Miami
Miller School of Medicine
at Florida Atlantic University

Secretary-elect
Leonel Vela, M.D.
University of Texas
School of Medicine at San Antonio

Past Chair
Jose Manuel De La Rosa, M.D.
Texas Tech University
Health Sciences Center–El Paso

Group on Research Advancement and Development (GRAND) Steering Committee

Chair
Brian Herman, Ph.D.
University of Texas Health Science Center

Chair-elect
Sally A. Shumaker, Ph.D.
Wake Forest University School of Medicine

Past Chair
Theodore J. Cicero, Ph.D.
Washington University in St. Louis
School of Medicine

Jeffrey R. Balser, M.D., Ph.D.
Vanderbilt University Medical Center

Richard J. Bookman, Ph.D.
University of Miami Miller School of Medicine

Alison M.J. Buchan, Ph.D.
University of British Columbia

Peter Davies, M.D., Ph.D.
University of Texas, Houston

Chi V. Dang, M.D., Ph.D.
Johns Hopkins Hospital

Robert P. Kimberly, M.D.
University of Alabama School of Medicine

Jay Moskowitz, Ph.D.
Health Sciences South Carolina

Robert A. Rizza, M.D.
Mayo Medical School

Richard Traystman, Ph.D.
University of Colorado School of Medicine

Group on Resident Affairs (GRA) Steering Committee

Chair
Linda M. Famiglio, M.D.
Geisinger Health System

Chair-elect
Lois L. Bready, M.D.
University of Texas
Medical School at San Antonio

Past Chair
Rosemarie L. Fisher, M.D.
Yale University School of Medicine

Term Expiring 2008
Diane M. Hartmann, M.D.
University of Rochester
School of Medicine and Dentistry

Jamie S. Padmore
MedStar Health

Term Expiring 2009
Marilane B. Bond, Ed.D.
Emory University School of Medicine

John R. Musich, M.D.
William Beaumont Hospital

Larry M. Opas, M.D.
Los Angeles County and U.S.C. Medical Center

Term Expiring 2010
Linda B. Andrews, M.D.
Baylor College of Medicine

Robin C. Newton, M.D.
Howard University College of Medicine

ORR Liaison
Laura Hobart-Porter, D.O.
University of Arkansas for Medical Services

GEA Liaison
James C. Norton, Ph.D.
University of Kentucky College of Medicine

VA Liaison
Elaine A. Muchmore, M.D.
VA San Diego Healthcare System

AAMC Staff
Sunny G. Yoder

Group on Student Affairs (GSA) Steering Committee

Chair
Molly L. Osborne, M.D., Ph.D.
Oregon Health & Science University
School of Medicine

Chair-elect
Michael G. Kavan, Ph.D.
Creighton University School of Medicine

Vice Chair
Maureen Garrity, M.D.
University of Colorado School of Medicine

Immediate Past Chair
Georgette A. Dent, M.D.
University of North Carolina at Chapel Hill
School of Medicine

Chair, GSA—MAS
Cynthia E. Boyd, M.D.
Medical College of Rush University
Medical Center

Central Region Chair
Linda Bissell
University of Iowa
Roy J. and Lucille A. Carver College of Medicine

Southern Region Chair
Marc J. Kahn, M.D.
Tulane University School of Medicine

Northeast Region Chair
Lori Alvord, M.D.
Dartmouth Medical School

Western Region Chair
Neil H. Parker, M.D.
University of California, Los Angeles,
David Geffen School of Medicine

Chair, COA
Robert A. Witzburg, M.D.
Boston University School of Medicine

Chair, COSA
Samuel K. Parrish, M.D.
Drexel University

Chair, COSFA
Carrie Steere-Salazar
University of California, San Francisco,
School of Medicine

Chair, COSR
Karen Lewis
Morehouse School of Medicine

COD Liaison
Jay Perman, M.D.
University of Kentucky College of Medicine

Steering Committees

Group on Student Affairs (GSA) Steering Committee, (con't)

OSR Past Chair
James Littlejohn
The Texas A&M University System

NAAHP Liaison
Jeremiah L. Putnam, Ph.D.
Davidson College

Group on Student Affairs-Minority Affairs Section (GSA-MAS) Coordinating Committee

Chair
Cynthia E. Boyd, M.D., M.B.A, F.A.C.P.
Rush Medical College
of Rush University Medical Center

Chair-Elect
Maria L. Soto-Greene, M.D.
University of Medicine and Dentistry of New Jersey-
New Jersey Medical School

Central Region
Chair
Gloria V. Hawkins, Ph.D.
University of Wisconsin
School of Medicine and Public Health

Chair-Elect
Wanda D. Lipscomb, Ph.D.
Michigan State University
College of Human Medicine

Northeast Region
Chair
Gary C. Butts, M.D.
Mount Sinai School of Medicine
of New York University

Chair-elect
Carlyle H. Miller, M.D.
Cornell University Weill Medical College

Southern Region
Chair
Karen A. Lewis
Meharry Medical College

Chair-elect
Brenda A. Latham-Sadler, M.D.
Wake Forest University
Health Sciences Medical Center

Western Region
Chair
Linda K. Don, M.Ed.
University of Arizona College of Medicine

Chair-elect
Valerie Romero-Leggott, M.D.
University of New Mexico School of Medicine

Ex-Officio Members
Past Chair
Marvin (Ted) Williams, Ph.D.
University of South Florida College of Medicine

GSA National Chair
Georgette A. Dent, M.D.
University of North Carolina at Chapel Hill
School of Medicine

GSA-MAS Liaison to GSA Committee on
Admissions (COA)
Sunny Nakae-Gibson
Northwestern University
Feinberg School of Medicine

GSA-MAS Liaison to GSA Committee on Student
Affairs (COSA)
Virginia D. Hardy, Ph.D.
The Brody School of Medicine
at East Carolina University

GSA-MAS Liaison to GSA Committee on Student
Financial Assistance (COSFA)
Martha C. Trujillo
Stanford University School of Medicine

GSA-MAS Liaison to GSA Committee on Student
Records (COSR)
Sonia Beasley
University of Maryland School of Medicine

OSR Liaison to the GSA-MAS
Nathan T. Chomilo
University of Minnesota Medical School

NAAHP Liaison to GSA-MAS
Michael Ellison, ED.D
Chicago State University

AAIP Liaison to MAS
Joycelyn Dorscher, M.D.
University of Minnesota Medical School

AAMC Staff Support
Charles Terrell, Ed.D.
Lily May Johnson
Juan Amador
Angela R. Moses

**Women in Medicine Coordinating
Committee**

Chair
J. Renee Navarro, Pharm.D., M.D.
University of California, San Francisco

Jocelyn D. Chertoff, M.D.
Dartmouth-Hitchcock Medical Center

Elisabeth Kunkel, M.D.
Thomas Jefferson University

Patricia A. Thomas, M.D., F.C.A.P.
University of Kansas Medical Center

Rebecca R. Pauly, M.D.
University of Florida College of Medicine

Diana L. Gray, M.D.
Washington University in St. Louis

Susan B. Gurley, Ph.D.
Duke University School of Medicine

OSR Liaison
Jennifer Weiss, M.D.
University of Wisconsin Hospitals & Clinics

GSA Representative
Lina Nayak

COD Liaison
Betty M. Drees, M.D.
University of Missouri-Kansas City

AAMC Staff Support
Diane Magrane, M.D.
Valarie Clark, M.P.A.

465

Organization of Student Representatives

2008–2009

Organization of Student Representatives Administrative Board, 2007-2008

Chair
Diane Reis
University of Wisconsin School of Medicine and Public Health

Chair-elect
Matt Rudy
Medical College of Georgia

Immediate Past Chair
James Littlejohn
Texas A&M University Health Science Center College of Medicine

Regional Chairs

Central
Jenny Guido
University of North Dakota School of Medicine and Health Sciences

Northeast
Janae Phelps
Howard University College of Medicine

Southern
Brittany Dawson
University of Alabama School of Medicine

Western
Antony Hazel
University of California, Irvine, College of Medicine

National Delegates

Communications
Sameer Vohra
Southern Illinois University School of Medicine

Community and Diversity
Dominique Arce
Meharry Medical College

Legislative Affairs
Bryan Harris
Vanderbilt University School of Medicine

Medical Education
Catherine Spina
Boston University School of Medicine

Student Affairs
Jennifer Olges
University of Kentucky College of Medicine

Organization of Resident Representatives

2008–2009

Organization of Resident Representatives Administrative Board, 2007-2008

Chair
Kelli Harding, M.D.
Columbia University Medical Center

Chair-elect
Jennifer Weiss, M.D.
Columbia University Medical Center

Immediate Past-Chair
Rachel Havyer, M.D.
Mayo Medical School

At-Large Members

Alan Anschel, M.D.
New York Presbyterian Hospital

Chiquitia Anderson, M.D.
Children's Hospital of Michigan

Emily Durkin, M.D.
University of Wisconsin Hospitals and Clinics

Laura Hobart-Porter, M.D.
University of Arkansas Medical Center

Mark Neuman, M.D.
Brigham & Women's Hospital

Marshall Kuremsky, M.D.
Carolinas Medical Center

Other Members

2008–2009

Distinguished Service Members

Distinguished Service Membership in the Association of American Medical Colleges recognizes significant contributions to the Association. Distinguished Service Members are elected by vote of the Executive Council upon recommendation of the Executive Committee.

Council of Deans

William G. Anlyan
Harry Beaty
Steven C. Beering
Stuart Bondurant
Peter P. Bosomworth
L. Thompson Bowles
George T. Bryan
William T. Butler
Joseph H. Ceithaml
David Challoner
Robert M. Daugherty
William B. Deal
Haile T. Debas

Robert J. Glaser
James A. Hallock
Jeffrey L. Houpt
John J. Hutton
Richard Janeway
Robert Kelch
Julius R. Krevans
Philip Lee
William Luginbuhl
Marion Mann
Sherman Mellinkoff
Stanley Olson
William Peck

Clayton Rich
Ralph Snyderman
Robert D. Sparks
Edward J. Stemmler
Robert Stone
Robert C. Talley
Daniel C. Tosteson
Robert L. Van Citters
Andrew G. Wallace
Donald E. Wilson
Emery A. Wilson
I. Dodd Wilson
Daniel H. Winship

Council of Academic Societies

Diana Beattie
Kenneth I. Berns
Alfred Jay Bollet
Rita A. Charon
Sam Clark
Carmine D. Clemente
David H. Cohen
Terrance G. Cooper

Joe D. Coulter
William H. Dantzler
Patrick J. Fitzgerald
Robert E. Forster
Paul J. Friedman
Myron Genel
Robert L. Hill

Robert O. Kelley
Frank G. Moody
Hiram C. Polk
George F. Sheldon
William B. Weil
Virginia V. Weldon
Frank C. Wilson

Council of Teaching Hospitals and Health Systems

Theresa Bischoff
J. Robert Buchanan
Frank A. Butler
John W. Colloton
David D'Eramo
Robert Derzon
N. Lynn Eckhert

Spencer Foreman
Gary Gambuti
Harvey Holzberg
R. Edward Howell
William B. Kerr
Paul L. McCarthy

Ralph W. Muller
Mitchell T. Rabkin
Barbara Schuster
Samuel O. Thier
Irvin G. Wilmot
Charles B. Womer

Emeritus

Emeritus Membership in the Association of American Medical Colleges was established in 1958 to recognize those individuals who had reached retirement age or had become emeritus members of their faculty and who, prior to retirement, had been active in the affairs of the Association. According to guidelines established by the Executive Council, Emeritus Members must be judged to have given outstanding service to the Association through membership on its Councils, Committees, or Task Forces. Emeritus Members are elected by vote of the Executive Council.

S. Craighead Alexander (1996)
DeWitt C. Baldwin Jr., M.D. (1983)
William B. Bean (1980)
Robert Blacklow (2003)
Giles G. Bole, M.D. (1996)
Arnold Brown (1991)
Stebbins B. Chandor, M.D. (2004)
John D. Chase, M.D. (1983)
Ira C. Clark (2003)
Robert M. D'Alessandri, M.D. (2005)
Walter J. Daly, M.D. (1996)
W. Dale Dauphinee, M.D. (2007)
Thomas Dublin (1986)
William E. Easterling, M.D. (1995)
John Eckstein (1991)
Ronald G. Evans, M.D. (2007)
Bernard J. Fogel, M.D. (1996)
Robert Frank (1991)
Earl J. Frederick *** (1992)
Daniel H. Funkenstein, M.D. (1983)
Wm. Ted Galey, M.D. (2003)
Neal L. Gault, M.D. (1987)
James R. Gay, M.D. (1986)
Irma E. Goertzen (2004)
David S. Greer, M.D. (1992)
Arthur P. Grollman, M.D. (2001)
E. Nigel Harris, M.D. (2005)

James W. Haviland, M.D. (1976)
Joseph E. Johnson III, M.D. (1991)
Treuman Katz (2007)
Thomas C. King, M.D. (1995)
John Lattimer (1981)
Donlin M. Long, M.D. (2001)
Ruy V. Lourenco, M.D. (2000)
Robert U. Massey, M.D. (1987)
Allen W. Mathies Jr., M.D. (1995)
Betty H. Mawardi, Ph.D. (1985)
Layton McCurdy, M.D. (2000)
Glenn Mitchell (1995)
Woodrow W. Morris, M.D. (1984)
Gerald S. Moss, M.D. (2005)
Richard H. Moy, M.D. (1993)
Eric B. Munson (2004)
Leonard M. Napolitano, M.D. (1994)
Len Presler (2007)
Malcolm Randall (2000)
Morton I. Rapoport, M.D. (2003)
Seymour L. Romney, M.D. (1987)
Richard Ross, M.D. (1992)
Irene Thompson (2007)
Gail L. Warden (2004)
Larry Warren (2006)
David S. Weiner (2003)
Donald Weston (1991)

Index

2008–2009

Index

Index

Index

Index

Index

Index

Index

Index

Index

Index

Index

Index

Index

Index

Index

Index

Index

Index

Index

Index

Index

Index

Index

Index

Index

Index

Index

Index

O

Index

Index

Index

Index

Index

Index

Index

Index

Index

Index

Index

Index

Index

Index